PARAMEDIC CARE: Principles & Practice &

SPECIAL CONSIDERATIONS/OPERATIONS

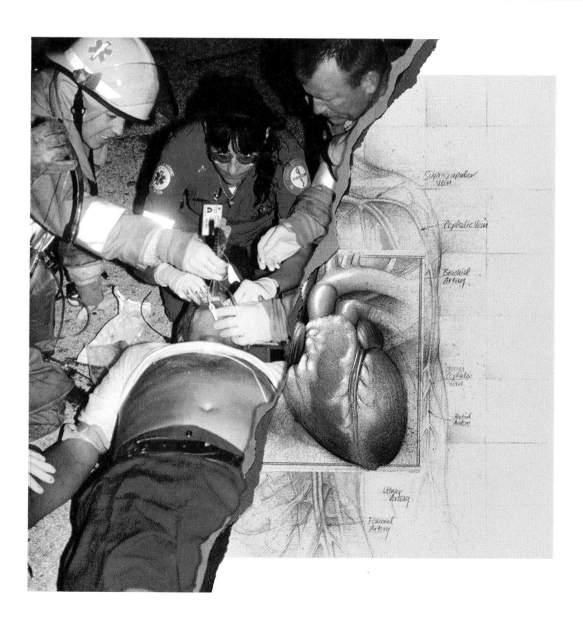

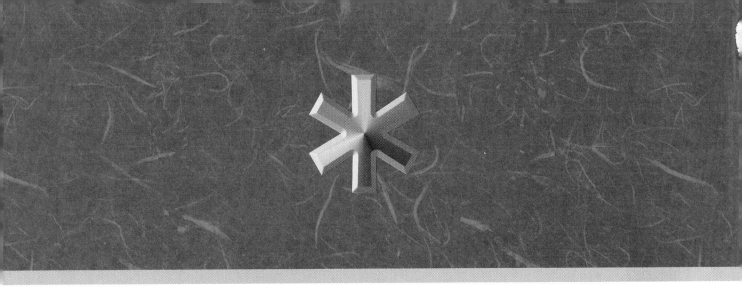

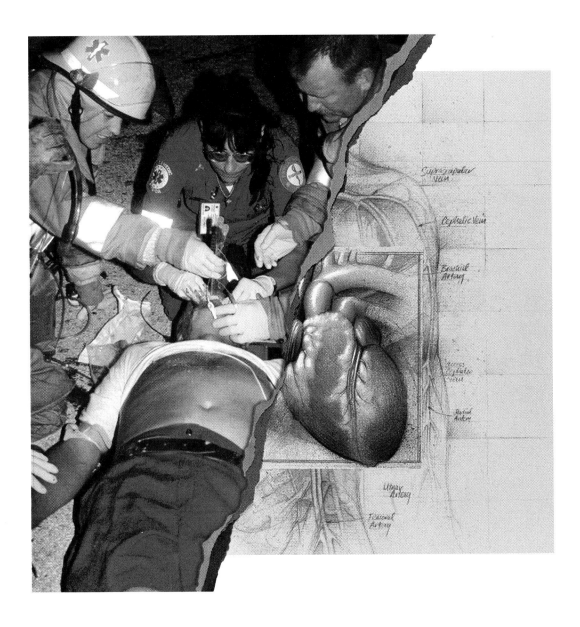

PARAMEDIC CARE: PRINCIPLES & PRACTICE

SPECIAL CONSIDERATIONS/OPERATIONS

BRYAN E. BLEDSOE, D.O., F.A.C.E.P., F.A.A.E.M., F.A.E.P., EMT-P

Emergency Department Staff Physician
Baylor Medical Center—Ellis County
Waxahachie, Texas
and
Clinical Associate Professor of Emergency Medicine
University of North Texas Health Sciences Center
Fort Worth, Texas

ROBERT S. PORTER, M.A., NREMT-P

Senior Advanced Life Support Educator
Madison County Emergency Medical Services
Canastota, New York
and
Flight Paramedic
AirOne, Onondaga County Sheriff's Department
Syracuse, New York

RICHARD A. CHERRY, M.S., NREMT-P

Clinical Assistant Professor of Emergency Medicine
Director of Paramedic Training
SUNY Upstate Medical University
Syracuse, New York

Prentice
Hall

Upper Saddle River, New Jersey 07458

Library of Congress Cataloging-in-Publication Data

Bledsoe, Bryan E., 1955-
    Paramedic care: principles & practice / Bryan E. Bledsoe, Robert S. Porter,
    Richard A. Cherry
        p. ; cm.
    Includes bibliographical references and index.
    Contents: vol. 5. Special Considerations/Operations
    ISBN 0-13-021599-6 (alk. paper)
        1. Emergency medicine. 2. Emergency medical technicians. I. Porter,
    Robert S., 1950- II. Title.

Publisher: Julie Alexander
Executive editor: Greg Vis
Managing development editor: Lois Berlowitz
Development editors: Sandra Breuer, Deborah A. Parks
Managing production editor: Patrick Walsh
Editorial/production supervision: Larry Hayden IV
Senior production manager: Ilene Sanford
Marketing manager: Tiffany Price
Marketing coordinator: Cindy Frederick
Interior design: Jill Yutkowitz
Cover design: Rob Richman
Cover photography: Eddie Sperling Photography
Cover illustration: Malcolm Farley
Managing photography editor: Michal Heron
Assistant photography editor: Theo Chewiwi
Interior photographers: Michael Gallitelli, Michal Heron,
    Richard Logan
Page makeup: Carlisle Communications, Inc.

©2001 by Prentice-Hall, Inc.
Upper Saddle River, New Jersey 07458

Printed in the United States of America
10   9   8   7   6

ISBN   0-13-021599-6

Prentice-Hall International (UK) Limited, *London*
Prentice-Hall of Australia Pty. Limited, *Sydney*
Prentice-Hall Canada Inc., *Toronto*
Prentice-Hall Hispanoamericana, S.A., *Mexico*
Prentice-Hall of India Private Limited, *New Delhi*
Prentice-Hall of Japan, Inc., *Tokyo*
Prentice-Hall (Singapore) Pte Ltd
Editora Prentice-Hall do Brasil, Ltda., *Rio de Janeiro*

Art Acknowledgments

Rolin Graphics, Plymouth, Minnesota

Photo Acknowledgments

All photographs not credited below as photo
sources were photographed on assignment for
Brady/Prentice Hall Pearson Education.

Photo Sources are credited as follows:

Harvy Eisner 8-3

Gamma Liason 9-2b

Craig Jackson/In The Dark Photography: 2-1,
3-5, 3-6, 3-7, 3-10, 7-2, 12-1

Mark Foster: Chapter 13 photos

Michal Heron Stock Photography: 3-4, 5-7,
5-9, 10-18d, 10-20

Glen Jackson: 7-4

Howard Paul: 10-23b, 10-24b

Photo Researchers/Vanessa Vick: 6-14

The Stock Market: 2-29 Charles Gupton; 3-2
Ariel Skelley; 3-15 Tom & DeeAnn McCarthy

Sygma/William Philpott: 9-2a; Sygma/Allen
Tannenbaum 9-1a

Woodfin Camp & Associates/Gerd
Ludwig: 6-5

SPECIAL NOTES

This book is respectfully dedicated to the EMTs and paramedics who toil each day in an environment that is unpredictable, often dangerous, and constantly changing. They risk their lives to aid the sick and the injured, driven only by their love of humanity and their devotion to this profession we call emergency medical services.

B.E.B.

To those who answer the call to care on cold, dark, and rainy nights.

R.S.P.

"At one time or another in everyone's lives the inner fire goes out. Then it is burst into flame by an encounter with another human being." Rudyard Kipling just described what my wife Sue has meant to me.

R.A.C.

Content Overview

Below is a brief content description of each chapter in
Special Considerations/Operations

Detailed Contents

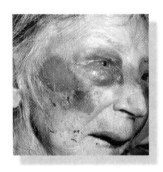

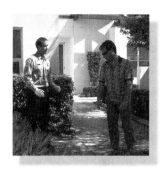

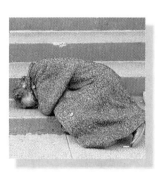

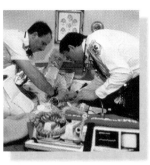

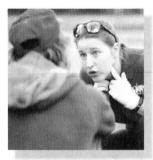

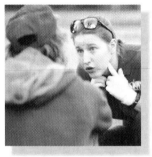

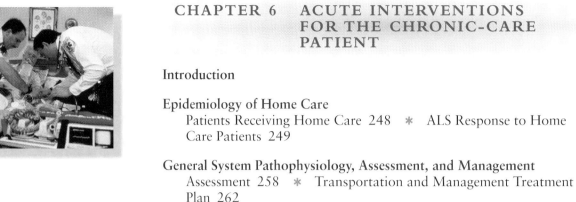

CHAPTER 9   MEDICAL INCIDENT COMMAND   338

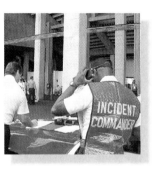

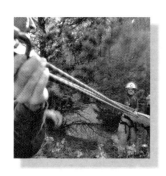

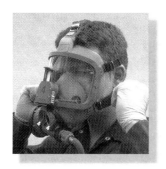

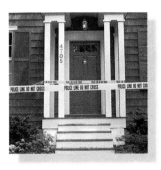

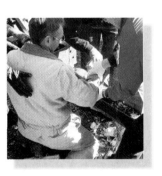

Series Preface

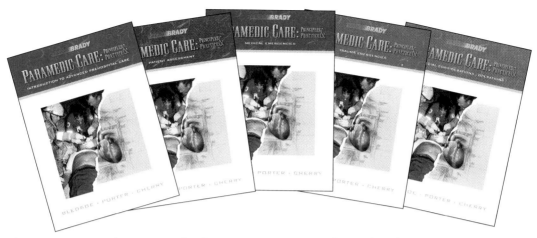

Congratulations on your decision to further your EMS career by undertaking the course of education required for certification as an Emergency Medical Technician-Paramedic! The world of paramedic emergency care is one that you will find both challenging and rewarding. Whether you will be working as a volunteer or paid paramedic, you will find the field of advanced prehospital care very interesting.

This textbook program will serve as your guide and reference to advanced out-of-hospital care. It is based upon the 1998 United States Department of Transportation *EMT-Paramedic: National Standard Curriculum* and is divided into five volumes. The first volume is entitled *Introduction to Advanced Prehospital Care* and addresses the fundamentals of paramedic practice, including pathophysiology, pharmacology, medication administration and advanced airway management. The second volume, *Patient Assessment*, builds on the assessment skills of the basic EMT with special emphasis on advanced patient assessment at the scene. The third volume of the series, *Medical Emergencies*, is the most extensive and addresses paramedic level care of medical emergencies. Particular emphasis is placed upon the most common medical problems as well as serious emergencies, such as respiratory and cardiovascular emergencies. *Trauma Emergencies*, the fourth volume of the text, discusses advanced prehospital care from the mechanism of injury analysis to shock/trauma resuscitation. The last volume in the series addresses *Special Considerations/Operations* including neonatal, pediatric, geriatric, home health care, and specially challenged patients, and incident command, ambulance service, rescue, hazardous material, and crime scene operations. These five volumes will help prepare you for the challenges of prehospital care.

SKILLS

The psychomotor skills of fluid and medication administration, advanced airway care, ECG monitoring and defibrillation, and advanced medical and trauma patient care are best learned in the classroom, skills laboratory, and then the clinical and field setting. Common advanced prehospital skills are discussed in the text as well as outlined in the accompanying procedure sheets. Review these before and while practicing the skill. It is important to point out that this or any other text cannot teach skills. Care skills are only learned under the watchful eye of a paramedic instructor and perfected during your clinical and field internship.

HOW TO USE THIS TEXTBOOK

Paramedic Care: Principles & Practice is designed to accompany a paramedic education program that follows the 1998 United States Department of Transportation *EMT-Paramedic: National Standard Curriculum*. The education program should include ample classroom, practical laboratory, in-hospital clinical, and prehospital field experience. These educational experiences must be guided by instructors and preceptors with special training and experience in their areas of participation in your program.

It is intended that your program coordinator will assign reading from *Paramedic Care: Principles & Practice* in preparation for each classroom lecture and discussion section. The knowledge gained from reading this text will form the foundation of the information you will need in order to function effectively as a paramedic in your EMS system. Your instructors will build upon this information to strengthen your knowledge and understanding of advanced prehospital care so that you may apply it in your practice. The in-hospital clinical and prehospital field experiences will further refine your knowledge and skills under the watchful eyes of your preceptors.

In preparing for each classroom session, read the assigned chapter carefully. First, review the chapter objectives. They will identify important concepts to be learned from the reading. Read the Case Study to get a feeling of why a chapter is important and how the knowledge it contains can be applied in the field. Read the chapter content carefully, while keeping the chapter objectives in mind. Read the You Make the Call feature and answer the questions to assure you understand the application of the knowledge presented in the chapter. Last, reread the chapter objectives and be sure that you are able to answer each one completely. If you cannot, reread the section of the chapter to which the objective relates. If you still do not understand the objective or any portion of what you have read, ask your instructor to explain it at your next class session.

Ideally, you should read this entire text series at least three times. The volume chapter should be read in preparation for the class session, the entire volume should be read before the division or course test, and the entire text series should be reread before the program final exam and/or certification testing. While this might seem like a lot of reading, it will improve your classroom performance, your knowledge of emergency care, and ultimately, the care you provide to emergency patients.

The workbook that accompanies this text can also assist in improving classroom performance. It contains information, sample test questions, and exercises designed to assist learning. Its use can be very helpful in identifying the important elements of paramedic education, in exercising the knowledge of prehospital care, and in helping you self-test your knowledge.

Paramedic Care: Principles & Practice presents the knowledge of emergency care in as accurate, standardized, and clear a manner as is possible. However, each EMS system is uniquely different, and it is beyond the scope of this text to address all differences. You must count heavily on your instructors, the program coordinator, and ultimately the program medical director to identify how specific emergency care procedures are applied in your system.

EMS in the third millennium involves a great deal more than simply transporting a patient to the hospital. The modern paramedic has tremendous responsibilities, both on the scene and in the community. In Volume 5, *Special Considerations/ Operations* of *Paramedic Care: Principles & Practice*, we have detailed important specialized information required of paramedics in the modern EMS system. In addition to a detailed discussion of special patients, we have provided crucial information on scene safety and operations as well as assessment-based patient management.

This text has been designed to serve as both an initial course textbook as well as a reference source for the practicing paramedic. In this final volume of *Paramedic Care: Principles & Practice*, we have addressed the last three divisions of the *1998 U.S. DOT EMT-Paramedic National Standard Curriculum*. These include:

Special Considerations—This section presents the essential information on special patient populations encountered in prehospital care including neonates, children, the elderly, the challenged, as well as chronically-ill patients.

Assessment-Based Management—The 1998 EMT-Paramedic curriculum was developed based upon the concept of assessment-based management. This division serves to tie together the various divisions of the curriculum previously presented (i.e., medical, trauma, and special patients) so that the paramedic can provide the necessary care based upon assessment findings.

Operations—Modern EMS is very comprehensive. The paramedic must have detailed knowledge of hazardous material scenes, rescue scenes, multiple casualty incidents, disasters, and other emergencies. This division provides essential information about these important aspects of prehospital care.

EMS is unique among the allied health professions. The modern paramedic, although functioning under the license and direction of the system medical director, is forced to make most patient care decisions in the field independently. Because of this, the modern paramedic must have a thorough knowledge of essential anatomy, physiology, and pathophysiology of the common emergencies encountered. Based on this knowledge, the paramedic must complete a detailed, yet focused patient assessment and determine the appropriate treatment plan. Although help is never more than a phone call or radio call away, the paramedic functions fairly autonomously in a dangerous environment that is constantly changing.

Chapters in this volume correspond to the *U.S. DOT 1998 EMT-Paramedic: National Standard Curriculum*. The following are short descriptions of each chapter:

Chapter 1 "Neonatology" introduces the paramedic student to the specialized world of neonatology. The neonate is a child less than one month of age. These patients have very different problems and their treatment must be modified to accommodate their size and anatomy. This chapter presents a detailed discussion of neonatology with a special emphasis on neonatal resuscitation in the field setting.

Chapter 2 "Pediatrics" presents a detailed discussion of pediatric emergencies. Children are not "small adults." They have special needs and must be approached and treated in a fashion different from adults. This chapter provides an overview of the common, and uncommon, pediatric emergencies encountered in prehospital care with a special emphasis on recognition and treatment. Specialized pediatric assessment techniques and emergency procedures are presented in detail.

Chapter 3 "Geriatric Emergencies" is a detailed presentation of emergencies involving the elderly. The elderly are the fastest growing aspect of our society. A significant number of EMS calls involve elderly patients. This chapter reviews the anatomy and physiology of aging. The chapter then presents a detailed discussion of the assessment and treatment of emergencies commonly seen in the elderly.

Chapter 4 "Abuse and Assault" presents a timely discussion of the needs of the abuse or assault victim. This chapter provides important information that will aid the paramedic in detecting abusive or dangerous situations. EMS personnel are often the first, and occasionally the only, personnel to encounter the abuse or assault victim. Because of this, it is essential that abusive situations be recognized early and the appropriate personnel notified.

Chapter 5 "The Challenged Patient" addresses patients with special needs. A medical emergency can be an extremely frightful event for the patient who is sensory or mentally challenged. Because of this, paramedics should be aware of strategies that reduce stress for patients with special challenges.

Chapter 6 "Acute Interventions for the Chronic-Care Patient" offers an important discussion of the role of EMS personnel in treating home-care patients and patients with chronic medical conditions. With declining hospital revenues, more and more patients are being cared for at home—either by family members or home care personnel. Paramedics are often summoned when a home care patient deteriorates or otherwise suffers a medical or trauma emergency. It is essential that prehospital personnel have a fundamental understanding of home health care as well as a basic knowledge of the medical devices and technology routinely used in home care. This chapter details the paramedic's role in assessing, treating, and managing the home care patient.

Chapter 7 "Assessment-Based Management" ties together the patient care material presented in this text. Paramedics are unique in that they function in an unstructured environment. They must often make field diagnoses and act upon these. This chapter details how to integrate the information learned from a comprehensive patient assessment and use that in formulating an appropriate treatment plan. This aspect of paramedic care is one of the fundamental differences between paramedicine and other allied health personnel. The paramedics of the 21st century are expected to not only have good patient care skills, they are also expected to have good field diagnostic skills. These skills are based upon the concept of assessment-based management.

Chapter 8 "Ambulance Operations" serves to present, and in some cases review, the special world of EMS and ambulance operations. Patient care begins long before the call is received. The paramedic is responsible for keeping the ambulance and medical equipment in a constant state of readiness. In addition, the paramedic must understand the various EMS system operations so that he or she may interact accordingly.

Chapter 9 "Medical Incident Command" provides a detailed discussion of the Incident Command System. The Incident Command System is a system for managing resources at the emergency scene, particularly at scenes involving multiple ambulances and multiple agencies. Paramedics must intimately understand the workings of the Incident Command System and apply them in daily operations.

Chapter 10 "Rescue Awareness and Operations" presents a comprehensive discussion of rescue operations. The level of EMS involvement with rescue operations varies significantly. In many EMS systems, paramedics are responsible for rescue operations. In others, paramedics are primarily responsible for patient care while rescue operations are carried out by specially trained and equipped rescue teams. Regardless, the modern paramedic must have a thorough understanding of rescue operations with an emphasis on scene safety.

Chapter 11 "Hazardous Materials Incidents" gives an overview of hazardous materials operations. More and more emergency scenes involve hazardous materials. Although most hazardous material scenes are handled by specialized "hazmat" teams, paramedics are responsible for patient care. The hazardous material scene can be extremely dangerous. Because of this, the modern paramedic must have a fundamental understanding of various hazardous materials and hazmat operations.

Chapter 12 "Crime Scene Awareness" details the importance of protecting the crime scene. EMS personnel are often the first to arrive at a crime scene. Although their principle responsibility is patient care, they should take great effort to avoid disturbing important aspects of the crime scene. This chapter provides an overview of crime scene operations so that EMS personnel will recognize and protect essential elements of the crime scene.

Chapter 13 "Rural EMS" provides an overview of the special needs of rural EMS. Although not a part of the 1998 U.S. DOT curriculum, this chapter has been added to enhance awareness of the challenges, such as distance, faced by rural EMS personnel and the creative problem-solving used to provide high-quality care to the nearly 53 million Americans who live in rural areas.

This volume, *Special Considerations/Operations*, describes important information that the modern paramedic needs in order to function effectively on the emergency scene. This information should prove beneficial both in initial paramedic education programs as well as in future refresher programs.

Brady's *Paramedic Care: Principles & Practice*, is a five-volume series designed to provide educational enrichment as prescribed by the 1998 U.S. D.O.T. *EMT–Paramedic: National Standard Curriculum*. Volume 1, *Introduction to Advanced Prehospital Care* presents the foundations of paramedic practice as well as an introduction to pathophysiology, pharmacology, medication administration, and airway management and ventilation. Volume 2, *Patient Assessment* adds the cognitive and psychomotor skills of patient assessment, communications, and documentation. This knowledge base expands as the series applies it to the medical patient in Volume 3, *Medical Emergencies* and to the trauma patient in Volume 4, *Trauma Emergencies*. Volume 5, *Special Considerations/Operations* enriches these general patient care concepts and principles with applications to special patients and circumstances we commonly see as paramedics. The product of this complete and integrated series is a set of principles of paramedic care you will be required to practice in the twenty-first century.

Acknowledgments

CHAPTER CONTRIBUTORS

We wish to acknowledge the remarkable talents and efforts of the following people who contributed to this volume of *Paramedic Care: Principles & Practice*. Individually, they worked with extraordinary commitment on this new program. Together, they form a team of highly dedicated professionals who have upheld the highest standards of EMS instruction.

Chapter 1 Neonatology
Jo Anne Schultz, B.A.; NREMT-P; Paramedic, Lifestar Ambulance, Inc., Salisbury, Maryland; Level II Instructor, Maryland Fire and Rescue Institute, University of Maryland; Paramedic Instructor, Maryland Institute of Emergency Medical Services, University of Maryland; ACLS, BTLS, and PALS Instructor

Chapter 2 Pediatrics
Bryan E. Bledsoe, D.O.; F.A.C.E.P.; F.A.A.E.M.; F.A.E.P.; EMT-P; Emergency Department Staff Physician, Baylor Medical Center—Ellis County, Waxahachie, Texas; Clinical Professor of Emergency Medicine, University of North Texas Health Sciences Center, Fort Worth, Texas.
Brenda Beasley, RN; BS; EMT-P; EMS Program Director, Calhoun College, Decatur, Alabama

Chapter 3 Geriatric Emergencies
Gail Weinstein, M.A.; EMT-P; Director of Paramedic Training, State University of New York Upstate Medical University, Syracuse, New York
Deborah Kufs, R.N.; B.S.; C.C.R.N.; C.E.N.; NREMT-P; Clinical Instructor, Hudson Valley Community College, Institute for Prehospital Emergency Medicine, Troy, New York

Chapter 4 Abuse and Assault
Matthew R. Streger, M.P.A.; NREMT-P; Deputy Commissioner, Cleveland Emergency Medical Services, Cleveland, Ohio

Chapter 5 The Challenged Patient
Marian D. Streger, R.N.; B.S.N.; C.E.N.; Cleveland, Ohio
Sandra Bradley, Pleasant Hill, California

Chapter 6 Acute Interventions for the Chronic-Care Patient
Matthew R. Streger, M.P.A.; NREMT-P; Deputy Commissioner, Cleveland Emergency Medical Services, Cleveland, Ohio
Chris Hendricks, NREMT-P; Field Instructor; Paramedic, Pridemark Paramedics, Boulder, Colorado

Chapter 7 Assessment-Based Management

Marian D. Streger, R.N.; B.S.N.; C.E.N.; Cleveland, Ohio.

Jo Anne Schultz, B.A.; NREMT-P; Paramedic, Lifestar Ambulance, Inc., Salisbury, Maryland; Level II Instructor, Maryland Fire and Rescue Institute, University of Maryland; Paramedic Instructor, Maryland Institute of Emergency Medical Services, University of Maryland; ACLS, BTLS, and PALS Instructor

Chapter 8 Ambulance Operations

Bob Elling, M.P.A.; REMT-P; Professor, American College of Prehospital Medicine; Faculty Member, Institute of Prehospital Emergency Medicine, Hudson Valley Community College, Troy, New York

Chapter 9 Medical Incident Command

Matthew R. Streger, M.P.A.; NREMT-P; Deputy Commissioner, Cleveland Emergency Medical Services, Cleveland, Ohio

Chapter 10 Rescue Awareness and Operations

Bob Elling, M.P.A.; REMT-P; Professor, American College of Prehospital Medicine; Faculty Member, Institute of Prehospital Emergency Medicine, Hudson Valley Community College, Troy, New York

Chapter 11 Hazardous Materials Incidents

Matthew R. Streger, M.P.A.; NREMT-P; Deputy Commissioner, Cleveland Emergency Medical Services, Cleveland, Ohio

Chapter 12 Crime Scene Awareness

Daniel Limmer, EMT-P, Frederick, Maryland; Police Investigator (Ret.), Colonie, New York

Chapter 13 Rural EMS

Mark Foster, AEMT-P, Greenport Rescue, Hudson, New York

Deborah McCoy, R.N.; NREMT-P; Regional EMS Coordinator, Altru Health System, Grand Forks, North Dakota

DEVELOPMENT AND PRODUCTION

The task of writing, editing, reviewing, and producing a textbook the size of *Paramedic Care: Principles & Practice* is complex. Many talented people at Brady have been involved in developing and producing this new program.

First, the authors would like to acknowledge the support of Julie Alexander and Laura Edwards. Their belief in us and support of EMS has allowed us to assure that *Paramedic Care: Principles & Practice* will be in the forefront of paramedic education. Special thanks go to Sandra Breuer, who served as Project Coordinator for this new paramedic series and Deborah Parks, Development Editor for this volume. The extraordinary efforts of these exceptionally dedicated editors are deeply appreciated.

The challenges of production were in the very capable hands of Patrick Walsh and Larry Hayden, who skillfully supervised all production stages to create the final product you now hold. In developing our art and photo program we were fortunate to work with yet additional talent, leaders within their professions. Most of the staged photographs are by Michal Heron of New York City, whose commitment to excellence never falters. The new art was drafted by Rolin Graphics of Plymouth, Minnesota.

REVIEW BOARDS

Our special thanks to Robert A. De Lorenzo, M.D., F.A.C.E.P.; Major, Medical Corps, U.S. Army; Associate Clinical Professor of Military and Emergency Medicine, Uniformed Services University of the Health Sciences. Dr. De Lorenzo's reviews were carefully prepared, and we appreciate the thoughtful advice and keen insight he shared with us.

INSTRUCTOR REVIEWERS

The reviewers of *Paramedic Care: Principles & Practice* have provided many excellent suggestions and ideas for improving the text. The quality of the reviews has been outstanding, and the reviews have been a major aid in the preparation and revision of the manuscript. The assistance provided by these EMS experts is deeply appreciated.

Stanley A. Bell, Jr.
MICP Lead Instructor
Trinitas Hospital Mobile ICU
Elizabeth, NJ

Michael D. Berg, NREMT-P
Medical Liaison Officer
Austin/Travis County EMS
Austin, TX

Robert Carter
Clinical Associate Pediatric Intensive
    Care Unit
Johns Hopkins Children's Center
Paramedic, Baltimore City Fire
    Department
Baltimore, MD

Edna Deacon, EMT
EMT Coordinator Sussex County
    Community College
Mine Hill First Aid Squad President
Newton, NJ

Robert De Lorenzo, MD, FACEP
Major, Medical Corps
United States Army
Associate Clinical Professor of
    Military and Emergency Medicine
Uniformed Services University of the
    Health Science
Bethesda, MD

Robert Dotterer, BSEd, MEd
    NREMT-P
Phoenix Fire Department
Phoenix College
Phoenix, AZ

Johnathon Hockman, Paramedic,
    ACLS, EMSIC
Goldrush Consulting
Detroit, MI

Darin Hoggatt, MS, FF/NREMT-P
Clarian Health and Greenwood Fire
    Department
Indianapolis, IN

Tony Hyre, BA, REMT-P
C.E. Officer
West Virginia EMS

James L. Jenkins, Jr.; BA, NREMT-P
Confidential Assistant to the
    Governor
Office of the Secretary of Public Safety
Virginia Department of Fire Programs
Richmond, VA

Anthony T. Kramer, RN, BSN,
    NREMT-P
Field Service Assistant Professor
Clinical Coordinator, Center for
    Prehospital Education
University of Cincinnati
Cincinnati, OH

Nick Meacher, NREMT-P
Instructor, Public Safety Center
Harrisburg Area Community College
York Springs, PA

Steven L. Poffenberger, BS, EMT-P
Paramedic Program Clinical
    Coordinator
Harrisburg Area Community College
Harrisburg, PA

Jackie L. Richey, RN, NREMT-P
Rural/Metro Ambulance
Indianapolis, IN

Michael G. Rubin, BS, NREMT-P
State University of New York at Stony
  Brook
Stony Brook, NY

Daniel L. Sponsler, BS, NREMT-P
Division Chair, Emergency Services
Northwest Technical College
East Grand Forks, MN

Andrew W. Stern, NREMT-P, MPA,
  MA
Senior Paramedic/Flightmedic
Town of Colonie Emergency Medical
  Services
Colonie, NY

Matthew R. Streger, MPA, NREMT-P
Deputy Commissioner
Cleveland Emergency Medical
  Services
Cleveland, OH

Anthony Tucci, EMT-P
Western Berks Ambulance Association
West Lawn, PA

Charles N. Zarrelli
Coordinator, EMT Training
Camden County College
Blackwood, NJ

About the Authors

BRYAN E. BLEDSOE, D.O., F.A.C.E.P., F.A.A.E.M., F.A.E.P., EMT-P

Dr. Bryan Bledsoe is an emergency physician with special interest in prehospital care. He received his B.S. degree from the University of Texas at Arlington and received his medical degree from the University of North Texas Health Sciences Center / Texas College of Osteopathic Medicine. He completed his internship at Texas Tech University and residency training at Scott and White Memorial Hospital / Texas A&M College of Medicine. Dr. Bledsoe is board-certified in emergency medicine and family practice. He is presently a Ph.D. candidate at Charles Sturt University at Wagga Wagga, New South Wales, Australia.

Prior to attending medical school, Dr. Bledsoe worked as an EMT, paramedic, and paramedic instructor. He completed EMT training in 1974 and paramedic training in 1976, and worked for 6 years as a field paramedic in Fort Worth, Texas. In 1979, he joined the faculty of the University of North Texas Health Sciences Center and served as coordinator of EMT and paramedic education programs at the university. Dr. Bledsoe is active in emergency medicine and serves as medical director for several EMS agencies and educational programs.

Dr. Bledsoe has authored several EMS books published by Brady including *Paramedic Emergency Care, Intermediate Emergency Care, Atlas of Paramedic Skills, Prehospital Emergency Pharmacology,* and *Pocket Reference for EMTs and Paramedics.* He is married to Emma Bledsoe. They have two children, Bryan and Andrea, and live in Midlothian, Texas, a suburb of Dallas. He enjoys saltwater fishing and listening to Jimmy Buffett.

ROBERT S. PORTER, M.A., NREMT-P

Robert Porter has been teaching in Emergency Medical Services for 25 years and currently serves as the Senior Advanced Life Support Educator for Madison County, New York, and as a Flight Paramedic with the Onondaga County Sheriff's Department helicopter service, AirOne. Mr. Porter is a Wisconsin native and received his Bachelor's degree in education from the University of Wisconsin. He completed his Paramedic training at Northeast Wisconsin Technical Institute in 1978 and earned a Master's Degree in Health Education at Central Michigan University in 1990.

Mr. Porter has been an EMT and EMS educator and administrator since 1973 and obtained his National Registration as an EMT-Paramedic in 1978. He has taught both basic and advanced level EMS courses in the states of Wisconsin, Michigan, Louisiana, Pennsylvania, and New York. Mr. Porter served for more than ten years as a paramedic program accreditation-site evaluator for the American Medical Association and is a past chair of the National Society of EMT Instructor/Coordinators. He has published numerous articles in EMS periodicals and has authored Brady's *Paramedic Emergency Care, Intermediate Emergency Care, Tactical Emergency Care,* and *Weapons of Mass Destruction: Emergency Care* as well as the workbooks accompanying this text, *Paramedic Emergency Care,* and *Intermediate Emergency Care.* When not writing or teaching, Mr. Porter enjoys offshore sailboat racing, historic home restoration, and listening to Dr. Bryan Bledsoe complain about the Texas heat.

RICHARD A. CHERRY, M.S., NREMT-P

Richard Cherry is Clinical Assistant Professor of Emergency Medicine and Director of Paramedic Training at SUNY Upstate Medical University in Syracuse, NY. His experience includes years of classroom teaching and emergency field work. A native of Buffalo, Mr. Cherry earned his Bachelor's degree and teaching certificate at nearby St. Bonaventure University in 1972. He taught high school for the next 10 years while he earned his Master's degree in Education from Oswego State University in 1977. He holds a permanent teaching license in New York State.

Mr. Cherry entered the emergency medical services field in 1974 with the De-Witt Volunteer Fire Department where he served his community as a firefighter and EMS provider for over 15 years. He took his first EMT course in 1977 and became an ALS provider two years later. He earned his paramedic certificate in 1985 as a member of the area's first paramedic class. He still answers emergency calls for Brewerton Ambulance.

Mr. Cherry has authored several books for Brady. Most notable is *EMT Teaching: A Common Sense Approach*. He has made presentations at many state, national, and international EMS conferences on a variety of teaching topics. In addition to his paramedic teaching, he is course director, instructor, and instructor trainer for ACLS, PALS, and PHTLS courses conducted for physicians, residents, nurses, medical students, and other house staff. He lives in Parish, New York with his wife Sue, a paramedic with Rural-Metro Medical Services, their children, and many pets.

Notices

It is the intent of the authors and publishers that this textbook be used as part of a formal paramedic education program taught by a qualified instructor and supervised by a licensed physician. The care procedures presented here represent accepted practices in the United States. They are not offered as a standard of care. Paramedic-level emergency care is to be performed only under the authority and guidance of a licensed physician. It is the reader's responsibility to know and follow local care protocols as provided by medical advisors directing the system to which he or she belongs. Also, it is the reader's responsibility to stay informed of emergency care procedure changes.

NOTICE ON DRUGS AND DRUG DOSAGES

Every effort has been made to ensure that the drug dosages presented in this textbook are in accordance with nationally accepted standards. When applicable, the dosages and routes are taken from the American Heart Association's Advanced Cardiac Life Support Guidelines. The American Medical Association's publication *Drug Evaluations*, the *Physician's Desk Reference*, and the Appleton & Lange *Health Professionals Drug Guide 2000* are followed with regard to drug dosages not covered by the American Heart Association's guidelines. It is the responsibility of the reader to be familiar with the drugs used in his or her system, as well as the dosages specified by the medical director. The drugs presented in this book should only be administered by direct order, whether verbally or through accepted standing orders, of a licensed physician.

NOTICE ON GENDER USAGE

The English language has historically given preference to the male gender. Among many words, the pronouns "he" and "his" are commonly used to describe both genders. Society evolves faster than language and the male pronouns still predominate in our speech. The authors have made great effort to treat the two genders equally, recognizing that a significant percentage of paramedics and patients are female. However, in some instances, male pronouns may be used to describe both male and female paramedics and patients solely for the purpose of brevity. This is not intended to offend any readers of the female gender.

NOTICE ON PHOTOGRAPHS

Please note that many of the photographs contained in this book are taken of actual emergency situations. As such, it is possible that they may not accurately depict current, appropriate, or advisable practices of emergency medical care. They have been included for the sole purpose of giving general insight into real-life emergency settings.

NOTICE ON CASE STUDIES

The names used and situations depicted in the case studies throughout this program are fictitious.

Precautions on Bloodborne Pathogens and Infectious Diseases

Prehospital emergency personnel, like all health care workers, are at risk for exposure to bloodborne pathogens and infectious diseases. In emergency situations it is often difficult to take or enforce proper infection control measures. However, as a paramedic, you must recognize your high-risk status. Study the following information on infection control before turning to the main portion of this book.

Infection control is designed to protect emergency personnel, their families, and their patients from unnecessary exposure to communicable diseases.

Laws, regulations, and standards regarding infection control include:

* *Centers for Disease Control (CDC) Guidelines.* The CDC has published extensive guidelines regarding infection control. Proper equipment and techniques that should be used by emergency response personnel to prevent or minimize risk of exposure are defined.
* *The Ryan White Act.* The Ryan White Act of 1990 allows emergency personnel to find out if they were exposed to an infectious disease while rendering patient care. Employers are required to name a "designated officer" to coordinate communications with the treating hospital.
* *Americans with Disabilities Act.* This act prohibits discrimination against individuals with disabilities including those with contagious diseases. It guarantees equal employment opportunities and job protection if the infected individual can perform essential job functions and does not pose a threat to the safety and health of patients and coworkers.
* *Occupational Safety and Health Administration (OSHA) Regulations.* OSHA recently enacted a regulation entitled Occupational Exposure to Bloodborne Pathogens that classifies emergency response personnel as being at the greatest risk of occupational exposure to communicable diseases. This regulation requires employers to provide hepatitis B (HBV) vaccinations free of charge, maintain a written exposure control plan, and provide personal protective equipment (PPE). These requirements primarily apply to private employers. Applicability to local and state governmental employees varies by locality. Many states have developed their own OSHA plans.
* *National Fire Protection Association (NFPA) Guidelines.* This is a national organization that has established specific guidelines and requirements regarding infection control for emergency response agencies, particularly fire departments and EMS services.

BODY SUBSTANCE ISOLATION PRECAUTIONS AND PERSONAL PROTECTIVE EQUIPMENT

Emergency response personnel should practice *Body Substance Isolation (BSI)*, a strategy that considers ALL body substances potentially infectious. To achieve this, all emergency personnel should utilize *Personal Protective Equipment (PPE)*.

Appropriate PPE should be available on every emergency vehicle. The minimum recommended PPE includes the following:

* *Gloves.* Disposable gloves should be donned by all emergency response personnel BEFORE initiating any emergency care. When an emergency incident involves more than one patient, you should attempt to change gloves between patients. When gloves have been contaminated, they should be removed as soon as possible. To remove gloves, first hook the gloved fingers of one hand under the cuff of the other glove. Then pull that glove off without letting your gloved fingers come in contact with bare skin. Then slide the fingers of the un-gloved hand under the remaining glove's cuff. Push that glove off, being careful not to touch the glove's exterior with your bare hand. Always wash hands after gloves are removed, even when the gloves appear intact.

* *Masks and Protective Eyewear.* Masks and protective equipment should be present on all emergency vehicles and used in accordance with the level of exposure encountered. Proper eyewear and masks prevent a patient's blood and body fluids from spraying into your eyes, nose, and mouth. Masks and protective eyewear should be worn together whenever blood spatter is likely to occur, such as arterial bleeding, childbirth, endotracheal intubation, invasive procedures, oral suctioning, and clean-up of equipment that requires heavy scrubbing or brushing. Both you and the patient should wear masks whenever the potential for airborne transmission of disease exists.

* *HEPA Respirators.* Due to the resurgence of tuberculosis (TB), prehospital personnel should protect themselves from TB infection through use of a high-efficiency particulate air (HEPA) respirator, a design approved by the National Institute of Occupational Safety and Health (NIOSH). It should fit snugly and be capable of filtering out the tuberculosis bacillus. The HEPA respirator should be worn when caring for patients with confirmed or suspected TB. This is especially true when performing "high hazard" procedures such as administration of nebulized medications, endotracheal intubation, or suctioning on such a patient.

* *Gowns.* Gowns protect clothing from blood splashes. If large splashes of blood are expected, such as with childbirth, wear impervious gowns.

* *Resuscitation Equipment.* Disposable resuscitation equipment should be the primary means of artificial ventilation in emergency care. Such items should be used once, then disposed of.

Remember, the proper use of personal protective equipment ensures effective infection control and minimizes risk. Use ALL protective equipment recommended for any particular situation to ensure maximum protection.

Consider ALL body substances potentially infectious and ALWAYS practice body substance isolation.

HANDLING CONTAMINATED MATERIAL

Many of the materials associated with the emergency response become contaminated with possibly infectious body fluids and substances. These include soiled linen, patient clothing, and dressings, and used care equipment, including intravenous needles. It is important that you collect these materials at the scene and dispose of them appropriately to assure your safety as well as that of your patients, their family members, bystanders, and fellow care-givers. Properly dispose of any contaminated materials according to the recommendations outlined below.

* Handle contaminated materials only while wearing the appropriate personal protective equipment.

* Place all blood- or body-fluid-contaminated clothing, linen, dressings and patient care equipment and supplies in properly marked biological hazard bags and assure they are disposed of properly.
* Assure all used needles, scalpels and other contaminated objects that have the potential to puncture the skin are properly secured in a puncture-resistant and clearly-marked sharps container.
* Do not recap a needle after use, stick it into a seat cushion or other object, or leave it lying on the ground. This increases the risk of an accidental needle stick.
* Always scan the scene before leaving to assure all equipment has been retrieved and all potentially infectious material has been bagged and removed.
* Should you be exposed to an infectious disease, have contact with body substances with a route for system entry (such as an open wound on your hand when a glove tears while moving a soiled patient), or receive a needle stick with a used needle, alert the receiving hospital and contact your service's infection control officer immediately.

Following these recommendations will help protect you and the people you care for from the dangers of disease transmission.

Welcome to Paramedic Care

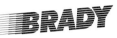

ONE LAKE STREET
UPPER SADDLE RIVER, NJ 07458

Dear Paramedic Instructor,

Brady, Your Partner in Education, is pleased to present *Paramedic Care: Principles & Practice*—a comprehensive series developed specifically to meet the new U.S. DOT National Standard Curriculum for EMT-Paramedics.

We recognize that for many of you the new curriculum represents a dramatic change in the way your paramedic course will be taught. *Paramedic Care: Principles & Practice* was developed specifically to help both you and your students succeed. Written in a student-friendly, easy-to-understand style, our new series consists of five volumes:

- Volume 1: *Introduction to Advanced Prehospital Care*
- Volume 2: *Patient Assessment*
- Volume 3: *Medical Emergencies*
- Volume 4: *Trauma Emergencies*
- Volume 5: *Special Considerations/Operations*.

The texts in this series are designed to work in tandem to cover all the objectives in the eight modules of the new U.S. DOT curriculum. However, each volume may also be used individually to help you tailor your course to state and local protocols.

Our high-quality instructor materials provide everything you need to help get your new curriculum course up and running. The Instructor's Resource Manual will contain lecture outlines and lesson plans that cover the new curriculum, along with student handouts and suggestions for class activities.

The *Paramedic Care* series also offers the latest multimedia technology to enhance and enrich your students' classroom experiences and to help you manage your classes more efficiently. The series' accompanying Companion Website contains chapter-by-chapter interactive student quizzes and links to related EMS sites for students. The Companion Website also offers downloadable instructor resources, teaching tips, links to curriculum-related websites, and an online syllabus builder. Our partnership with Victory Technology brings you *MedMedic*, an interactive CD-ROM tied chapter by chapter to each of the books. These new CDs include video, interactive student quizzes, and animations.

We wish you the best of luck as you transition to the new paramedic curriculum.

Sincerely,

Julie Levin Alexander
Vice President and Publisher

BRADY
Your Partner in Education

EMPHASIZING PRINCIPLES

Chapter Objectives with Page References

Each chapter begins with clearly stated **Objectives** that follow the new DOT Paramedic curriculum. Students can refer to these objectives while studying to make sure they understand the material fully. Page references after each objective indicate where relevant content is covered in the chapter.

Content Review

Content Review summarizes important content and gives students a format for quick review.

Key Points

Key Points in the margins help students identify and learn the fundamental principles of paramedic practice.

Key Terms

Reinforcement of **Key Terms** helps students master new terminology.

CHAPTER 6

Documentation

Objectives

After reading this chapter, you should be able to:

1. Identify the general principles regarding the importance of EMS documentation and ways in which documents are used. (pp. 212–214)
2. Identify and properly use medical terminology, medical abbreviations, and acronyms. (pp. 215–218)
3. Explain the role of documentation in agency reimbursement. (pp. 219–220)
4. Identify and eliminate extraneous or nonprofessional information. (pp. 222–224)
5. Describe the differences between subjective and objective elements of documentation. (pp. 225–227)
6. Evaluate a finished document for errors and omissions and proper use and spelling of abbreviations and acronyms. (p. 230)
7. Evaluate the confidential nature of an EMS report. (pp. 234–236)
8. Describe the potential consequences of illegible, incomplete, or inaccurate documentation. (pp. 239–242)

Continued

Content Review

FACILITATING BEHAVIORS
- Stay calm
- Plan for the worst
- Work systematically
- Remain adaptable

Be like the duck—cool and calm on the water's surface, while paddling feverishly underneath.

Except for safety concerns, never allow anything to distract you from your most important job—assessing and caring for your patient.

★ **reflective** acting thoughtfully, deliberately, and analytically.

★ **impulsive** acting instinctively without stopping to think.

★ **divergent** taking into account all aspects of a complex situation.

USEFUL THINKING STYLES

As a paramedic, you will face confusing emergencies that would challenge even the most knowledgeable, analytical care provider. You must be able to stay calm and not panic. Your self-control in the face of extreme chaos will set the example for other team members to follow. Even when you are struggling to maintain your composure—especially then—never let others know. The key is focusing on the task and blocking out the distractions. Be like the duck—cool and calm on the water's surface, while paddling feverishly underneath.

Assume and plan for the worst, and always err on the side of benefitting your patient. For example, if you are deliberating whether to immobilize your patient, initiate advanced life support procedures, or administer oxygen, just do it! It is better to err by providing care than by withholding it. Be pessimistic! Anticipate all potential bad side effects of your treatments and prepare "plan B." For example, as you deliver a bronchodilating drug to your severe asthmatic patient, anticipate that it will not work and mentally prepare to intubate him and perform positive pressure ventilation. Or while you are administering atropine to your patient with symptomatic bradycardia, plan ahead for external cardiac pacing and dopamine, if atropine therapy fails to restore adequate circulation.

Establish and maintain a systematic assessment pattern. Practice your assessments until they become second nature, and you will avoid skipping and missing steps. Be disciplined and stay focused, especially when you are confronted with a complex emergency scene. For example, your patient lies moaning on the ground in a pool of blood. Bystanders are screaming at you to help him; others are trying to tell you what happened. The police are gathering the story and trying unsuccessfully to talk with your patient. You must gain control of this scene. You do so by focusing on your patient and performing a systematic assessment. Use common acronyms (MS-ABC, OPQRST, SAMPLE) or make up your own to help you remember the key elements of your assessment. Except for safety concerns, never allow anything to distract you from your most important job—assessing and caring for your patient.

The different situations you encounter will require a variety of management styles. Adapting your styles of situation analysis (reflective vs. impulsive), data processing (convergent vs. divergent), and decision making (anticipatory vs. reactive) to each situation will enable you to provide the best possible care in every case.

Reflective vs. Impulsive Some situations call for you to be **reflective**, take your time, and figure out what is wrong with your patient. You have a patient who complains of "not feeling well." She has a long history of cardiac, renal, respiratory, and diabetic problems. Since she is in no real distress and is hemodynamically stable, you can take your time to determine her primary problem. Other situations call for immediate action. They require you to make an instinctive, **impulsive** decision and manage your patient's life-threatening condition. For example, if your patient presents apneic and pulseless, you will immediately begin CPR and prepare for rapid defibrillation. If he presents with a spurting artery, you will at once take measures to control the hemorrhage. If he is choking and has a weak, ineffective cough, you will quickly perform the Heimlich maneuver. You have to think fast in these situations.

Divergent vs. Convergent To process the data you receive from your patient and the scene, you can use either a divergent approach or a convergent approach. The **divergent** approach considers all aspects of a situation before arriving at a solution. It is insightful and works well when you are confronted with complex

communicating with other emergency care professionals.

...try ha... with ...
...5-1). These wo... ...orten air time and transmit thoughts and ideas quickly. For example, *copy*, *10-4*, and *roger* mean "I heard you and I understand what you said." Using industry terminology appropriately is an important part of effective communication. It provides a common means of communicating with other emergency care professionals.

Tables and Illustrations

Tables and **illustrations** offer visual support to enhance students' understanding of paramedic principles and practice.

Table 5-1	COMMON RADIO TERMINOLOGY
Term	**Meaning**
Copy, 10-4, roger	I understand
Affirmative	Yes
Negative	No
Stand by	Please wait
Repeat	Please repeat what you said
Land-line	Telephone communications
Rendezvous	Meet with
LZ	Landing zone (helicopter)
ETA	Estimated time of arrival
Over	I am finished with my transmission
Mobile status	On the air, driving around
Stage	Wait before entering a scene
Clear	End of transmission
Unfounded	We cannot find the incident/patient
Be advised	Listen carefully to this

Thyroid gland · Trachea · First rib (cut) · Right lung · Left lung · Superior vena cava · Aorta · Base of heart · Pulmonary artery · Diaphragm · Parietal pericardium (cut) · Apex of heart

FIGURE 1-3 If the patient cannot provide useful information, gather it from family members or bystanders.

BLINDNESS

Blind patients present special problems. They need you to identify yourself immediately, since they cannot see your uniform. Always announce yourself and explain who you are and why you are there. If possible, take your patient's hand to establish a personal contact and to show him where you are. Remember that nonverbal communication such as hand gestures, facial expressions, and body language, are useless in these cases. Your voice is your only tool for effective communication.

TALKING WITH FAMILIES OR FRIENDS

You will often encounter patients who cannot give you any useful information. In these cases, find a third party who can augment the patient history and offer a useful adjunct to the patient's answers (Figure 1-3). The typical case is the postictal patient who cannot describe his seizure activity to you. Another example is learning from his friend that your patient's wife died in an automobile accident just three weeks ago. Now you better understand why your patient appears depressed and suicidal. Make sure that patient confidentiality is a priority when you accept personal information from a family member, friend, or bystander.

SUMMARY

This chapter dealt with taking a good history. While it presented the patient history in its entirety, common sense will determine which parts are appropriate for a given situation. Most of a paramedic's work is patient contact. It is making a connection with people in crisis. Patients most often comment on the attitudes of their paramedics. How well did they relate to them? Did they make them feel at ease? Did they care for them? Patients rarely comment on a paramedic's technical skills. Top-notch paramedics are technically skillful and treat all their patients with dignity and compassion. This begins with the history.

Good patient interaction can lead to good patient outcomes, improved patient satisfaction, and better adherence to treatment. As a paramedic you have

Summa...

End-of-Chapter Summary

Each end-of-chapter **Summary** reviews the main topics covered.

c) Past H...
c) Current H...
d) Review of Systems

FURTHER READING

Bates, Barbara, Lynn S. Bickley, and Robert A. Hoekelman. *A Guide to Physical Examination and History Taking.* 6th ed. Philadelphia: J.B. Lippincott, 1995.
Coulehan, John L. and Marian R. Block. *The Medical Interview: Mastering Skills for Clinical Practice.* 3rd ed. Philadelphia: F.A. Davis, 1997.
Epstein, Owen, et al. *Clinical Examination.* St. Louis: Mosby, 1997.
Lipkin, Mack Jr., Samuel M. Putnam, and Aaron Lazare. *The Medical Interview: Clinical Care, Education, and Research.* New York: Springer, 1994.
Seidel Henry M. *Mosby's Guide to Physical Examination.* 3rd ed. St. Louis: Mosby, 1994.
Willms, Janice L., Henry Schniederman, and Paula S. Algranati. *Physical Diagnosis: Bedside Evaluation of Diagnosis and Function.* Baltimore: Williams & Wilkins, 1994.

ON THE WEB

Visit Brady's Paramedic Website through www.brady books.com/paramedic.

Further Reading and On the Web

Each chapter ends with recommendations for books and journal articles. Links to relevant websites plus a link to the text's Companion Website can be found at **www.bradybooks.com/paramedic.**

EMPHASIZING PRACTICE

Objectives Continued

8. Identify and differentiate among the following communications systems:
   - Simplex (pp. 101–102)
   - Multiplex (pp. 102–103)
   - Duplex (p. 104)
   - Trunked (pp. 104–106)
   - Digital communications (pp. 110–113)
   - Cellular telephone (p. 114)
   - Facsimile (pp. 114–115)
   - Computer (pp. 116–118)

9. Describe the functions and responsibilities of the Federal Communications Commission. (pp. 120–122)

10. Describe the role of emergency medical dispatch and the importance of prearrival instructions in a typical EMS response. (pp. 122–124)

11. List appropriate caller information gathered by the emergency medical dispatcher. (pp. 124–125)

12. Describe the structure and importance of verbal patient information communication to the hospital and medical direction. (pp. 128–131)

13. Diagram a basic communications system. (pp. 130–133)

14. Given several narrative patient scenarios, organize a verbal radio report for electronic transmission to medical direction. (pp. 138–142)

CASE STUDY

On a dry, warm Sunday afternoon, a 31-year-old male loses control of his motorcycle and strikes a highway sign. Several people witness the incident. The first bystander to reach the patient rushes to his automobile to dial 911 on his cellular telephone. Emergency medical dispatcher Vern Holland takes the necessary information and dispatches a basic life support engine company and an advanced life support ambulance. As Holland dispatches the emergency units, his partner, paramedic dispatcher Fred Hughes, instructs the caller in basic emergency care. The units receive the call via a computer printout of essential information.

They quickly arrive at the scene and initiate the appropriate care. Because the patient has a severe head injury, the paramedic performs only a limited assessment and immediately initiates transport. As the ambulance departs, he relays the following to Dr. Doyle, the medical direction physician:

Paramedic: Depew Ambulance to Mercy Hospital.

Dr. Doyle: Go ahead, Depew.

Paramedic: We are leaving the scene of a motorcycle accident on I-90. We have one patient, a male who is in his 30s, the rider of a motorcycle that went off the roadway and struck a sign. He responds to pain only, with obvious facial and chest

Case Study

Case Studies draw students into the reading and create a link between text content and real-life situations and experiences.

...of injury may a...up rehabilitation ...provide better therapy. Your PCR becomes an important document th...helps ensure your patient's continuous effective care.

Prehospital Care Report

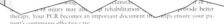

FIGURE 6-1   The run data in a prehospital care report is vital to your agency's efforts to improve patient care.

Documentation

Covered thoroughly throughout the text, **proper documentation techniques** are critical to ensuring provider protection on the job as well as patient safety during the transition of care.

You Make the Call

Promoting critical thinking skills, each **You Make the Call** presents a hypothetical situation that requires students to apply principles to actual practice. Suggested responses are found at the back of the text.

YOU MAKE THE CALL

A call comes into your unit for a "possible heart attack" on State Route 11. You and your partner climb into Palermo Rescue, a nontransport first-response vehicle. Your response time is about ten minutes. Upon arrival, a family member meets you. He leads you into the den of a small farm house. Here you see your patient sitting in an overstuffed chair. You note that your patient is a 69-year-old male in obvious distress.

You begin questioning your patient to develop a history. As he speaks, you immediately notice that he has difficulty breathing. He complains of severe chest pain, which began about 30 minutes ago. With his hand, he indicates that the pain is pressure-like and substernal. He also indicates that it radiates to his left arm and jaw. He describes a history of heart disease, including two prior heart attacks. Three years ago, he had cardiac bypass surgery. He currently takes Lanoxin, Lasix, Capoten, and an aspirin a day. He is allergic to Mellaril.

You and your partner complete your assessment. Your patient says he weighs about 250 pounds. He is alert, but anxious. He exhibits jugular venous distention and bibasilar crackles. His abdomen is nontender. His distal pulses are good. Vital signs include: blood pressure 210/110 mmHg, pulse of 70 per minute and regular, and respirations of 20 breaths per minute and mildly labored. Pulse oximetry is 93% on supplemental oxygen. During your assessment, your patient becomes progressively more dyspneic. The transporting ambulance arrives and the paramedic asks you to give a radio report to the receiving hospital based on your assessment while she prepares her patient for transport.

- Based on the information above, organize and prepare your radio report to inform the receiving hospital of your patient's condition.

See Suggested Responses at the back of this book.

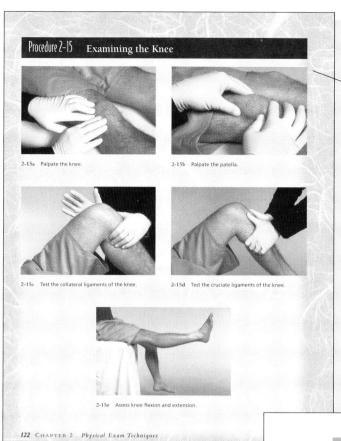

2-15a   Palpate the knee.

2-15b   Palpate the patella.

2-15c   Test the collateral ligaments of the knee.

2-15d   Test the cruciate ligaments of the knee.

2-15e   Assess knee flexion and extension.

122   CHAPTER 2   *Physical Exam Techniques*

Procedure Scans

Newly photographed **Procedure Scans** provide step-by-step visual support on how to perform skills included in the DOT curriculum.

Patient Care Algorithms

Clearly presented **algorithms** provide graphic "pathways" that integrate assessment and care for medical or trauma emergencies. These visual summaries give students a step-by-step flow of assessment and emergency care procedures.

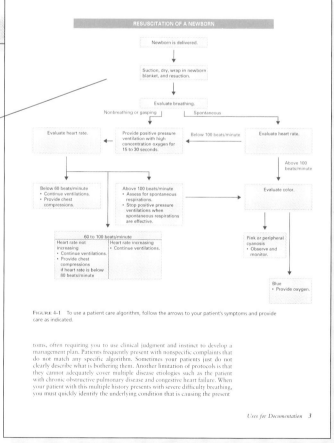

FIGURE 4-1   To use a patient care algorithm, follow the arrows to your patient's symptoms and provide care as indicated.

toms, often requiring you to use clinical judgment and instinct to develop a management plan. Patients frequently present with nonspecific complaints that do not match any specific algorithm. Sometimes your patients just do not clearly describe what is bothering them. Another limitation of protocols is that they cannot adequately cover multiple disease etiologies such as the patient with chronic obstructive pulmonary disease and congestive heart failure. When your patient with this multiple history presents with severe difficulty breathing, you must quickly identify the underlying condition that is causing the present

Uses for Documentation   *3*

Teaching & Learning Package

FOR THE INSTRUCTOR

Instructor's Resource Manual

The Instructor's Resource Manual for each volume contains everything needed to teach the 1998 U.S. DOT National Standard Curriculum for Paramedics. It fully covers the DOT curriculum with:

• time estimates for various topics
• listing of additional resources
• lecture outlines
• student activities handouts
• answers to student review questions
• case study discussion questions.

The manual is also available on disk so instructors can customize resources to their individual needs.

PowerPoint® Presentations on CD-ROM

This CD-ROM offers PowerPoint® presentations that contain word slides and images organized by chapter. The entire presentation is fully customizable.

Computerized Test Bank

The Computerized Test Bank contains textbook-based questions in a format that enables instructors to select questions based on topic area and degree of difficulty.

FOR THE STUDENT

Student Workbook

A student workbook with review and practice activities accompanies each volume of the *Paramedic Care* series. The workbooks include multiple-choice questions, fill-in-the-blank questions, labeling exercises, case studies, and special projects, along with an answer key with text page references.

ONLINE RESOURCES

Paramedic Care Companion Website: www.bradybooks.com/paramedic

This free site, tied chapter-by-chapter to the five texts, reinforces student learning through interactive online study guides, quizzes based on the new curriculum, and case studies, as well as links to important EMS-related Internet resources. The *Paramedic Care* Companion Website also includes instructor resources, such as a bridge guide to help instructors transition to the new curriculum, links to EMS-related sites (including a site to download the new curriculum), and teaching tips. Instructors can also use the site to create a customized syllabus.

EMS Supersite: www.bradybooks.com/ems

Brady's EMS Supersite is a free, one-stop Web resource for both students and instructors offering:

• Online Brady catalog
• Links to all Brady Companion Websites
• Interactive case studies
• Case Study of the Month
• Useful EMS-related links
• Games, puzzles, and activities
• Test-taking tips
• Test-writing and teaching tips
• Sample chapters and multimedia demos.

For information on additional media to support the series, please contact your Brady representative:
1-800-638-0220

OTHER TITLES OF INTEREST

ANATOMY & PHYSIOLOGY

GUY, Learning Human Anatomy, Second Edition (0-8385-5657-4)

Organized by body regions, this popular text helps students learn human anatomy. Its outline format and easy-to-remember illustrations make it ideal for review and a perfect introductory gross anatomy text.

MARTINI et al., Essentials of Anatomy and Physiology, Second Edition (0-13-082192-6)

A one-semester/one-quarter anatomy and physiology text for students in allied health, physical education, and other programs requiring an overview of the human body's systems. An extensive instructor support package is available.

CARDIAC/EKG

BEASLEY, Understanding EKGs (0-8359-8571-7)

This text is a direct, basic approach to EKG interpretation that presents all the essential concepts for mastering the basics of this challenging field, while assuming no prior knowledge of EKGs.

BEASLEY, Understanding 12-Lead EKGs (0-13-027281-7)

This comprehensive, reader-friendly text teaches beginning students basic 12-lead EKG interpretation.

MISTOVICH et al., Advanced Cardiac Life Support (0-8359-5050-6)

Straightforward and easy to follow, this text offers clear explanations, a colorful design, and covers all of the core concepts covered in an advanced cardiac life support course.

PAGE, 12-Lead ECG for the Acute Care Provider (0-13-022460-X)

This full-color text presents EKG interpretation in a practical, easy-to-understand and user-friendly manner. Practice cases are included throughout the text.

For a complete listing of additional Brady titles, visit us on the Web: www.bradybooks.com

WALRAVEN, Basic Arrhythmias, Fifth Edition (0-8359-5305-X)

This classic bestseller covers all the basics of EKG and includes appendices on Clinical Implications of Arrhythmias, Cardiac Anatomy & Physiology, 12-Lead EKG, Basic 12-Lead Interpretation and Pacemakers.

MATHEMATICS

BENJAMIN-CHUNG, Math Principles and Practice: Preparing for Health Career Success (0-8359-5272-X)

This easy-to-follow text provides basic math skills for students or practicing health care professionals. It employs a common sense approach that builds on basic math skills to facilitate the understanding of more complex math calculations.

TIGER, Mathematical Concepts for Clinical Sciences (0-13-011549-5)

This book is geared for all entry-level clinical science curricula and presents material in a step-by-step approach that emphasizes the understanding of concepts, not the memorization of numbers and formulas.

MEDICAL

DALTON et al., Advanced Medical Life Support (0-8359-5179-0)

This groundbreaking text offers a practical approach to adult medical emergencies. Each chapter discusses realistic methods that a seasoned EMS practitioner would use.

MEDICAL TERMINOLOGY

FREMGEN, Medical Terminology: An Anatomy & Physiology Systems Approach (0-8359-4991-5)

In this full-color text-workbook, Bonnie F. Fremgen uses an integrated body systems approach and reader-friendly writing style to teach medical terminology.

LILLIS, A Concise Introduction to Medical Terminology (0-8385-4321-9)

A basic introduction to over 700 commonly used medical terms and word elements to help students learn the terminology they need to succeed.

(continued on next page)

OTHER TITLES OF INTEREST

MEDICAL TERMINOLOGY *(continued)*

RICE, Medical Terminology with Human Anatomy, Fourth Edition (0-8385-6274-4)

Providing comprehensive coverage of all aspects of medical terminology, the Fourth Edition of this popular text is arranged by body systems and specialty areas. Rice makes learning easy and interesting by presenting important prefixes, roots, and suffixes as they relate to each specialty or system.

RICE, The Terminology of Health and Medicine (0-8385-6260-4)

This self-study text presents learning concepts in numbered frames—with a series of statements on the right side of the page and the answers provided in a column on the outside. Terms are arranged by body system.

PATHOPHYSIOLOGY

BURNS, Pathophysiology (0-8385-8084-X)

Students will master the basics of general disease processes—as well as major diseases of the body system—by using the only pathophysiology text that offers a programmed approach with questions within each frame that test comprehension, and self-tests at the end of each section.

KENT/HART, Introduction to Human Disease, Fourth Edition (0-8385-4070-8)

This is the perfect text for any student seeking a reliable and concise overview of human disease. Each chapter contains most frequently encountered and serious problems, symptoms, signs and tests, specific diseases, and review questions.

MULVIHILL, Human Disease, Fourth Edition (0-8385-3928-9)

This popular book comprehensively covers mechanisms of disease and health problems, as well as commonly occurring diseases. Normal anatomy and physiology is reviewed at the beginning of each chapter.

For a complete listing of additional Brady titles, visit us on the Web:
www.bradybooks.com

PEDIATRICS

EICHELBERGER, Pediatric Emergencies, Second Edition (0-8359-5123-5)

This text was developed to provide a standard of prehospital pediatric emergency care for both basic and advanced providers.

MARKENSON et al., Pediatric Prehospital Care (0-13-022618-1)

Written for all levels of EMS providers, this text presents a physiological approach to rapid and accurate pediatric assessment, identification of potential problems, establishing treatment priorities with effective on-going assessment, and rapid and safe transport.

PHARMACOLOGY

GRAJEDA-HIGLEY, Pharmacology (0-8385-8136-6)

This pharmacology handbook combines a systems approach with cartoon-type illustrations for a unique and user-friendly physiological presentation of pharmacological concepts.

MIKOLAJ, Drug Dosage Calculations (0-8359-4994-X)

This practical volume gives readers all the tools needed to solve virtually every type of dosage and calculation problem they will encounter in the workplace.

SHANNON, The Health Professional's Drug Guide 2000 (0-8385-0424-8)

This drug guide provides health care professionals with accurate, easily accessible information about their patients' medications. Comprehensive yet user-friendly, this handy resource includes important clinical implications for hundreds of drugs, including adverse reactions, interactions and side effects.

TRAUMA

CAMPBELL, Basic Trauma Life Support for Paramedics and Advanced Providers, Fourth Edition (0-13-084584-1)

Brady's best selling BTLS text provides a complete course that covers all the skills necessary for rapid assessment, resuscitation, stabilization and transportation of the trauma patient.

BRADY

PARAMEDIC CARE: Principles & Practice

SPECIAL CONSIDERATIONS/OPERATIONS

CHAPTER 1

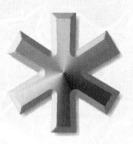

Neonatology

Objectives

After reading this chapter, you should be able to:

1. Define newborn and neonate. (p. 4)
2. Identify important antepartum factors that can affect childbirth. (p. 5)
3. Identify important intrapartum factors that can determine high-risk newborn patients. (p. 6)
4. Identify the factors that lead to premature birth and low-birth-weight newborns. (pp. 23, 25, 29–30)
5. Distinguish between primary and secondary apnea. (p. 6)
6. Discuss pulmonary perfusion and asphyxia. (p. 6)
7. Identify the primary signs utilized for evaluating a newborn during resuscitation. (p. 8)
8. Identify the appropriate use of the APGAR scale. (pp. 8–9)
9. Calculate the APGAR score given various newborn situations. (pp. 8–9)
10. Formulate an appropriate treatment plan for providing initial care to a newborn. (p. 9)

Continued

Objectives Continued

11. Describe the indications, equipment needed, application, and evaluation of the following management techniques for the newborn in distress:
    a. Blow-by oxygen (pp. 19–20)
    b. Ventilatory assistance (pp. 20–21)
    c. Endotracheal intubation (pp. 17–18)
    d. Orogastric tube (p. 21)
    e. Chest compressions (p. 21)
    f. Vascular access (pp. 21–23)
12. Discuss the routes of medication administration for a newborn. (pp. 21–24)
13. Discuss the signs of hypovolemia in a newborn. (pp. 30–31)
14. Discuss the initial steps in resuscitation of a newborn. (pp. 15–17)
15. Discuss the effects of maternal narcotic usage on the newborn. (p. 23)
16. Determine the appropriate treatment for the newborn with narcotic depression. (pp. 23, 25)
17. Discuss appropriate transport guidelines for a newborn. (p. 25)
18. Determine appropriate receiving facilities for low- and high-risk newborns. (pp. 6, 25)

19. Describe the epidemiology, including the incidence, morbidity/mortality, risk factors and prevention strategies, pathophysiology, assessment findings, and management for the following neonatal problems:
    a. Meconium aspiration (pp. 26–27)
    b. Apnea (p. 27)
    c. Diaphragmatic hernia (pp. 27–28)
    d. Bradycardia (p. 29)
    e. Prematurity (pp. 29–30)
    f. Respiratory distress/cyanosis (p. 30)
    g. Seizures (p. 31)
    h. Fever (pp. 31–32)
    i. Hypothermia (pp. 32–33)
    j. Hypoglycemia (p. 33)
    k. Vomiting (p. 34)
    l. Diarrhea (p. 35)
    m. Common birth injuries (pp. 36–37)
    n. Cardiac arrest (p. 36)
    o. Post-arrest management (p. 36)
20. Given several neonatal emergencies, provide the appropriate procedures for assessment, management, and transport. (pp. 4–36)

CASE STUDY

A storm rages outside, making travel dangerous. Around midnight you receive a call from the dispatcher. A woman has just gone into labor. She lives about 20 minutes from the hospital, but her husband is worried about the weather conditions and requests help from your EMS unit.

Upon arrival, you find a 24-year-old female who is about to deliver her second baby. You quickly determine that there is not enough time to transport the patient to the hospital. You and your partner begin to prepare the equipment needed for a field delivery.

The delivery goes beautifully, and you announce the arrival of the couple's new daughter. Following the birth, however, the baby remains blue and limp—even after you suction the airway. You quickly dry the baby and then wrap her in a dry blanket. You stimulate the baby by rubbing her back and flicking the soles of her feet gently. Once again, you suction the baby, first the mouth and then the nose.

When the baby stays blue and limp, you push aside a very normal urge to panic and deliver "blow-by" oxygen. When her heart rate remains less than 100, you grab the bag-valve-mask unit and apply artificial ventilation. The baby "pinks up" almost immediately and begins to cry.

Using the pulse oximeter, you determine that the oxygen saturation is 95 percent and increasing. You prepare the baby for transport, making sure her head is covered. You ask the mother to hold her new daughter and then load both of your patients into the ambulance.

En route to the hospital, you continue to administer blow-by oxygen and assign a five-minute APGAR score of 9. The trip is uneventful. The baby leaves the hospital only one day after the mother. The parents later pay a surprise visit to your EMS unit. They proudly introduce a healthy baby daughter named after you!

INTRODUCTION

Babies pass through stages of physical and emotional development. This chapter concerns itself with babies one month old and under. Babies less than one month old are called **neonates**. Recently born neonates—those in the first few hours of their lives—may also be called **newborns** or *newly born infants* (Figure 1-1).

After an unscheduled delivery in the field, you have two patients to manage—the mother and the baby. You can review information on care of the mother in Volume 3, Chapter 14. The present chapter describes the initial care of newborns, focusing on the special needs of distressed and premature newborns.

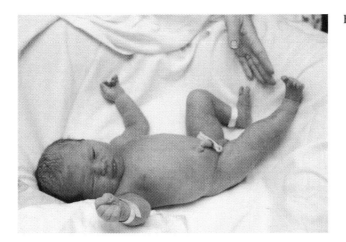

FIGURE 1-1 Term newborn.

GENERAL PATHOPHYSIOLOGY, ASSESSMENT, AND MANAGEMENT

The care of newborns follows the same priorities as for all patients. You should complete the initial assessment first. Correct any problems detected during the initial assessment before proceeding to the next step. The vast majority of newborns require no resuscitation beyond suctioning the airway, mild stimulation, and maintenance of body temperature. However, for newborns that require additional care, your quick actions can make the difference between life and death.

EPIDEMIOLOGY

Approximately 6 percent of field deliveries require life support. The incidence of complications increases as the birth weight decreases. About 80 percent of newborns weighing less than 1,500 grams (3 pounds, 5 ounces) at birth require resuscitation. Determine at-risk newborns by considering the **antepartum** and **intrapartum** factors that may indicate complications at the time of delivery (Table 1-1).

Your success in resuscitating these at-risk infants increases with training, ongoing practice, and proper stocking of equipment on board the ambulance. Make sure your ambulance carries a basic OB kit and resuscitation equipment for newborns of various sizes. (See the list under "Resuscitation," later in this chapter.)

For newborns that require additional care, your quick actions can make the difference between life and death.

∗ antepartum before the onset of labor.

∗ intrapartum occurring during childbirth.

Your success in treating at-risk newborns increases with training, ongoing practice, and proper stocking of equipment on board the ambulance.

Table 1-1	RISK FACTORS INDICATING POSSIBLE COMPLICATIONS IN NEWBORNS	
Antepartum Factors	**Intrapartum Factors**	
Multiple gestation	Premature labor	
Inadequate prenatal care	Meconium-stained amniotic fluid	
Mother's age (<16 or >35)	Rupture of membranes more than 24 hours prior to delivery	
History of perinatal morbidity or mortality	Use of narcotics within four hours of delivery	
Post-term gestation		
Drugs/medications	Abnormal presentation	
Toxemia, hypertension, diabetes	Prolonged labor or precipitous delivery	
	Prolapsed cord or bleeding	

Plan transport in advance. Know the type of facilities available in your locality and local protocols governing use of these facilities. A nearby neonatal intensive care unit (NICU) makes the best choice for at-risk newborns. However, if you must transport to a distant NICU, determine whether it might be in the best interests of the infant to transport him or her to the nearest facility for stabilization. Follow local protocols and consult medical direction as needed.

PATHOPHYSIOLOGY

 extrauterine outside the uterus.

Upon birth, dramatic changes take place within the newborn to prepare it for extrauterine life.

 ductus arteriosus channel between the main pulmonary artery and the aorta of the fetus.

The time of a newborn's first breath is unrelated to the cutting of the umbilical cord.

Upon birth, dramatic changes occur within the newborn to prepare it for **extrauterine** life. The respiratory system, which is essentially nonfunctional when the fetus is in the uterus, must suddenly initiate and maintain respirations. While in the uterus, fetal lung fluid fills the fetal lungs. The capillaries and arterioles of the lungs are closed. Most blood pumped by the heart bypasses the nonfunctional respiratory system by flowing through the **ductus arteriosus.**

Approximately one-third of fetal lung fluid is removed through compression of the chest during vaginal delivery. Under normal conditions, the newborn takes its first breath within the first few seconds after delivery. The timing of the first breath is unrelated to the cutting of the umbilical cord. Factors that stimulate the baby's first breath include:

- Mild acidosis
- Initiation of stretch reflexes in the lungs
- Hypoxia
- Hypothermia

With the first breaths, the lungs rapidly fill with air, which displaces the remaining fetal fluid. The pulmonary arterioles and capillaries open, decreasing pulmonary vascular resistance. At this point, the resistance to blood flow in the lungs is now less than the resistance of the ductus arteriosus. Because of this pressure difference, blood flow is diverted from the ductus arteriosus to the lungs, where it picks up oxygen for transport to the peripheral tissues (Figure 1-2).

Soon, there is no need for the ductus arteriosus, and it eventually closes. However, if hypoxia or severe acidosis occurs, the pulmonary vascular bed may constrict again and the ductus may reopen. This will retrigger fetal circulation with its attendant shunting and ongoing hypoxia. (This condition is called **persistent fetal circulation.**) To help the newborn make its transition to extrauterine life, it is very important for the paramedic to facilitate its first few breaths and to prevent ongoing hypoxia and acidosis.

 persistent fetal circulation condition in which blood continues to bypass the fetal respiratory system, resulting in ongoing hypoxia.

Remain alert at all times to signs of respiratory distress. Infants are susceptible to hypoxemia, which can lead to permanent brain damage. After initial hypoxia, the infant rapidly gasps for breath. If the asphyxia continues, respiratory movements cease altogether, the heart rate begins to fall, and neuromuscular tone gradually diminishes. The infant then enters a period of apnea known as *primary apnea.* In most cases, simple stimulation and exposure to oxygen will reverse bradycardia and assist in the development of pulmonary perfusion.

With ongoing asphyxia, however, the infant will enter a period known as *secondary apnea.* During secondary apnea, the infant takes several last deep gasping respirations. The heart rate, blood pressure, and oxygen saturation in the blood continue to fall. The infant becomes unresponsive to stimulation and will not spontaneously resume respiration on its own. Death will occur unless you promptly initiate resuscitation. For this reason, always assume that apnea in the newborn is secondary apnea and rapidly treat it with ventilatory assistance with oxygen and, when appropriate, chest compressions.

Always assume that apnea in the newborn is secondary apnea and rapidly treat it with ventilatory assistance.

FIGURE 1-2 Hemodynamic changes in the newborn at birth.

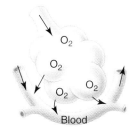

Air

Fetal lung fluid

Air

1st 2nd 3rd
Breaths

Following birth, the lungs expand as they are filled with air. The fetal lung fluid gradually leaves the alveoli.

Arterioles dilate and blood flow increases

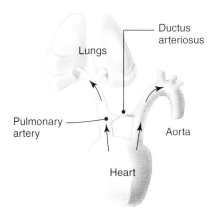

O_2
O_2
O_2 O_2
Blood

At the same time as the lungs are expanding and the fetal lung fluid is clearing, the arterioles in the lung begin to open, allowing a considerable increase in the amount of blood flowing through the lungs.

Pulmonary blood flow increases

Ductus arteriosus

Lungs

Pulmonary artery

Aorta

Heart

Blood previously diverted through the ductus arteriosus flows through the lungs where it picks up oxygen to transport to tissues throughout the body. Soon there is no need for the ductus and it eventually closes.

Congenital Anomalies

Approximately 2 percent of infants are born with some sort of congenital problem. Congenital problems typically arise from a problem in fetal development. Most fetal development occurs during the first trimester of pregnancy. It is during this time that the developing fetus is most sensitive to environmental factors and substances that can affect normal development.

There are many types of congenital anomalies. These may affect a single organ or structure or may affect many organs or structures. There are several recognized patterns, called *syndromes*, that can occur. It is not within the scope of this text to discuss all the various congenital anomalies. However, there are a few congenital anomalies that can make resuscitation more difficult. For example, some children may be born with a defect in the diaphragm that allows some of the abdominal contents to enter the chest. This abnormality is referred to as a **diaphragmatic hernia.** If you suspect a diaphragmatic hernia, do not treat the infant with bag-valve-mask ventilation. This procedure will distend the stomach, which protrudes into the chest cavity, thus decreasing ventilatory capacity. Instead, immediately intubate the infant. (Diaphragmatic hernia will be discussed in more detail later in this chapter.)

Newborns may have congenital anomalies that make resuscitation more difficult.

* **diaphragmatic hernia** protrusion of abdominal contents into the thoracic cavity through an opening in the diaphragm.

Some infants are born with a defect in their spinal cords. In some cases, the spinal cord and associated structures may be exposed. This abnormality is called a **meningomyelocele.** Infants born with a meningomyelocele should not be placed on their backs. Instead, place them on their stomachs or sides and conduct resuscitation in this position, if possible. Cover the spinal defect with sterile gauze pads soaked in warm sterile saline and inserted in a plastic covering.

A newborn may exhibit a defect in the area of the umbilicus. In some cases, the abdominal contents will fill this defect, resulting in an **omphalocele.** If you encounter a newborn with an omphalocele, cover the defect with an occlusive plastic covering to decrease water and heat loss.

Since newborns are obligate nose breathers, **choanal atresia** can cause upper airway obstruction and respiratory distress. Choanal atresia is the most common birth defect involving the nose and is due to the presence of a bony or membranous septum between the nasal cavity and the pharynx. Suspect this condition if you are unable to pass a catheter through either nare into the oropharynx. An oral airway will usually bypass the obstruction.

A fairly common congenital anomaly is cleft lip and cleft palate. During fetal development, the lip and palate come together in the middle forming the oral cavity. Failure of the palate to completely close during fetal development can result in a defect known as **cleft palate.** Cleft palate may also be associated with failure of the upper lip to close. This condition, referred to as **cleft lip,** can make it difficult to obtain an adequate seal for effective mask ventilation. If a child with a cleft lip or cleft palate will require more than brief mechanical ventilation, you should place an endotracheal tube.

Pierre Robin Syndrome is a congenital condition characterized by a small jaw and large tongue in conjunction with a cleft palate. In this condition, the tongue is likely to obstruct the upper airway. A nasal or oral airway usually bypasses the obstruction. If the obstruction cannot be bypassed with a simple airway, then intubation will be necessary, although it can be very difficult to carry out on newborns with this condition.

ASSESSMENT

Assess the newborn immediately after birth. (Ideally, if two paramedics are available, one paramedic attends the mother, while the other attends the newborn.) Make a mental note of the time of birth and then quickly obtain vital signs. Remember that newborns are slippery and will require both hands to support the head and torso. Position yourself so that you can work close to the surface where you have placed the infant.

The newborn's respiratory rate should average 40–60 breaths per minute. If respirations are not adequate or if the newborn is gasping, immediately start positive-pressure ventilation.

Expect a normal heart rate of 150–180 beats per minute at birth, slowing to 130–140 beats per minute thereafter. A pulse rate of less than 100 beats per minute indicates distress and requires emergency intervention.

Evaluate the skin color as well. Some cyanosis of the extremities is common immediately after birth. However, cyanosis of the central part of the body is abnormal, as is persistent peripheral cyanosis. In such cases, administer 100% oxygen until the cause is determined or the condition is corrected.

THE APGAR SCALE

As soon as possible, assign the newborn an **APGAR score** (Table 1-2). Ideally, try to do this at 1 and 5 minutes after birth. However, if the newborn is not breathing, DO NOT withhold resuscitation in order to determine the APGAR score.

Table 1-2	THE APGAR Score				Score	
Sign	0	1	2	1 min	5 min
Appearance (Skin color)	Blue, pale	Body pink, extremities blue	Completely pink		
Pulse Rate (Heart rate)	Absent	Below 100	Above 100		
Grimace (Irritability)	No response	Grimace	Cries		
Activity (Muscle tone)	Limp	Some flexion of extremities	Active motion		
Respiratory Effort	Absent	Slow and irregular	Strong cry		
			TOTAL SCORE =		

The APGAR scoring system helps distinguish between newborns who need only routine care and those who need greater assistance. The system also predicts long-term survival. An anesthesiologist named Dr. Virginia Apgar developed the system in 1952, and her name forms an acronym for its parameters. The parameters for APGAR scoring include:

- Appearance
- Pulse rate
- Grimace
- Activity
- Respiratory effort

A score of 0, 1, or 2 is given for each of the above parameters. The minimum total score is 0 and the maximum is 10. A score of 7–10 indicates an active and vigorous newborn that requires only routine care. A score of 4–6 indicates a moderately distressed newborn that requires oxygenation and stimulation. Severely distressed newborns, those with APGAR scores of less than 4, require immediate resuscitation. By determining the APGAR score at 1 and 5 minutes, you can determine whether intervention has caused a change in the newborn's status.

Severely distressed newborns, those with APGAR scores of less than 4, require immediate resuscitation.

TREATMENT

Treatment starts prior to delivery. Begin care by preparing the environment and assembling the equipment needed for delivery and immediate care of the newborn. The initial care of a newborn follows the same priorities as for all patients. Complete the initial assessment first. Correct any problems detected during the initial assessment before proceeding to the next step. The vast majority of term newborns—approximately 80 percent—require no resuscitation beyond suctioning of the airway, mild stimulation, and maintenance of body temperature by drying and warming with blankets.

Airway management is one of the most critical steps in caring for the newborn.

Establishing the Airway

Airway management is one of the most critical steps in caring for the newborn. During delivery, fluid is forced out of the baby's lungs, into the oropharynx, and out through the nose and mouth. Fluid drainage occurs independently of gravity. As soon as you deliver the newborn's head, suction the mouth and then the nose, using a bulb suction. Always suction the mouth first so that there is nothing for the infant to aspirate if he or she gasps when the nose is suctioned.

Always suction the mouth first so that there is nothing for the infant to aspirate if he or she gasps when the nose is suctioned.

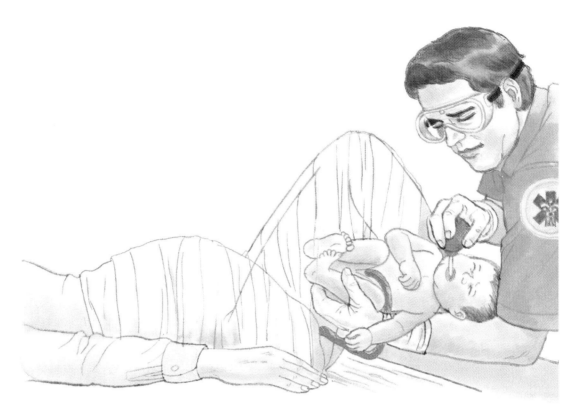

FIGURE 1-3   Position of newborn when first suctioning upon delivery.

If the newborn does not cry immediately, stimulate it by gently rubbing its back or flicking the soles of its feet. DO NOT spank or vigorously rub a newborn baby.

Cold infants quickly become distressed infants.

Immediately following delivery, maintain the newborn at the same level as the mother's vagina, with the head approximately 15 degrees below the torso (Figure 1-3). This facilitates the drainage of secretions and helps to prevent aspiration. If there appears to be a large amount of secretions, attach a **DeLee suction trap** to a suction source. As previously explained, suction the mouth first and then the nose (Figure 1-4a). Repeat these steps until the airway is clear. If you detect **meconium,** prepare intubation equipment and a meconium aspirator (Figure 1-4b). (Meconium staining will be discussed in more detail in several later sections of this chapter.)

Drying and suctioning produce enough stimulation to initiate respirations in most newborns. If the newborn does not immediately cry, stimulate it by flicking the soles of its feet or gently rubbing its back (Figure 1-5). DO NOT spank or vigorously rub a newborn baby.

Prevention of Heat Loss

Heat loss can be a life-threatening condition in newborns. Cold infants quickly become distressed infants. Heat loss occurs through evaporation, convection, conduction, and radiation. Most heat loss in newborns results from evaporation. The newborn comes into the world wet, and the amniotic fluid quickly evaporates. Immediately after birth, the newborn's core temperature can drop 1° C (1.8°F) or more from its birth temperature of 38° C (100.4° F).

Loss of heat can also occur through convection, depending upon the temperature of the room and the movement of the air around the newborn. The newborn can lose additional heat through contact with surrounding surfaces (convection) or by radiating heat to colder objects nearby.

FIGURE 1-4a Suctioning of the mouth using flexible suction catheter.

When head is delivered

As soon as the baby's head is delivered (prior to delivery of the shoulders) *the mouth, oropharynx, and hypopharynx should be thoroughly suctioned*, using a 10 Fr. DeLee suction catheter or other flexible suction catheter. Any catheter used should be no smaller than a 10 Fr.

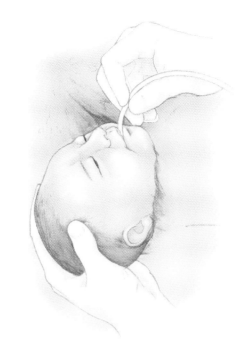

FIGURE 1-4b Intubation for removal of residual meconium.

Following delivery

After delivery of the infant, if a great deal of meconium is present, the trachea should be intubated and any residual meconium removed from the lower airway.

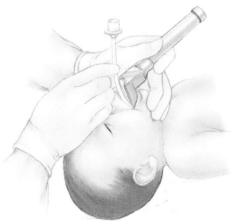

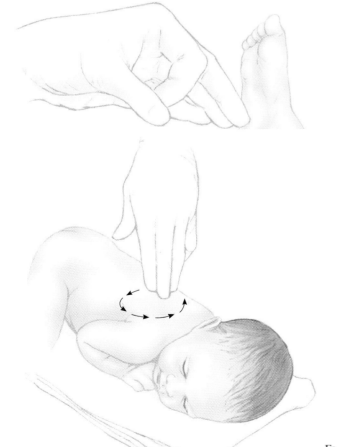

FIGURE 1-5 Stimulate the newborn as required.

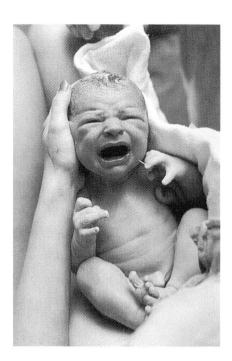

FIGURE 1-6   Dry the infant to prevent loss of evaporative heat.

To prevent heat loss, take these steps.

- Dry the newborn immediately to prevent evaporative cooling (Figure 1-6).
- Maintain the ambient temperature—the temperature in the delivery room or ambulance—at a *minimum* of 23–24° C (74–76° F).
- Close all windows and doors.
- Discard the towel used to dry the newborn and swaddle the infant in a warm, dry receiving blanket or other suitable material. Cover the head.
- In colder areas, place well-insulated water bottles or rubber gloves filled with warm water (40°C or 104°F) around the newborn to help maintain a warm body temperature. To avoid burns, do not place these items against the skin. Be sure the newborn is wrapped in a blanket and place the water bottle or rubber glove against the blanket.

Cutting the Umbilical Cord

After you have stabilized the newborn's airway and minimized heat loss, clamp and cut the umbilical cord. You can prevent over- and under-transfusion of blood by maintaining the baby at the same level as the vagina, as previously described. Do not "milk" or strip the umbilical cord, since this increases blood viscosity, or **polycythemia.** Polycythemia can cause cardiopulmonary problems. It can also contribute to excessive red blood cell destruction, which may in turn lead to **hyperbilirubinemia**—an increased level of bilirubin in the blood that causes jaundice.

Apply the umbilical clamps within 30–45 seconds after birth. Place the first clamp approximately 10 cm (4 inches) from the newborn. Place the second clamp

Do not "milk" or strip the umbilical cord.

✳ **polycythemia** an excess of red blood cells. In a newborn, the condition may reflect hypovolemia or prolonged intrauterine hypoxia.

✳ **hyperbilirubinemia** an excessive amount of bilirubin—the orange-colored pigment associated with bile—in the blood. In newborns, the condition appears as jaundice. Precipitating factors include maternal Rh or ABO incompatibility, neonatal septis, anoxia, hypoglycemia, and congenital liver or gastrointestinal defects.

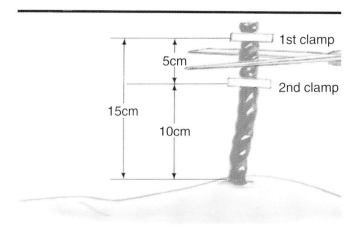

FIGURE 1-7   Clamping and cutting the cord.

about 5 cm (2 inches) farther away than the first. Then cut the cord between the two clamps (Figure 1-7). After the cord is cut, inspect it periodically to make sure there is no additional bleeding.

THE DISTRESSED NEWBORN

The distressed newborn can be either full term or premature. (See "Premature Infants" later in this chapter.) The presence of fetal meconium at birth indicates that fetal distress has occurred at some point during pregnancy. If the newborn is simply meconium stained, then distress may have occurred at a remote time. If you see *particulate* meconium, however, distress may have occurred recently and the newborn should be managed accordingly.

Aspiration of meconium can cause significant respiratory problems and should be prevented. Whenever you spot meconium during delivery, do not induce respiratory effort until you have removed the meconium from the trachea by suctioning under direct visualization with the laryngoscope. (There will be more about this topic under "Meconium Stained Amniotic Fluid" later.) Be sure to report the presence of meconium to the medical direction physician.

The most common problems experienced by newborns during the first minutes of life involve the airway. For this reason, resuscitation usually consists of ventilation and oxygenation. Except in special situations, the use of IV fluids, drugs, or cardiac equipment is usually not indicated. (See "Inverted Pyramid for Resuscitation" on the next page.) The most important procedures include suctioning, drying, and stimulating the distressed newborn.

Of the vital signs, fetal heart rate is the most important indicator of neonatal distress. The newborn has a relatively fixed stroke volume. Thus, cardiac output depends more on heart rate. Bradycardia, as caused by hypoxia, results in decreased cardiac output and, ultimately, poor perfusion. A pulse rate of less than 60 beats per minute in a distressed newborn should be treated with chest compressions. In distressed newborns, monitor the heart rate manually. Do not depend on external electronic monitors.

Of the vital signs, fetal heart rate is the most important indicator of neonatal distress.

RESUSCITATION

The vast majority of newborns do not require resuscitation beyond stimulation, maintenance of the airway, and maintenance of body temperature. Unfortunately, it is difficult to predict which newborns ultimately will require resuscitation. Each EMS unit, therefore, should contain a neonatal resuscitation kit with the following items:

- Neonatal bag-valve-mask unit
- Bulb syringe
- DeLee suction trap
- Meconium aspirator
- Laryngoscope with size 0 and 1 blades
- Uncuffed endotracheal tubes (2.5, 3.0, 3.5, 4.0) with appropriate suction catheters
- Endotracheal tube stylet
- Tape or device to secure endotracheal tube
- Umbilical catheter and 10 mL syringe
- Three-way stopcock
- 20 mL syringe and 8 french feeding tube for gastric suction
- Glucometer
- Assorted syringes and needles
- Towels (sterile)
- Medications:
  - Epinephrine 1:10,000 and 1:1,000
  - Neonatal naloxone (Narcon)
  - Volume expander (lactated Ringer's solution or saline)
  - Sodium bicarbonate (10 mEq in 10 mL)

INVERTED PYRAMID FOR RESUSCITATION

Resuscitation of the newborn follows an inverted pyramid (Figure 1-8). As this pyramid indicates, most distressed newborns respond to relatively simple maneuvers. Few require CPR or advanced life support measures.

FIGURE 1-8   The inverted pyramid of neonatal resuscitation showing approximate relative frequencies of neonatal care and resuscitative efforts. Note that a majority of infants respond to the simple measures noted at the top, wide part of the pyramid.

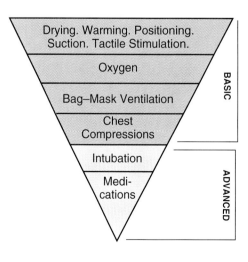

NORMAL NEWBORN ASSESSMENT AND SUPPORT

Temperature: Dry, warm
Airway: Position, suction
Breathing: Gentle stimulation to cry
Circulation: Pulse rate, color

ASSISTANCE SOME NEWBORNS MAY REQUIRE
(Note: Moving down the list, progressively
fewer patients will require the listed interventions.)

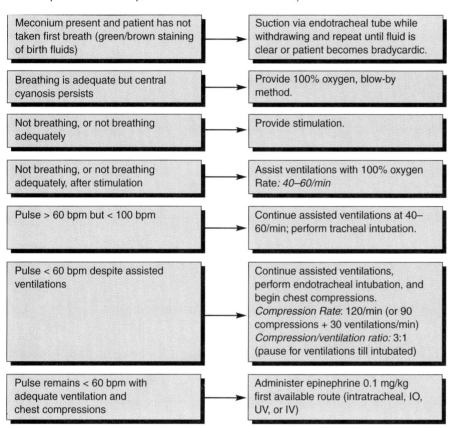

Meconium present and patient has not taken first breath (green/brown staining of birth fluids)	Suction via endotracheal tube while withdrawing and repeat until fluid is clear or patient becomes bradycardic.
Breathing is adequate but central cyanosis persists	Provide 100% oxygen, blow-by method.
Not breathing, or not breathing adequately	Provide stimulation.
Not breathing, or not breathing adequately, after stimulation	Assist ventilations with 100% oxygen Rate: *40–60/min*
Pulse > 60 bpm but < 100 bpm	Continue assisted ventilations at 40–60/min; perform tracheal intubation.
Pulse < 60 bpm despite assisted ventilations	Continue assisted ventilations, perform endotracheal intubation, and begin chest compressions. *Compression Rate*: 120/min (or 90 compressions + 30 ventilations/min) *Compression/ventilation ratio*: 3:1 (pause for ventilations till intubated)
Pulse remains < 60 bpm with adequate ventilation and chest compressions	Administer epinephrine 0.1 mg/kg first available route (intratracheal, IO, UV, or IV)

FIGURE 1-9   Resuscitation of the newborn. (Adapted from David S. Markenson, *Pediatric Prehospital Care,* Prentice Hall, 2002.)

The following are steps for the initial care of the newborn. Also see the resuscitation steps illustrated in Figure 1–9 and in Procedure 1-1.

Step 1: Drying, Warming, Positioning, Suctioning, and Tactile Stimulation

Resuscitation begins with drying, warming, positioning, suctioning, and stimulating the newborn. Immediately upon delivery, minimize heat loss by drying the newborn. Next, place the newborn in a warm, dry blanket. Make sure the environment is warm and free of drafts.

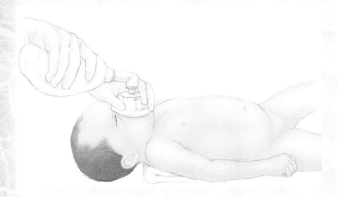

1-1a   Ventilate with 100% oxygen for 15–30 seconds.

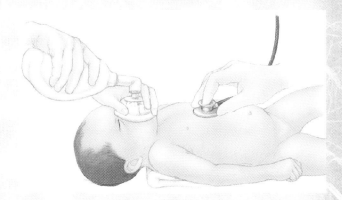

1-1b   Evaluate heart rate.

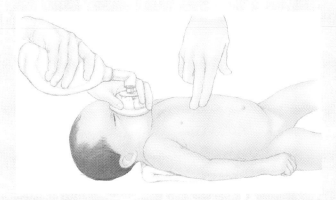

1-1c   Initiate chest compressions if: HR less than 60, or between 60 and 80 and **not** increasing.

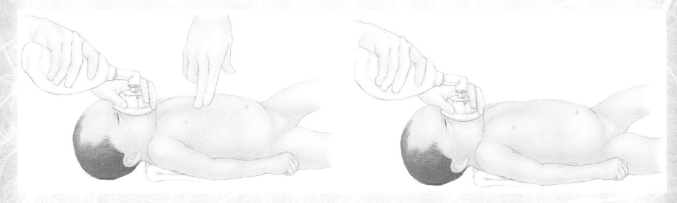

1-1d   Evaluate heart rate: Below 80—Continue chest compressions, 80 or above—Discontinue chest compressions

CORRECT

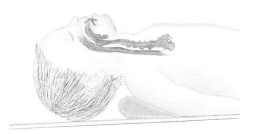

Neck slightly extended

Care should be taken to prevent hyperextension or underextension of the neck since either may decrease air entry.

INCORRECT

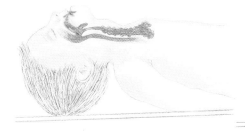 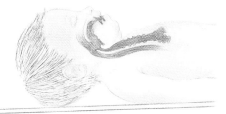

Neck hyperextended   Neck underextended

FIGURE 1-10   Positioning the newborn to open the airway.

After you have dried the newborn, place the infant on its back with its head slightly below its body and its neck slightly extended (Figure 1-10). This facilitates drainage of secretions and fluids from the lungs. Place a small blanket, folded to a 2 cm (3/4 inch) thickness, under the newborn's shoulders to help maintain this position.

Next, suction the newborn again, using a bulb syringe or DeLee suction trap. Deep suctioning can cause a **vagal response,** resulting in bradycardia. Because of this, suctioning should last no longer than 10 seconds. If meconium is present, avoid stimulating the infant and visualize the airway with a laryngoscope. Suction the meconium, preferably with a DeLee suction trap. If there is a great deal of meconium, place an appropriately-sized endotracheal tube (Table 1-3) and suction the meconium directly through the tube. Remove the tube and discard. Do not use the same tube for mechanical ventilation. (See Procedure 1-2.) Following adequate tracheal suctioning, stimulate the newborn by flicking the soles of its feet or rubbing its back.

✽ **vagal response** stimulation of the vagus nerve causing a parasympathetic response.

Suctioning of a newborn should last no longer than 10 seconds.

Table 1-3	GUIDELINES FOR TRACHEAL TUBE SIZES AND DEPTH OF INSERTION IN THE NEWBORN		
Tube Size, mm ID	Depth of Insertion from Upper Lip, cm	Weight, g	Gestation, wk
2.5	6.5–7	<1000	<28
3.0	7–8	1000–2000	28–34
3.5	8–9	2000–3000	34–38
3.5–4.0	> 9	>3000	>38

American Heart Association: *2000 Handbook of Cardiovascular Care for Healthcare Providers*
© 2000, American Heart Association

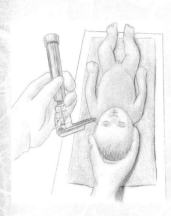

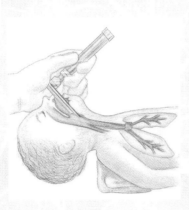

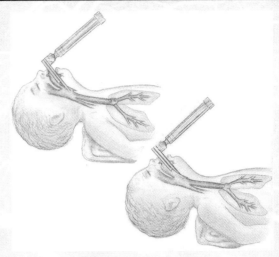

1-2a   Position the infant.

1-2b   Insert the laryngoscope.

1-2c   Elevate the epiglottis by lifting.

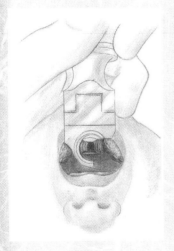

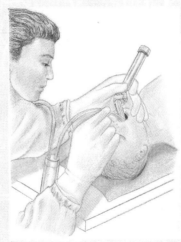

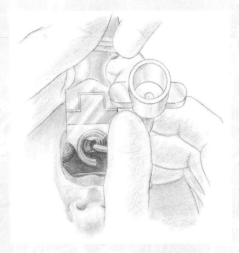

1-2d   Visualize the cords.

1-2e   Suction any meconium present.

1-2f   Insert a fresh tube for ventilation.

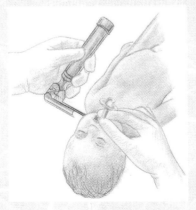

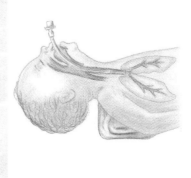

1-2g   Remove the laryngoscope.

1-2h   Check proper tube placement.

After carrying out the preceding procedures, assess the newborn as noted below.

Newborn Assessment Parameters

- *Respiratory effort.* The rate and depth of the newborn's breathing should increase immediately with tactile stimulation. If the respiratory response is adequate, evaluate the heart rate next. If the respiratory rate is inadequate, begin positive-pressure ventilation (see Step 3).
- *Heart rate.* As noted earlier, heart rate is critical in the newborn. Check the heart rate by listening to the apical area of the heart with a stethoscope, feeling the pulse by lightly grasping the umbilical cord, or feeling either the brachial or femoral pulse. If the heart rate is greater than 100 and spontaneous respirations are present, continue the assessment. If the heart rate is less than 100, immediately begin positive-pressure ventilation (see Step 3).
- *Color.* A newborn may be cyanotic despite a heart rate greater than 100 and spontaneous respirations. If you note central cyanosis, or cyanosis of the chest and abdomen, in a newborn with adequate ventilation and a pulse rate greater than 100, administer supplemental oxygen (see Step 2). Newborns with peripheral cyanosis do not usually need supplemental oxygen UNLESS the cyanosis is prolonged.
- *APGAR score.* Unless resuscitation is required, obtain 1- and 5-minute APGAR scores.

Step 2: Supplemental Oxygen

If central cyanosis is present or the adequacy of ventilation is uncertain, administer supplemental oxygen by blowing oxygen across the newborn's face (Figure 1-11). If possible, the oxygen should be warmed and humidified. Continue oxygen administration until the newborn's color has improved. Although oxygen toxicity

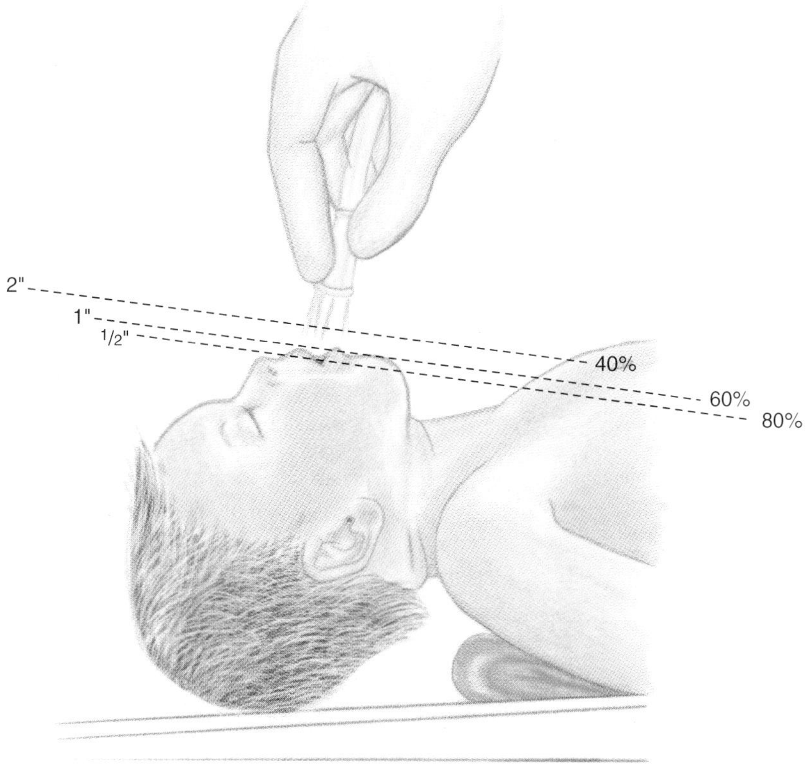

> **Content Review**
>
> **NEWBORN ASSESSMENT PARAMETERS**
> - Respiratory effort
> - Heart rate
> - Color
> - APGAR Score

> **Content Review**
>
> **NORMAL NEWBORN VITAL SIGNS**
> - Respirations 30–60
> - Heart rate 100–180
> - Blood pressure 60–90 systolic
> - Temperature 36.7°–37.8° C (98°–100° F)

FIGURE 1-11 Guidelines for estimating oxygen concentration. Based in oxygen flow rate of 5 liters per minute.

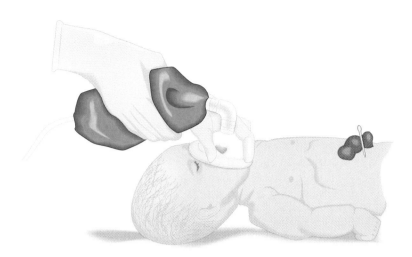

FIGURE 1-12   Use of a bag-valve mask to provide positive pressure ventilation. Maintain a good mask seal and use just enough force to raise the infant's chest. Ventilate at a rate of 60 per minute for 30 seconds. Then reassess.

is a concern, this condition usually results from prolonged usage over several days. Administration of blow-by oxygen in the prehospital setting will not cause problems. NEVER DEPRIVE A NEWBORN OF OXYGEN IN THE PREHOSPITAL SETTING FOR FEAR OF OXYGEN TOXICITY.

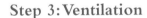

Never deprive a newborn of oxygen in the prehospital setting for fear of oxygen toxicity.

Step 3: Ventilation

Begin positive-pressure ventilation if *any* of the following conditions is present:

- Heart rate less than 100 beats per minute
- Apnea
- Persistence of central cyanosis after administration of supplemental oxygen

A ventilatory rate of 40–60 breaths per minute is usually adequate. A bag-valve-mask unit is the device of choice (Figure 1-12). A self-inflating bag of an appropriate size (450 mL is optimal) should be used. Many self-inflating bags have a pressure-limiting pop-off valve that is preset at 30–45 cm H_2O. However, since the initial pressures required to ventilate a newborn may be as high as 60cm/H_2O, you may have to depress the pop-off valve to deactivate it and ensure adequate ventilation. If prolonged ventilation is required, it may be necessary to disable the pop-off valve.

Face masks in various sizes must be available. The most effective ones are designed to fit the contours of the newborn's face and have a low dead space volume (less than 5 mL). When a mask is correctly sized and positioned, it covers the newborn's nose and mouth, but not the eyes.

Endotracheal intubation of a newborn should be carried out in the following situations:

- The bag-valve-mask unit does not work.
- Tracheal suctioning is required (such as in cases of thick meconium).
- Prolonged ventilation will be required.
- A diaphragmatic hernia is suspected.
- Inadequate respiratory effort is found.

Because of the narrowness of the neonatal airway at the level of the cricoid cartilage, always use an *uncuffed* endotracheal tube. (Review Table 1-3.) After inserting it, ensure proper placement by noting symmetrical chest wall motion and equal breath sounds. (Review Procedure 1-2.)

Intubation has several effects in the newborn. First, it bypasses **glottic function.** Second, it eliminates **PEEP**—the physiologic positive end-expiratory pressure created during normal coughing and crying. To maintain adequate functional residual capacity, a PEEP of 2–4 cm/H_2O should be provided when mechanical ventilation is initiated by adding a magnetic-disk PEEP valve to the bag-valve outlet.

Gastric distention, caused by a leak around an uncuffed endotracheal tube, may compromise ventilation of a newborn. This can be minimized by using a properly sized endotracheal tube. If there is significant gastric distension, a **nasogastric tube** or **orogastric tube** should be inserted (through the nose or mouth, then through the esophagus into the stomach) as soon as the airway is controlled. It is recommended that the endotracheal tube be in place before the gastric tube is placed to avoid misplacing the gastric tube into the trachea.

Make sure the newborn is well oxygenated before attempting to insert a gastric tube. To determine the depth of insertion, measure a nasogastric tube from the tip of the nose, around the ear, to below the xiphoid process. Measure an orogastric tube from the lips to below the xiphoid process. Lubricate the end of the tube and pass it gently along the nasal floor or the mouth and into the esophagus. Confirm that the tube is in the stomach by injecting 10 cc of air into the tube and auscultating a bubbling sound, or sound of rushing air, over the epigastrium.

✱ glottic function opening and closing of the glottic space.

✱ PEEP positive end-expiratory pressure.

✱ nasogastric tube/orogastric tube a tube that runs through the nose or mouth and esophagus into the stomach, used for administering liquid nutrients or medications or for removing air or liquids from the stomach.

Step 4: Chest Compressions

Initiate chest compressions if *either* of the following conditions exists:

- The heart rate is less than 60 beats per minute.
- The heart rate is between 60 and 80, *but does not increase* with 30 seconds of positive-pressure ventilation and supplemental oxygenation.

Perform chest compressions by following these steps.

- Encircle the newborn's chest, placing both of your thumbs on the lower one-third of the sternum. If the newborn is very small, you may need to overlap your thumbs. If the newborn is very large, you may need to place the ring and middle fingers of one hand just below the nipple line and perform two-finger compression (Figure 1-13).
- Compress the sternum 1.5–2.0 cm ($\frac{1}{2} - \frac{1}{3}$ inch) at a rate of 120 times per minute. Accompany compressions with positive-pressure ventilation. Maintain a ratio of 3 compressions to 1 ventilation.
- Reassess the newborn after 20 cycles of compressions and ventilations, or at approximately one-minute intervals.
- Discontinue compressions if the spontaneous heart rate exceeds 80 per minute.

Step 5: Medications and Fluids

Most cardiopulmonary arrests in newborns result from hypoxia. Because of this, initial therapy consists of ventilation and oxygenation. However, when these measures fail, fluid and medications should be administered. They may also be

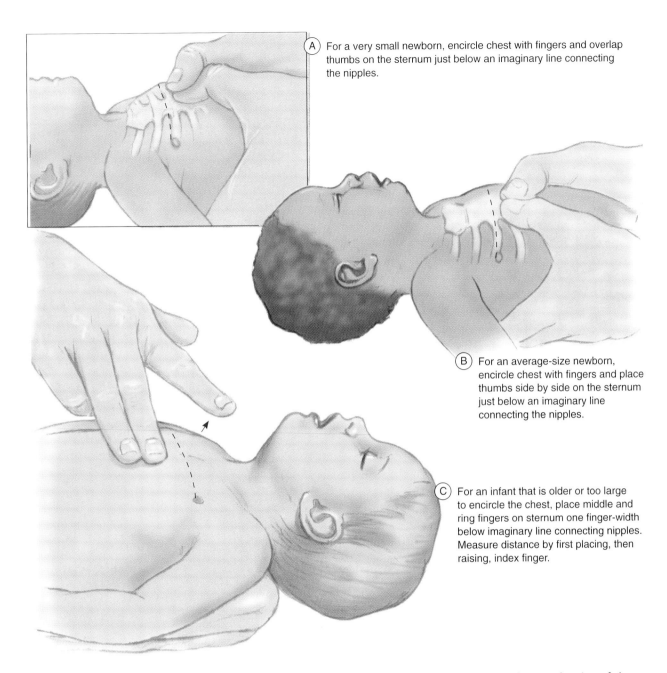

(A) For a very small newborn, encircle chest with fingers and overlap thumbs on the sternum just below an imaginary line connecting the nipples.

(B) For an average-size newborn, encircle chest with fingers and place thumbs side by side on the sternum just below an imaginary line connecting the nipples.

(C) For an infant that is older or too large to encircle the chest, place middle and ring fingers on sternum one finger-width below imaginary line connecting nipples. Measure distance by first placing, then raising, index finger.

FIGURE 1-13   Position fingers for chest compressions according to the size of the infant.

Vascular access for the administration of fluids and drugs can most readily be managed by using the umbilical vein.

necessary in cases of persistent bradycardia, hypovolemia, respiratory depression secondary to narcotics, and metabolic acidosis.

Vascular access for the administration of fluids and drugs can most readily be managed by using the umbilical vein. The umbilical cord contains three vessels—two arteries and one vein. The vein is larger than the arteries and has a thinner wall (Figure 1-14). To establish venous access, follow these procedures.

- Trim the umbilical cord with a scalpel blade to 1 cm above the abdomen. Be sure to save enough of the umbilical cord stump in case neonatal personnel have to place additional lines.

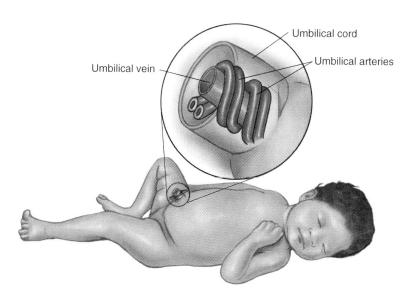

FIGURE 1-14 The umbilical cord contains two arteries and one vein. The umbilical vein can be accessed for vascular administration of fluids and drugs. The vein is larger than the arteries and has a thinner wall.

- Insert a 5 French umbilical catheter into the umbilical vein. Connect the catheter to a three-way stopcock and fill it with saline.
- Insert the catheter until the tip is just below the skin and you note the free flow of blood. (If the catheter is inserted too far, it may become wedged against the liver, and it will not function.)
- After the catheter is in place, secure it with umbilical tape.

If an umbilical vein catheter cannot be placed, some medications can be given via the endotracheal tube. They include atropine, epinephrine, lidocaine, and naloxone. Other options for vascular access are peripheral vein cannulation and intraosseous cannulation. Table 1-4 lists recommended medications and doses for the newborn. Fluid therapy should consist of 10 mL/kg of saline or lactated Ringer's solution given by syringe as a slow IV push.

MATERNAL NARCOTIC USE

Maternal abuse of narcotics—either illegal or prescribed—can complicate field deliveries. Maternal narcotic use has been shown to produce low-birth-weight infants. Such infants may demonstrate withdrawal symptoms—tremors, startles, and decreased alertness. They also face a serious risk of respiratory depression at birth.

Naloxone (Narcan), which is extremely safe even at high doses, is the treatment of choice for respiratory depression secondary to maternal narcotic use *within four hours of delivery.* Ventilatory support must be provided prior to administration of naloxone. Because the duration of the narcotics may exceed that of the naloxone, repeat administration as necessary.

Keep in mind, however, that the naloxone may induce a withdrawal reaction in an infant born to *a narcotic-addicted* mother. Medical direction may advise that naloxone NOT be administered if the mother is drug addicted, advising that prolonged ventilatory support be provided instead.

Keep in mind that naloxone may induce a withdrawal reaction with an infant born to a narcotic-addicted mother.

Table 1-4 NEONATAL RESUSCITATION DRUGS

Medication	Concentration to Administer	Preparation	Dosage/Route*	Total Dose/Infant	Rate/Precautions
Epinephrine	1:10,000	1 mL	0.1–0.3 mL/kg I.V. or I.T.	*weight . . . total mLs* 1 kg 0.1–0.3 mL 2 kg 0.2–0.6 mL 3 kg 0.3–0.9 mL 4 kg 0.4–1.2 mL	Give rapidly.
Volume Expanders	Whole Blood 5% Albumin Normal Saline Lactated Ringer's	40 mL	10 mL/kg I.V.	*weight . . . total mLs* 1 kg 10 mL 2 kg 20 mL 3 kg 30 mL 4 kg 40 mL	Give over 5–10 min.
Sodium Bicarbonate	0.5 mEq/mL	20 mL or two 10-mL prefilled syringes	2 mEq/kg I.V.	*weight . . . total dose . . . mLs* 1 kg 2 mEq 4 mL 2 kg 4 mEq 8 mL 3 kg 6 mEq 12 mL 4 kg 8 mEq 16 mL	Give slowly, over at least 2 min. Give only if infant is being effectively ventilated.
Narcan Neonatal	1.0 mg/mL or 0.4 mg/mL (dilute 1.0 mg in 9 mL of saline)	2 mL	0.1 mg/kg I.V., I.M., S.Q., I.T.	*weight . . . total mLs (0.1 mg/mL)* 1 kg 1.0 mL 2 kg 2.0 mL 3 kg 3.0 mL 4 kg 4.0 mL	Give rapidly.
Dopamine	$6 \times \dfrac{\text{weight} \times \text{desired dose}}{(\text{kg}) \quad (\text{mcg/kg/min})}{\text{desired fluid (mL/hr)}} = \dfrac{\text{mg of dopamine per 100 mL of solution}}{}$		Begin at 5 mcg/kg/min (may increase to 20 mcg/kg/min if necessary) I.V.	*weight . . . total mcg/min* 1 kg 5–20 mcg/min 2 kg 10–40 mcg/min 3 kg 15–60 mcg/min 4 kg 20–80 mcg/min	Give as continuous infusion using an infusion pump. Monitor HR and BP closely. Seek consultation.

From Textbook of Neonatal Resuscitation © 2001, American Heart Association

* I.M. = Intramuscular
  I.T. = Intratracheal
  I.V. = Intravenous
  S.Q. = Subcutaneous

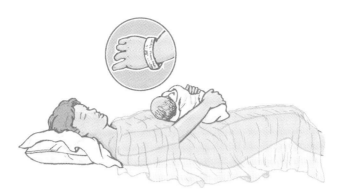

FIGURE 1-15 A healthy newborn can be placed on the mother's abdomen. Write the mother's last name and time of delivery on a tape and place it around the infant's wrist. (Do not allow adhesive to contact the infant's skin.)

The dosage of naloxone is 0.1 mg/kg. The initial dose may be repeated every 2 to 3 minutes as needed. Naloxone may be given by intravenous, intraosseous, endotracheal, subcutaneous, or intramuscular routes.

As with other newborns, continue all resuscitative measures until the newborn is resuscitated or until the emergency staff assumes care.

NEONATAL TRANSPORT

Healthy newborns should be allowed to begin the bonding process with the mother as soon as possible (Figure 1-15). Distressed newborns, however, must be positioned on their side to prevent aspiration and rapidly transported.

In addition to field deliveries, paramedics are frequently called upon to transport a high-risk newborn from a facility where stabilization has occurred to a neonatal intensive care unit (NICU). The trip may be across the street or across the state. Usually, a pediatric nurse, respiratory therapist, and, often, a physician accompany the newborn. During transport, a paramedic crew will help maintain a newborn's body temperature, control oxygen administration, and maintain ventilatory support. Often, a transport **isolette** with its own heat, light, and oxygen source is available (Figure 1-16). In such cases, intravenous medications are usually infused through the umbilical vein. The umbilical artery is catheterized as well.

If a self-contained isolette is not available for transport, it is important to keep the ambulance warm. Wrap the newborn in several blankets, keep the infant's head covered, and place hot-water bottles containing water heated to no more than 40° C (104° F) near, but not touching, the newborn. Do not use chemical packs to keep the newborn warm. These can generate excessive heat and may burn the infant.

✳ **isolette** also known as an *incubator*; a clear plastic enclosed bassinet used to keep prematurely born infants warm. The temperature of an isolette can be adjusted regardless of the room temperature. Some isolettes also provide humidity control.

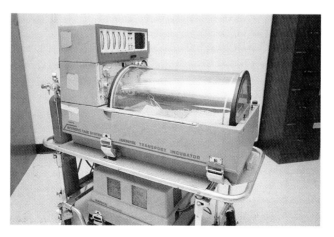

FIGURE 1-16 Neonatal transport isolette.

SPECIFIC NEONATAL SITUATIONS

Rapid assessment and treatment of a distressed newborn is the key to the infant's survival. The following information will help you to formulate treatment plans for specific emergencies involving newborns. Remember that, unless otherwise directed, it will be necessary to transport these infants to a facility that is able to handle high-risk neonates. A reference card should be available in the ambulance and in the dispatch office that tracks the availability of neonatal unit beds. Whenever possible, keep the parents advised of what is happening and the reason for any treatments being given to the infant. However, do not discuss "chances of survival" with the family or caregivers.

Do not discuss "chances of survival" with a newborn's family or caregivers.

MECONIUM-STAINED AMNIOTIC FLUID

Meconium-stained amniotic fluid occurs in approximately 10–15 percent of deliveries, mostly in post-term or in small-for-gestational-age (SGA) newborns. The mortality rate for meconium-stained infants is considerably higher than the mortality rate for non-stained infants, and meconium aspiration accounts for a significant proportion of neonatal deaths.

Fetal distress and hypoxia can cause the passage of meconium into the amniotic fluid. Meconium is a dark green substance found in the digestive tract of full-term newborns. It arises from secretions of the various digestive glands and amniotic fluid. Either *in utero*, or more often with the first breath, thick meconium is aspirated into the lungs, resulting in small-airway obstruction and aspiration pneumonia. This may produce respiratory distress within the first hours, or even minutes, of life as evidenced by tachypnea, retraction, grunting, and cyanosis in severely affected newborns.

The partial obstruction of some airways may lead to pneumothorax. A pneumothorax may occur in an infant, cause no distress, and require no active treatment. If, however, the infant has significant respiratory distress, then the pneumothorax must be evacuated. If tension pneumothorax has occurred, needle decompression may be required.

An infant born through thin meconium may not require treatment, but depressed infants born through thick, particulate (pea-soup) meconium-stained fluid should be intubated immediately, prior to the first ventilation (Figure 1-17). Aspiration of meconium by a newborn can result in either partial or complete

FIGURE 1-17 Intubate the infant born through particulate, thick meconium immediately—prior to the first ventilation.

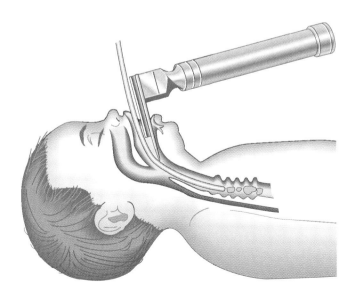

airway obstruction. Complete airway obstruction causes atelectasis (collapsed or airless lungs). In addition, some aspects of fetal blood flow resume a right-to-left shunt of blood across the foramen ovale (the opening between the atria of the fetal heart). This results from increased pulmonary pressures. Incomplete obstruction can act as a ball-valve in the smaller airways, thus preventing exhalation. Also, the newborn is at increased risk of developing a pneumothorax.

Before stimulating the infant to breathe, apply suction with a meconium aspirator attached to an endotracheal tube. Connect to suction at 100 cm/H_2O or less to remove meconium from the airway. Withdraw the endotracheal tube as suction is applied.

Repeat intubation and suction until the meconium clears, usually not more than two times. Once the airway is clear and the infant is able to breathe on its own, ventilate with 100% oxygen. If the infant is found to be hypotensive, consider a fluid challenge. Remember to warm the infant to prevent hypothermia. The parents will probably question the treatment being performed on the infant. Explain what you are doing and why, without discussing chances of survival. Stress the need for rapid transport to a facility able to handle high-risk infants.

APNEA

Apnea is a common finding in pre-term infants, infants weighing under 1,500 grams (3 pounds, 5 ounces), infants exposed to drugs, or infants born after prolonged or difficult labor and delivery. Typically, the infant fails to breathe spontaneously after stimulation, or the infant experiences respiratory pauses of greater than 20 seconds.

While apnea is usually due to hypoxia or hypothermia, there may be other causative factors. These include:

- Narcotic or central nervous depressants
- Weakness of the respiratory muscles
- Septicemia
- Metabolic disorders
- Central nervous system disorders

Begin management of apnea with tactile stimulation. Flick the soles of the infant's feet or gently rub its back. If necessary, ventilate using a bag-valve mask with the pop-off valve disabled. If the infant still does not breathe on its own, or if it has a heart rate of less than 60 with adequate ventilation and chest compressions, perform tracheal intubation with direct visualization. Gain circulatory access, and monitor the heart rate continuously. If the apnea is due to narcotics administered within the previous four hours, consider naloxone. As noted earlier, however, the use of narcotic antagonists is generally contraindicated if the mother is a drug abuser.

Early and aggressive treatment of apnea usually results in a good outcome. Throughout treatment, keep the infant warm to prevent hypothermia. Also explain procedures to parents and the need for rapid transport.

DIAPHRAGMATIC HERNIA

Diaphragmatic hernias rarely occur. They are seen in approximately 1 out of every 2,200 live births. When they do appear, the **herniation** takes place most often in the posterolateral segments of the diaphragm, and most commonly (90 percent) on the left side. The defect is caused by the failure of the pleurperitoneal canal (foramen of Bochdalek) to close completely. The survival rate for infants

Content Review

CAUSES OF APNEA IN NEWBORNS

- Hypoxia
- Hypothermia
- Narcotics
- Respiratory muscle weakness
- Septicemia
- Metabolic disorder
- Central nervous system disorder

DO NOT utilize narcotic antagonists if the mother is a drug abuser.

✱ **herniation** protrusion or projection of an organ or part of an organ through the wall of the cavity that normally contains it.

who require mechanical ventilation in the first 18 to 24 hours is approximately 50 percent. However, if there is no respiratory distress in the first 24 hours of life, the survival rate approaches 100 percent.

Protrusion of abdominal viscera through the hernia into the thoracic cavity occurs in varying degrees. In severe cases, the stomach and a large part of the intestines and the spleen, liver, and kidneys displace the lungs and heart to the opposite side. The lung on the affected side is compressed, causing diminished total lung volume. In at least one-third of patients, pulmonary hypertension is present. With a patent ductus arteriosus, there may be severe right-to-left shunting, further aggravating tissue hypoxia.

Assessment findings may include:

- Little to severe distress present from birth
- Dyspnea and cyanosis unresponsive to ventilations
- Small, flat (scaphoid) abdomen
- Bowel sounds in the chest
- Heart sounds displaced to the right

As soon as you suspect a diaphragmatic hernia, position the infant with its head and thorax higher than the abdomen and feet (Figure 1-18). This will help facilitate the downward displacement of the abdominal organs. Place a nasogastric or orogastric tube and apply low, intermittent suctioning. This will decrease the entrapment of air and fluid within the herniated viscera and will lessen the degree of ventilatory compromise. DO NOT use bag-valve-mask ventilation, which can worsen this condition by causing gastric distention. If necessary, cautiously administer positive-pressure ventilation through an endotracheal tube.

This condition usually requires surgical repair. Explain the possible need for surgery to parents, assuring them that their newborn child will be transported quickly to the facility best able to handle this procedure.

If you suspect a diaphragmatic hernia, DO NOT use bag-valve-mask ventilation, which can worsen the condition by causing gastric distention.

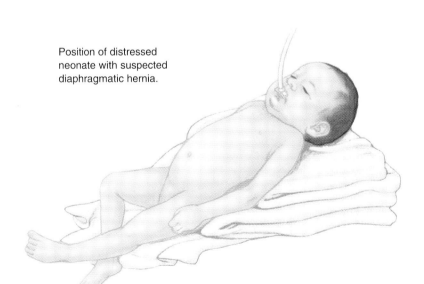

Position of distressed neonate with suspected diaphragmatic hernia.

FIGURE 1-18   If a diaphragmatic hernia is suspected, position the infant with its head and thorax higher than the abdomen and feet to facilitate downward displacement of abdominal organs.

BRADYCARDIA

Bradycardia in the newborn is most commonly caused by hypoxia. However, it may also be due to several other factors, including increased intracranial pressure, hypothyroidism, or acidosis.

In cases of hypoxia, the infant experiences minimal risk if the hypoxia is corrected quickly. In providing treatment, follow the procedures in the inverted pyramid, as discussed earlier. Check for secretions in the airway, check tongue and soft tissue positioning, and check for possible foreign body obstruction. Resist the inclination to treat the bradycardia with pharmacological measures alone. While epinephrine may be necessary, in all likelihood you will be able to correct the problem with suctioning, positioning, administration of oxygen (blow-by or bag-valve mask), or tracheal intubation. Throughout treatment, keep the newborn warm and transport to the nearest facility.

Resist the temptation to treat bradycardia in a newborn with pharmacological measures alone.

PREMATURE INFANTS

A premature newborn is an infant born prior to 37 weeks of gestation or with weight ranging from 0.6 to 2.2 kg (1 pound, 5 ounces to 4 pounds, 13 ounces). Healthy premature infants weighing more than 1,700 grams (3 pounds, 12 ounces) have a survivability and outcome approximately that of full-term infants. The mortality rate decreases weekly as the gestational age surpasses the age of fetal viability. With the technology currently available, fetal viability is considered to be 23–24 weeks of gestation.

Premature newborns are at greater risk of respiratory suppression, head or brain injury caused by hypoxemia, changes in blood pressure, intraventricular hemorrhage, and fluctuations in serum osmolarity. They are also more susceptible to hypothermia than full-term newborns. Reasons premature newborns lose heat more readily include:

- The premature newborn has a relatively large body surface area and comparatively small weight.
- The premature newborn has not sufficiently developed the various control mechanisms needed to regulate body temperature.
- The premature newborn has smaller subcutaneous stores of insulating fat.
- Newborns cannot shiver and must maintain body temperature through other mechanisms.

The degree of immaturity determines the physical characteristics of a premature newborn (Figure 1-19). Premature newborns often appear to have a

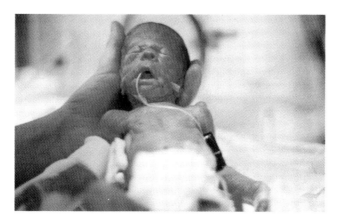

FIGURE 1-19 The premature newborn.

larger head relative to body size. They may have large trunks and short extremities, transparent skin, and few wrinkles.

Prematurity should not be a factor in short-term treatment. Resuscitation should be attempted if there is any sign of life.

Prematurity should not be a factor in short-term treatment. Resuscitation should be attempted if there is any sign of life, and the measures of resuscitation should be the same as those for newborns of normal weight and maturity. Maintain a patent airway and avoid potential aspiration of gastric contents. Medical direction may advise administration of epinephrine. Throughout treatment, maintain the newborn's body temperature and transport to a facility with special services for low-birth-weight newborns.

RESPIRATORY DISTRESS/CYANOSIS

Prematurity is the single most common factor causing respiratory distress and cyanosis in the newborn. The problem occurs most frequently in infants less than 1,200 grams (2 pounds, 10 ounces) and 30 weeks of gestation. Premature infants have an immature central respiratory control center and are easily affected by environmental or metabolic changes. Multiple gestations or prenatal maternal complications may also increase the risk of respiratory distress and cyanosis.

The severely ill newborn with respiratory distress and cyanosis presents a difficult diagnostic challenge. There may be many contributing factors, including lung or heart disease, central nervous system disorders, meconium aspiration, metabolic problems, obstruction of the nasal passages, shock and sepsis, diaphragmatic hernia, and more. Assessment findings include:

- Tachypnea
- Paradoxical breathing
- Intercostal retractions
- Nasal flaring
- Expiratory grunt

Follow the inverted pyramid of treatment, paying particular attention to airway and ventilation. Suction as needed and provide a high concentration of oxygen. Ventilate, as needed, with a BVM. If prolonged ventilation will be required, consider placing an endotracheal tube. Perform chest compressions, if indicated. Sodium bicarbonate may be helpful for prolonged resuscitation. Consider dextrose ($D_{10}W$ or $D_{25}W$) solution if the newborn is hypoglycemic. Maintain body temperature and transport. Be sure to keep the parents informed and provide needed psychological support.

HYPOVOLEMIA

Hypovolemia is the leading cause of shock in newborns. It may result from dehydration, hemorrhage, or third-spacing of fluids. Dehydration is by far the most common cause. Signs of hypovolemia include:

- Pale color
- Cool skin
- Diminished peripheral pulses
- Delayed capillary refill, despite normal ambient temperature
- Mental status changes
- Diminished urination (oliguria)

When you observe these signs, administer a fluid bolus and assess the infant's response. If signs of shock continue, administer a second bolus. Additional boluses should be infused as indicated by repeated assessments. A hypovolemic infant may often need 40 to 60 mL/kg of fluid during the first hour of resuscitation.

Fluid bolus resuscitation consists of 10 mL/kg of an isotonic crystalloid solution, such as Ringer's lactate or normal saline. Administer the bolus over 5 to 10 minutes as soon as intravascular or intraosseous access is obtained. Do not use solutions containing dextrose, as they can produce hypokalemia or worsen ischemic brain injury.

> *In treating hypovolemia in a newborn, do not use solutions containing dextrose, as they can produce hypokalemia or worsen ischemic brain injury.*
>

SEIZURES

Although seizures occur in a very small percentage of all newborns, they usually indicate a serious underlying abnormality and represent a medical emergency. Prolonged and frequent multiple seizures may result in metabolic changes and cardiopulmonary difficulties.

Neonatal seizures differ from seizures in a child or an adult, because generalized tonic-clonic convulsions normally do not occur during the first month of life. Seizures in neonates include:

- *Subtle seizures.* These seizures consist of chewing motions, excessive salivation, blinking, sucking, swimming movements of the arms, pedaling movements of the legs, apnea, and changes in color.

- *Tonic seizures.* These seizures are characterized by rigid posturing of the extremities and trunk. They are sometimes associated with fixed deviation of the eyes. They occur more commonly in premature infants, especially those with an intraventricular hemorrhage.

- *Focal clonic seizures.* These seizures consist of rhythmic twitching of muscle groups, particularly the extremities and face. They may occur in both full-term and premature infants.

- *Multi focal seizures.* These seizures are similar to focal clonic seizures, except that multiple muscle groups are involved. Clonic activity randomly migrates. These seizures occur primarily in full-term newborns.

- *Myoclonic seizures.* These seizures involve brief focal or generalized jerks of the extremities or parts of the body that tend to involve distal muscle groups. They may occur singly or in a series of repetitive jerks.

Causes of neonatal seizures include sepsis, fever, hypoglycemia, hypoxic-ischemic encephalopathy, metabolic disturbances, meningitis, developmental abnormalities, or drug withdrawal. Assessment findings include a decreased level of consciousness and seizure activities such as those described above. Treatment focuses on airway management and oxygen saturation. With medical direction, consider administration of an anti-convulsant. You might also administer a benzodiazepine (usually lorazepam) for status epilepticus or dextrose ($D_{10}W$ or $D_{25}W$) for hypoglycemia. As with all distressed newborns, maintain body temperature and transport rapidly.

FEVER

Average normal temperature in a newborn is 37.5° C (99.5°F). A rectal temperature of 38.0° C (100.4° F) or higher is considered fever. Neonates do not develop fever as readily as older children. Thus, any fever in a neonate requires extensive evaluation, because it may be caused by life-threatening conditions

Any neonate with a fever should be considered to have meningitis until proven otherwise.

In assessing a neonate with fever, remember that infants have a limited ability to control their body temperature. As a result, fever can be a serious condition.

such as pneumonia, sepsis, or meningitis. Fever may be the only sign of meningitis in a neonate. Because of their immature development, they do not develop the classic symptoms such as a stiff neck. Thus, any neonate with a fever should be considered to have meningitis until proven otherwise.

In assessing a neonate with fever, remember that infants have a limited ability to control their body temperature. As a result, fever can be a serious problem. Assessment findings will probably include the following:

- Mental status changes (irritability/somnolence)
- Decreased feeding
- Skin warm to the touch
- Rashes or *petechia* (small, purplish, hemorrhagic spots on the skin)

Term infants may produce beads of sweat on their brow, but not on the rest of their body. Premature infants will have no visible sweat at all.

Treatment of a neonate with fever will, for the most part, be limited to assuring a patent airway and adequate ventilation. Do not use cold packs, which may drop the temperature too quickly and may also cause seizures. If the newborn becomes bradycardic, provide chest compressions. In the prehospital setting, administration of an antipyretic agent to a neonate is of questionable benefit and should be avoided. Select the appropriate treatment facility, and explain the need for transport to the parents or caregivers.

HYPOTHERMIA

As previously noted, hypothermia presents a common and life-threatening condition for newborns. Adults sometimes fail to realize that a newborn may die because of exposure to temperatures that adults find comfortable. The increased surface-to-volume relationship in newborns makes them extremely sensitive to environmental temperatures, especially right after delivery when they are wet. As a result, it is important to control the four methods of heat loss—evaporation, conduction, convection, and radiation.

In treating hypothermia—a body temperature below 35°C (95° F)—keep in mind that it can also be an indicator of sepsis in the newborn. Regardless of the cause, the increased metabolic demands created by hypothermia can produce a variety of related conditions including metabolic acidosis, pulmonary hypertension, and hypoxemia.

In assessing a hypothermic newborn, remember that they do not shiver. Instead, expect these findings:

- Pale color
- Skin cool to the touch, particularly in the extremities
- **Acrocyanosis**
- Respiratory distress
- Possible apnea
- Bradycardia
- Central cyanosis
- Initial irritability
- Lethargy in later stages

Management focuses on assuring adequate ventilations and oxygenation. Chest compressions may be performed, if necessary. With medical direction, you

✱ **acrocyanosis** cyanosis of the extremities.

might administer warm fluids through an IV fluid heater. Do not microwave fluids, as there can be a great variation in fluid temperature. Dextrose ($D_{10}W$ or $D_{25}W$) may also be given if the newborn is hypoglycemic. Above all, the newborn must be kept warm. Set the ambulance temperature at 24–26°C (75.2°F–78.8°F). Also remember to warm your hands before touching the newborn. Select the appropriate receiving facility and transport rapidly.

Remember to warm your hands before touching a neonate.

HYPOGLYCEMIA

Newborns are the only age group that can develop severe hypoglycemia and not have diabetes mellitus. Hypoglycemia may be due to inadequate glucose intake or increased glucose utilization. Stress and other factors can also cause the blood sugar to fall, sometimes to a critical level.

Hypoglycemia is more common in premature or small-for-gestational-age (SGA) infants, the smaller twin, and newborns of a diabetic mother, as these infants often have decreased glycogen stores. Hypoglycemia can also develop due to increased glucose utilization. Causes include respiratory illnesses, hypothermia, toxemia, CNS hemorrhage, asphyxia, meningitis, and sepsis. In an older infant, hypoglycemia may be due to an inadequate glucose intake or increased utilization of glucose. Infants receiving glucose infusions can develop hypoglycemia if the infusion is suddenly stopped.

Infants with hypoglycemia may be asymptomatic or they may exhibit symptoms such as apnea, color changes, respiratory distress, lethargy, seizures, acidosis, and poor myocardial contractility.

Persistent hypoglycemia can have catastrophic effects on the brain. The normal newborn's glycogen stores are sufficient to meet glucose requirements for only 8–12 hours. This time frame is diminished in infants with decreased glycogen stores or the presence of other problems where glucose utilization increases. As a result, you should determine the blood glucose on all sick infants. A blood glucose screening test of less than 45 mg/dl indicates hypoglycemia.

Because hypoglycemia can have a catastrophic effect on a neonate's brain, you should determine the blood glucose on all sick infants.

In response to hypoglycemia, the newborn's body will release counter-regulatory hormones such as glucagon, epinephrine, cortisol, and growth hormone. These hormones help raise the blood glucose level by mobilizing glucose stores. In fact, this hormone response may cause transient symptoms of hyperglycemia that may last for several hours. However, when the infant's glucose stores are depleted, the glucose level will again fall.

In assessing hypoglycemic newborns, expect these findings:

- Twitching or seizures
- Limpness
- Lethargy
- Eye-rolling
- High-pitched cry
- Apnea
- Irregular respirations
- Possible cyanosis

Treatment begins with management of the airway and ventilations. Assure adequate oxygenation. Perform chest compressions, if indicated. With medical direction, administer dextrose ($D_{10}W$ or $D_{25}W$). Maintain a normal body temperature in the newborn and transport to the appropriate facility.

VOMITING

Vomiting in a neonate may result from a variety of causes and rarely presents as an isolated symptom. Vomiting (a forceful ejection of stomach contents) is uncommon during the first weeks of life and may be confused with regurgitation (a simple backflow of stomach contents into the mouth, or "spitting up"). Vomiting in the neonate usually occurs because of an anatomic abnormality such as a tracheoesophageal fistula or upper gastrointestinal obstruction. More often, it may be a symptom of some disease such as increased intracranial pressure or an infection. Vomitus containing dark blood often signals a life-threatening illness. Keep in mind, however, that vomiting of mucus—which may occasionally be blood streaked—in the first few hours after birth is not uncommon.

Assessment findings may include a distended stomach, signs of infection, increased ICP, or drug withdrawal. Because vomitus can be aspirated, management considerations focus on assuring a patent airway. If you detect respiratory difficulties or obstruction of the airway, suction or clear vomitus from the airway and assure adequate oxygenation. Fluid administration may be needed to prevent dehydration. Also remember that, as with older patients, vagal stimulation may cause bradycardia in the neonate.

After you have protected the airway, place the infant on its side and transport to an appropriate facility. As with all other situations involving distressed neonates, advise parents or caregivers of steps taken and why.

DIARRHEA

Diarrhea in a neonate can cause severe dehydration and electrolyte imbalances. Although diarrhea may be harder to assess in neonates than in other patients, consider five to six stools per day as normal, especially in breast-fed infants.

Causes of diarrhea in a neonate include:

- Bacterial or viral infection
- Gastroenteritis
- Lactose intolerance
- **Phototherapy**
- **Neonatal abstinence syndrome (NAS)**
- **Thyrotoxicosis**
- Cystic fibrosis

In treating neonates with diarrhea, remember to take appropriate BSI precautions, just as you would do in any situation involving body fluids. Expect to find loose stools, decreased urinary output, and other signs of dehydration such as prolonged capillary refill time, cool extremities, and listlessness or lethargy. It is often difficult for the parents to estimate the number of stools. In such cases, it might be better to inquire about the number of diapers the baby is using.

Management consists of maintenance of airway and ventilations, adequate oxygenation, and chest compressions, if indicated. With medical direction, you might also consider fluid therapy. Explain all treatments to parents or caregivers, and transport the neonate to a facility able to handle high-risk infants.

COMMON BIRTH INJURIES

A **birth injury** occurs in an estimated 2 to 7 of every 1,000 live births in the United States. About 5 to 8 of every 100,000 infants die of birth trauma and 25

✱ phototherapy exposure to sunlight or artificial light for therapeutic purposes. In newborns, light is used to treat hyperbilirubinemia or jaundice.

✱ neonatal abstinence syndrome (NAS) a generalized disorder presenting a clinical picture of CNS hyperirritability, gastrointestinal dysfunction, respiratory distress, and vague autonomic symptoms. It may be due to intrauterine exposure to heroin, methadone, or other less potent opiates. Non-opiate central nervous system depressants may also cause NAS.

✱ thyrotoxicosis toxic condition characterized by tachycardia, nervous symptoms, and rapid metabolism due to hyperactivity of the thyroid gland.

In treating a neonate with diarrhea, remember to take appropriate BSI precautions.

✱ birth injury avoidable and unavoidable mechanical and anoxic trauma incurred by the newborn during labor and delivery.

of every 100,000 die of anoxic injuries. Such injuries account for 2–3 percent of infant deaths. Risk factors for birth injury include:

- Prematurity
- Postmaturity
- Cephalopelvic disproportion
- Prolonged labor
- Breech presentation
- Explosive delivery
- Diabetic mother

Birth injuries take various forms. Cranial injuries may include molding of the head and overriding of the parietal bones, erythema (reddening of the skin), abrasions, ecchymosis (black-and-blue discoloration) and subcutaneous fat necrosis, subconjunctival and retinal hemorrhage, subperiosteal hemorrhage, and fracture of the skull. Intracranial hemorrhage may result from trauma or asphyxia. Often the infant will develop a large scalp hematoma during the birth process. This injury, called *caput succedaneum*, will usually resolve over a week's time. There may be damage to the spine and spinal cord from strong traction exerted when the spine is hyperextended or there is a lateral pull. Other birth injuries include peripheral nerve injury, injury to the liver, rupture of the spleen, adrenal hemorrhage, fractures of the clavicle or extremities, and, of course, hypoxia-ischemia.

Assessment findings may include:

- Diffuse, sometimes ecchymotic, edematous swelling of soft tissues around the scalp
- Paralysis below the level of the spinal cord injury
- Paralysis of the upper arm with or without paralysis of the forearm
- Diaphragmatic paralysis
- Movement on only one side of the face when crying
- Inability to move the arm freely on the side of the fractured clavicle
- Lack of spontaneous movement of the affected extremity
- Hypoxia
- Shock

Management of a newborn or newborn with birth injuries usually centers on protection of the airway, provision of adequate ventilation and oxygen, and, if needed, chest compressions. With medical direction, you may administer medications or take other non-pharmacological steps to support the specific injury. Newborns with birth injuries usually require treatment at specialized facilities. As in the management of other neonatal emergencies, provide professional and compassionate communication to parents or caregivers.

> *In treating distressed neonates with birth injuries or other critical conditions, provide professional and compassionate communication to the parents or caregivers.*

CARDIAC RESUSCITATION, POST RESUSCITATION, AND STABILIZATION

The incidence of neonatal cardiac arrest is related primarily to hypoxia. As previously explained, the outcome will be poor unless you immediately initiate appropriate interventions. As you might expect, cases involving cardiac arrest have an increased chance of brain and organ damage. Risk factors for cardiac arrest in newborns include:

- Bradycardia
- Intrauterine asphyxia
- Prematurity
- Drugs administered to or taken by the mother
- Congenital neuromuscular diseases
- Congenital malformations
- Intrapartum hypoxemia

Cardiac arrest can be caused by primary or secondary apnea, bradycardia, persistent fetal circulation, or pulmonary hypertension. Assessment findings may include peripheral cyanosis, inadequate respiratory effort, and ineffective or absent heart rate.

In managing neonatal cardiac arrest, follow the inverted pyramid for resuscitation. Administer drugs or fluids according to medical direction. Maintain normal body temperature while you transport the distressed newborn to the appropriate facility. This situation will require delicate handling of the parents or caregivers. Explain what is being done for the infant, without entering into the possibilities of survival.

SUMMARY

After a woman gives birth, you must care for two patients—the mother and her newborn child. The newborn has several special needs, the most important of which are protection of the airway and support of ventilations. The newborn must be kept warm at all times. If assessment reveals a distressed newborn, you should initiate ventilatory support, stimulation, and, if required, CPR. If possible, newborns should be transported to a facility with an NICU. Maintain communications with family members or caregivers, explaining all procedures performed on the newborn.

YOU MAKE THE CALL

You are called to assist a BLS unit with a difficult delivery. When you arrive at the scene, the EMTs report that the patient is a 35-year-old female who is two weeks past full term. Her amniotic sac has just ruptured, and there is thick meconium staining. The infant is crowning. Just after your arrival at the scene, the mother begins to scream that the baby is coming.

1. Should you stimulate this baby to breathe as soon as it is delivered? Why or why not?
2. What is the major danger associated with this type of problem?
3. Once you have stabilized this infant, where should it be transported?

See Suggested Responses at the back of this book.

FURTHER READING

American Heart Association: *Guidelines 2000 for Cardiopulmonary Resuscitation and Emergency Cardiovascular Care*. Dallas, TX. American Heart Association. 2000.

American Heart Association and American Academy of Pediatrics: *Textbook of Neonatal Resuscitation*. Dallas, TX. American Heart Association. 1995.

American Heart Association and American Academy of Pediatrics: *Textbook of Pediatric Advanced Life Support*. Dallas, TX. American Heart Association. 1997.

Behrman, R.E., *et. al.: Nelson Textbook of Pediatrics*, 16th ed. Philadelphia, PA. W.B. Saunders Company. 2000.

Kattwinkel, J., *et. al.:* "Resuscitation of the Newly Born Infant: An Advisory Statement From the Pediatric Working Group of the International Committee on Resuscitation." *Circulation*, 1999 (pp 1927–1938).

Tintinalli, J.E., R.L. Krome, E. Ruiz: *Emergency Medicine: A Comprehensive Guide*, 5th ed. New York, NY. McGraw-Hill, Inc. 1999.

Rosen, P, *et. al.: Emergency Medicine: Concepts and Clinical Practice*, 4th ed. St. Louis, MO. Mosby. 1998.

ON THE WEB

Visit Brady's Paramedic Website at www.bradybooks.com/paramedic.

CHAPTER 2

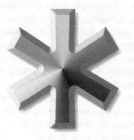

Pediatrics

Objectives

After reading this chapter, you should be able to:

1. Discuss the paramedic's role in the reduction of infant and childhood morbidity and mortality from acute illness and injury. (pp. 41–43)
2. Identify methods/mechanisms that prevent injuries to infants and children. (pp. 42–43)
3. Describe Emergency Medical Services for Children (EMSC) and how it can affect patient outcome. (p. 42)
4. Identify the common family responses to acute illness and injury of an infant or child. (pp. 44–45)
5. Describe techniques for successful interaction with families of acutely ill or injured infants and children. (pp. 44–45)
6. Identify key anatomical, physiological, growth, and developmental characteristics of infants and children and their implications. (pp. 45–49)
7. Outline differences in adult and childhood anatomy, physiology, and "normal" age-group-related vital signs. (pp. 50–55)
8. Describe techniques for successful assessment and treatment of infants and children. pp. 55–68)

Continued

9. Discuss the appropriate equipment used to obtain pediatric vital signs. (pp. 65–68)
10. Determine appropriate airway adjuncts, ventilation devices, and endotracheal intubation equipment; their proper use; and complications of use for infants and children. (pp. 68–80)
11. List the indications and methods of gastric decompression for infants and children. (pp. 80–81, 82)
12. Define pediatric respiratory distress, failure, and arrest. (pp. 90–92)
13. Differentiate between upper airway obstruction and lower airway disease. (pp. 93–99)
14. Describe the general approach to the treatment of children with respiratory distress, failure, or arrest from upper airway obstruction or lower airway disease. (pp. 93–99)
15. Discuss the common causes and relative severity of hypoperfusion in infants and children. (pp. 99–105)
16. Identify the major classifications of pediatric cardiac rhythms. (pp. 105–108)
17. Discuss the primary etiologies of cardiopulmonary arrest in infants and children. (pp. 90–92, 99)
18. Discuss age-appropriate sites, equipment, techniques, and complications of vascular access for infants and children. (pp. 81, 83–85)
19. Describe the primary etiologies of altered level of consciousness in infants and children. (pp. 89–117, 122–123, 133–134)
20. Identify common lethal mechanisms of injury in infants and children. (pp. 117–120)
21. Discuss anatomical features of children that predispose or protect them from certain injuries. (pp. 123–126)
22. Describe aspects of infant and child airway management that are affected by potential cervical spine injury. (pp. 120–121)
23. Identify infant and child trauma patients who require spinal immobilization. (p. 86)
24. Discuss fluid management and shock treatment for infant and child trauma patients. (pp.100–105, 122)
25. Determine when pain management and sedation are appropriate for infants and children. (p. 122)
26. Define child abuse, child neglect, and sudden infant death syndrome (SIDS). (pp. 126–130)
27. Discuss the parent/caregiver responses to the death of an infant or child. (p. 127)
28. Define children with special health care needs and technology-assisted children. (pp. 131–134)
29. Discuss basic cardiac life support (CPR) guidelines for infants and children. (pp. 68–75)
30. Integrate advanced life support skills with basic cardiac life support for infants and children. (pp. 75–86, 105–108)
31. Discuss the indications, dosage, route of administration, and special considerations for medication administration in infants and children. (pp. 84–86)
32. Discuss appropriate transport guidelines for low- and high-risk infants and children. (p. 89)
33. Describe the epidemiology, including the incidence, morbidity/mortality, risk factors, prevention strategies, pathophysiology, assessment, and treatment of infants and children with:
    a. Respiratory distress/failure (pp. 90–99)
    b. Hypoperfusion (pp. 99–104)
    c. Cardiac dysrhythmias (pp. 105–108)
    d. Neurological emergencies (pp. 107, 109–110)
    e. Trauma (pp. 86–89, 117–126)
    f. Abuse and neglect (pp. 127–130)
    g. Special health-care needs, including technology-assisted children (pp. 131–134)
    h. SIDS (pp. 126–127)
34. Given several pre-programmed simulated pediatric patients, provide the appropriate assessment, treatment, and transport. (pp. 41–134)

CASE STUDY

Three tones sound on the paramedic radios in the ED. A message crackles: "LA 54, I need you to be 10-8." The crew of LA 54 transfers care of the patient in Bed #6 to the hospital staff. Within 60 seconds, they depart from the hospital parking lot. En route to the emergency, they review information provided by the dispatcher. They will be treating a 5-month-old female who is described as "not breathing" by the father.

The response time is 4 minutes. Upon arrival, the parents lead the paramedics into the patient's bedroom. The little girl is lying in a crib. Immediately, paramedics note that she has pale, cool, clammy skin. Her anterior fontanelle is noticeably sunken. The respiratory rate and quality is 20 and shallow. Upon mild painful stimuli, the infant cries vigorously, increasing her tidal rate and volume. However, no tears appear. After taking appropriate BSI precautions, the paramedics check the diaper and find that it is dry. "She hasn't kept any food down for three days," explains the mother. "She hasn't wet her diaper in hours."

The crew places the patient on 15 LPM supplemental oxygen via a nonrebreather mask. The infant responds to the mask by crying, but she makes no effort to remove it. Capillary refill is borderline (2.5 seconds). The paramedics prepare to transport the infant to the ED, informing the parents of all the steps that will be taken to help their daughter.

En route to the hospital, the crew establishes an IV and administers a fluid bolus of 20 mL/kg of normal saline. By the time they pull up to the ambulance ramp at the ED, the patient's color and respiratory rate have improved greatly. Capillary refill time and pulse rate move toward normal limits. The ED staff evaluates the patient and admits her for 24-hour observation and IV fluid therapy. She returns home the following day. The paramedics later learn that she had contracted a viral gastroenteritis that was going around her day care. Within 48 hours she was back to her usual playful self.

INTRODUCTION

The ill or injured child presents special concerns for prehospital personnel. Current research indicates that more than 20,000 pediatric deaths occur each year in the United States. The leading causes of death are age specific. They include motor vehicle collisions, burns, drownings, suicides, and homicides. These alarming facts become even more troublesome when experts theorize that many of them could have been prevented by early intervention. Tragedies involving children—neonates to adolescents—account for some of the most stressful incidents that you will encounter in EMS practice.

Treatment of pediatric patients presents a number of challenges for the paramedic. Children, especially young ones, often cannot describe what is bothering them or what has happened to them. In addition to the child patient, you must deal with the parents or caregivers. Finally, a child's size often makes routine procedures more difficult. Keep in mind that children are not simply small adults. They have special considerations and needs. This chapter will present the topic of pediatric emergencies as it applies to advanced prehospital care.

ROLE OF PARAMEDICS IN PEDIATRIC CARE

When considering the reduction of pediatric morbidity and mortality, your role as a paramedic centers around two key concepts. First, you must realize that pediatric injuries have become a major health concern. Second, you should remember that children are at a higher risk of injury than adults and that they are more likely to be adversely affected by the injuries that they suffer.

Numerous factors account for the high pediatric injury rates. Some factors, such as geography and weather, cannot be altered. However, other factors, particularly dangers within the home and community, can be eliminated or minimized. As health care professionals, we must all get involved in identifying and implementing methods and mechanisms that prevent injuries to infants and children. Those of us who deliver prehospital care must do more than simply enter the picture after an injury has taken place.

In addition to pediatric injuries, paramedics are often responsible for treating the ill child. There are many aspects of disease and disease processes that are unique to children. It is important that the paramedic be familiar with these, as early intervention is often the key to reduced morbidity and mortality.

CONTINUING EDUCATION AND TRAINING

Your role in improving the health care offered to pediatric patients begins with your own training. Because you will encounter pediatric patients less frequently than adult patients, you have a professional responsibility to maintain and improve upon your pediatric knowledge, particularly your clinical skills. Continuing education programs include:

- Pediatric Advanced Life Support (PALS)
- Pediatric Basic Trauma Life Support (PBTLS)
- Advanced Pediatric Life Support (APLS)
- Prehospital Pediatric Care (PPC)

Tragedies involving children account for some of the most stressful incidents that you will encounter in EMS practice.

Children are not simply small adults.

Because you will encounter pediatric patients less frequently than adult patients, you have a professional responsibility to maintain and improve upon your pediatric knowledge, particularly your clinical skills.

In addition to these programs, you can also attend regional conferences and seminars designed to increase your knowledge of pediatric care. These are often conducted by regional children's hospitals. You can further enhance your clinical skills by spending time in pediatric emergency departments, pediatric hospitals, or pediatric departments in local hospitals. You might also visit the offices of pediatricians or talk with Pediatric Nurse Practitioners—registered nurses who provide primary health care to children.

For self-study, you can choose among many excellent pediatric textbooks currently available or read articles on pediatric care in the various EMS journals. Many good pediatric educational sites are available on the Internet. A particularly useful source of information is the Center for Pediatric Medicine (CPEM), established in 1985 at the New York University Medical Center and Bellevue Hospital. This federally funded center promotes education, research, and development of systems aimed at improving emergency medical services for children in the United States. CPEM has made available the *Teaching Resource for Instructors in Prehospital Pediatrics* (TRIPP), a progressive and comprehensive resource for instructors of prehospital providers. This resource contains a thorough review of prehospital pediatric emergencies.

IMPROVED HEALTH CARE AND INJURY PREVENTION

✱ **Emergency Medical Services for Children (EMSC)** federally funded program aimed at improving the health of pediatric patients who suffer from life-threatening illnesses and injuries.

Funding for CPEM comes largely from a group known as the **Emergency Medical Services for Children (EMSC).** This federally funded program falls under the management of the Maternal and Child Health Bureau—an agency of the U.S. Department of Health and Human Services. The EMSC was formed for the express purpose of improving the health of pediatric patients who suffer potentially life-threatening illnesses or injuries. This nationally coordinated effort has identified a number of pediatric health care concerns, including:

- Community education
- Data collection
- Quality improvement
- Injury prevention
- Access
- Prehospital care
- Emergency care
- Definitive care
- Finance
- Rehabilitation
- A systems approach to pediatric care
- Ongoing health care from birth to young adulthood

As a paramedic, you can take part in this national effort by actively participating in programs that promote injury prevention. Let's face it—as prehospital care providers, we see the consequences of pediatric trauma all too often. You can help reduce the rate of injury by taking advantage of opportunities to share "teaching points" in your daily life, both personally and professionally. Take part in, or offer to organize, school or community programs in injury prevention or health care (Figure 2-1). Engage student interest in the EMS profession by volunteering to speak at "career days," emphasizing those aspects of your job that relate to young people. Use non-urgent ambulance calls as a chance to educate family members or caregivers on the importance of "child-proofing" a home or

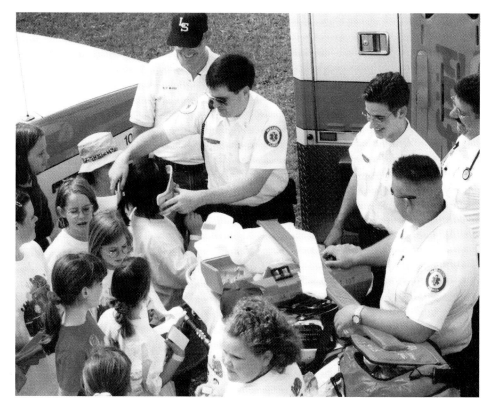

FIGURE 2-1   It is important to organize or participate in programs that educate children about injury prevention and health care.

neighborhood. Work with appropriate agencies in initiating or conducting safety inspections, block watches, and more.

There has been an increased effort to identify the severity and nature of pre-hospital pediatric emergencies. Many regions now have both pediatric and trauma registries. These, in addition to standard epidemiological research conducted by local health departments, are dependent on quality prehospital documentation. If your area is participating in a registry program or research study, be sure to obtain and record all required data. Information gained from these registries will help identify the need for more or specialized resources.

GENERAL APPROACH TO PEDIATRIC EMERGENCIES

The approach to the pediatric patient varies with the age of the patient and with the problem being treated. Foremost in approaching any pediatric emergency is consideration of the patient's emotional and physiological development. Care also involves the family members or caregivers responsible for the child. They will demand information, express fears, and, ultimately, give or refuse consent for treatment and/or transport.

COMMUNICATION AND PSYCHOLOGICAL SUPPORT

Treatment of an infant, child, or teenager begins with communication and psychological support. Interaction with pediatric patients and related adults continues throughout assessment and management. When obtaining the medical history

Treatment of an infant, child, or teenager begins with communication and psychological support.

of the pediatric patient, you should gather information as quickly and as accurately as possible. The parents and caregivers are often the primary source of information, especially in the case of infants. However, as children become older, they can also be a good source of information. Older children, for example, can often give accurate descriptions of symptoms or other details. Treat pediatric patients with respect, allowing them to express opinions and ask questions. Your listening skills will play an important role in alleviating the fears of child patients. You can even communicate a calm and caring attitude to infants, who respond to touch and voice just like any other human being.

Responding to Patient Needs

As previously mentioned, a child's response to an emergency will vary, depending on the age and emotional maturity of the child. The child's most common response to illness or injury is fear. Common fears of children include:

- Fear of being separated from the parents or caregivers
- Fear of being removed from a family place, such as home, and never returning
- Fear of being hurt
- Fear of being mutilated or disfigured
- Fear of the unknown

These fears may be intensified if the child detects fear or anxiety from the parents or caregivers. The general chaos and panic that often surround pediatric emergency situations may further distress the child.

Remember that children have the right to know what is being done to them. Be as honest as possible.

Remember that children have the right to know what is being done to them. You should be as honest as possible with them. If a procedure such as an IV needle stick will hurt, tell them so. Tell them immediately before performing a procedure. Do not say that a procedure will be painful and then take 5 minutes to prepare the equipment, allowing time for the child's anticipation of pain to build.

Always use language that is appropriate for the age of the child. Medical and anatomical terms that we routinely use may be completely foreign to children. Telling a child that you are going to "apply a cervical collar" means nothing. Instead, tell the child: "I'm going to put this collar around your neck to keep it from moving." "Try to hold your head still." "Tell me if it is too tight." Communication such as this will involve children in their own care and reduce their feelings of helplessness.

Responding to Parents or Caregivers

As you might expect, the reaction of parents or caregivers to a pediatric emergency will vary. Initial reactions might include shock, grief, denial, anger, guilt, fear, or complete loss of control. Their behavior may change during the course of the emergency. Communication is the key. Preferably only one paramedic will speak with adults at the scene. This will avoid any chance of conflicting information and allow a second paramedic to focus on the child. If parents or caregivers sense your confidence and professionalism, they will regain control and trust your suggestions for care. As with the child, most parents and caregivers feel overwhelmed by fear. They often express their fears in questions such as the following:

"Is my child going to die?"
"Did my child suffer brain damage?"

"Is my child going to be all right?"

"What are you doing to my child?"

"Will my child be able to walk?"

It may be difficult to answer these questions in the prehospital setting. However, the following actions may help allay parents' fears:

- Tell them your name and qualifications.
- Acknowledge their fears and concerns.
- Reassure them that it is all right to feel the way they do.
- Redirect their energies toward helping you care for the child.
- Remain calm and appear in control of the emergency.
- Keep the parents or caregivers informed as to what you are doing.
- Don't "talk down" to them.
- Assure parents or caregivers that everything possible is being done for their child.

If conditions permit, you should allow one of the parents or caregivers to remain with the child at all times. Some family members may be extremely emotional in emergency situations. The child will react more positively to a family member who appears calm and reassuring. If a parent or caregiver is "out of control," have another person take him or her away from the immediate area to settle down. Maintain a reasonable level of suspicion if a child shows a pattern of injuries, some old and some new. In such cases, the parent or caregiver may try to cover up what may be an abusive situation. They may also try to block examination and treatment. (There will be more on potential abuse or neglect later in this chapter.)

GROWTH AND DEVELOPMENT

Children progress through developmental stages on their way to adulthood. You should tailor your approach to the developmental level of your pediatric patient, as discussed in the following segments.

Newborns (First Hours after Birth)

Although the terms "newborn" and "neonate" are often used interchangeably, "newborn" refers to a baby in the first hours of extrauterine life. The term "neonate" describes infants from birth to 1 month of age. The method most frequently used to assess newborns is the *APGAR scoring system*, which was described in Chapter 1. Resuscitation of the newborn generally follows the inverted pyramid described in Chapter 1 and the guidelines established in the Neonatal Advanced Life Support (NALS) curriculum.

Neonates (Ages Birth to 1 Month)

The neonate, as noted above (and described in Chapter 1), is an infant up to 1 month of age. This is a major stage of development. Soon after birth, the neonate typically loses up to 10 percent of its birth weight as it adjusts to extrauterine life. This lost weight, however, is ordinarily recovered within 10 days. Gestational age affects early growth. Children born at term (40 weeks) should follow accepted developmental guidelines. Infants born prematurely will not be as developed, either neurologically or physically, as their term counterparts.

The neonatal stage of development centers on reflexes. The neonate's personality also begins to form. The infant is close to the mother and may stare at faces and smile. The mother, and occasionally the father, can comfort and quiet the child. Obviously, the history must be obtained from the parents or caregivers. However, it is also important to observe the child. Common illnesses in this age group include jaundice, vomiting, and respiratory distress. Serious illnesses, such as meningitis, are difficult to distinguish from minor illnesses in neonates. Often, fever is the only sign, although the majority of neonates with fever have minor illnesses (96–97 percent). The few that are seriously ill can be easily missed. For this reason, any fever in a neonate requires extensive evaluation.

The approach to this age group should include several factors. First, the child should always be kept warm. Observe skin color, tone, and respiratory activity. The absence of tears when crying may indicate dehydration. The lungs should be auscultated early during the exam, while the infant is quiet. You might find it helpful to have the child suck on a pacifier during the examination. Allowing the infant to remain in a parent's or caregiver's lap may help keep the child calm.

Infants (Ages 1 to 5 Months)

Infants should have doubled their birth weight by 5 to 6 months of age. They should be able to follow the movements of others with their eyes. Muscle control develops in a cephalo-caudal progression. This means, literally, that development of muscular control begins at the head (cephalo) and moves toward the tail (caudal). Muscular control also spreads from the trunk toward the extremities during this period. The infant's personality at this stage still centers closely on the parents or caregivers. The history must be obtained from these individuals, with close attention to possible illnesses and accidents, including SIDS, vomiting, dehydration, meningitis, child abuse, and household accidents.

Concentrate on keeping these patients warm and comfortable. Allow the infant to remain in the parent's or caregiver's lap. A pacifier or bottle can be used to help keep the baby quiet during the examination.

Infants (Ages 6 to 12 Months)

Infants in this age group may stand or even walk with assistance. They are quite active and enjoy exploring the world with their mouths. In this stage of development, the risk of **foreign body airway obstruction (FBAO)** becomes a serious concern.

Infants 6 months and older have more fully formed personalities and express themselves more readily. They have considerable anxiety toward strangers. They don't like lying on their backs. Children in this age group tend to cling to the mother, though the father "will do" in many cases. Common illnesses and accidents include febrile seizures, vomiting, diarrhea, dehydration, bronchiolitis, car accidents, croup, child abuse, poisonings, falls, airway obstructions, and meningitis.

These children should be examined while sitting in the lap of the parent or caregiver (Figure 2-2). The exam should progress in a toe-to-head order, since starting at the face may upset the child. If time and conditions permit, allow the child to become familiar with you before beginning the examination.

Toddlers (Ages 1 to 3 Years)

Great strides occur in gross motor development during this stage. Children tend to run underneath or stand on almost everything. They seem to always be on the move. As they grow older, toddlers become braver and more curious or stubborn. They begin to stray away from the parents or caregivers more frequently. Yet

* **foreign body airway obstruction (FBAO)** blockage or obstruction of the airway by an object that impairs respiration; in the case of pediatric patients, tongues, abundant secretions, and deciduous (baby) teeth are more likely to block airways.

Examine infants and toddlers in a toe-to-head order.

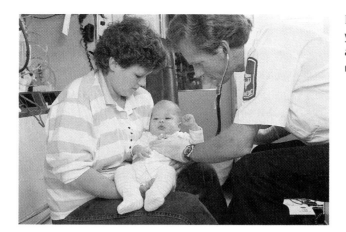

these remain the only people who can comfort them quickly, and most children will cling to a parent or caregiver if frightened.

At ages 1 to 3 years, language development begins. Often children can understand better than they can speak. Therefore, the majority of the medical history will still come from the parents or caregivers. Remember, however, that you can ask toddlers simple and specific questions.

Accidents of all types are the leading cause of injury deaths in pediatric patients ages 1 to fifteen years. Common accidents in this age group include motor vehicle collisions, homicides, burn injuries, drownings, and pedestrian accidents. Common illnesses and injuries in the toddler age group include vomiting, diarrhea, febrile seizures, poisonings, falls, child abuse, croup, and meningitis. Keep in mind that FBAO is still a high risk for toddlers.

Be cautious when treating toddlers. Approach toddlers slowly and try to gain their confidence. Conduct the exam in a toe-to-head order. The child may be difficult to examine and may resist being touched. Speak quietly and use only simple words. Avoid asking questions that allow the child to say "no." If the situation permits, allow toddlers to hold transitional objects such as a favorite blanket or toy. Be sure to tell the child if something will hurt. If at all possible, avoid procedures on the dominant arm/hand, which the child will try to pull away.

Preschoolers (Ages 3 to 5 Years)

Children in this age group show a tremendous increase in fine and gross motor development. Language skills increase greatly. Children in this age group know how to talk. However, if frightened, they often refuse to speak, especially to strangers. They often have vivid imaginations and may see monsters as part of their world. Preschoolers may have tempers and will express them. During this stage of development, children fear mutilation and may feel threatened by treatment. Avoid frightening or misleading comments.

Preschoolers often run to a particular parent or caregiver, depending upon the occasion. They stick up for the people they love and are openly affectionate. They still seek support and comfort from within the home.

When evaluating children in this age group, question the child first, keeping in mind that imagination may interfere with the facts. The child often has a distorted sense of time, and thus you must rely on the parents or caregivers to fill in the gaps. Common illnesses and accidents in this age group include croup,

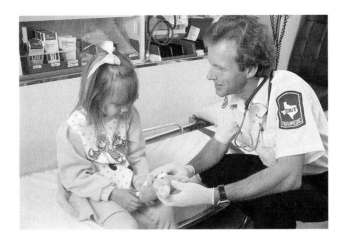

FIGURE 2-3 A small toy may calm a child in the 6–10 year age range.

asthma, poisonings, auto accidents, burns, child abuse, ingestion of foreign bodies, drownings, epiglottitis, febrile seizures, and meningitis.

Treatment of preschoolers requires tact. Avoid baby talk. If time and situation permit, give the child health care choices. Often the use of a doll or stuffed animal will assist in the examination. Allow the child to hold a piece of equipment, such as a stethoscope, and to use it. Let the child sit on your lap. Start the examination with the chest and evaluate the head last. Avoid misleading comments. Do not trick or lie to the child, and always explain what you are going to do.

Do not trick or lie to the child, and always explain what you are going to do.

School-Age Children (Ages 6–12 Years)

Children in this age group are active and carefree. Growth spurts sometimes lead to clumsiness. The personality continues to develop. School-age children are protective and proud of their parents or caregivers and seek their attention. They value peers, but also need home support.

When examining school-age children, give them the responsibility of providing the history. However, remember that children may be reluctant to provide information if they sustained an injury while doing something forbidden. The parents or caregivers can fill in the pertinent details. When assessing children in this age group, it is important to respect their modesty. Be honest and tell the child what is wrong. A small toy may help to calm the child (Figures 2-3 and 2-4). Common illnesses and injuries for this age group include drownings, auto collisions, bicycle accidents, falls, fractures, sports injuries, child abuse, and burns.

Adolescents (Ages 13 to 18)

Adolescence covers the period from the end of childhood to the start of adulthood (age 18). It begins with puberty, roughly age 13 for male children and age 11 for female children. (For this reason, adolescence is often defined as including ages 11 to 18, rather than 13 to 18.) Puberty is highly child specific and can begin at various ages. A female child, for example, may experience her first menstrual period as early as age 7 or 8.

Adolescents vary significantly in their development. Those over age 15 are physically nearer to adults in terms of their vital signs but emotionally may still be children. Regardless of physical maturity, remember that teenagers as a group are "body conscious." They worry about their physical image more than any

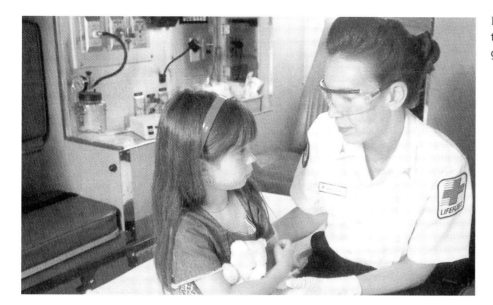

other pediatric age group. You should tactfully address their stated concerns about body integrity or disfigurement. The slightest possibility of a lasting scar may be a tremendous issue to the adolescent patient.

Although patients in this age are not yet legally adults, most consider themselves to be grown up. They take offense at the use of the word "child." They have a strong desire to be liked by their peers and to be included. Relationships with parents and caregivers may at times be strained as the adolescent demands greater independence. They value the opinions of other adolescents, especially members of the opposite sex. Generally, these patients make good historians. Do not be surprised, however, if their perception of events differs from that of their parents or caregivers.

Common illnesses and injuries in this age group include mononucleosis, asthma, auto collisions, sports injuries, drug and alcohol problems, suicide gestures, sexual abuse. Remember that pregnancy is also possible in female adolescents. When assessing teenagers, remember that vital signs will approach those of adults. In gathering a history, be factual and address the patient's questions. It may be wise to interview the patient away from the parents or caregivers. Listen to what the teenager is saying, as well as what he or she is *not* saying. If you suspect substance abuse or endangerment of the patient or others, approach the subject with tact and compassion. If you must perform a detailed physical exam, respect the teenager's sense of privacy. If the patient exhibits modesty or bodily shame, have a paramedic of the same sex as the teenager conduct the examination, if possible. Regardless of the situation, provide psychological support and reassurance.

It may be wise to interview the adolescent patient away from the parents or caregivers.

ANATOMY AND PHYSIOLOGY

The differences between the anatomy and physiology of infants and children and that of adults form the basis for the differences in the emergency medical care offered to the two groups (Table 2-1). As previously mentioned, children are not simply small adults. They possess bodies well suited to growth. As a rule, they have

Table 2-1 — ANATOMICAL AND PHYSIOLOGICAL CHARACTERISTICS OF INFANTS AND CHILDREN

Differences in Infants and Children as Compared to Adults	Potential Effects That May Impact Assessment and Care
Tongue proportionately larger	More likely to block airway
Smaller airway structures	More easily blocked
Abundant secretions	Can block the airway
Deciduous (baby) teeth	Easily dislodged; can block the airway
Flat nose and face	Difficult to obtain good face mask seal
Head heavier relative to body and less-developed neck structures and muscles	Head may be propelled more forcefully than body producing a higher incidence of head injury in trauma
Fontanelle and open sutures (soft spots) palpable on top of young infant's head	Bulging fontanelle can be a sign of increased intracranial pressure (but may be normal if infant is crying); shrunken fontanelle may indicate dehydration
Thinner, softer brain tissue	Susceptible to serious brain injury
Head larger in proportion to body	Tips forward when supine; possible flexion of neck, which makes neutral alignment of airway difficult
Shorter, narrower, more elastic (flexible) trachea	Can close off trachea with hyperextension of neck
Short neck	Difficult to stabilize or immobilize
Abdominal breathers	Difficult to evaluate breathing
Faster respiratory rate	Muscles easily fatigue, causing respiratory distress
Newborns breathe primarily through the nose (obligate nose breathers)	May not automatically open mouth to breathe if nose is blocked; airway more easily blocked
Larger body surface relative to body mass	Prone to hypothermia
Softer bones	More flexible, less easily fractured; traumatic forces may be transmitted to internal organs, causing injuring without fracturing the ribs; lungs easily damaged with trauma
Spleen and liver more exposed	Organ injury likely with significant force to abdomen

healthier organs, a greater ability to compensate for most illnesses, and softer, more flexible tissues. Because you will probably have infrequent contact with pediatric patients, you need to regularly review the physical characteristics that distinguish them from the adult patients that you encounter more often (Figure 2-5).

Head

The pediatric patient's head is proportionally larger than an adult's and the occipital region is significantly larger. In comparison to their head size, most pediatric patients have small faces and flat noses, which makes it difficult to obtain a good face mask seal.

With infants, pay special attention to the fontanelles—areas of the skull that have not yet fused. The fontanelles allow for compression of the head during childbirth and for rapid growth of the brain during early life. The posterior fontanelle generally closes by 4 months of age. The anterior fontanelle diminishes after 6 months of age and usually closes between 9 and 18 months.

During assessment, always inspect the anterior fontanelle. Normally, it should be level with the surface of the skull or slightly sunken. It also may pulsate. With increased intracranial pressure, as with meningitis or head trauma, the

In assessing infants, pay special attention to the fontanelles, especially the anterior fontanelle.

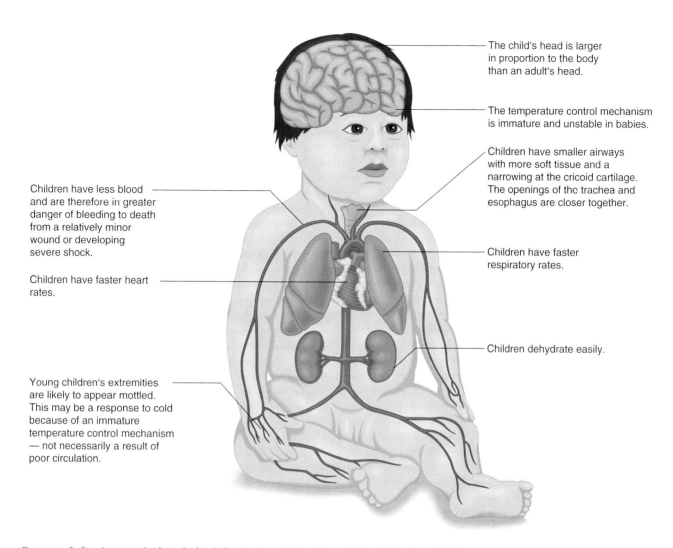

The child's head is larger in proportion to the body than an adult's head.

The temperature control mechanism is immature and unstable in babies.

Children have smaller airways with more soft tissue and a narrowing at the cricoid cartilage. The openings of the trachea and esophagus are closer together.

Children have less blood and are therefore in greater danger of bleeding to death from a relatively minor wound or developing severe shock.

Children have faster heart rates.

Children have faster respiratory rates.

Children dehydrate easily.

Young children's extremities are likely to appear mottled. This may be a response to cold because of an immature temperature control mechanism — not necessarily a result of poor circulation.

FIGURE 2-5   Anatomical and physiological considerations in the infant and child.

fontanelle may become tight and bulging and pulsations may diminish or disappear. In the presence of dehydration, the anterior fontanelle often falls below the level of the skull and appears sunken.

The heavy head relative to body size places an infant or child at risk of blunt head trauma. In accidents, the head may be propelled more forcefully than the body, resulting in a higher incidence of brain injury. Head size also affects the airway positioning techniques you should use in treating pediatric patients. In general, follow these guidelines:

- In treating seriously injured patients less than 3 years of age, place a thin layer of padding under their back to obtain a neutral position. This will prevent the head from tipping forward when supine, causing flexion of the neck (Figure 2-6).

- In treating medically ill children over 3 years of age, place a folded sheet or towel under the occiput to obtain a sniffing position (neck flexed slightly forward, head extended slightly backward to align pharynx and trachea).

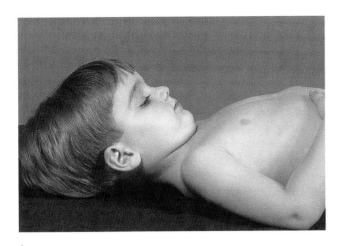
a.

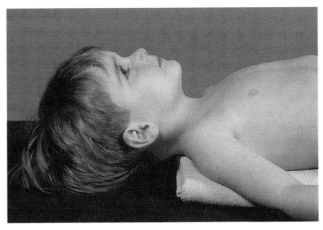
b.

FIGURE 2-6   a. In the supine position, an infant's or child's larger head tips forward, causing airway obstruction. b. Placing padding under the patient's back and shoulders will bring the airway to a neutral or slightly extended position.

Airway

In managing the airway of an infant or child, keep in mind these anatomical and physiological considerations:

- Pediatric patients have narrower airways at all levels and these are more easily blocked by secretions or obstructions.
- Infants are obligate nose breathers. If their noses are blocked by secretions, for example, they may not automatically "know" to open their mouths to breathe.
- The tongue takes up more space proportionately in a child's mouth and can more easily obstruct breathing in an unconscious patient.
- The trachea is softer and more flexible in a child and can collapse if the neck and head are hyperextended.
- A child's larynx is higher (C-3–C-4) and extends into the pharynx.
- In young children, the cricoid ring is the narrowest part of the airway.
- Infants have an omega-shaped (horseshoe-shaped) epiglottis that extends at a 45-degree angle into the airway. Because epiglottic folds in pediatric patients have softer cartilage than in adults, they can be more floppy, especially in infants.

Take these anatomic and physiological differences into account by following these general procedures: Always keep the nares clear in infants less than 6 months of age. Do not overextend the neck, which may collapse the trachea. Open the airway gently to avoid soft-tissue injury. Because any device placed in the infant's or child's airway further narrows the passage's diameter and may result in localized swelling, consider use of an oral or a nasal airway only after other manual maneuvers have failed to keep the airway open. (There will be more information on pediatric airway management later in this chapter.)

Consider use of an oral or nasal airway in a pediatric patient only after other manual maneuvers have failed to keep the airway open.

Chest and Lungs

In evaluating the chest and lungs of an infant or child, remember that tissues and muscles are more immature than in adults. Chest muscles tire easily, and lung tissues are more fragile. The soft, pliable ribs offer less protection to organs. Expect the ribs to be positioned horizontally and the mediastinum to be more mobile.

Take into account the following anatomical and physiological considerations when assessing the chest and lungs of a pediatric patient:

- Infants and children are diaphragmatic breathers.
- Pediatric patients, especially young infants, are prone to gastric distention.
- Although rib fractures occur less frequently in children, they are not uncommon in cases of child abuse.
- Because of the softness of a child's ribs, greater energy can be transmitted to underlying organs following trauma. As a result, significant internal injury can be present without external signs.
- Pulmonary contusions are more common in pediatric patients who have been subjected to major trauma.
- An infant's or child's lungs are more prone to pneumothorax following barotrauma.
- The mediastinum of a child or infant will shift more with tension pneumothorax than in an adult.
- Thin chest walls in infants and children allow for easily transmitted breath sounds. This may result in perception of breath sounds from elsewhere in the chest, which may cause you to miss a pneumothorax or misplaced intubation.

Abdomen

Note that the liver and spleen, both very vascular organs, are proportionally larger in the pediatric patient than in the adult patient. Abdominal organs lie closer together. Because of the immature abdominal muscles in an infant or child, expect to find more frequent damage to the liver and spleen and more multiple organ injuries than in an adult.

Extremities

Until pediatric patients reach adolescence, they have softer and more porous bones than adults. Therefore, you should treat "sprains" and "strains" as fractures and immobilize them accordingly.

During early stages of development, injuries to the **growth plate** may also disrupt bone growth. Keep this in mind when inserting an intraosseous needle, which could mistakenly pierce the plate. (Intraosseous infusion is discussed later in this chapter.)

* **growth plate** the area just below the head of a long bone in which growth in bone length occurs; the epiphyseal plate.

During the early stages of development, injuries to the growth plate by an intraosseous needle may disrupt bone growth.

Skin and Body Surface Area (BSA)

There are three distinguishing features of the pediatric patient's skin and BSA. First, the skin of an infant or child is thinner than that of an adult. Second, infants and children generally have less subcutaneous fat. Finally, they have a larger body-suface-area-to-weight ratio.

As a result of these features, children risk greater injury from extremes in temperature or thermal exposure. They lose fluids and heat more quickly than adults and have a greater likelihood of dehydration and hypothermia. They also burn more easily and deeply than adults, explaining why burns account for one of the leading causes of death among pediatric trauma patients.

Respiratory System

Although infants and children have a tidal volume proportionately similar to that of adolescents and adults, they require double the metabolic oxygen. They also have proportionately smaller oxygen reserves. The combination of increased oxygen requirements and decreased oxygen reserves makes infants and children especially susceptible to hypoxia.

Cardiovascular System

Infants and children increase their cardiac output by increasing their heart rate. They have a very limited capacity to increase their stroke volume.

Cardiac output is rate dependent in infants and small children. They possess vigorous, but limited, cardiovascular reserves. Although infants and children have a circulating blood volume proportionately larger than adults, their absolute blood volume is smaller. As a result, they can maintain blood pressure longer than an adult but still be at risk of shock (hypoperfusion). In assessing a pediatric patient for shock, keep in mind the following points:

- A smaller absolute volume of fluid/blood loss is needed to cause shock in infants and children.
- A larger proportional volume of fluid/blood loss is needed to cause shock in these same patients.
- As with all categories of patients, hypotension is a late sign of shock. In pediatric patients, it is an ominous sign of imminent cardiopulmonary arrest.
- A child may be in shock despite a normal blood pressure.
- Shock assessment in children and infants is based upon clinical signs of tissue perfusion. (See the later discussion of circulation assessment.)
- Suspect shock if tachycardia is present.
- Monitor the pediatric patient carefully for the development of hypotension.

Bleeding that would not be dangerous in an adult may be life-threatening in an infant or child.

Once again, remember that children are not small adults. Bleeding that would not be dangerous in an adult may be a serious and life-threatening condition in an infant or child. Shock can develop in the small child who has a laceration to the scalp (with its many blood vessels), or in the 3-year-old who loses as little as a cup of blood. (Management of shock in pediatric patients will be discussed in detail later in the chapter.)

Nervous System

The nervous system develops continually throughout childhood. Even so, the neural tissue remains more fragile than in adults. The skull and spinal column, which are softer and more pliable than in adults, offer less protection of the brain and spinal cord. Therefore, greater force can be transmitted to a child's neural tissue with more devastating consequences. These injuries can occur without injury to the skull or to the spinal column. (Treatment of head and neck trauma will be discussed later in the chapter.)

Metabolic Differences

You may have noticed the repeated emphasis on the need to keep neonatal and pediatric patients warm during treatment and transport. The emphasis on warming techniques is based upon the following metabolic considerations:

- Infants and children have a limited store of glycogen and glucose.
- Pediatric patients are prone to hypothermia because of their greater BSA-to-weight ratio.
- Significant volume loss can result from vomiting and diarrhea.
- Newborns and neonates lack the ability to shiver.

To prevent heat loss, always cover the patient's head and maintain adequate temperature controls in the ambulance. Ensure that the ambulance is always stocked with an adequate supply of blankets and, if you live in a cold area, hot water bottles.

GENERAL APPROACH TO PEDIATRIC ASSESSMENT

Priorities in the management of the pediatric patient, as with all patients, are established on a threat-to-life basis. If life-threatening problems are not present, you will complete each of the general steps discussed in the following sections.

BASIC CONSIDERATIONS

Many of the components of the initial patient assessment can be done during a visual examination of the scene. (This is sometimes called the "assessment from the doorway," during which you quickly note signs of an ill child such as lethargy.) Whenever possible, involve the parent or caregiver in efforts to calm or comfort the child. Depending on the situation, you may decide to allow the parent or caregiver to remain with the child during treatment and transport. As previously mentioned, the developmental stage of the patient and the coping skills of the parents or guardians will be key factors in making this decision.

When interacting with parents or other responsible adults, keep in mind the communication techniques suggested earlier. Pay attention to the way in which parents or caregivers interact with the child. Are the interactions appropriate to the emergency? Are family members concerned? Are they angry? Are they overly emotional or entirely indifferent?

From the time of dispatch, you will continually acquire information relative to the patient's condition. As with all patients, personal safety must be your first priority. In treating pediatric patients, follow the same guidelines in approaching the scene as you would with any other patient. Observe for potentially hazardous situations, and make sure you take appropriate BSI precautions. Remember that infants and young children are at especially high risk of an infectious process.

Remember to take appropriate BSI precautions when treating infants and children.

SCENE SIZE-UP

Upon arrival, conduct a quick scene size-up. Dispatch information received en route, as well as your own observations, can provide critical indicators of scene safety. Be aware of the increased anxiety and stress in any situation involving an infant or child. Try to set aside thoughts of your own children and adopt the professional, systematic approach to assessment necessary for scene safety and effective patient management. If you find yourself getting angry or upset, temporarily turn over care to another paramedic until you compose yourself.

As you survey the scene, look for clues to the mechanism of injury (MOI) or the nature of the illness (NOI). These clues will help guide your assessment and determine appropriate interventions. Note the presence of dangerous substances—e.g., medicine bottles, household chemicals, or poisonous plants—that the child may have ingested. Spot environmental hazards such as unprotected stairwells, kerosene heaters, and so on. Identify possible causes of trauma, especially in motor vehicle collisions. Remain alert for evidence of child abuse, particularly in cases in which the injury and history do not coincide. As already mentioned, pay attention to the way parents or caregivers respond to the child and the way the child responds to them.

Keep the child in mind while conducting your scene size-up. Pace your approach to give the child time to adjust to your presence. Speak in a soft voice, using simple words. As soon as you reach the child, position yourself at eye level with the patient and make every effort to win his trust. If the child bonds more readily with one member of the team than another, allow that person to remain with the child and, if possible, to conduct most of the physical exam.

INITIAL ASSESSMENT

The patient's condition determines the course of your initial assessment. An active and alert child will allow for a more comfortable approach, with more time spent on communication with the child and appropriate adults. A critically ill or injured child, however, may require quick intervention and rapid transport. Your choice of action depends upon your general impression of the patient. (For a summary of the initial assessment of a pediatric patient, see Figure 2-7.)

General Impression

The major points in forming your general impression are outlined in an assessment tool called the *pediatric assessment triangle* (included in Figure 2-7). Many experts recommend this assessment tool as a way of quickly evaluating the level of severity and the need for immediate intervention. It is a rapid "eyes-open, hands-on" approach that allows you to detect a life-threatening situation without the use of a stethoscope, blood pressure cuff, pulse oximeter, or other medical device. The triangle's three components are:

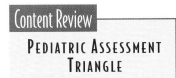

Content Review

PEDIATRIC ASSESSMENT TRIANGLE
• Appearance
• Breathing
• Circulation

- *Appearance*—focuses on the child's mental status and muscle tone
- *Breathing*—directs attention to respiratory rate and respiratory effort
- *Circulation*—uses skin signs and color as well as capillary refill as indicators of the patient's circulatory status

Vital Functions

After quickly applying the pediatric assessment triangle to form a general impression, you will evaluate vital functions—mental status (level of consciousness) and the ABCs—as they apply to infants and children. Although assessment steps are basically the same as for adults, certain modifications must be made to collect accurate data.

Level of Consciousness Employ the AVPU method (*a*lert, responds to *v*erbal stimuli, responds to *p*ainful stimuli, *u*nresponsive) to evaluate the pediatric patient's level of consciousness. Adjust the techniques for the child's age. With an infant, you may

Initial Assessment

↓

Forming a general impression. Elements to consider:
- Skin color
- Quality of cry or speech
- Interaction with surroundings
- Emotional state
- Response to the EMT
- Body tone and positioning.

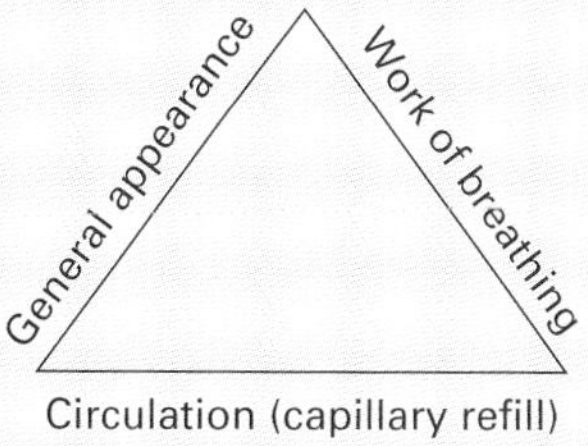

General appearance / Work of breathing

Circulation (capillary refill)

↓

Determining Mental Status
- AVPU scale

↓

Assessing ABCs
- Observe the respiratory rate.
- Observe for full and symmetrical chest rise with inspiration.
- Note the effort or work of breathing. Look for:
  —Retractions
  —Nasal flaring
  —"Seesaw" breathing
- Listen for audible abnormal breathing sounds.
  —Grunting
  —Stridor
  —Crowing
  —Other noisy breathing.
- Listen with a stethoscope to both sides of the chest.
- Assess peripheral perfusion.
  —Feel for brachial, femoral, and peripheral pulses.
  —Check capillary refill in children 5 years of age or younger.
- Assess the skin for color, moisture, and temperature.
- Take a blood pressure reading in children older than 3 years.

↓

History and Physical Exam

↓   ↓

Common Medical Problems
- Airway obstruction
- Respiratory emergencies
- Seizures
- Altered mental status
- Fever
- Poisonings
- Shock
- Near drowning
- Sudden infant death syndrome (SIDS)

Common Trauma Situations
- Seat belt injuries
- Bicycle-related injuries
- Car vs. pedestrian injuries
- Head and neck injuries
- Burns
- Abuse and neglect

FIGURE 2-7   The basic steps in pediatric assessment. Notice the components and signs in the Pediatric Assessment Triangle.

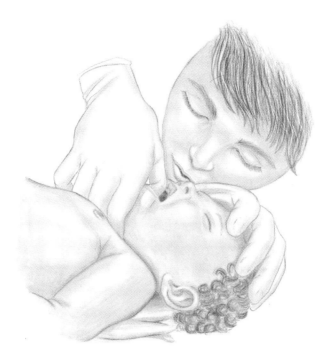

FIGURE 2-8   Opening the airway in a child.

Never shake an infant or child.

Airway and respiratory problems are the most common cause of cardiac arrest in infants and young children.

need to shout to elicit a response (perhaps crying) to verbal stimulus. An infant should withdraw from a noxious stimulus. *Never shake an infant or child.*

Airway   Assess the airway using the techniques shown in Figures 2-8 to 2-11. If at any point the patient shows little or no movement of air, intervene immediately. Keep this fact in mind: *Airway and respiratory problems are the most common cause of cardiac arrest in infants and young children.*

As you inspect the airway, ask yourself the following questions:

- Is the airway patent?
- Is the airway maintainable with head positioning, suctioning, or airway adjuncts?

FIGURE 2-9   Head-tilt/chin-lift method.

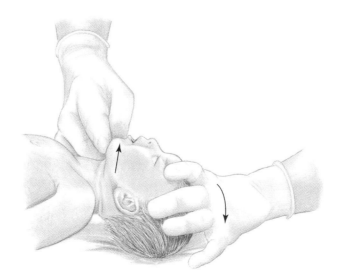

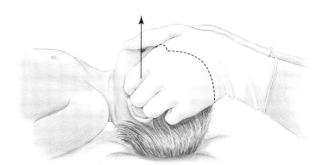

FIGURE 2-10   Jaw-thrust method.

- Is the airway *not* maintainable? If so, what action is required? (Airway management techniques are discussed later in this chapter.)

Breathing   In assessing the breathing of a pediatric patient, recall the CPR certification courses in which you learned to "Look, Listen, and Feel." *Look* at the patient's chest and abdomen for movement. *Listen* for breath sounds—both normal and abnormal. *Feel* for air movement at the patient's mouth.

Keep in mind that pediatric patients have small chests. For this reason, place the stethoscope near each of the armpits in order to minimize transmitted breath sounds. When considering the respiratory rate, remember that pain or fear can increase a child's respiratory efforts. Tachypnea, an abnormally rapid rate of breathing, may indicate fear, pain, inadequate oxygenation, or, in the case of neonates, exposure to cold.

FIGURE 2-11   Assessing breathing.

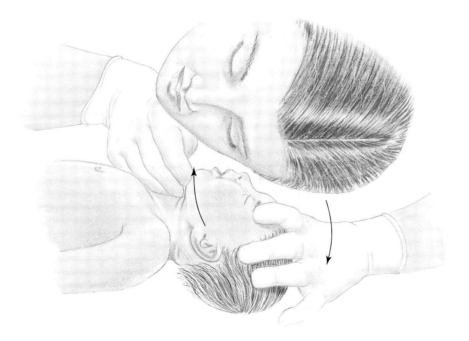

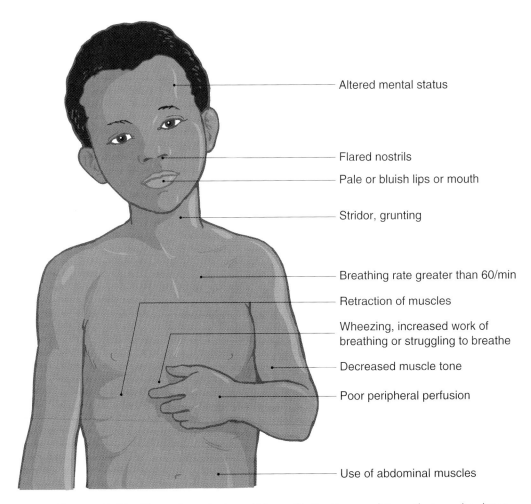

Altered mental status

Flared nostrils
Pale or bluish lips or mouth

Stridor, grunting

Breathing rate greater than 60/min
Retraction of muscles
Wheezing, increased work of
breathing or struggling to breathe
Decreased muscle tone
Poor peripheral perfusion

Use of abdominal muscles

FIGURE 2-12   Signs of respiratory distress. Notice the conditions that can be determined by quick observation.

If you suspect trauma, check the infant or child for life-threatening chest injuries. Keep in mind that even a minor injury to the chest can interfere with a child's breathing efforts. A chest injury can also interfere with your effort to provide adequate oxygenation or ventilation.

Your goal is to identify any evidence of compromised breathing (Figure 2-12). Evaluation of breathing includes assessment of the following conditions:

- *Respiratory Rate.* Tachypnea is often the first manifestation of respiratory distress in infants. Regardless of the cause, an infant breathing at a rapid rate will eventually tire. Keep in mind that a decreasing respiratory rate may be a result of tiring and is not necessarily a sign of improvement. A slow respiratory rate in an acutely ill infant or child is an ominous sign. (Normal respiratory rates are listed in Table 2-2.) In short, be alert for a respiratory rate that is *either* abnormally fast *or* abnormally slow.

- *Respiratory Effort.* The quality of air entry can be assessed by observing for chest rise, breath sounds, stridor, or wheezing. An increased respiratory effort in the infant or child is also evidenced by

Table 2-2 — NORMAL VITAL SIGNS: INFANTS AND CHILDREN*

Normal Pulse Rates (Beats per Minute, at Rest)

Newborn	100 to 180
Infant (0–5 Months)	100 to 160
Infant (6–12 Months)	100 to 160
Toddler (1–3 Years)	80 to 110
Preschooler (3–5 Years)	70 to 110
School Age (6–10 Years)	65 to 110
Early Adolescence (11–14 Years)	60 to 90

Normal Respiration Rates (Breaths per Minute, at Rest)

Newborn	30 to 60
Infant (0–5 Month)	30 to 60
Infant (6–12 Months)	30 to 60
Toddler (1–3 Years)	24 to 40
Preschooler (3–5 Years)	22 to 34
School Age (6–10 Years)	18 to 30
Early Adolescence (11–14 Years)	12 to 26

Normal Blood Pressure Ranges (mmHg, at Rest)

	Systolic Approx. 90 plus 2 × age	Diastolic Approx. 2/3 systolic
Preschooler (3–5 Years)	average 98 (78 to 116)	average 65
School age (6–10 Years)	average 105 (80 to 122)	average 69
Early Adolescence (11–14 Years)	average 114 (88 to 140)	average 76

*Adolescents ages 15 to 18 approach the vital signs of adults.

Note: A high pulse in an infant or child is not as great a concern as a low pulse. A low pulse may indicate imminent cardiac arrest. Blood pressure is usually not taken in a child under 3 years of age. In cases of blood loss or shock, a child's blood pressure will remain within normal limits until near the end, then fall swiftly.

nasal flaring and the use of accessory respiratory muscles. (Signs of respiratory effort are listed in Table 2-3.)

- *Color.* Cyanosis is a fairly late sign of respiratory failure and is most frequently seen in the mucous membranes of the mouth and the nail beds. Cyanosis of the extremities alone is more likely due to circulatory failure (shock) than to respiratory failure.

Circulation As mentioned earlier, you should assess a pediatric patient's circulation by first checking the child's color. Keep in mind that the pediatric patient tends to become hypothermic; therefore, you should check the capillary refill time in an area of central circulation, such as the sternum or forehead. (Note that capillary refill time, as discussed later in this chapter, is considered reliable as a sign of perfusion primarily in children less than 6 years of age.) In general, evaluate the following conditions when assessing circulation during the initial assessment:

- *Heart Rate.* As previously mentioned, infants develop sinus tachycardia in response to stress. Thus any tachycardia in an infant or child

Table 2-3	SIGNS OF INCREASED RESPIRATORY EFFORT
Retraction	Visible sinking of the skin and soft tissues of the chest around and below the ribs and above the collarbone
Nasal flaring	Widening of the nostrils; seen primarily on inspiration
Head bobbing	Observed when the head lifts and tilts back as the child inhales and then moves forward as the child exhales
Grunting	Sound heard when an infant attempts to keep the alveoli open by building back pressure during expiration
Wheezing	Passage of air over mucous secretions in bronchi; heard more commonly upon expiration; a low- or high-pitched sound
Gurgling	Coarse, abnormal bubbling sound heard in the airway during inspiration or expiration; may indicate an open chest wound
Stridor	Abnormal, musical, high-pitched sound, more commonly heard on inspiration

requires further evaluation to determine the cause. Bradycardia in a distressed infant or child may indicate hypoxia and is an ominous sign of cardiac arrest. (Normal heart rates are listed in Table 2-2.)

- *Peripheral Circulation.* The presence of peripheral pulses is a good indicator of the adequacy of end-organ perfusion. Loss of central pulses is an ominous sign.
- *End-Organ Perfusion.* End-organ perfusion is most evident in the skin, kidneys, and brain. Decreased perfusion of the skin is an early sign of shock. A capillary refill time of greater than 2 seconds is indicative of low cardiac output. Impairment of brain perfusion is usually evidenced by a change in mental status. The child may become confused or lethargic. Seizures may occur. Failure of the child to recognize the parents' faces is often an ominous sign. Urine output directly relates to kidney perfusion. Normal urine output is 1–2 mL/kg/hr. Urine flow of less than 1 mL/kg/hr is an indicator of poor renal perfusion.

Remember that evaluation of mental status and ABCs during the initial assessment is rapid and not detailed—aimed at discovering and correcting immediate life threats. More thorough measurements will be performed during the focused history and physical exam.

Anticipating Cardiopulmonary Arrest

At each stage of evaluating vital functions, ask yourself "Does this child have pulmonary or circulatory failure that may lead to cardiopulmonary arrest?"

Your initial assessment—and the repeated assessments that follow—help you to recognize and prevent cardiopulmonary arrest. At each stage of evaluating vital functions, ask yourself this question: *"Does this child have pulmonary or circulatory failure that may lead to cardiopulmonary arrest?"* Early recognition of the physiologically unstable child is one of the main goals of pediatric advanced life support (PALS). Conditions that place a pediatric patient at risk of cardiopulmonary arrest include:

- Respiratory rate greater than 60
- Heart rate greater than 180 or less than 80 (under 5 years)
- Heart rate greater than 180 or less than 60 (over 5 years)

- Respiratory distress
- Trauma
- Burns
- Cyanosis
- Altered level of consciousness
- Seizures
- Fever with petechiae (small purple spots resulting from skin hemorrhages)

Evaluate the patient for these conditions throughout assessment and transport. Cardiopulmonary arrest in infants and children is usually not a sudden event. Instead, it is the end result of progressive deterioration in respiratory and cardiac function. Therefore, you need to determine whether the patient's condition is deteriorating or improving. Any decompensation or change in the patient's status will prompt you to perform basic or advanced life support measures, as appropriate.

Transport Priority

Based on your initial assessment, you will assign the patient one of the following transport priorities:

- *Urgent*—Proceed with the rapid trauma assessment, if trauma is suspected, then transport immediately with further assessment and treatment performed en route.
- *Non-urgent*—Complete the focused history and physical exam at the scene, then transport.

Transitional Phase

The way in which the pediatric patient is transferred to EMS care depends entirely on the seriousness of the patient's condition. A transitional phase is intended for the conscious, non-acutely ill child. This phase of assessment allows the infant or child to become familiar with you and the equipment that you will be using. When dealing with the unconscious or acutely ill patient, however, you will skip this phase and proceed directly to the treatment and transport phases of assessment. In essence, you assign the patient an "urgent" status.

FOCUSED HISTORY AND PHYSICAL EXAM

After you have prioritized patient care at the end of the initial assessment, you will obtain a history and perform a physical exam. If the patient has a medical illness, the history will precede the physical exam. If the patient is suffering from trauma, the physical exam will take precedence. If partners are working together, the history and physical exam may be performed simultaneously. (For a summary of conditions that may be found during the focused history and physical exam, review Figure 2-7.)

History

Whenever a patient is identified as a priority patient, then the focused history will occur en route to the hospital, after essential treatments or interventions for life-threatening conditions have been performed.

To obtain a history for a pediatric patient, you will probably need to involve a family member or caregiver. Remember, however, that school-age children and adolescents like to take part in their own care. As previously mentioned, you can elicit valuable information from even very young patients. As a general precaution, question older adolescent patients in private, especially about issues such as sexual activity, pregnancy, or illicit drug and alcohol use. If you question adolescents about these subjects in the presence of an adult, they will probably be more reticent for fear of later repercussions.

As with any patient, you will use the history to uncover additional pertinent injuries or medical conditions. The history should center on the chief complaint and past medical history.

To evaluate the nature of the chief complaint, determine each of the following:

- Nature of the illness/injury
- Length of time the patient has been sick/injured
- Presence of fever
- Effects of the illness/injury on patient behavior
- Bowel/urine habits
- Presence of vomiting/diarrhea
- Frequency of urination

The past medical history identifies chronic illnesses, use of medications, and allergies. Be sure to inquire whether the infant or child is currently under a doctor's care. If so, obtain the name of the physician and present it at the receiving hospital. In the case of trauma patients, reconsider the mechanism of injury and the results of your on-scene physical examination (which, as noted earlier, will precede the history in the case of trauma).

Physical Exam

Focused Exam Carry out the physical exam after all life-threatening conditions have been identified and addressed. If there is a significant mechanism of injury or if the patient is unresponsive, perform a complete rapid trauma assessment or rapid medical assessment. Use the toe-to-head approach with the younger child (or begin with the chest and examine the head last) and the head-to-toe approach in the older child. If the injury is minor or if the ill patient is responsive, perform a physical exam that is focused on the affected areas and systems.

Perform the physical exam as described in Volume 2. Depending upon the particular situation, some or all of the following assessment techniques may be appropriate to include in the exam:

- *Pupils.* Inspect the patient's pupils for equality and reaction to light.
- *Capillary Refill.* As noted earlier, this technique is valuable for pediatric patients less than 6 years of age. Blanch the nail bed, base of the thumb, or sole of one of the feet. Remember that normal capillary refill is 2 seconds or less. Recall that this technique is less reliable in cold environments.
- *Hydration.* Note skin turgor, presence of tears and saliva and, with infants, the condition of the fontanelles.
- *Pulse Oximetry.* Use this mechanical device on moderately injured or ill infants and children. Readings will give you immediate information regarding peripheral oxygen saturation and allow you to

Table 2-4	GLASGOW COMA SCALE MODIFICATIONS FOR INFANTS		
Category	Response		Score
Verbal	Happy, coos, babbles, or cries spontaneously		5
	Irritable crying, but consolable		4
	Cries to pain, weak cry		3
	Moans to pain		2
	None		1
Motor	Spontaneous movement		6
	Withdraws to touch		5
	Withdraws to pain		4
	Abnormal flexion		3
	Abnormal extension		2
	None		1
Eye Opening (same as adult)	Spontaneous		4
	To speech		3
	To pain		2
	None		1

Source: *Adapted from James, H.E., (1986): "Neurological evaluation and support in the child with acute brain insult,"* Pediatric Annals, 15(1): 17.

follow trends in the patient's pulse rate and oxygenation status. Keep in mind, however, that hypothermia or shock can affect readings.

Glasgow Coma Scale In cases of trauma, you may need to apply the Glasgow coma scale (GCS)—a scoring system for monitoring the neurological status of patients with possible head injuries. The Glasgow coma scale assigns scores based on verbal responses, motor functions, and eye movements.

In using the Glasgow coma scale with pediatric patients, you will have to make certain modifications. The younger the patient, the more adjustments you will need to make. Verbal responses, for example, will not be possible for neonates and infants. However, motor function may be assessed in very young children by observing voluntary movement. Infants under 4 months of age should have a grasp reflex when an object is placed on the palmar surface of their hand. The grasp should be immediate. Children over 3 years of age will follow directions, when encouraged. Sensory function can be observed by the withdrawal reaction from "tickling" the patient. (See Table 2-4 for a modified GCS for infants.)

After you score the GCS for the patient, prioritize the patient according to severity. Guidelines are:

- *Mild*—GCS 13 to 15
- *Moderate*—GCS 9 to 12
- *Severe*—GCS less than or equal to 8

Vital Signs Remember that poorly taken vital signs are of less value than no vital signs at all. The following guidelines will help you obtain accurate pediatric readings. (Review Table 2-2 for normal pediatric vital signs.)

- Take vital signs with the patient in as close to a resting state as possible. If necessary, allow the child to calm down before attempting vital signs. Vital signs in the field should include pulse, respiration, blood pressure, and temperature.

In using the Glasgow coma scale with pediatric patients, you will have to make certain modifications. The younger the patient, the more adjustments you will need to make.

Remember that poorly taken vital signs are of less value than no vital signs at all.

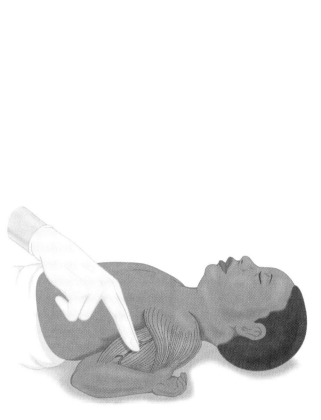

FIGURE 2-13a   Taking the brachial pulse.

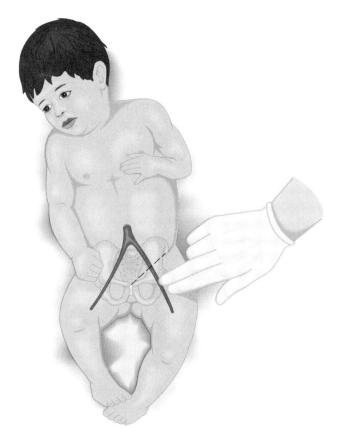

FIGURE 2-13b   Taking the femoral pulse.

- Obtain blood pressure with an appropriate-sized cuff. The cuff should be two-thirds the width of the upper arm. Note that the pulse pressure (the difference between the systolic and diastolic blood pressure) narrows as shock develops. *Note that hypotension is a late and often sudden sign of cardiovascular decompensation.* Even mild hypotension should be taken seriously and treated quickly and vigorously, since cardiopulmonary arrest is probably imminent.

- Feel for peripheral, brachial, or femoral pulses (Figures 2-13 a and b). There is often a significant variation in pulse rate in children due to varied respirations. Therefore, it is important to monitor the pulse for at least 30 seconds, a full minute if possible.

- It is generally not possible to weigh the child. However, if medications are required, make a good estimate of the child's weight. Often the parents or caregivers can provide a fairly reliable weight from a recent visit to the doctor. Table 2-5 lists the average weights by age for pediatric patients. (Remember that these are only averages.)

- Observe respiratory rate before beginning the examination. After the examination is started, the child will often begin to cry. It will then be impossible to determine respiratory rate. For an estimate of the upper limit of respiratory rate, subtract the child's age from 40. It is also important to identify respiratory pattern, as well as retractions, nasal flaring, or paradoxical chest movement.

- Measure temperature early in the patient encounter and repeat toward the end. IV fluid and exposure to the environment can cause a drop in core temperature.

Age	Weight (lb)	Weight (kg)
Birth	7	3.5
3 Months	10	5
6 Months	15	7
9 Months	18	8
1 Year	22	10
2 Years	26	12
3 Years	33	15
4 Years	37	17
5 Years	40	18
6 Years	44	20
7 Years	50	23
8 Years	56	25
9 Years	60	28
10 Years	70	33
11 Years	75	35
12 Years	85	40
13 Years	98	44

Table 2-5 PEDIATRIC WEIGHTS AND POUND-KILOGRAM CONVERSION

- Continue to observe the child for level of consciousness. There may be a wide variety in levels of consciousness and activity during treatment.

Noninvasive Monitoring Modern noninvasive monitoring devices all have their application in pediatric emergency care (Figure 2-14). These may include the pulse oximeter, automated blood pressure devices, self-registering thermometers, and ECGs. To promote the goal of early recognition of cardiopulmonary arrest, every seriously ill or injured child should receive continuous pulse oximetry. This will provide you with essential information regarding the patient's heart rate and peripheral O_2 saturation. It will also help you to monitor the effects of any medications administered. ECG and automated blood pressure/pulse monitor should also be considered. However, these devices may frighten the child. Before applying any monitoring device, explain what you are going to do. Demonstrate the display or

Every seriously ill or injured child should receive continuous ECG monitoring.

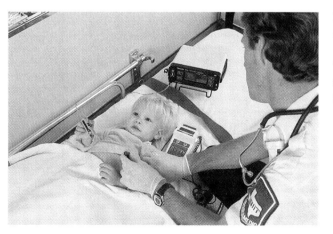

FIGURE 2-14   If available, noninvasive monitoring, including pulse oximetry and temperature measurement, should be used in prehospital pediatric care.

lights. If the monitoring device makes noise, allow the child to hear the noise before you apply it. Reassure the child that the device will not hurt him.

ONGOING ASSESSMENT

Because a pediatric patient's condition can rapidly change for the better or the worse, it is necessary to repeat relevant portions of the assessment. (For this reason, ongoing assessment is sometimes called "reassessment.") You should continually monitor the patient's respiratory effort, skin color, mental status, temperature, and pulse oximetry. Retake vital signs and compare them with baseline vitals. In general, reassess stable patients every 15 minutes, critical patients every 5 minutes.

GENERAL MANAGEMENT OF PEDIATRIC PATIENTS

The same ABCs that guide the management of adult patients apply to pediatric patients: Your top priorities in treating an infant or child are airway, breathing, and circulation. However, because of the special anatomical and physiological considerations that influence the management of pediatric patients, you need to practice these skills on an ongoing and regular basis.

BASIC AIRWAY MANAGEMENT

In treating the pediatric patient, basic life support (BLS) should be applied according to current standards and protocols. BLS should include maintenance of the airway, artificial ventilation, and if required, chest compressions. (See Table 2-6.) As with all patients, your priority is to assure an open airway. The following modifications of BLS airway skills will ensure that you take into account the clinical implications of the pediatric airway.

Table 2-6	SUMMARY OF BLS MANEUVERS IN INFANTS AND CHILDREN		
Target of Maneuver	**Infant (< 1 year)**	**Child (1 to 8 years)**
Airway		
Open airway	Head tilt/chin lift (unless trauma present)	Head tilt/chin lift (unless trauma present)
	Jaw thrust	Jaw Thrust
Clear foreign body obstruction	Back blows/chest thrusts	Heimlich maneuver
Breathing		
Initial	2 breaths at 1 to 1½ seconds/breath	2 breaths at 1 to 1½ seconds/breath
Subsequent	20 breaths/minute	20 breaths/minute
Circulation		
Pulse check	Brachial/femoral	Carotid
Compression area	Lower third of sternum	Lower third of sternum
Compression width	2 or 3 fingers	Heel of 1 hand
Depth	Approximately ½ to 1 inch (Newborn ½ to ¾ inch)	Approximately 1 to 1½ inches
Rate	At least 100/minute (Newborn 120/minute)	100/minute
Compression-ventilation ratio	5:1 (Newborn 3:1)	5:1

Manual Positioning

Allow the pediatric patient to assume a position of comfort, if possible. When placing the patient in a supine position, avoid hyperextension of the neck. As previously mentioned, infants and small children risk collapsed tracheas from hyperextension of the neck. For trauma patients less than 3 years old, place support under the torso. For supine medical patients 3 years old and older, provide occipital elevation.

Foreign Body Airway Obstruction (FBAO)

Before administering treatment, determine if an airway obstruction is partial or complete. Infants or children with a partial airway obstruction will have a cough, hoarse voice or cry, stridor, or some other evidence that at least some air is passing through the airway. Avoid any maneuvers that will turn a partial obstruction into a complete obstruction. Instead, place the patient in a position of comfort and transport immediately.

In the case of complete airway obstruction, take one of the following age-specific maneuvers:

- *Children.* For children older than 1 year of age, perform a series of abdominal thrusts (Figures 2-15 a and b).
- *Infants.* For infants less than 1 year old, deliver a series of 5 back blows followed by 5 chests thrusts. Inspect the infant's mouth upon completion of each series (Procedure 2-1).

As you recall from the basic CPR courses, never check a pediatric patient's mouth with blind finger sweeps.

Never use blind finger sweeps in a pediatric patient.

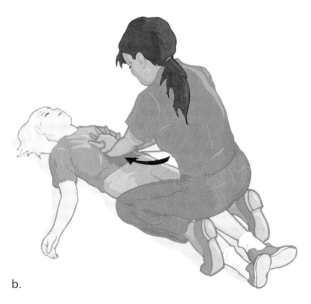

b.

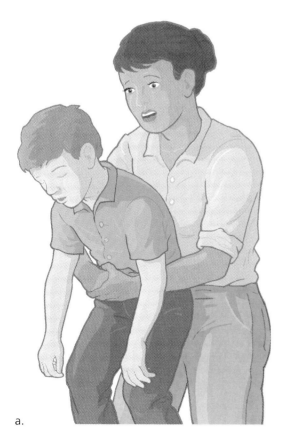

a.

FIGURE 2-15   Delivering abdominal thrusts (a) on a responsive child and (b) on an unresponsive child.

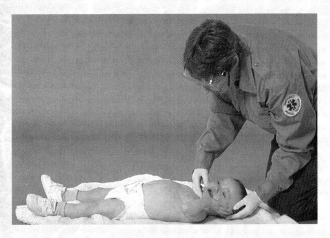

2-1a   Recognize and assess for choking. Look for breathing difficulty, ineffective cough, and lack of a strong cry.

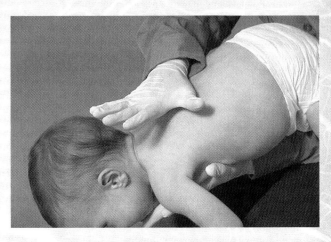

2-1b   Give up to 5 back blows.

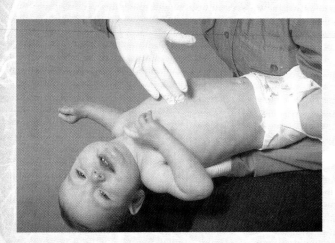

2-1c   Then administer 5 chest thrusts

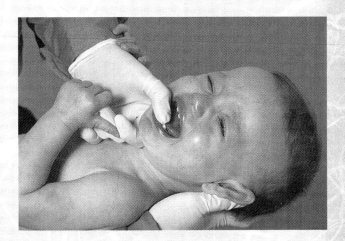

2-1d   If the infant becomes unresponsive, perform a tongue-jaw lift and look for a foreign body. If you see one, use a finger sweep to remove it. (*Never do blind finger sweeps in an infant or child.*) Attempt to ventilate. If this fails, reposition the head and try again. If you are not successful, repeat the sequence shown above. If the infant remains unresponsive, transport immediately, continuing airway clearance and ventilation efforts.

Note: For realism, the photo sequence above shows airway clearance procedures performed on a real infant. The infant is awake. In practice, of course, the infant with an airway obstruction is likely to be unresponsive

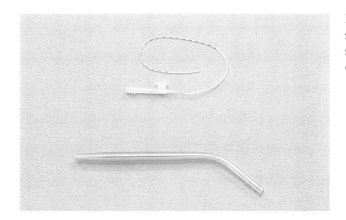

FIGURE 2-16 Pediatric-size suction catheters. Top: soft suction catheter. Bottom: rigid or hard suction catheter.

Suctioning

Apply suctioning whenever you detect heavy secretions in the nose or mouth of a pediatric patient, especially if the patient has a diminished level of consciousness. You can use a bulb syringe, flexible suction catheter, or rigid-tip suction catheter, depending upon the patient's age or size (Figure 2-16). Make sure that flexible catheters are correctly sized (Table 2-7).

Although pediatric suctioning techniques vary very little from adult suctioning techniques, keep the following modifications in mind:

- Decrease suction pressure to less than 100 mm/Hg in infants.
- Avoid excessive suctioning time (suction less than 10 seconds) in order to decrease the possibility of hypoxia.
- Avoid stimulation of the vagus nerve, which may produce bradycardia. As a general rule, suction no deeper than you can see and for no more than 15 seconds per attempt.
- Frequently check the patient's pulse. If bradycardia occurs, stop suctioning immediately and oxygenate.

Oxygenation

Adequate oxygenation is the hallmark of pediatric patient management. Methods of oxygen delivery include "blow-by" techniques (especially for neonates) and pediatric-sized nonrebreather masks. Although nonrebreather masks provide the highest concentration of supplemental oxygen, children may resist their

Adequate oxygenation is the hallmark of pediatric patient management.

Table 2-7	SUCTION CATHETER SIZES FOR INFANTS AND CHILDREN	

Age	Suction Catheter Size (French)
Up to 1 Year	8
2 to 6 Years	10
7 to 15 Years	12
16 Years	12 to 14

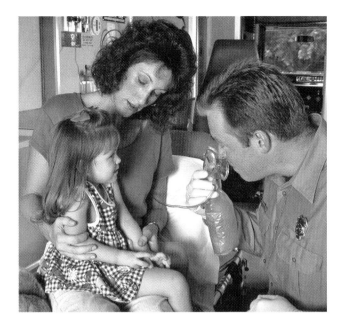

FIGURE 2-17 To overcome the child's fear of the nonrebreather mask, try it on yourself or have the parent try it on before attempting to place it on the child.

use. Try to overcome their fear by demonstrating the use of the mask on yourself (Figure 2-17). Better yet, enlist the support of a parent or caregiver, and ask them to demonstrate the mask. As an alternative, you might place the mask over the face of a stuffed animal.

If the child refuses to accept the nonrebreather mask, resort to high-flow, blow-by oxygen. Some units place oxygen tubing through the bottom of a colorful paper cup and use it to deliver the blow-by supplemental oxygen. Children often find a familiar object less frightening than complicated medical equipment.

Airway Adjuncts

As a general rule, use airway adjuncts in pediatric patients only if prolonged artificial ventilations are required. There are two reasons for this. First, infants and children often improve quickly through the administration of 100 percent oxygen. Second, airway adjuncts may create greater complications in children than in adults. Pediatric patients risk soft-tissue damage, vomiting, and stimulation of the vagus nerve.

Use airway adjuncts in pediatric patients only if prolonged artificial ventilations are required.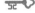

Oropharyngeal Airways Oropharyngeal airways should be used only in pediatric patients who lack a gag reflex. (Patients with a gag reflex risk vomiting and bradycardia.) Size the airway by measuring from the corner of the mouth to the front of the earlobe. Remember: Oropharyngeal airways that are too small can obstruct breathing; ones that are too large can both block the airway and cause trauma. (For general sizing suggestions, see Table 2-8.)

In placing an oropharyngeal airway, use a tongue blade to depress the tongue and jaw (Figure 2-18). If you detect a gag reflex, continue to maintain an open airway with a manual maneuver (jaw-thrust or head tilt/chin lift) and consider the use of a nasal airway. Remember that with a pediatric patient, the oral airway is

	Table 2-8	**EQUIPMENT GUIDELINES ACCORDING TO AGE AND WEIGHT**					
		Age (50th Percentile Weight)					
Equipment		**Premie (1–2.5 kg)**	**Neonate (2.5–4.0 kg)**	**6 Months (7.0 kg)**	**1–2 Years (10–12 kg)**	**5 Years (16–18 kg)**	**5–10 Years (24–30 kg)**
Airway *Oral*		infant (00)	infant (small) (0)	small (1)	small (2)	medium (3)	medium large (4.5)
Breathing *Self-inflating bag*		infant	infant	child	child	child	child/adult
O₂ ventilation mask		premature	newborn	infant/child	child	child	small adult
Endotracheal tube		2.5–3.0 (uncuffed)	3.0–3.5 (uncuffed)	3.5–4.0 (uncuffed)	4.0–4.5 (uncuffed)	5.0–5.5 (uncuffed)	5.5–6.5 (uncuffed)
Laryngoscope blade		0 (straight)	1 (straight)	1 (straight)	1–2 (straight)	2 (straight or curved)	2–3 (straight or curved)
Suction/stylet (F)		6–8/6	8/6	8–10/6	10/6	14/14	14/14
Circulation *BP cuff*		newborn	newborn	infant	child	child	child/adult
Venous access *Angiocath*		22–24	22–24	22–24	20–22	18–20	16–20
Butterfly needle		25	23–25	23–25	23	20–23	18–21
Intracath		—	—	19	19	16	14
Arm board		6″	6″	6″–8″	8″	8″–15″	15″
Orogastric tube (F)		5	5–8	8	10	10–12	14–18
Chest tube (F)		10–14	12–18	14–20	14–24	20–32	28–38

Reproduced with permission of the American Heart Association.

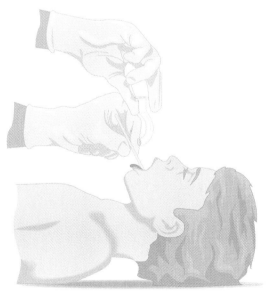

FIGURE 2-18 Inserting an oropharyngeal airway in a child with the use of a tongue blade.

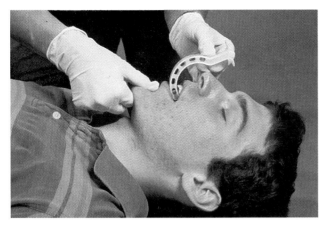
a.

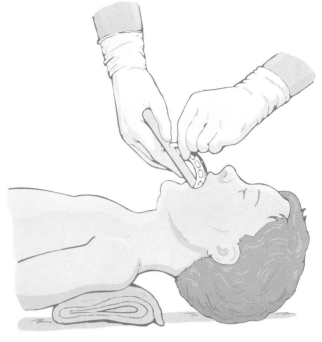
b.

FIGURE 2-19   a. In an adult, the airway is inserted with the tip pointing to the roof of the mouth, then rotated into position. b. In an infant or small child, the airway is inserted with the tip pointing toward the tongue and pharynx, in the same position it will be in after insertion.

inserted with the tip pointing toward the tongue and pharynx. For a comparison with insertion in the adult patient, see Figure 2-19 a and b.

Nasopharyngeal Airways Use nasopharyngeal airways for those children who possess a gag reflex and who require prolonged artificial ventilations. DO NOT use them on any child with midface or head trauma. You might mistakenly pass the airway through a fracture into the sinuses or the brain.

Size a nasal airway in the same fashion as for adult patients. (Use the outside diameter of the patient's little finger as a measure.) Although nasopharyngeal airways come in a variety of sizes, they are not readily available for infants less than 1 year old. Equipment required for insertion of a nasal airway includes:

- Appropriately sized soft, flexible latex tubing
- Water-based lubricant

When inserting the nasal airway, follow the same basic method as you would in an adult patient. It is important to remember that younger children often have enlarged adenoids (lymphatic tissues in the nasopharynx) which can be easily lacerated when inserting a nasopharyngeal airway. Because of this, always use care when inserting a nasopharyngeal airway in a younger child. If resistance is met, do not force the airway as significant bleeding can result.

DO NOT use nasal airways on a child with midface or head trauma.

Ventilation

Adequate tidal volume and ventilatory rate provide more than just a high oxygen saturation for your patient. Ventilation is a two-way physiological street: Maintenance of appropriate oxygen levels results in appropriate carbon dioxide levels as well. However, you will achieve neither of these clinically important events without tailoring the ventilatory device and technique to your pediatric patient. Important points to remember include the following:

- Avoid excessive bag pressure and volume. Ventilate at an age-appropriate rate, using only enough ventilation to make the chest rise.

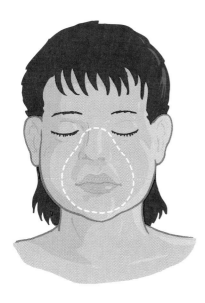

FIGURE 2-20 In placing a mask on a child, it should fit on the bridge of the nose and the cleft of the chin.

- Use a properly sized mask to ensure a good fit. In general, the mask should fit on the bridge of the nose and the cleft of the chin (Figure 2-20).
- Obtain a chest rise with each breath.
- Allow adequate time for exhalation.
- Assess BVM ventilation. (Provide 100 percent oxygen by using a reservoir attached to the BVM.)
- Remember that flow-restricted, oxygen-powered ventilation devices are contraindicated in pediatric resuscitation.
- Do not use BVMs with pop-off valves unless they can be readily occluded, if necessary. (Ventilatory pressures required during pediatric CPR may exceed the limit of the pop-off valve.)
- Apply cricoid pressure through application of the Sellick maneuver to minimize gastric inflation and passive regurgitation (Figure 2-21).
- Ensure correct positioning to avoid hyperextension of the neck.

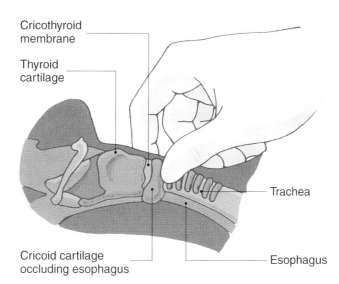

Cricothyroid membrane

Thyroid cartilage

Trachea

Cricoid cartilage occluding esophagus

Esophagus

FIGURE 2-21 In the Sellick maneuver, pressure is placed on the cricoid cartilage, compressing the esophagus. This reduces regurgitation and helps bring the vocal cords into view, which is useful if intubation is to be performed.

ADVANCED AIRWAY AND VENTILATORY MANAGEMENT

As a paramedic, you will be expected to master the advanced life support (ALS) procedures that make you a leader in the EMS system. Your clinical skills will help save the lives of pediatric patients whose respiratory systems have failed so severely that BLS measures are insufficient. When signs of impending cardiopulmonary arrest have been identified (as discussed earlier), you may be called upon to implement the following pediatric advanced life support (PALS) techniques, either in your own unit or in a transfer of care from a BLS unit. The success of these techniques requires knowledge of the procedures that set pediatric skills apart from the advanced life support skills used on adults. (Review the advanced airway skills for adults discussed in Volume 1, Chapter 13.)

Foreign-Body Airway Obstruction

One advantage of being able to perform endotracheal intubation is that it gives you another treatment modality for children with foreign-body airway obstructions. If a child's airway cannot be cleared by basic airway procedures, visualize the airway with the laryngoscope. Often, the obstructing foreign body can be seen. Once visualized, grasp the foreign body with the Magill forceps and remove it. If you cannot remove the foreign body with Magill forceps, try to intubate around the obstruction. This often requires using an endotracheal tube smaller than you would normally choose. However, this will provide an adequate airway until the foreign body can be removed at the hospital. Finally, if the foreign body cannot be removed with Magill forceps, and it is impossible to intubate around it, then you should consider placing a cricothyrotomy needle. This should only be done as a last resort. Be sure to follow local protocols regarding needle cricothyrotomy.

Needle Cricothyrotomy

The only indication for cricothyrotomy is failure to obtain an airway by any other method.

Needle cricothyrotomy in children is the same as for adult patients (as discussed in Volume 1, Chapter 13). It is important to remember that the anatomical landmarks are smaller and more difficult to identify. For years it was taught that needle cricothyrotomy was contraindicated in children less than one year of age. However, current thinking is that the possible benefit (life) exceeds the risks (bleeding, local tissue damage). Remember, the only indication for cricothyrotomy is failure to obtain an airway by any other method.

Endotracheal Intubation

Remember: An endotracheal tube that is mistakenly sized or misplaced, especially in the apneic patient, can quickly lead to hypoxia and death.

Endotracheal intubation allows direct visualization of the lower airway through the trachea, bypassing the entire upper airway. It is the most effective method of controlling a patient's airway, whether it be an adult or a child. However, endotracheal intubation is not without complications. It is an invasive technique with little room for error. A tube that is mistakenly sized or misplaced, especially in an apneic patient, can quickly lead to hypoxia and death.

Alternative airways (EOA, PtL, ETC) cannot be used in children. A properly sized laryngeal mask airway (LMA) can be used in the pediatric patient. However, you should remember that LMAs do not protect the airway from aspiration.

Anatomical and Physiological Concerns Although endotracheal intubation of a child and an adult follow the same basic procedures, the special features of the pediatric airway complicate placement of any orotracheal tube. In fact, variations in the airway size of children discourage the use of certain airways, including esophageal obturator airways (EOA), pharyngeotracheal lumen airways (PtL), and esophageal-tracheal combitubes (ETC). In using an endotracheal tube, keep in mind these points:

- In infants and small children, it is often more difficult to create a single clear visual plane from the mouth, through the pharynx, and

Table 2-9	INFANT/CHILD ENDOTRACHEAL TUBES
Age of Patient	**Measurement of the Endotracheal Tube at the Teeth**
6 Months to 1 Year	12 cm—teeth to mid-trachea
2 Years	14 cm—teeth to mid-trachea
4 to 6 Years	16 cm—teeth to mid-trachea
6 to 10 Years	18 cm—teeth to mid-trachea
10 to 12 Years	20 cm—teeth to mid-trachea

into the glottis. A straight-blade laryngoscope is preferred, since it provides greater displacement of the tongue and better visualization of the relatively cephalad and anterior glottis. For larger children, a curved blade may sometimes be used. (Review Table 2-8.)

- Variations in the sizes of pediatric airways, coupled with the fact that the narrowest portion of the airway is at the level of the cricoid ring, makes proper sizing of the endotracheal tube crucial. To determine correct size, apply any of the following methods:
  – Use a resuscitation tape, such as the Broselow™ tape, to estimate tube size based on height.
  – Estimate the correct tube size by using the diameter of the patient's little finger or the diameter of the nasal opening.
  – Calculate the correct tube size by using this simple numerical formula:
    (Patient's age in years + 16) ÷ 4 = Tube size
- The depth of insertion can be estimated based on age (Table 2-9). However, the best method of determining depth is direct visualization. Due to the distance between the mouth and the trachea, a stylet is rarely needed to position the tube properly. When a stylet is used, select a malleable yet rigid style.
- Because the pediatric airway narrows at the level of the cricoid cartilage, uncuffed tubes should be used in children younger than 8 years old. The tubes should display a vocal cord marker to ensure correct placement.
- Infants and small children may have greater vagal response than adults. Therefore, laryngoscopy and passage of an endotracheal tube are likely to cause a vagal response, dramatically slowing the child's heart rate and decreasing the cardiac output and blood pressure. As a result, pediatric intubations must be carried out swiftly, accurately, and with continuous monitoring.

Pediatric intubation must be carried out swiftly, accurately, and with continuous monitoring.

Indications The indications for endotracheal intubation in a pediatric patient are the same as those for an adult. They include:

- Need for prolonged artificial ventilations
- Inadequate ventilatory support with a bag-valve mask
- Cardiac or respiratory arrest
- Control of an airway in a patient without a cough or gag reflex
- Necessary for providing a route for drug administration
- Need to gain access to the airway for suctioning

Additionally, if local protocols allow it, endotracheal intubation may be used in a child who is suffering croup or epiglottitis and an increasingly compromised airway.

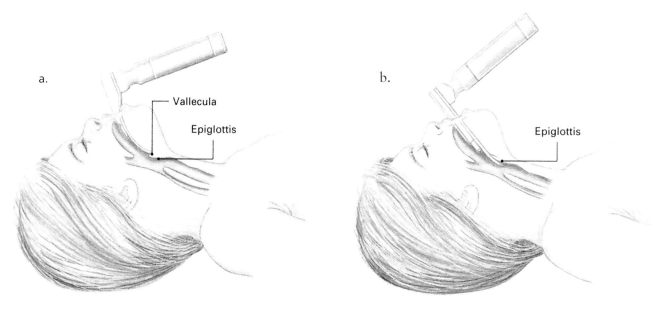

a.

Vallecula

Epiglottis

b.

Epiglottis

FIGURE 2-22   Placement of the laryngoscope: a. MacIntosh (curved) blade, b. Miller (straight) blade.

Techniques for Pediatric Intubation   To perform endotracheal intubation on a pediatric patient, follow the basic steps in Procedure 2-2. Detailed steps include:

1. While maintaining ventilatory support, hyperventilate the patient with 100 percent oxygen. If time allows, hyperventilate for a full 2 minutes.

2. Assemble and check your equipment. As stated earlier, a straight-blade laryngoscope is preferred. Assorted sizes of endotracheal tubes, both cuffed and uncuffed, should be stocked in the pediatric kit aboard your ambulance.

3. Place the patient's head and neck into an appropriate position. With a pediatric patient, the head should be maintained in a sniffing position.

4. Hold the laryngoscope in your left hand.

5. Insert your laryngoscope blade into the right side of the patient's mouth. With a sweeping action, displace the tongue to the left.

6. Move the blade slightly toward the midline, and then advance it until the distal end is positioned at the base of the tongue (Figure 2-22).

7. Look for the tip of the epiglottis, and place the laryngoscope blade into its proper position. Keep in mind that a child—particularly an infant—has a shorter airway and a higher glottis than an adult. Because of this, you'll see the cords much sooner than you may expect.

8. With your left wrist straight, use your shoulder and arm to lift the mandible and tongue at a 45-degree angle to the floor until the glottis is exposed. Use the little finger of your left hand to apply gentle downward pressure to the cricoid cartilage. This will permit easier visualization of the cords.

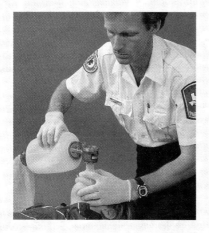

2-2a   Hyperventilate the child.

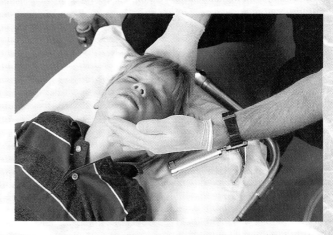

2-2b   Position the head.

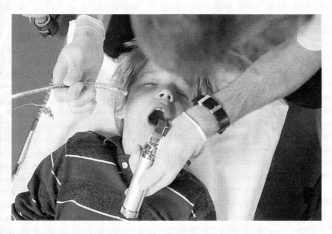

2-2c   Insert the laryngoscope and visualize the airway.

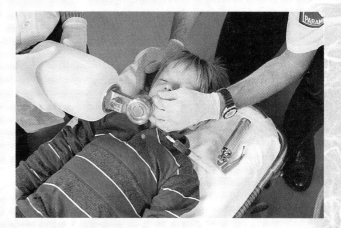

2-2d   Insert the tube and ventilate the child.

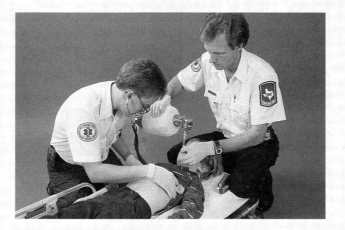

2-2e   Confirm tube placement.

9. Grasp the endotracheal tube in your right hand. To pass the tube into your patient's mouth, it may be helpful to hold it so that its curve is in a horizontal plane (bevel sideways). Insert the tube through the right corner of the child's mouth.

10. Under direct observation, insert the endotracheal tube into the glottic opening and pass it through until its distal cuff disappears past the vocal cords—approximately 5 to 10 cm. As a tube is advanced, it should be rotated into the proper plane. In some cases, it will be difficult to advance an endotracheal tube at the level of the cricoid. DO NOT force the tube through this region, as it may cause laryngeal edema.

11. Hold the tube in place with your left hand. Attach an infant- or child-size bag-valve device to the 15/22 mm adapter and deliver several breaths.

12. Check for proper tube placement. Watch for chest rise and fall with each ventilation and listen for equal, bilateral breath sounds. There should also be an absence of sounds over the epigastrium with ventilations. Confirm placement with an $ETCO_2$ detector.

13. If the tube has a distal cuff, inflate it with the recommended amount of air.

14. Recheck for proper placement of the tube, and hyperventilate the patient with 100% oxygen.

15. Secure the endotracheal tube with umbilical tape while maintaining ventilatory support.

16. Continue supporting the tube manually while maintaining ventilations. Check periodically to ensure proper tube position. As with adults, allow no more than 30 seconds to pass without ventilating your patient.

DO NOT force an endotracheal tube through the cricoid region, as it may cause laryngeal edema.

Nasogastric Intubation

If gastric distention is present in a pediatric patient, you may consider placing a nasogastric tube (NG tube). In infants and children, gastric distention may result from overly aggressive artificial ventilations or from air swallowing. Placement of an NG tube will allow you to decompress the stomach and proximal bowel of air. An NG tube can also be used to empty the stomach of blood or other substances. Indications for use of a nasogastric intubation include:

- Inability to achieve adequate tidal volumes during ventilation due to gastric distention
- Presence of gastric distention in an unresponsive patient

As with nasopharyngeal airways, an NG tube is contraindicated in pediatric patients who have sustained head or facial trauma. Because the NG tube might migrate into the cranial sinuses, consider the use of an orogastric tube instead. Other contraindications include possible soft-tissue damage in the nose and inducement of vomiting.

Equipment for placing an NG tube includes:

- Age-appropriate NG tubes
- 20 mL syringe
- Water-soluble lubricant
- Emesis basin
- Tape

- Suctioning equipment
- Stethoscope

In sizing the NG tube, keep in mind the following recommended guidelines:

- Newborn/infant: #8.0 French
- Toddler/preschooler: #10 French
- School-age children: #12 French
- Adolescents: #14-16 French

In determining the correct length, measure the tube from the top of the nose, over the ear, to the tip of the xiphoid process. The steps for inserting the tube can be followed in Procedure 2-3. Keep in mind as you examine these steps that many experts believe that an NG tube should only be inserted when an endotracheal tube is in place. This precaution will prevent misplacement of the tube into the trachea instead of the esophagus. Consult protocols in your area on the use of NG tubes.

NG tube insertion is safest when the airway is protected with an ET tube.

Rapid Sequence Intubation

Advanced airway management may sometimes be indicated in pediatric patients with a significant level of consciousness and the presence of a gag reflex. Examples may include a combative child with head trauma or an adolescent with a drug overdose. In such cases, clenched teeth and resistance may make intubation difficult or impossible. As a result, medical direction may authorize the use of "paralytics" to induce a state of neuromuscular compliance. All skeletal muscles, including the muscles of respiration, respond to these drugs, known as neuromuscular blocking agents. Following their administration, the patient will require mechanical ventilation.

An example of a commonly used neuromuscular blocker is succinylcholine (Anectine). Typically, it is administered at 1–2 mg/kg IV push. It acts in 60–90 seconds and lasts approximately 3–5 minutes. Remember that succinylcholine has no effect on consciousness or pain. Thus, a sedative agent must be used for all children except those who are unconscious. Commonly used drugs include midazolam (Versed), diazepam (Valium), thiopental, and fentanyl. A bite block should be placed to prevent the patient from biting the endotracheal tube. Medical direction may authorize sedation to minimize the emotional trauma to the patient or drugs such as pancuronium or vecuronium if longer paralysis is required.

CIRCULATION

As mentioned earlier, the respiratory and cardiovascular systems are interdependent. In pediatrics, you are encouraged to look at the total child. You should assess the child by assessing the various body systems. For example, instead of simply checking a pulse, you should look for end-organ changes that indicate the effectiveness of respiratory and cardiovascular function. These include such things as mental status, skin color, skin temperature, urine output, and others. There are two problems that lead to cardiopulmonary arrest in children: shock and respiratory failure. Both must be identified and corrected early. The following section will address assessment of the cardiovascular system. Particular emphasis is placed on venous access and fluid resuscitation, as these are essential skills for prehospital ALS personnel who treat pediatric patients.

There are two problems that lead to cardiopulmonary arrest in children: shock and respiratory failure.

Vascular Access

Intravenous techniques for children are basically the same as for adults. (See Volume 1, Chapter 10.) However, additional veins may be accessed in the infant. These include veins of the neck and scalp, as well as of the arms, hands, and feet. The external jugular vein, however, should only be used for life-threatening situations.

In obtaining venous access, the external jugular vein should only be used for life-threatening situations.

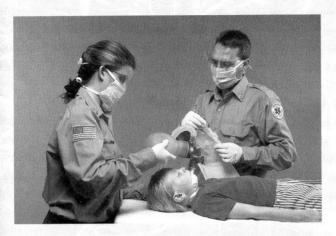

2-3a   Oxygenate and continue to ventilate, if possible.

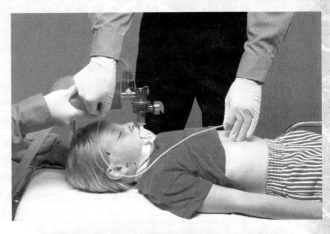

2-3b   Measure the NG tube from the tip of the nose, over the ear, to the tip of the xiphoid process.

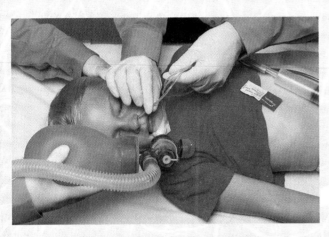

2-3c   Lubricate the end of the tube. Then pass it gently downward along the nasal floor to the stomach.

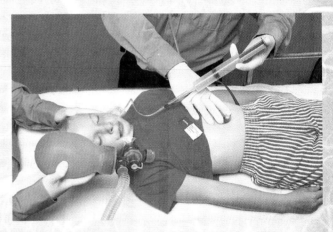

2-3d   Ausculate over the epigastrium to confirm correct placement. Listen for bubbling while injecting 10–20 cc of air into the tube.

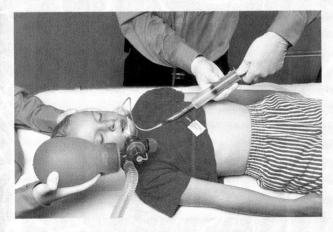

2-3e   Use suction to aspirate stomach contents.

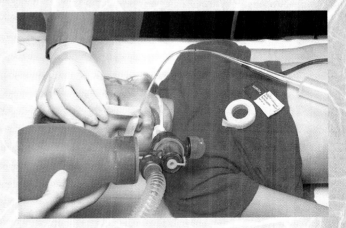

2-3f   Secure the tube in place.

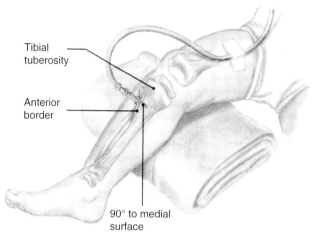

Tibial
tuberosity

Anterior
border

90° to medial
surface

a.

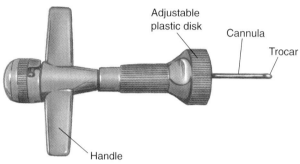

Adjustable
plastic disk

Cannula

Trocar

Handle

b.

FIGURE 2-23   a. Intraosseous administration in the pediatric patient.
b. An intraosseous needle.

Intraosseous Infusion

The use of intraosseous (IO) infusion has become popular in the pediatric patient. (See Figure 2-23a.) This is especially true when large volumes of fluid must be administered, as occurs in hypovolemic shock, and when other means of venous access are unavailable. Certain drugs can be administered intraosseously, including epinephrine, atropine, dopamine, lidocaine, sodium bicarbonate, and dobutamine. Indications for intraosseous infusion include:

- Children less than 6 years old
- Existence of shock or cardiac arrest
- An unresponsive patient
- Unsuccessful attempts at peripheral IV insertion

The primary contraindications for IO infusion include:

- Presence of a fracture in the bone chosen for infusion
- Fracture of the pelvis or extremity fracture in the bone proximal to the chosen site

In performing IO perfusion, you can use a standard 16- or 18-gauge needle (either hypodermic or spinal). However, an intraosseous needle is preferred and significantly better (Figure 2-23b). The anterior surface of the leg below the knee

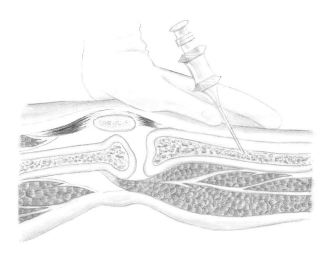

FIGURE 2-24 Correct needle placement for intraosseous administration. Note that the needle tip is in the marrow cavity.

should be prepped with antiseptic solution such as povidone iodine. The needle is then inserted, in a twisting fashion, 1–3 centimeters below the tuberosity. Insertion should be slightly inferior in direction (to avoid the growth plate) and perpendicular to the skin (Figure 2-24). Placement of the needle into the marrow cavity can be determined by noting a lack of resistance as the needle passes through the bony cortex. Other indications include the needle standing upright without support, the ability to aspirate bone marrow into a syringe, or free flow of the infusion without infiltration into the subcutaneous tissues. (See also the discussion of intraosseous infusion in Volume 1, Chapter 10.)

Fluid Therapy

The accurate dosing of fluids in children is crucial. Too much fluid can result in heart failure and pulmonary edema. Too little fluid can be ineffective.

DO NOT allow a full liter bag of fluid to be directly connected to a small child or infant without having a flow limiter attached.

The accurate dosing of fluids in children is crucial. Too much fluid can result in heart failure and pulmonary edema. Too little fluid can be ineffective. The initial dosage of fluid in hypovolemic shock should be 20 mL/kg of an isotonic solution such as lactated Ringer's or normal saline, as soon as IV access is obtained. After the infusion, the child should be reassessed. If perfusion is still diminished, then a second bolus of 20 mL/kg should be administered. A child with hypovolemic shock may require 40–60 mL/kg, while a child with septic shock may require at least 60–80 mL/kg. Fluid therapy should be guided by the child's clinical response.

Intravenous infusions in children should be closely monitored with frequent patient reassessment. Minidrip administration sets, flow limiters, or infusion pumps should be routinely used in pediatric cases.

Medications

Cardiopulmonary arrest in infants and children is almost always due to a primary respiratory problem, such as drowning, choking, or smoke inhalation. The major aim in pediatric resuscitation is airway management and ventilation, as well as replacement of intravascular volume, if indicated. In certain cases, medications may be required. The objectives of medication therapy in pediatric patients include:

- Correction of hypoxemia
- Increased perfusion pressure during chest compressions
- Stimulation of spontaneous or more forceful cardiac contractions
- Acceleration of the heart rate
- Correction of metabolic acidosis

- Suppression of ventricular ectopy
- Maintenance of renal perfusion

The dosages of medications must be modified for the pediatric patient. Tables 2-10 and 2-11 illustrate recommended pediatric drug dosage in advanced cardiac life support.

ELECTRICAL THERAPY

You are less likely to use electrical therapy on pediatric patients than adult patients. This is due to the fact that ventricular fibrillation is much less common

Table 2-10 DRUGS USED IN PEDIATRIC ADVANCED LIFE SUPPORT*

Drug	Dose	Remarks
Adenosine	0.1 to 0.2 mg/kg Maximum strength dose 12 mg	Rapid IV bolus
Amiodarone	5 mg/kg IV/IO	Rapid IV bolus
Atropine sulfate	0.02 mg/kg per dose	Minimum dose 0.1 mg Maximum single dose: 0.5 mg in child; 1.0 mg in adolescent
Calcium chloride 10 percent	20 mg/kg per dose	Give slowly
Dopamine hydrochloride	2–10 mcg/kg per minute	Adrenergic action dominates at $\geq$ 15–20 mcg/kg per minute
Epinephrine *for bradycardia*	IV/IO 0.01 mg/kg (1:10,000) ET: 0.1 mg/kg (1:1,000)	Be aware of effective dose of preservatives administered (if preservatives are present in epinephrine preparation) when high doses are used
for asystolic or pulseless arrest	*First dose:* IV/IO: 0.01 mg/kg (1: 10,000) ET: 0.1 mg/kg (1:1,1000) Doses as high as 0.2 mg/kg may be effective *Subsequent doses:* IV/IO/ET: 0.1 mg/kg (1:1,000) Doses as high as 0.2 mg/kg may be effective	Be aware of effective dose of preservatives administered (if preservatives are present in epinephrine preparation) when high doses are used
Epinephrine infusion	Initial at 0.1 mcg/kg per minute Higher infusion dose used if asystole present	Titrate to desired effect (0.1–1.0 mcg/kg per minute)
Lidocaine	1 mg/kg per dose	Rapid bolus
Lidocaine infusion	20–50 mcg/kg per minute	
Sodium bicarbonate	1 mEq/kg per dose or 0.3 $\times$ kg $\times$ base deficit	Infuse slowly and only if ventilation is adequate

*IV indicates intravenous route; IO, intraosseous route; ET, endotracheal route.

Table 2-11 PREPARATION OF INFUSIONS

Drug	Preparation*	Dose
Epinephrine	0.6 × body weight (kg) equals milligrams added to diluent[†] to make 100 mL	Then 1 mL/h delivers 0.1 mcg/kg per minute; titrate to effect
Dopamine/ dobutamine	0.6 × body weight (kg) equals milligrams added to diluent[†] to make 100 mL	Then 1 mL/h delivers 0.3 mcg/kg per minute; titrate to effect
Lidocaine	120 mg of 40 mg/mL solution added to 97 mL of 5 percent dextrose in water, yielding 1200 mcg/mL solution	Then 1 mL/kg per hour delivers 20 mcg/kg per minute

*Standard concentration may be used to provide more dilute or more concentrated drug solution, but then individual dose must be calculated for each patient and each infusion rate:

$$\text{Infusion Rate (mL/h)} = \frac{\text{Weight (kg)} \times \text{Dose (mcg/kg/min)} \times 60 \text{ min/h}}{\text{Concentration (mcg/mL)}}$$

[†]Diluent may be 5 percent dextrose in water, 5 percent dextrose in half-normal, normal saline, or Ringer's lactate.

in children than adults. However, you should review and keep the following principles in mind for times when these emergencies arise:

- Administer an initial dosage of 2 joules per kilogram of body weight. (Keep in mind the estimated body weights in Table 2-5.)
- If this is unsuccessful, increase the dosage to 4 joules per kilogram.
- If this is unsuccessful, focus your attention on correcting hypoxia and acidosis.
- Transport to a pediatric critical care unit, if possible.

C-SPINE IMMOBILIZATION

Any time an infant or child sustains a head injury, assume that a neck injury may also be present.

Spinal injuries in children are not as common as in adults. However, because of a child's disproportionately larger and heavier head, the cervical spine (C-spine) is vulnerable to injury. Any time an infant or child sustains a significant head injury, assume that a neck injury may also be present. Children can suffer a spinal cord injury with no noticeable damage to the vertebral column as seen on cervical spine X-rays. Thus, negative cervical spine X-rays do not necessarily assure that a spinal cord injury does not exist. Because of this, children should remain immobilized until a spinal cord injury has been excluded by hospital personnel. As previously noted, even children secured in a car safety seat can suffer neck injuries if the heads are propelled forward during an accident or sudden stop.

Always make sure that you use the appropriate-sized pediatric immobilization equipment. These supplies may include rigid cervical collars, towel or blanket rolls, foam head blocks, commercial pediatric immobilization devices, vest-type or short wooden backboards, and long boards with the appropriate padding. For pediatric patients found in car seats, you can also use the seat for immobilization (Procedure 2-4). The Kendrick Extrication Device (KED) can be quickly modified to immobilize a pediatric patient. Because of the significant variations in the size of children, you must be creative in devising a plan for pediatric immobilization.

In securing the pediatric patient to the backboard, use appropriate amounts of padding to secure infants, toddlers, and preschoolers in a supine, neutral position. Never use sandbags when immobilizing a pediatric patient's head. If you must tip the board to manage vomiting, the weight of the sand bag may worsen the head injury. For steps in applying a pediatric immobilization system, see Procedure 2-5.

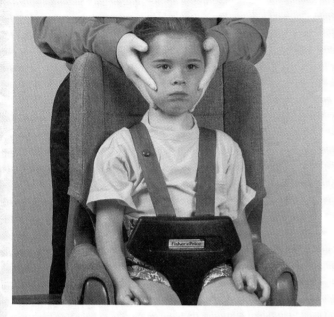

2-4a One paramedic stabilizes the car seat in an upright position and applies and maintains manual in-line stabilization throughout the immobilization process.

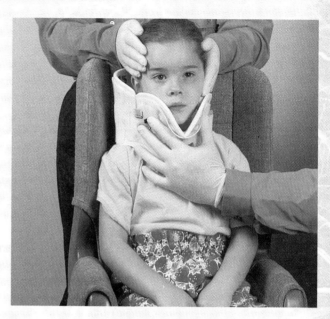

2-4b A second paramedic applies an appropriately sized cervical collar. If one is not available, improvise using a rolled hand towel.

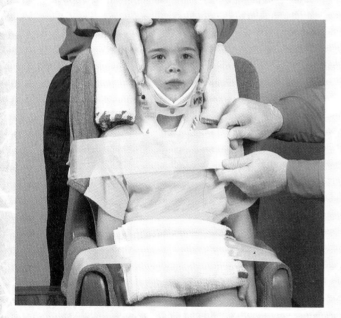

2-4c The second paramedic places a small blanket or towel on the child's lap, then uses straps or wide tape to secure the chest and pelvic areas to the seat.

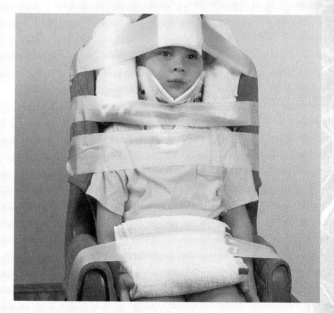

2-4d The second paramedic places towel rolls on both sides of the child's head to fill voids between the head and seat. The medic tapes the head into place, taping across the forehead and the collar, but avoiding taping over the chin, which would put pressure on the neck. The patient and seat can be carried to the ambulance and strapped to the stretcher, with the stretcher head raised.

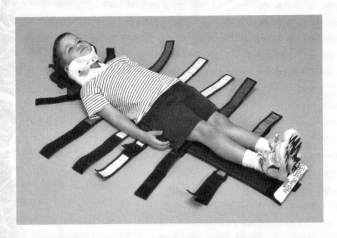

2-5a   Position the patient on the immobilization system.

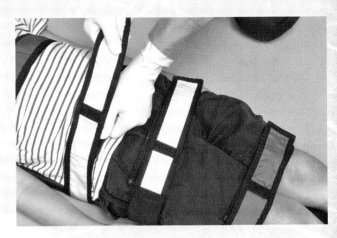

2-5b   Adjust the color-coded straps to fit the child.

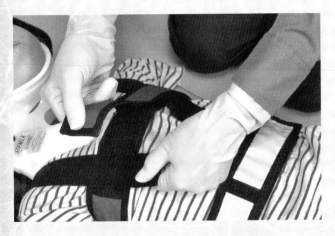

2-5c   Attach the four-point safety system.

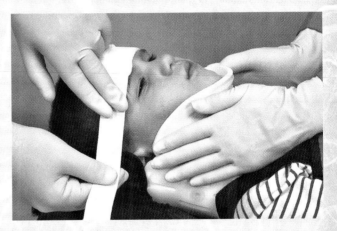

2-5d   Fasten the adjustable head-support system.

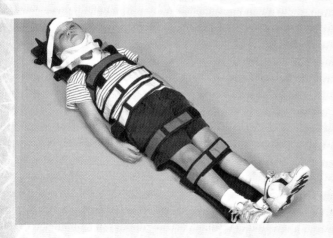

2-5e   The patient fully immobilized to the system.

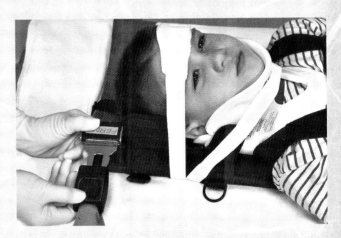

2-5f   Move the immobilized patient onto the stretcher and fasten the loops at both ends to connect to the stretcher straps.

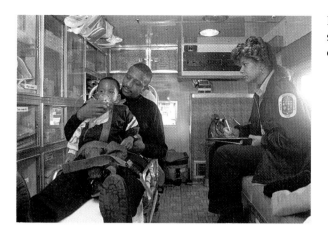

FIGURE 2-25 Emotional support of the infant or child continues during transport.

Any time you immobilize a pediatric patient, remember that many children, especially those under age 5, will protest or fight restraint. Try to minimize the emotional stress by having a parent or caretaker stand near or touch the child. Often the child will quit struggling when secured totally in an immobilization device. Ideally, a rescuer or family member should remain with the child at all times to reassure and calm the child, if possible.

TRANSPORT GUIDELINES

In managing a pediatric patient, never delay transport to perform a procedure that can be done en route to the hospital. After deciding upon necessary interventions—first BLS, then ALS—determine the appropriate receiving facility. In reaching your decision, consider three factors:

In managing a pediatric patient, never delay transport to perform a procedure that can be done en route to the hospital.

- Time of transport
- Specialized facilities
- Specialized personnel

If you live in an area with specialized prehospital crews such as Critical Care Crews and Neonatal Nurses, their availability should weigh in your decision as well. Consider whether the patient would benefit by transfer by one of these crews. If so, request support. If not, determine the closest definitive care facility for the infant or child placed in your care. If time allows, continue to reduce the fear involved in transition of care from the family to the hospital. If you have won the trust of the child, and conditions permit, you might allow the patient to sit on your lap en route to the hospital (Figure 2-25). Think of what you would do or say to calm your own child or the child of a close relative or friend.

SPECIFIC MEDICAL EMERGENCIES

As you already realize from your earlier training and experience, a variety of pediatric medical problems can activate the EMS system. Although the majority of childhood medical emergencies involve the respiratory system, other body systems can be involved as well. To help you recognize and treat pediatric medical emergencies, the following sections cover some of the specific conditions you may encounter.

INFECTIONS

Infectious diseases account for the majority of pediatric illnesses.

Childhood is a time of frequent illnesses because of the relative immaturity of the pediatric immune system. Infectious diseases may be caused by the infection or infestation of the body by an infectious agent such as a virus, bacterium, fungus, or parasite. Most infections are minor and self limiting. There are, however, several infections that can be life-threatening. These include meningitis, pneumonia, and septicemia—a systemic infection (usually bacterial) in the bloodstream.

The impact of an infection upon physiological processes depends upon the type of infectious agent and the extent of the infection. Signs and symptoms also vary, depending upon the type of infection and the time since exposure. Any of the following conditions may indicate the presence of an infection: fever, chills, tachycardia, cough, sore throat, nasal congestion, malaise, tachypnea, cool or clammy skin, petechiae, respiratory distress, poor appetite, vomiting, diarrhea, dehydration, hypoperfusion (especially with septicemia), purpura (purple blotches resulting from hemorrhages into the skin that do not disappear under pressure), seizures, severe headache, irritability, stiff neck, or bulging fontanelle (infants).

The management of infections depends upon the body system or systems affected. Treatment of some of the most common and serious infections will be found in the sections that follow. As a general rule, you should adhere to these guidelines when treating an infectious illness:

- Take all BSI precautions, due to the unknown cause of the infection.
- Become familiar with the common pediatric infections encountered in your area.
- If possible, try to determine which, if any, pediatric infections you have not been exposed to or vaccinated for. For example, if you did not have chicken pox (varicella) or measles (rubeola) as a child, and were not vaccinated for them, then you should consider receiving vaccination for these illnesses. If you encounter a child suspected of having an infectious disease to which you may be susceptible, consider allowing another rescuer to be the primary person to care for the child.

RESPIRATORY EMERGENCIES

Respiratory emergencies constitute the most common reason EMS is summoned to care for a pediatric patient. Respiratory illnesses can cause respiratory compromise due to their affect on the alveolar/capillary interface. Some illnesses are quite minor, causing only mild symptoms, while others can be rapidly fatal. Your approach to the child with a respiratory emergency will depend upon the severity of respiratory compromise. If the child is alert and talking, then you can take a more relaxed approach. However, if the child is ill-appearing and exhibiting marked respiratory difficulty, then you must immediately intervene to prevent respiratory arrest and possible cardiopulmonary arrest.

Severity of Respiratory Compromise

The severity of respiratory compromise can be quickly classified into the following categories:

- Respiratory distress
- Respiratory failure
- Respiratory arrest

Content Review

STAGES OF RESPIRATORY COMPROMISE
- Respiratory distress
- Respiratory failure
- Respiratory arrest

Respiratory emergencies in pediatric patients may quickly progress from respiratory distress to respiratory failure to respiratory arrest. You must learn to recognize the phase your patient is in and take the appropriate interventions. Prompt recognition and treatment can literally mean the difference between life and death for an infant or child suffering from respiratory compromise.

Respiratory Distress The mildest form of respiratory impairment is classified as respiratory distress. The most noticeable finding is an increased work of breathing. One of the earliest indicators of respiratory distress is an increase in respiratory rate. Unfortunately, respiratory rate is one of the vital signs that is most often "estimated." As mentioned previously, it is essential to obtain an accurate respiratory rate in children. Ideally, the respiratory rate should be measured for an entire minute. If time does not allow it, or if the child is deteriorating, then the respiratory rate should be measured for at least 30 seconds and multiplied by two to obtain the respiratory rate.

In addition to an increased work of breathing, the child in respiratory distress will initially have a slight decrease in the arterial carbon dioxide tension as the respiratory rate increases. However, as respiratory distress increases, the carbon dioxide tension will gradually increase.

The signs and symptoms of respiratory distress include:

- Normal mental status deteriorating to irritability or anxiety
- Tachypnea
- Retractions
- Nasal flaring (in infants)
- Good muscle tone
- Tachycardia
- Head bobbing
- Grunting
- Cyanosis that improves with supplemental oxygen

If not corrected immediately, respiratory distress will lead to respiratory failure.

Respiratory Failure Respiratory failure occurs when the respiratory system is not able to meet the demands of the body for oxygen intake and for carbon dioxide removal. It is characterized by inadequate ventilation and oxygenation. During respiratory failure, the carbon dioxide level begins to rise as the body is not able to remove carbon dioxide. This ultimately leads to respiratory acidosis.

The signs and symptoms of respiratory failure include:

- Irritability or anxiety deteriorating to lethargy
- Marked tachypnea later deteriorating to bradypnea
- Marked retractions later deteriorating to agonal respirations
- Poor muscle tone
- Marked tachycardia later deteriorating to bradycardia
- Central cyanosis

Respiratory failure is a very ominous sign. If immediate intervention is not provided, the child will deteriorate to full respiratory arrest.

Respiratory Arrest The end result of respiratory impairment, if untreated, is respiratory arrest. The cessation of breathing typically follows a period of bradypnea and agonal respirations.

Prompt recognition of a respiratory emergency in an infant or child can literally mean the difference between life and death.

It is essential that you carefully count the pediatric's respiratory rate for at least 30 seconds, preferably 1 minute.

Signs and symptoms of respiratory arrest include:

- Unresponsivenes deteriorating to coma
- Bradypnea deteriorating to apnea
- Absent chest wall motion
- Bradycardia deteriorating to asystole
- Profound cyanosis

Respiratory arrest will quickly deteriorate to full cardiopulmonary arrest if appropriate interventions are not made. The child's chances of survival markedly decrease when cardiopulmonary arrest occurs.

Management of Respiratory Compromise

The management of respiratory compromise should be based upon the severity of the problem. The goals of management include increasing ventilation and increasing oxygenation. You should try to identify the signs and symptoms of respiratory distress early so that you can intervene before the child deteriorates.

Your initial attention should be directed at the airway. Is it patent? Is it maintainable with simple positioning? Is endotracheal intubation required?

After assessing the airway, assure continued maintenance of the airway by positioning, placement of an airway adjunct (oropharyngeal or nasopharyngeal airway), or endotracheal intubation.

For children in respiratory distress or early respiratory failure, administer oxygen at high flow. Some children will tolerate a nonrebreather mask. Others may not and may require that someone (perhaps a parent) hold blow-by oxygen for them to breathe. If the child fails to improve with supplemental oxygen administration, the patient should be treated more aggressively. Oftentimes it is necessary to separate the parents from the child so that you can provide the necessary care without interruption or distraction.

Pediatric patients with late respiratory failure or respiratory arrest require aggressive treatment. This includes:

- Establishment of an airway
- High-flow supplemental oxygen administration
- Mechanical ventilation with a bag-valve-mask device attached to a reservoir delivering 100% oxygen
- Endotracheal intubation if mechanical ventilation does not rapidly improve the patient's condition
- Consideration of gastric decompression with an orogastric or nasogastric tube if abdominal distension is impeding ventilation
- Consideration of needle decompression of the chest if a tension pneumothorax is thought to be present
- Consideration of cricothyrotomy if complete airway obstruction is present and the airway cannot be obtained by any other method.

In addition to the above, you should obtain venous access. The child should be promptly transported to a facility staffed and equipped to handle critically ill children. While en route, continue to reassess the child. Signs of improvement include an improvement in skin color and temperature. As end-organ perfusion improves, the child will exhibit an increase in pulse rate, an increase in oxygen saturation, and an improvement in mental status. Provide emotional and psychological support to the parents and keep them abreast of the results of your care.

SPECIFIC RESPIRATORY EMERGENCIES

Respiratory problems typically arise from obstruction of a part of the respiratory tract or impairment of the mechanics of respiration. In the following discussion we will present the common pediatric respiratory emergencies based upon the part of the airway they most affect.

Upper Airway Obstruction

Obstruction of the upper airway can be caused by many factors. As previously mentioned, upper airway obstruction may be partial or complete. It can be caused by inflamed or swollen tissues caused by infection or by an aspirated foreign body. Appropriate care depends on prompt and immediate identification of the disorder and its severity. Whenever you find an infant, toddler, or young child in respiratory or cardiac arrest, assume complete upper airway obstruction until proven otherwise.

Croup Croup, medically referred to as *laryngotracheobronchitis*, is a viral infection of the upper airway. It most commonly occurs in children 6 months to 4 years of age and is prevalent in the fall and winter. Croup causes an inflammation of the upper respiratory tract involving the subglottic region. The infection leads to edema beneath the glottis and larynx, thus narrowing the lumen of the airway. Severe cases of croup can lead to complete airway obstruction. Another form of croup called *spasmodic croup* occurs mostly in the middle of the night without any prior upper respiratory infection.

Assessment The history for croup is fairly classic. Often, the child will have a mild cold or other infection and be doing fairly well until evening. After dark, however, a harsh, barking or brassy cough develops. The attack may subside in a few hours but can persist for several nights.

The physical exam will often reveal inspiratory stridor. There may be associated nasal flaring, tracheal tugging, or retraction. You *should never* examine the oropharynx. Often, in the prehospital setting, it is difficult to distinguish croup from **epiglottitis**. (See Table 2-12 and Figure 2-26.) If epiglottitis is present, examination of the oropharynx may result in laryngospasm and complete airway obstruction. If the attack of croup is severe and progressive, the child may develop restlessness, tachycardia, and cyanosis. Although croup can result in complete airway obstruction and respiratory arrest, this is a rare event.

Management Management of croup consists of appropriate airway maintenance. Place the child in a position of comfort and administer cool mist oxygen at 4–6 L/minute. Oxygen can be delivered by face mask or blow-by method. If the attack is severe, the medical direction physician may order the administration of racemic epinephrine or albuterol. Some physicians also advocate the use of steroids, because they feel these drugs will shorten the course of the illness.

> *Whenever you find an infant, toddler, or young child in respiratory or cardiac arrest, assume complete upper airway obstruction until proven otherwise.*
>
>

✱ **croup** laryngotracheobronchitis; a common viral infection of young children, resulting in edema of the sub-glottic tissues; characterized by barking cough and inspiratory stridor.

✱ **epiglottitis** bacterial infection of the epiglottis, usually occurring in children older than age four; a serious medical emergency.

Table 2-12	SYMPTOMS OF CROUP AND EPIGLOTTITIS	

Croup	Epiglottitis
Slow onset	Rapid onset
Generally wants to sit up	Prefers to sit up
Barking cough	No barking cough
No drooling	Drooling; painful to swallow
Fever approx. 100–101° F	Fever approx. 102–104° F
	Occasional stridor

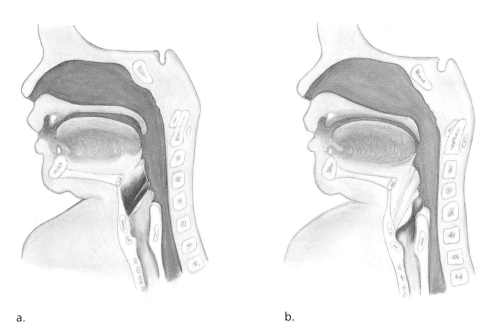

a.   b.

FIGURE 2-26   a. Epiglottitis is characterized by inflammation of the epiglottis and supraglottic tissues. b. Croup is characterized by subglottic edema.

In preparing the patient for transport, remember that the journey from the house to the ambulance will often allow the child to breathe cool air. Because cool air causes a decrease in subglottic edema, the child may be clinically improved by the time you reach the ambulance. If appropriate, keep the parent or caregiver with the infant or child. Do not agitate the patient, which could worsen the croup, by administering nonessential measures such as IVs or blood pressure readings.

Epiglottitis Epiglottitis is an acute infection and inflammation of the epiglottis and is potentially life-threatening. (Recall that the epiglottis is a flap of cartilage that protects the airway during swallowing.) Epiglottitis, unlike croup, is caused by a bacterial infection, usually *Hemophilus influenza* type B. Due to the availability of the *H. flu* vaccination, epiglottitis has become an uncommon occurrence. When it does occur, it tends to strike preschool and school-age children ages 3–7 years.

Assessment   Epiglottitis presents similarly to croup. Often the child will go to bed feeling relatively well, usually with what parents or caregivers consider to be a mild infection of the respiratory tract. Later, the child awakens with a high temperature and a brassy cough. The progression of symptoms can be dramatic. There is often pain upon swallowing, sore throat, high fever, shallow breathing, dyspnea, inspiratory stridor, and drooling (Figure 2-27).

On physical examination, the child will appear acutely ill and agitated. *Never attempt to visualize the airway.* If the child is crying, the tip of the epiglottis can be seen posterior to the base of the tongue. In epiglottitis, the epiglottis is cherry red and swollen. As airway obstruction develops, the child will exhibit retractions, nasal flaring, and pulmonary hyperexpansion. As the epiglottis swells, he may not be able to swallow his saliva and will begin to drool. Often the child will want to remain seated. Patients will often assume the "tripod position" to help maximize their airway. If they lean backward or lie flat, the epiglottis can fall back and completely obstruct the airway.

Management   Management of epiglottitis consists of appropriate airway maintenance and oxygen administration by face mask (Figure 2-28) or the blow-

Never attempt to visualize the airway in patients with epiglottitis.

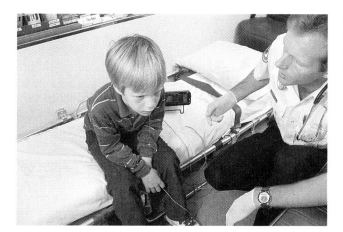

FIGURE 2-27   Posturing of the child with epiglottitis. Often, there will be excessive drooling.

by technique. Ideally, the oxygen should be humidified to minimize drying of the epiglottis and airway. To reduce the child's anxiety, you might ask the parent or caregiver to administer the oxygen. If the airway becomes obstructed, two-rescuer ventilation with BVM is almost always effective. Make sure that all intubation equipment is available, including an appropriate-sized endotracheal tube. Remember, however, that intubation is contraindicated unless complete obstruction has occurred.

Also, do not intubate in settings with short transport times. If endotracheal intubation is required, it may be necessary to use a smaller endotracheal tube because of narrowing of the glottic opening. If you perform chest compression upon glottic visualization during intubation, a bubble at the tracheal opening may form. This may help to establish upper airway landmarks that are distorted by the disease. As a last resort, consider needle cricothyrotomy per medical direction.

Pediatric patients with epiglottitis require immediate transport. Handle the child gently, since stress could lead to total airway obstruction from spasms of the larynx and swelling tissues. Avoid IV sticks, do not take a blood pressure, and do not attempt to look into the mouth. During transport, allow the child to sit on the lap of the parent or caregiver, if appropriate. Constantly monitor the child, and notify the hospital of any changes in status. Remember, if the patient is maintaining his airway, *do not put anything in the child's mouth*, including a thermometer. At all times, consider epiglottitis a critical condition.

Do not put anything in the mouth of an epiglottitis patient, including a thermometer.

At all times, consider epiglottitis a critical condition.

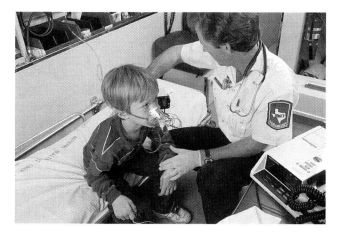

FIGURE 2-28   The child with epiglottitis should be administered humidified oxygen and transported in a comfortable position.

Bacterial Tracheitis Bacterial tracheitis is a bacterial infection of the airway, subglottic region. Although the condition is very uncommon, it is most likely to appear following episodes of viral croup. It afflicts mainly infants and toddlers 1–5 years of age.

Assessment In assessing this condition, parents or caregivers will typically report that the child has experienced an episode of croup in the preceding few days. They will also indicate the presence of a high-grade fever accompanied by coughing up of pus and/or mucus. The patient may exhibit a hoarse voice and, if able to talk, the child may complain of a sore throat. A physical examination may reveal inspiratory or expiratory stridor.

Management As with all respiratory emergencies, the child must be carefully monitored since respiratory failure or arrest may be an end result. Carefully manage airway and breathing, providing oxygenation by face mask or blow-by technique. Keep in mind that ventilations may require high pressure in order to adequately ventilate the patient. This may require depressing the pop-off valve of the pediatric bag-valve-mask device, if the valve is present. Consider intubation only in cases of complete airway obstruction. Transport guidelines are similar to those for cases of epiglottitis.

Foreign Body Aspiration Children—especially toddlers and preschoolers ages 1–4—like to put objects into their mouths. As a result, these children are at increased risk of aspirating foreign bodies, especially when they run or fall. In fact, foreign body aspiration is the number one cause of in-home accidental deaths in children under 6 years of age. In addition, many children choke on, or aspirate, food given to them by their parents or other well-meaning adults. Young children have not yet developed coordinated chewing motions in their mouth and pharynx and cannot adequately chew food. Common foods associated with aspiration and airway obstruction in children include hard candy, nuts, seeds, hot dogs, sausages, and grapes. Non-food items include coins, balloons, and other small objects.

Assessment The child with a suspected aspirated foreign body may present in one of two ways. If the obstruction is complete, the child will have minimal or no air movement. If the obstruction is partial, the child may exhibit inspiratory stridor, a muffled or hoarse voice, drooling, pain in the throat, retractions, and cyanosis.

Management Whenever you suspect that a child has aspirated a foreign body, immediately assess the patient's respiratory efforts. If the obstruction is partial, make the child as comfortable as possible and administer humidified oxygen. If old enough, place the child in a sitting position. Do not attempt to look in the mouth. Intubation equipment should be readily available since complete airway obstruction can occur. Transport the child to a hospital, where the foreign body can be removed by hospital personnel in a controlled environment.

If the obstruction is complete, clear the airway with accepted basic life support techniques. Sweep visible obstructions with your gloved finger. Do not perform blind finger sweeps, as this can push a foreign body deeper into the airway. Following BLS foreign body removal procedures, attempt ventilation with a BVM. If unsuccessful, visualize the airway with a laryngoscope. If the foreign body is seen and readily accessible, try to remove it with Magill forceps. Intubate if possible. Continue BLS foreign body removal procedures. If the airway cannot be cleared by routine measures, consider needle cricothyrotomy per medical direction and only as a last resort. Transport following appropriate guidelines, avoiding further agitation of the child.

> ## Content Review
> ### COMMON CAUSES OF UPPER AIRWAY OBSTRUCTIONS
> - Croup
> - Epiglottitis
> - Bacterial tracheitis
> - Foreign body aspiration

Lower Airway Distress

As already discussed, suspect lower airway distress when the following conditions exist: an absence of stridor, presence of wheezing during exhalation, and increased work of breathing. Common causes of lower airway distress include respiratory diseases such as asthma, bronchiolitis, and pneumonia. Although infrequent, you may also encounter cases of foreign body lower airway aspiration, especially in toddlers and preschoolers.

Asthma Asthma is a chronic inflammatory disorder of the lower respiratory tract. The disease affects more than 6 million Americans. It occurs before age 10 in approximately 50 percent of the cases, and before age 30 in another 33 percent of cases. The disease tends to run in families. It is also commonly associated with atopic conditions, such as eczema and allergies. Although deaths from other respiratory conditions have been steadily declining, asthmatic deaths have risen significantly in recent decades. Hospitalization of children for treatment of asthma has increased by more than 200 percent over the past 20 years. Because children can readily succumb to asthma, prompt prehospital recognition and treatment are essential.

Pathophysiology Asthma is a chronic inflammatory disorder of the airways, characterized by bronchospasm and excessive mucus production. In susceptible children, this inflammation causes widespread, but variable, airflow obstruction. In addition to airflow obstruction, the airways become hyperresponsive.

Asthma may be induced by one of many different factors, commonly called "triggers." The triggers vary from one child to the next. Common triggers include environmental allergens, cold air, exercise, foods, irritants, emotional stress, and certain medications.

Within minutes of exposure to the trigger, a two-phase reaction occurs. The first phase of the reaction is characterized by the release of chemical mediators such as histamine. These cause bronchoconstriction and bronchial edema that effectively decreases expiratory airflow, causing the classic "asthmatic attack." If treated early, asthma may respond to inhaled bronchodilators. If the attack is not aborted, or does not resolve spontaneously, a second phase may occur. The second phase is characterized by inflammation of the bronchioles as cells of the immune system invade the respiratory tract. This causes additional edema and further decreases expiratory airflow. The second phase is typically unresponsive to inhaled bronchodilators. Instead, antiinflammatory agents, such as corticosteroids, are often required.

As the attack continues, and swelling of the mucous membranes lining the bronchioles worsens, there may be plugging of the bronchi by thick mucus. This further obstructs airflow. As a result, there is an increase in sputum production. In addition, the lungs become progressively hyperinflated, since airflow is more restricted in exhalation. This effectively reduces vital capacity and results in decreased gas exchange by the alveoli, resulting in hypoxemia. If allowed to progress untreated, hypoxemia will worsen, and unconsciousness and death may ensue.

Assessment Asthma can often be differentiated from other pediatric respiratory illnesses by the history. In many cases, there is a prior history of asthma or reactive airway disease. The child's medications may also be an indicator. Children with asthma often have an inhaler or take a theophylline or oral beta agonist preparation.

On physical examination, the child is usually sitting up, leaning forward, and tachypneic. Often, there is an associated unproductive cough. Accessory respiratory muscle usage is usually evident. Wheezing may be heard. However, in a severe attack, the patient may not wheeze at all. This is an ominous finding. Some children will not wheeze, but will cough—often continuously. Generally there is associated tachycardia, and this should be monitored, since virtually all medications used to treat asthma increase the heart rate.

Management The primary therapeutic goals in the asthmatic are to correct hypoxia, reverse bronchospasm, and decrease inflammation. First, it is imperative that you establish an airway. Next, administer supplemental, humidified

Content Review

ASTHMA TRIGGERS
- Environmental allergens
- Cold air
- Exercise
- Foods
- Irritants
- Emotional stress
- Certain medications

If an asthmatic attack is allowed to progress untreated, hypoxemia will worsen, and unconsciousness and death may result.

In severe asthmatic attacks, the patient may not wheeze at all. This is an ominous finding.

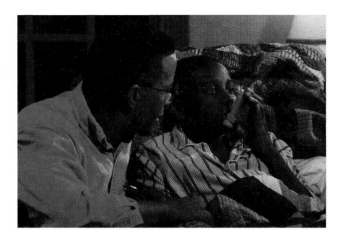

FIGURE 2-29 The young asthma patient may be making use of a prescribed inhaler to relieve symptoms. (© The Stock Market Photo Agency.)

oxygen as necessary. Initial pharmacological therapy is the administration of an inhaled beta agonist (Figure 2-29). All paramedic units should have the capability of administering nebulized bronchodilator medications, such as albuterol, metaproterenol, or isoetharine. Alternatively, a metered-dose inhaler (MDI) may be used. If there is a prolonged transport time, the medical direction physician may also request administration of a steroid preparation.

Status Asthmaticus   Status asthmaticus is defined as a severe, prolonged asthma attack that cannot be broken by aggressive pharmacological management. This is a serious medical emergency and prompt recognition, treatment, and transport are required. Often, the child suffering status asthmaticus will have a greatly distended chest from continued air trapping. Breath sounds, and often wheezing, may be absent. The patient is usually exhausted, severely acidotic, and often dehydrated. The management of status asthmaticus is basically the same as for asthma. However, you should recognize that respiratory arrest is imminent and remain prepared for endotracheal intubation. Transport should be immediate, with aggressive treatment continued en route.

Bronchiolitis   Bronchiolitis is a respiratory infection of the medium-sized airways—the bronchioles—that occurs in early childhood. It should not be confused with bronchitis, which is an infection of the larger bronchi. Bronchiolitis is caused by a viral infection, most commonly *respiratory syncytial virus (RSV)*, that affects the lining of the bronchioles.

Bronchiolitis is characterized by prominent expiratory wheezing and clinically resembles asthma. It most commonly occurs in winter in children less than 2 years of age. Bronchiolitis often spreads quickly through day care and preschool facilities. Most children will develop life-long immunity to *RSV* following infection. The exception is the very young infant who has an immature immune system.

Assessment   A history is necessary to distinguish bronchiolitis from asthma. Often, with bronchiolitis, there is a family history of asthma or allergies although neither is yet present in the child. In addition, there is often a low-grade fever. A major distinguishing factor is age. Asthma rarely occurs before the age of 1 year, where bronchiolitis is more frequent in this age group.

Your physical examination should be systematic. Pay particular attention to the presence of crackles or wheezes. Also, note any evidence of infection or respiratory distress.

Management   Prehospital management of suspected bronchiolitis is much the same as with asthma. Place the child in a semi-sitting position, if old enough, and administer humidified oxygen by mask or blow-by method. Ventilations should be supported as necessary. Equipment for intubation should be readily

Subcutaneous epinephrine or terbutaline may be used when inhaled medications are poorly tolerated or are unavailable.

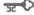

Status asthmaticus requires immediate transport with aggressive treatment administered en route.

✱ **bronchiolitis** viral infection of the medium-sized airways, occurring most frequently during the first year of life.

available. If respiratory distress is present, consider administration of a bronchodilator such as albuterol (Ventolin, Proventil) by small-volume nebulizer. The cardiac rhythm should be constantly monitored. Pulse oximetry, if available, should be used continuously.

Pneumonia Pneumonia is an infection of the lower airway and lungs. It may be caused by either a bacterium or a virus. Pneumonia can occur at any age, but in pediatric patients, it most commonly appears in infants, toddlers, and preschoolers ages 1–5 years. Most cases of pneumonia in children are viral and self-limited. As children get older, they can contract bacterial pneumonias like adults. A pneumonia vaccine is available. However, its use is reserved for patients with an immune system problem or who are asplenic.

Assessment Persons with pneumonia often have a history of a respiratory infection, such as a severe cold or bronchitis. Signs and symptoms include a low-grade fever, decreased breath sounds, crackles, rhonchi, and pain in the chest area. Conduct a systematic assessment of a patient with suspected pneumonia, paying particular attention to evidence of respiratory distress.

Management Prehospital management of pneumonia is supportive. Place the patient in a position of comfort. Assure a patent airway and administer supplemental oxygen via a nonrebreather device. If respiratory failure is present, support ventilations with a bag-valve-mask device. If prolonged ventilation will be required, perform endotracheal intubation. Transport the patient in a position of comfort. Provide emotional and psychological support to the parents.

Foreign Body Lower Airway Obstruction The same pediatric patients that are at risk from upper airway obstruction are at risk for lower airway obstruction. A foreign body can enter the lower airway if it is too small to lodge in the upper airway. The object is often food (nuts, seeds, candy), small toys, or parts of toys. The child will take a deep breath or will fall and accidentally aspirate the foreign body. The foreign body will fall into the lower airway until it reaches the airway that is smaller than the foreign body. Depending upon positioning, the foreign body can act as a one-way valve either trapping air in distal lung tissues or preventing aeration of distal lung tissues, causing a ventilation/perfusion mismatch.

Assessment There will often be a history of the child having a foreign body in the mouth and then it is gone. The parents may be unsure whether the child swallowed it, aspirated it, or simply lost the object. If the object is fairly large and aspirated, then respiratory distress may be present. There is often considerable, often intractable, coughing. The child will be anxious and may have diminished breath sounds in the part of the chest affected by the foreign body. There may be crackles or rhonchi, usually unilateral. In some cases, there may be unilateral wheezing where some air is getting past the object. Unilateral wheezing should be considered to be due to an aspirated foreign body until proven otherwise.

Management The management of an aspirated foreign body is supportive. Place the child in a position of comfort and avoid agitation. Provide supplemental oxygen. Transport the child to a facility that has the capability of performing pediatric fiber-optic bronchoscopy. The bronchoscope can be used to visualize the airway and remove any foreign objects detected.

> **Content Review**
>
> **COMMON CAUSES OF LOWER AIRWAY DISTRESS**
> - Asthma
> - Bronchiolitis
> - Pneumonia
> - Foreign body lower airway obstruction

SHOCK (HYPOPERFUSION)

The second major cause of pediatric cardiopulmonary arrest—after respiratory impairment—is shock. Shock can most simply be defined as inadequate perfusion of the tissues with oxygen and other essential nutrients and inadequate removal of metabolic waste products. This ultimately results in tissue hypoxia and metabolic acidosis. Ultimately, if untreated, cellular death will occur.

The definitive care of shock takes place in the emergency department of a hospital. However, early detection of shock by EMS personnel makes sure the patient gets to the hospital.

A slight increase in the heart rate is one of the earliest signs of shock.

When compared with the incidence of shock in adults, shock is an unusual occurrence in children because their blood vessels constrict so efficiently. However, when blood pressure does drop, it drops so far and so fast that the child may quickly develop cardiopulmonary arrest. A number of factors place infants and young children at risk of shock. As mentioned in Chapter 1, newborns and neonates can develop shock as a result of a loss of body heat. Other causes include dehydration (from vomiting and/or diarrhea), infection (particularly septicemia), trauma (especially from abdominal injuries), and blood loss. Less common causes of shock in infants and children include allergic reactions, poisoning, and cardiac events (rare).

The definitive care of shock takes place in the emergency department of a hospital. Because shock is a life-threatening condition in pediatric patients, it is important to recognize early signs and symptoms—or even the possibility of shock in a situation where signs and symptoms have not yet developed. In a situation in which you suspect a possibility of shock, provide oxygen to boost tissue perfusion and transport as quickly as possible. Also, keep the patient in a supine position and take steps to protect the child from hypothermia and agitation that might worsen the condition.

Severity of Shock

Shock is classified by degrees of severity as compensated, decompensated, and irreversible. The child responds to decreased perfusion by increasing heart rate and by increasing peripheral vascular resistance. The child has very little capacity to increase stroke volume. The key to early identification of shock is detecting the subtle signs that result from the body's various compensatory mechanisms.

Compensated Shock Early shock is known as *compensated shock* because the body is able to compensate for decreased tissue perfusion through various physiological mechanisms. In compensated shock, the patient exhibits a normal blood pressure. The signs and symptoms of compensated shock include:

- Irritability or anxiety
- Tachycardia
- Tachypnea
- Weak peripheral pulses, full central pulses
- Delayed capillary refill (more than 2 seconds in children less than 6 years of age)
- Cool, pale extremities
- Systolic blood pressure within normal limits
- Decreased urinary output

Compensated shock is generally reversible if appropriate treatment measures are instituted. Again, the key to a good outcome is prompt detection of the early signs and symptoms and initiation of therapy based upon this. Management is directed at correcting the underlying problem. High-flow oxygen should be administered and venous access obtained. If the patient is hypovolemic, then fluid replacement should be initiated. If the cause is cardiogenic, then medications should be administered to support cardiac output and increase peripheral vascular resistance. Sometimes definitive care of shock is surgical. However, in these cases, fluid therapy and oxygen administration will help buy time until the patient can be taken to surgery.

Decompensated Shock *Decompensated shock* develops when the body can no longer compensate for decreased tissue perfusion. The hallmark of decompen-

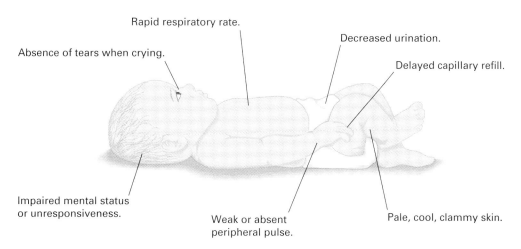

Rapid respiratory rate.

Absence of tears when crying.

Decreased urination.

Delayed capillary refill.

Impaired mental status or unresponsiveness.

Weak or absent peripheral pulse.

Pale, cool, clammy skin.

FIGURE 2-30   Signs and symptoms of shock (hypoperfusion) in a child.

sated shock is a fall in blood pressure (an ominous sign in children). This results in hypoperfusion and inadequate end-organ perfusion. It is important to remember that a child's compensatory mechanisms are quite efficient. Thus, when a child develops decompensated shock, there has been a significant loss of fluid or a significant impairment of cardiac output. The signs and symptoms of decompensated shock (Figure 2-30) include:

The hallmark of decompensated shock is a fall in blood pressure (an ominous sign in children).

- Lethargy or coma
- Marked tachycardia or bradycardia
- Absent peripheral pulses, weak central pulses
- Markedly delayed capillary refill
- Cool, pale, dusky, mottled extremities
- Hypotension
- Markedly decreased urinary output
- Absence of tears

Decompensated shock can become irreversible if aggressive treatment measures are not undertaken. In some cases, it may be irreversible despite the fact that aggressive treatment measures have been provided. Management is directed at treatment of the underlying cause. You should have a low threshold for initiating mechanical ventilation with a bag-valve-mask device and 100% oxygen. Consider intubating the patient if mechanical ventilation will be prolonged.

The child in decompensated shock is critically ill and will rapidly die without aggressive intervention.

Irreversible Shock   *Irreversible shock* occurs when treatment measures are inadequate or too late to prevent significant tissue damage and death. Sometimes, blood pressure and pulse can be restored. However, the patient later succumbs due to organ failure. The best treatment for irreversible shock is prevention.

Categories of Shock

There are a number of ways of categorizing shock. Shock can be categorized as *cardiogenic* (caused by impaired pumping power of the heart), *hypovolemic* (caused by decreased blood or water volume), *obstructive* (caused by an obstruction that interferes with return of blood to the heart, such as a pulmonary embolism, cardiac tamponade, or tension pneumothorax), and *distributive* (caused by abnormal distribution and return of blood resulting from vasodilation, vasopermeability, or both, as in septic, anaphylactic, or neurogenic shock).

Often, shock is classified into two general categories—cardiogenic and noncardiogenic. As noted above, **cardiogenic shock** results from an inability of the heart to maintain an adequate cardiac output to the circulatory system and tissues. Cardiogenic shock in a pediatric patient is ominous and often fatal. **Noncardiogenic shock** includes types of shock that result from causes other than inadequate cardiac output. Causes may include hemorrhage, abdominal trauma, systemic bacterial infection, spinal cord injury, and others.

Noncardiogenic Shock

Noncardiogenic shock is more frequently encountered in prehospital pediatric care than cardiogenic shock. (Recall that children have a much lower incidence of cardiac problems than adults.) The forms that you will most commonly assess and manage are hypovolemic and distributive shock. (See also the discussion of metabolic problems in children later in the chapter.)

Hypovolemic Shock Hypovolemic shock results from loss of intravascular fluids. In pediatric patients, the most common causes include severe dehydration from vomiting and/or diarrhea and blood loss, usually as a result of trauma. Trauma may include blood loss into a body cavity (particularly the abdomen) or frank external hemorrhage. Children are also at risk of fluid loss as a result of burns, the second leading cause of pediatric deaths in the United States.

Treatment of hypovolemic shock involves administration of supplemental oxygen and establishment of intravenous access. This should be followed by a 20 mL/kg bolus of lactated Ringer's or normal saline. Following the bolus, the child should be reassessed. If signs and symptoms of compensated shock still exist, then administer a second bolus. Some children may require 80–100 mL/kg of fluid, depending upon the volume of fluid lost.

Distributive Shock Distributive shock presents with a marked decrease in peripheral vascular resistance, usually due to a loss of vasomotor tone. In pediatric patients, causes include septicemia from bacterial infection, anaphylactic reaction, and damage to the brain and/or spinal cord. Cardiac output and fluid volume are adequate.

Septic Shock   This condition is caused by sepsis, an infection of the bloodstream by some pathogen, usually bacterial. Sepsis commonly occurs as a complication of an infection at some other site such as pneumonia, an ear infection, or a urinary tract infection. Meningitis is frequently associated with sepsis. The etiology can be varied, as can be the signs and symptoms.

The septic child is critically ill. Septic shock may develop when the pathogen causing the infection releases deadly toxins. These toxins cause peripheral vasodilatation, leading to a drop in blood pressure and decreased tissue perfusion. Sepsis can be rapidly fatal if not promptly identified and treated.

Signs of sepsis include:

- Ill appearance
- Irritability or altered mental status
- Fever
- Vomiting and diarrhea
- Cyanosis, pallor, or mottled skin

✳ **cardiogenic shock** the inability of the heart to meet the metabolic needs of the body, resulting in inadequate tissue perfusion.

✳ **noncardiogenic shock** types of shock that result from causes other than inadequate cardiac output.

✳ **hypovolemic shock** decreased amount of intravascular fluid in the body; often due to trauma that causes blood loss into a body cavity or frank external hemorrhage; in children, can be the result of vomiting and diarrhea.

✳ **distributive shock** marked decrease in peripheral vascular resistance with resultant hypotension; examples include septic shock, neurogenic shock, and anaphylactic shock.

Sepsis can be rapidly fatal if not promptly identified and treated. Your goal in treating sepsis is to prevent the development of septic shock.

- Nonspecific respiratory distress
- Poor feeding

Signs and symptoms of septic shock include:

- Very ill appearance
- Altered mental status
- Tachycardia
- Capillary refill time greater than 2 seconds
- Hyperventilation, leading to respiratory failure
- Cool and clammy skin
- Inability of child to recognize parents

Your goal in treating sepsis is to prevent the development of septic shock. Supplemental oxygen should be administered and intravenous access obtained. Administer a 20 mL/kg bolus of lactated Ringer's or normal saline. Consider initiating pressor therapy with dopamine. Begin at 2 mcg/kg/minute and gradually increase the dose until the blood pressure improves or there is evidence of improved end-organ perfusion. Definitive treatment includes antibiotics and other therapy. Transport should be rapid with care provided en route.

Septic shock kills!

The child in septic shock may require pressor therapy (dopamine or epinephrine).

Anaphylactic Shock   Anaphylactic shock results from exposure to an antigen to which the patient has been previously exposed. Milder cases may simply result in an allergic reaction. More severe reactions can impair tissue perfusion. This primarily occurs as a result of the release of histamine and other similar chemicals. Histamine causes peripheral vasodilation and leakage of fluid from the intravascular space into the interstitial space. Anaphylactic shock can be differentiated from a severe allergic reaction by the presence of signs and symptoms of impaired end-organ perfusion. These include:

- Tachycardia
- Tachypnea
- Wheezing
- Urticaria (hives)
- Anxiousness
- Edema
- Hypotension

Treatment of a severe allergic reaction includes administration of subcutaneous epinephrine 1:1,000 and an antihistamine. Treatment of anaphylactic shock includes supplemental oxygen administration and intravenous access. If the patient is exhibiting decompensated shock, administer epinephrine 1:10,000 intravenously and diphenhydramine (Benadryl) intravenously. Patients not exhibiting hypotension may be given an initial dose of epinephrine subcutaneously. If this does not rapidly improve the situation, then an intravenous dose of epinephrine should be considered. Contact medical direction for additional assistance. EMS systems with long transport times may be asked to administer an initial dose of a corticosteroid such as methylprednisolone (Solu-Medrol).

Allergic reactions can usually be managed with subcutaneous epinephrine 1:1,000, while severe allergic reactions require intravenous spinephrine 1:10,000.

Neurogenic Shock   Neurogenic shock is due to sudden peripheral vasodilation resulting from interruption of nervous control of the peripheral vascular system. The most common cause is injury to the spinal cord. Cardiac output and intravascular fluid volume are usually adequate.

Treatment is directed at increasing peripheral vascular resistance. This is primarily through administration of a pressor agent such as dopamine. Care should also include stabilization of the injury and administration of supplemental oxygen.

Cardiogenic Shock

Cardiogenic shock results from inadequate cardiac output. In children, cardiogenic shock usually results from a secondary cause such as near-drowning or a toxic ingestion. Children, unlike adults, rarely have primary cardiac disease. The exceptions are congenital heart disease and cardiomyopathy.

Congenital heart disease is an abnormality or defect in the heart that is present at birth. Many congenital cardiac problems are detected at birth. However, some may not be detected until later in life. Cardiomyopathy causes a decrease in cardiac output due to impairment of cardiac muscle contraction. Dysrhythmias, although rare in children, can cause a decrease in cardiac output. Rapid dysrhythmias may impair ventricular filling and thus cause a decrease in cardiac output. Likewise, slow dysrhythmias may cause decreased cardiac output simply due to their slow rate.

In the following sections we will discuss in more detail congenital heart disease, cardiomyopathy, and dysrhythmias which, as noted, are primary causes of pediatric cardiogenic shock. Remember, however, cardiogenic shock in children most often results from secondary causes.

* congenital present at birth.

Congenital Heart Disease

Congenital heart disease is the primary cause of heart disease in children. As noted above, although most congenital heart problems are detected at birth, some problems may not be discovered until later in childhood. A common symptom of congenital heart disease is cyanosis. This occurs when blood going to the lungs for oxygenation mixes with blood bound for other parts of the body. This may result from holes in the internal walls of the heart or from abnormalities of the great vessels.

The child with congenital heart disease may develop respiratory distress, congestive heart failure, or a "cyanotic spell." *Cyanotic spells* occur when oxygen demand exceeds that provided by the blood. They begin as irritability, inconsolable crying, or altered mental status, and progressive cyanosis in conjunction with severe dyspnea. In severe and prolonged cases, seizures, coma, or cardiac arrest may result. Non-cyanotic problems associated with congenital heart disease include respiratory distress, tachycardia, decreased end-organ perfusion, drowsiness, fatigue, and pallor.

Treatment includes the standard primary assessment. Administer oxygen at a high concentration. If necessary, provide ventilatory support. If the patient is having a cyanotic spell, place the child in the knee-chest position facing downward. This will help increase the cardiac return. Apply the ECG monitor, and start an intravenous line at a keep-open rate. Transport immediately.

Tetralogy of Fallot, a type of congenital heart disease with a right-to-left shunt, is often characterized by cyanotic episodes ("tet" spells) which are relieved by the child squatting.

Cardiomyopathy

Cardiomyopathy is a disease or dysfunction of the cardiac muscle. Although fairly rare, cardiomyopathy can result from congenital heart disease or infection. A frequent cause of infectious cardiomyopathy is Coxsackie virus. Cardiomyopathy causes mechanical pump failure, which is usually biventricular. It often develops slowly and is not detectable until heart failure develops.

The signs and symptoms of cardiomyopathy include early fatigue, crackles, jugular venous distension, engorgement of the liver, and peripheral edema. Later, as the disease progresses, the signs and symptoms of shock can develop.

The prehospital treatment of cardiomyopathy is supportive. Supplemental oxygen should be administered via a nonrebreather mask. Fluids should be restricted. If possible, IV access should be obtained. Severe cases resulting in the development of severe dyspnea should be treated with furosemide and pressor agents (dobutamine, dopamine). The child should be transported to a facility capable of managing critically ill children. Most cases of cardiomyopathy are managed with medication. Definitive care in severe cases may include cardiac transplantation.

Dysrhythmias

Dysrhythmias in children are uncommon. When dysrhythmias occur, bradydysrhythmias are the most common. Supraventricular tachydysrhythmias are uncommon and ventricular tachydysrhythmias are very uncommon. Dysrhythmias can cause pump failure ultimately leading to cardiogenic shock. Children have a very limited capacity to increase stroke volume. The primary mechanism through which they increase cardiac output is through changes in the heart rate. The treatment of dysrhythmias is specific for the dysrhythmia in question.

Tachydysrhythmias Tachydysrhythmias are dysrhythmias in which the rate is greater than the estimated maximum normal heart rate for the child. These can result from primary cardiac disease or from secondary causes. Tachydysrhythmias from any cause are relatively uncommon in children.

Supraventricular Tachycardia   True supraventricular tachycardia is a narrow complex tachycardia with a heart rate of 220 per minute or greater. Supraventricular tachycardia is typically due to a problem in the cardiac conductive system. Rarely, it can be due to a secondary cause such as drug ingestion. It is occasionally seen in infants with no prior history. The cause is uncertain but may be due to immaturity of the cardiac conductive system. Rapid heart rates often do not allow time for adequate cardiac filling, eventually causing congestive heart failure and cardiogenic shock.

The signs and symptoms of supraventricular tachycardia include irritability, poor feeding, jugular venous distension, hepatomegaly (enlarged liver), and hypotension. The ECG will show a narrow complex (supraventricular) tachycardia with a rate greater than 220 per minute. Children can often tolerate the rapid rate well.

Prehospital treatment of supraventricular tachycardia depends upon the clinical findings. Children who are tolerating the heart rate (normal blood pressure) and are stable should receive supplemental oxygen and transport. Adenosine should be considered if the child is stable. If the child is exhibiting signs of decompensation (hypotension, mental status change, poor skin color) then synchronized cardioversion should be attempted at initial dose of 0.5 to 1.0 Joules per kilogram of body weight. This can be increased to 2 Joules per kilogram if the initial shock is unsuccessful. The child should be transported to the appropriate facility.

Ventricular Tachycardia with a Pulse   Ventricular tachycardia and ventricular fibrillation are exceedingly rare in children. They are occasionally seen following drowning or following a prolonged resuscitation attempt. Unlike adults, where ventricular tachydysrhythmias result from primary heart disease, ventricular tachydysrhythmias in children are almost always due to a secondary cause. The exception is structural, congenital heart disease.

The signs and symptoms of ventricular tachycardia with a pulse include poor feeding, irritability, and a rapid, wide complex tachycardia. Children are unable to tolerate this dysrhythmia very long. They soon develop signs of shock.

The prehospital management of ventricular tachycardia with a pulse include supplemental oxygen and intravenous access. Stable patients who are not hypotensive should be transported. Unstable patients (hypotension) should be aggressively treated. Initially, amiodarone, procainamide, or lidocaine should be administered. However, ventricular tachycardia due to structural heart disease often does not respond to antidysrhythmic drugs. If the patient is unstable or deteriorating, administer synchronized cardioversion at 0.5—1.0 Joules/kilogram. This can be increased to 2 Joules/kilograms if needed. Transport emergently and provide care en route.

Bradydysrhythmias Bradydysrhythmias are the most common type of pediatric dysrhythmia. They most frequently result from hypoxia. Although rare, they can also result from vagal stimulation from such causes as marked gastric distension.

The signs and symptoms of bradycardia include a slow, narrow complex rhythm. The child may be lethargic or exhibiting early signs of congestive heart failure.

Stable children with bradydysrhythmias should receive supportive care. Unstable children should be ventilated with a bag-valve-mask unit and 100% oxygen. If the heart rate does not readily increase, consider endotracheal intubation. Perform chest compressions if oxygenation and ventilation do not increase the heart rate. Consider administering epinephrine or atropine down the endotracheal tube until intravenous access can be obtained. Transport emergently with care provided en route. (See the algorithm for treatment of pediatric bradycardia, Figure 2-31.)

Absent Rhythm The absence of a cardiac rhythm is an ominous finding. Most cases are asystole. However, some cases may be a very fine ventricular fibrillation. If necessary, turn up the gain on the ECG to distinguish between the two.

Asystole Asystole is the absence of a rhythm and may be the initial rhythm seen in cardiopulmonary arrest. (Remember, children rarely develop ventricular fibrillation, which is often the precursor to arrest in adults.) Bradycardias can degenerate to asystole if appropriate intervention is not provided. The mortality rate associated with asystole in children is very high.

The child with asystole is pulseless and apneic. The cardiac rhythm is a straight line that should be confirmed in two leads. Treatment is often futile. However, CPR should be initiated. The patient should be intubated and ventilated with 100% oxygen. Chest compressions should be continued. Emergency resuscitative drugs (epinephrine, atropine) should be administered through the endotracheal tube until intravenous access can be obtained. (See the algorithm for pediatric asystole and cardiac arrest, Figure 2-32.)

Ventricular Fibrillation/Pulseless Ventricular Tachycardia Ventricular fibrillation and pulseless ventricular tachycardia are functionally the same rhythm. They are exceedingly rare in children. Causes include electrocution and drug overdoses. The mortality rate is very high.

The child with ventricular fibrillation/pulseless ventricular tachycardia will be pulseless and apneic. The ECG will exhibit a wide complex tachycardia or fibrillation. In unmonitored patients, provide CPR. If the patient was monitored at the time of the arrest, then defibrillate 3 times (2 Joules/kg, then 4 Joules/kg, then repeat at 4 Joules/kg). Ventilate the patient with 100% oxygen and intubate. Continue chest compressions. Resuscitative medications (epinephrine, lidocaine, amiodarone) can be administered down the endotracheal tube until intravenous access can be obtained. Transport as soon as possible.

Pulseless Electrical Activity Pulseless electrical activity (PEA) is the presence of a cardiac rhythm without an associated pulse. This is due to noncardiogenic causes such as hypoxia, pericardial tamponade, tension pneumothorax, trauma, acidosis, hypothermia, hypoglycemia, and others.

The patient with PEA is pulseless and apneic. Resuscitation should be directed toward correcting the underlying cause. The patient should receive CPR, be intubated and ventilated, and given the standard resuscitative medications (epinephrine). Transport should be prompt with care provided en route.

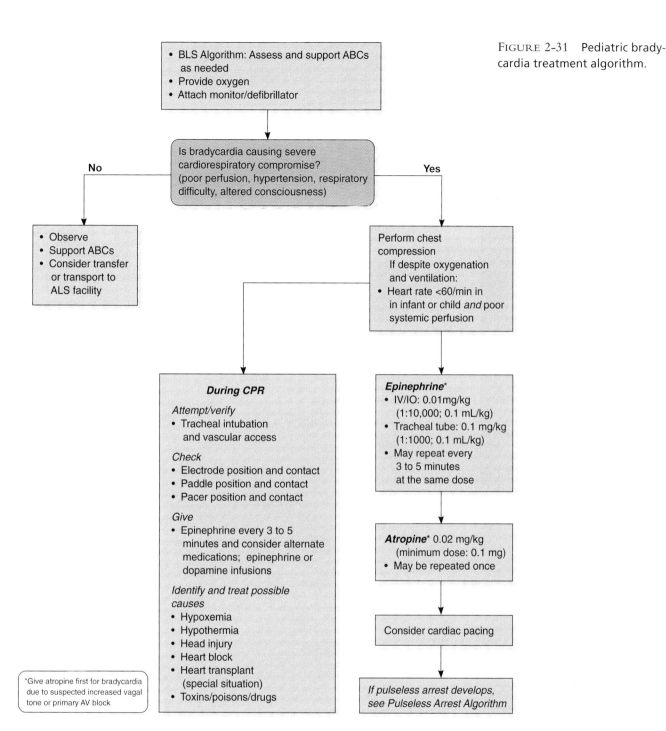

FIGURE 2-31 Pediatric brady-cardia treatment algorithm.

- BLS Algorithm: Assess and support ABCs as needed
- Provide oxygen
- Attach monitor/defibrillator

Is bradycardia causing severe cardiorespiratory compromise? (poor perfusion, hypertension, respiratory difficulty, altered consciousness)

No

Yes

- Observe
- Support ABCs
- Consider transfer or transport to ALS facility

Perform chest compression
  If despite oxygenation and ventilation:
- Heart rate <60/min in in infant or child *and* poor systemic perfusion

During CPR

Attempt/verify
- Tracheal intubation and vascular access

Check
- Electrode position and contact
- Paddle position and contact
- Pacer position and contact

Give
- Epinephrine every 3 to 5 minutes and consider alternate medications; epinephrine or dopamine infusions

Identify and treat possible causes
- Hypoxemia
- Hypothermia
- Head injury
- Heart block
- Heart transplant (special situation)
- Toxins/poisons/drugs

*Epinephrine**
- IV/IO: 0.01mg/kg (1:10,000; 0.1 mL/kg)
- Tracheal tube: 0.1 mg/kg (1:1000; 0.1 mL/kg)
- May repeat every 3 to 5 minutes at the same dose

*Atropine** 0.02 mg/kg (minimum dose: 0.1 mg)
- May be repeated once

Consider cardiac pacing

If pulseless arrest develops, see Pulseless Arrest Algorithm

*Give atropine first for bradycardia due to suspected increased vagal tone or primary AV block

NEUROLOGICAL EMERGENCIES

Neurological emergencies in childhood are fairly uncommon. However, seizures can and do occur in children. In fact, they are a frequent reason for summoning EMS. In addition to seizures, meningitis tends to show up more often in children than in adults. Although your chances of encountering either of these two conditions are small, both are life threatening and should be promptly identified and treated.

Seizures

Seizures result from an abnormal discharge of neurons in the brain. Many people suffer seizures and it is a common reason why EMS is summoned. People with

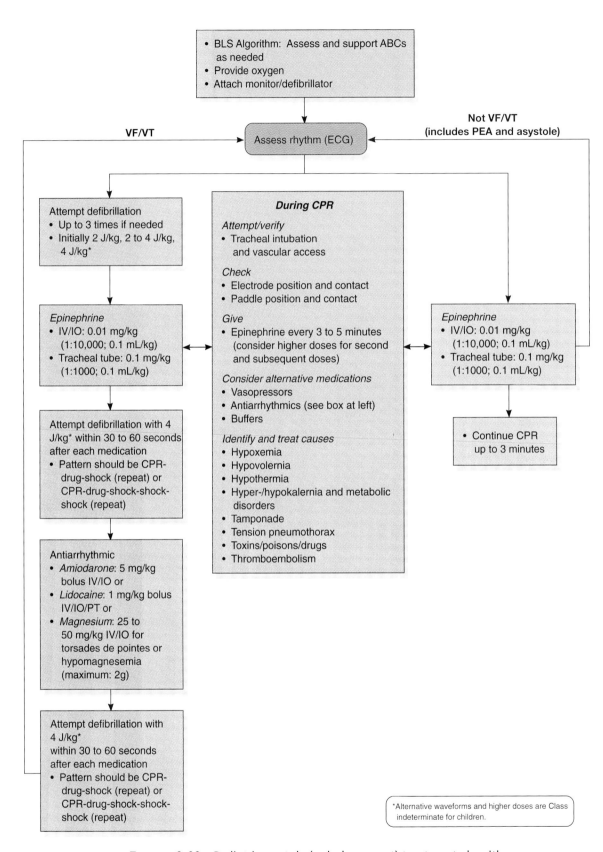

FIGURE 2-32   Pediatric asystole (pulseless arrest) treatment algorithm.

chronic seizure disorders can often control their seizures with medications. A seizure can be an exceptionally scary event for both the parents and the child. This is especially true if the child has never had a seizure before.

Although the etiology for seizures is often unknown, several risk factors have been identified. They include:

- Fever
- Hypoxia
- Infections
- Idiopathic epilepsy (epilepsy of unknown origin)
- Electrolyte disturbances
- Head trauma
- Hypoglycemia
- Toxic ingestions or exposure
- Tumor
- CNS malformations

Seizures in pediatric patients may be either partial or generalized. (Recall that generalized seizures normally do not occur during the first month of life.) Simple partial seizures, sometimes called focal motor seizures, involve sudden jerking of a particular part of the body, such as an arm or a leg. Other characteristics include lip smacking, eye blinking, staring, confusion, and lethargy. There is usually no loss of consciousness. Generalized seizures involve sudden jerking of both sides of the body, followed by tenseness and relaxation of the body. In a generalized seizure, patients typically experience a loss of consciousness.

Keep in mind that children can have **status epilepticus**—a series of one or more generalized seizures without any intervening periods of consciousness. Status epilepticus is a serious medical emergency because it involves a prolonged period of apnea, which in turn can cause hypoxia of vital brain tissues. (For more on seizures and status epilepticus, see Volume 3, Chapter 3.)

Most of the pediatric seizures that you will probably encounter are febrile seizures. **Febrile seizures** are those seizures that occur as a result of a sudden increase in body temperature. They occur most commonly between the ages of 6 months and 6 years. Febrile seizures seem related to the rate at which the body temperature increases, not to the degree of fever. Often, the parents or caregivers will report the recent onset of fever or cold symptoms. The diagnosis of febrile seizure should not be made in the field. All pediatric patients suffering a seizure must be transported to the hospital so that other etiologies can be excluded.

Assessment The history is a major factor in determining seizure type. Febrile seizure should be suspected if the temperature is above 103°F (39.2° C). The history of a previous seizure may suggest idiopathic epilepsy or another CNS problem. However, there is also a tendency for recurrence of febrile seizures in children.

When confronted with a seizing child, determine whether there is a history of seizures or seizures with fever. Has the child had a recent illness? Also, determine how many seizures occurred during the incident. If the child is not seizing upon arrival, elicit a description of the seizure activity. Note the condition and position of the child when found. Question parents, caregivers, or bystanders about the possibility of head injury. A history of irritability or lethargy prior to the seizure may indicate CNS infection. If possible, find out whether the child suffers from diabetes or has recently complained of a headache or a stiff neck. Note any current medications, as well as possible ingestions.

The physical examination should be systematic. Pay particular attention to the adequacy of respirations, the level of consciousness, neurological evaluation,

✱ **status epilepticus** prolonged seizure or multiple seizures with no regaining of consciousness between them.

Status epilepticus is a serious medical emergency because it involves a prolonged period of apnea, which in turn can cause hypoxia of vital brain tissues.

✱ **febrile seizures** seizures that occur as a result of a sudden increase in body temperature; occur most commonly between ages 6 months and 6

The diagnosis of febrile seizure should not be made in the field.

and signs of injury. Also inspect the child for signs of dehydration. Dehydration may be evidenced by the absence of tears or, in an infant, by the presence of a sunken fontanelle.

Management Management of pediatric seizures is essentially the same as for seizing adults. Place patients on the floor or on the bed. Be sure to lay them on their side, away from the furniture. Do not restrain patients, but take steps to protect them from injury. Maintain the airway, but do not force anything, such as a bite stick, between the teeth. Administer supplemental oxygen. Then take and record all vital signs. If the patient is febrile, remove excess layers of clothing, while avoiding extreme cooling. If status epilepticus is present, institute the following steps:

- Start an IV of normal saline or lactated Ringer's and perform a glucometer evaluation.
- Administer diazepam as follows:
  - *Children 1 month to 5 years:* 0.2–0.5 mg slowly IV push every 2–5 minutes up to a maximum of 2.5 milligrams.
  - *Children 5 years and older:* 1 mg slowly IV push every 2–5 minutes to a maximum of 5 milligrams.
- Contact medical direction for additional dosing. Diazepam can be administered rectally if an IV cannot be established.
- If the seizure appears to be due to fever and a long transport time is anticipated, medical direction may request the administration of acetaminophen to lower the fever. Acetaminophen is supplied as an elixir or as suppositories. The dose should be 15 mg/kg body weight.

As mentioned previously, all pediatric patients should be transported. Reassure and support the parents or caregivers, since this is a very stressful and frightening situation for them.

Some medical directors prefer lorazepam (Ativan) as the anticonvulsant of choice for pediatrics.

Meningitis

Meningitis is an infection of the meninges, the lining of the brain and spinal cord. Meningitis can result from both bacteria and viruses. Viral meningitis is frequently called *aseptic meningitis*, since an organism cannot be routinely cultured from CSF fluid. Aseptic meningitis is generally less severe than bacterial meningitis and self-limiting. Bacterial meningitis most commonly results from *Streptococcus pneumoniae, Haemophilus influenza,* and *Neisseria meningitides.* These infections can be rapidly fatal if they are not promptly recognized and treated appropriately.

Assessment Meningitis is more common in children than in adults. Findings in the history that may suggest meningitis include a child who has been ill for one day to several days, recent ear or respiratory tract infection, high fever, lethargy or irritability, a severe headache, or a stiff neck. Infants generally do not develop a stiff neck. They will generally become lethargic and will not feed well. Some babies may simply develop a fever.

On physical examination, the child with meningitis will appear very ill. With an infant, the fontanelle may be bulging or full unless accompanied by dehydration. Extreme discomfort with movement, due to irritability of the meninges, may be present.

Be alert for rapid cardiopulmonary collapse in the child with fulminant meningitis, or severe meningitis with a rapid onset.

Management Prehospital care of the pediatric patient with meningitis is supportive. Rapidly complete the primary assessment and transport the child to the emergency department. If shock is present, treat the child with intravenous fluids (20 mL/kg) and oxygen.

Table 2-13 SIGNS AND SYMPTOMS OF DEHYDRATION

Signs/Symptoms	Mild	Moderate	Severe
Vital Signs			
Pulse	normal	increased	markedly increased
Respirations	normal	increased	tachypneic
Blood pressure	normal	normal	hypotensive
Capillary refill	normal	2–3 seconds	> 2 seconds
Mental Status	alert	irritable	lethargic
Skin	normal	dry and ashen	dry, cool, mottled
Mucous Membranes	dry	very dry	very dry/no tears

GASTROINTESTINAL EMERGENCIES

Childhood gastrointestinal problems almost always present with nausea and vomiting as a chief complaint. As a child gets older, other gastrointestinal system emergencies, such as appendicitis, become more common.

Nausea and Vomiting

Nausea and vomiting are not diseases themselves, but are symptoms of other disease processes. Virtually any medical problem can cause these conditions in an infant or child. The most common causes include fever, ear infections, and respiratory infections. In addition, many viruses and certain bacteria can infect the gastrointestinal system. These infections—collectively known as *gastroenteritis*—readily cause vomiting, diarrhea, or both.

The biggest risks associated with nausea and vomiting in children are dehydration and electrolyte abnormalities. Infants and toddlers can quickly become dehydrated from bouts of vomiting. If diarrhea or fever is also present, fluid loss is further accelerated, worsening the situation. Dehydration in infants and toddlers is more difficult to detect than in older children. (See Table 2-13 for a description of the signs and symptoms of dehydration.)

Treatment of pediatric nausea and vomiting is primarily supportive. If the child is dehydrated and unable to keep oral fluids down, intravenous fluid therapy may be indicated. Severe dehydration, as evidenced by prolonged capillary refill time, should be treated by 20 mL/kg fluid boluses of lactated Ringer's solution or 0.9 percent sodium chloride solution (normal saline).

Vomiting and diarrhea carry the potential for dehydration and electrolyte abnormalities—serious conditions in the pediatric patient.

Diarrhea

Diarrhea is a common occurrence in childhood. Often, what parents call diarrhea is actually loose bowel movements. Generally, 10 or more stools per day is considered diarrhea. As with nausea and vomiting, the main concern associated with diarrhea is dehydration. Most diarrhea is due to viral infections of the gastrointestinal system or secondary to infections elsewhere in the body. However, certain bacterial infections can cause significant, even life-threatening, diarrhea.

Treatment of the child suffering from diarrhea is primarily supportive. If dehydration is evident, administer fluids. Severe dehydration should be treated with 20 mL/kg boluses of intravenous fluids (lactated Ringer's or normal saline).

METABOLIC EMERGENCIES

Metabolic problems are uncommon in children. However, diabetes can occur in very young children. It is rarely diagnosed until the child comes to the hospital in diabetic ketoacidosis. Diabetic children can have great swings in their blood glucose levels due to diet, growth, and physical activity. Because of this, hypoglycemia and hyperglycemia are possible. It is important to remember that very young children, unlike adults, can develop hypoglycemia without having diabetes. This can occur with severe illnesses such as meningitis and pneumonia. The following section will present the prehospital treatment of pediatric hypoglycemia and hyperglycemia.

Hypoglycemia

✱ hypoglycemia abnormally low concentration of glucose in the blood.

Hypoglycemia is a true medical emergency that must be treated immediately.
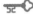

Hypoglycemia is an abnormally low concentration of sugar (glucose) in the blood. It is a true medical emergency that must be treated immediately. Without treatment, a low blood sugar may progress to unconsciousness and convulsions.

In the prehospital setting, hypoglycemia in pediatric patients usually occurs in newborn infants and children with Type I diabetes. Diabetic children increase their risk of hypoglycemia through overly strenuous exercise, too much insulin, and dehydration from illness. Non-diabetic children can develop hypoglycemia from physical activity, diet changes, illness, and growth.

In known diabetics or hypoglycemics, preventive steps include:

- Taking extra snacks for extra activity
- Eating immediately after taking insulin if the blood sugar is less than 100 mg/dl
- Eating regular meals
- Regularly monitoring blood sugar
- Eating an extra snack of carbohydrate and protein if the blood sugar is less than 120 mg/dl at bedtime
- Replacing carbohydrates in the meal plan with things like regular soda pop or regular popsicles on days when the child is sick

Assessment Suspect hypoglycemia when the patient exhibits the signs and symptoms listed in Table 2-14. Measure blood glucose with a glucometer, and elicit a history of conditions known to cause hypoglycemia in infants and children. Treatment should be initiated whenever you have a high index of suspicion and/or blood sugar drops below 70 mg/dl.

Management As with all patients, continually monitor the ABCs. Be sure to find out if parents or caregivers have given the patient any glucose tablets, gels, foods (cake icing, honey, maple syrup, sugar, raisins), or drinks (juice, regular

Table 2-14 SIGNS AND SYMPTOMS OF HYPOGLYCEMIA

Mild	Moderate	Severe
Hunger	Sweating	Decreased level of consciousness
Weakness	Tremors	Seizure
Tachypnea	Irritability	Tachycardia
Tachycardia	Vomiting	Hypoperfusion
Shakiness	Mood swings	
Yawning	Blurred vision	
Pale skin	Stomach ache	
Dizziness	Headache	
	Dizziness	
	Slurred speech	

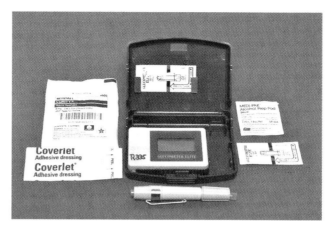

FIGURE 2-33   Many diabetic children have home glucometers to test their blood glucose levels. Older children know what the readings mean and will be curious about any glucose testing device that you may use.

soda pop, milk) to correct the situation. If so, find out what was given, how much was given, and when it was given. Take a blood glucose test, if possible.

In the conscious, alert patient, administer oral fluids with sugar or oral glucose. (Amounts are age and/or weight specific, so check with medical direction.) If there is no response, or if the patient exhibits an altered mental status, transport immediately. Consult your medical direction physician on orders for the administration of dextrose or IM glucagon. Twenty-five percent dextrose solution ($D_{25}W$) can be prepared by diluting fifty percent dextrose solution 1:1 with sterile water or saline. It is easier to dose children with this concentration and does not cause as much discomfort as with intravenous administration. Repeat blood glucose tests within 10–15 minutes of infusion or the administration of glucose.

In treating diabetic pediatric patients, remember that most children have been taught about their condition and can participate, in varying degrees, in their care. Most understand how glucometers work, for example, and can hand you a test strip (Figure 2-33). Also, they may be sensitive to their condition. So avoid labeling any tests as "good" or "bad."

Hyperglycemia

Hyperglycemia is an abnormally high concentration of blood sugar. For patients with Type I diabetes, hyperglycemia may lead to dehydration and **diabetic ketoacidosis,** a very serious medical emergency. Left untreated, the condition will deteriorate to coma. Hyperglycemia and diabetic ketoacidosis are the most common findings in new-onset diabetics.

In the prehospital setting, pediatric hyperglycemia is commonly associated with Type I diabetes. Causes include:

* Eating too much food relative to injected insulin
* Missing an insulin injection
* Defective insulin pump, blockage of tubing, or disconnection of insulin pump infusion set
* Illness or stress

Hyperglycemia can occur with other severe illnesses and not necessarily mean that the child is developing diabetes mellitus.

Assessment In cases of hyperglycemia, glucose is spilled into the urine, taking water with it through osmotic diuresis. This can result in a signficant fluid loss with resultant dehydration.

✱ **hyperglycemia** abnormally high concentration of glucose in the blood.

✱ **diabetic ketoacidosis** complication of diabetes due to decreased insulin secretion or intake; characterized by high levels of blood glucose, metabolic acidosis, and, in advanced stages, coma; often referred to as diabetic coma.

Diabetic ketoacidosis is a very serious medical emergency, which may quickly deteriorate into coma.

Table 2-15 SIGNS AND SYMPTOMS OF HYPERGLYCEMIA

Early	Late	Ketoacidosis
Increased thirst	Weakness	Continued decreased level of consciousness progressing to coma
Increased urination	Abdominal pain	
Weight loss	Generalized aches	Kussmaul respirations (deep and slow)
	Loss of appetite	Signs of dehydration
	Nausea	
	Vomiting	
	Signs of dehydration, except increased urinary output	
	Fruity breath odor	
	Tachypnea	
	Hyperventilation	
	Tachycardia	

Keep in mind that acidosis results from the accumulation of ketones, a by-product of fat metabolism. A continual increase in the ketones eventually leads to metabolic acidosis, which produces the fruity breath odor commonly associated with hyperglycemia. For other signs and symptoms, see Table 2-15.

As with hypoglycemia, elicit a history to determine causes linked with hyperglycemia. If possible, confirm your suspicions with blood glucose test. A blood sugar reading of greater than 200 mg/dl typically indicates hyperglycemia.

Management Carefully monitor the ABCs and vital signs. If you cannot confirm the presence of hyperglycemia with a blood glucose test, consider administering oral fluids with sugar or oral glucose in case the patient is hypoglycemic. If intravenous access is possible, consider initiating an IV of either normal saline or lactated Ringer's. Administer an IV bolus of 20 mL/kg, and repeat the bolus if the patient's vital signs do not change. Monitor the patient's mental status and be prepared to intubate if the respirations continue to decrease.

Remember this is a potentially life-threatening situation. Consult with medical direction on all actions taken and transport immediately.

POISONING AND TOXIC EXPOSURE

Accidental poisoning or toxic exposure is a common reason for summoning EMS. Pediatric patients account for the majority of poisonings treated by EMS. Most poisonings result from accidental ingestion of a toxic substance, usually by a young child. Toddlers and preschoolers like to taste things, especially colorful objects and substances that look like food or beverages (Figure 2-34). They also mimic their parents or caregivers, swallowing pills or drinking alcohol "just like Mommy and Daddy." Teenagers on antidepressants are also at risk of misusing or abusing their prescriptions, especially if given a one- or two-month supply of a medication.

Poisonings are the leading cause of preventable death in children under age 5. Because of their immature respiratory and cardiovascular systems, even a single pill can poison or, in some cases, kill a child. Of all the substances ingested by young children, iron-containing supplements are the leading cause of poisonings, especially in toddlers and preschoolers.

The most dangerous rooms in a house in terms of poisons are the kitchen, where household cleaners are stored, and the bathroom, where many people

INGESTION

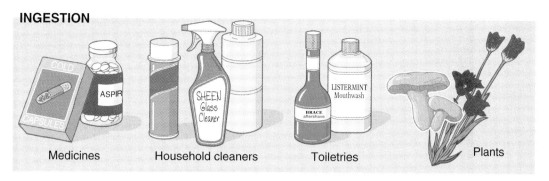

Medicines   Household cleaners   Toiletries   Plants

FIGURE 2-34   Some of the poisons commonly ingested by children.

keep their over-the-counter and prescription medications. Garages and utility rooms also contain toxic substances, made more attractive to children when they are poured into everyday containers such as coffee cans, soda bottles, or plastic cups. Living rooms may have poisonous plants and liquor bottles.

The best way to prevent pediatric poisonings is by helping the families in your communities learn how to "poison proof" their homes. If your EMS system does not have information available on this topic, you can obtain guidelines from the Food and Drug Administration located in Rockville, Maryland. Poisoning prevention should be a major goal of EMS prevention and community education programs. Many EMS systems will dedicate a specific month out of the year to poisoning awareness and prevention.

Assessment   Assessment of a pediatric poisoning depends upon the type of poison ingested or the extent to which a child was exposed to a toxic substance (Figure 2-35). Common substances involved in pediatric poisonings include:

- Alcohol, barbiturates, sedatives
- Amphetamines, cocaine, hallucinogens
- Anticholinergic agents (jimson weed, belladonna products)
- Aspirin, acetaminophen
- Lead
- Vitamins and iron-containing supplements
- Corrosives
- Digitalis and beta blockers
- Hydrocarbons
- Narcotics
- Organic solvents (inhaled)
- Organophosphates (insecticides)

Poisoning can cause many different signs and symptoms depending upon the poison ingested, the route of exposure, and the time since exposure. Narcotics and some of the hydrocarbons can cause respiratory system depression. Digitalis, beta blockers, and many of the antihypertensive agents can cause circulatory depression or collapse. The central nervous system can be impaired by a great many agents. These include alcohol, barbiturates, narcotics, cocaine and others. Thought and behavior can be affected by virtually any substance. Common agents include the anticholinergics, alcohol, narcotics, hydrocarbons, and many others. Aspirin, corrosives, and hydrocarbons can irritate or destroy the gastrointestinal system. Acetaminophen can cause liver necrosis and eventually liver failure.

POSSIBLE INDICATORS OF INGESTED POISONING IN CHILDREN

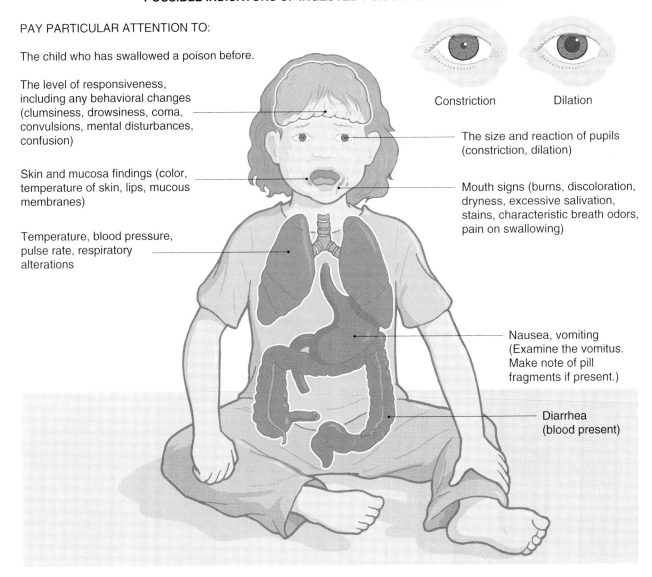

PAY PARTICULAR ATTENTION TO:

The child who has swallowed a poison before.

The level of responsiveness, including any behavioral changes (clumsiness, drowsiness, coma, convulsions, mental disturbances, confusion)

Skin and mucosa findings (color, temperature of skin, lips, mucous membranes)

Temperature, blood pressure, pulse rate, respiratory alterations

Constriction   Dilation

The size and reaction of pupils (constriction, dilation)

Mouth signs (burns, discoloration, dryness, excessive salivation, stains, characteristic breath odors, pain on swallowing)

Nausea, vomiting (Examine the vomitus. Make note of pill fragments if present.)

Diarrhea (blood present)

FIGURE 2-35   Possible indicators of ingested poisoning in children.

Management Although scenarios vary, take these general steps in managing a pediatric poisoning patient:

Responsive poisoning patient

- Administer oxygen.
- Contact medical direction and/or the poison control center.
- Consider the need for activated charcoal.
- Transport. (Be sure to take all pills, substances, and containers to the hospital.)
- Monitor the patient continuously in case the child suddenly becomes unresponsive.

Unresponsive poisoning patient

- Assure a patent airway. Apply suctioning, if necessary.
- Administer oxygen.
- Be prepared to provide artificial ventilations if respiratory failure or cardiac arrest is present.
- Contact medical direction and/or the poison control center.
- Transport.
- Monitor the patient continuously, and rule out trauma as a cause of altered mental status.

For more on poisonings and toxic exposure, see Volume 3 Chapter 8.

TRAUMA EMERGENCIES

Trauma is the number one cause of death in infants and children. Most pediatric injuries result from blunt trauma. As previously mentioned, children have thinner body walls that allow forces to be more readily transmitted to body contents, increasing the possibility of injury to internal tissues and organs. If you serve in an urban area, you can expect to see a higher incidence of penetrating trauma, mostly intentional and mostly from gunfire or knife wounds. There is also a significant incidence of penetrating trauma outside the cities, mostly unintentional from hunting accidents and agricultural accidents.

MECHANISMS OF INJURY

Although pediatric patients can be injured in the same way as adults, children tend to be more susceptible to certain types of injuries than grownups. The following categories describe the most common mechanisms of injury among infants and children.

Falls

Falls are the single most common cause of injury in children (Figure 2-36). Fortunately, serious injury or death from accidental falls is relatively uncommon unless from a significant height. Falls from bicycles account for a significant number of injuries. The incidence of head injuries is declining, primarily because of bicycle safety helmets.

Motor Vehicle Collisions

Approximately 25,000 American children die annually from trauma. Approximately one-third of these die from motor vehicle collisions, making motor vehicle collisions the leading cause of traumatic death in children. In addition, motor vehicle collisions are the leading cause of permanent brain injury and the new-onset of epilepsy. Improperly seated children are at increased risk of sustaining injury or death from automobile air bags when they deploy (Figure 2-37). This is an area where EMS prevention strategies can make a difference. Public education programs on drunk driving, safe driving, air bags, and proper use of children's car seats can be a major focus of EMS personnel. Some states have given paramedics the ability to issue citations for persons who do not correctly buckle their children or place them in child safety seats.

> **Content Review**
>
> **MOST COMMON PEDIATRIC MECHANISMS OF INJURY**
> - Falls
> - Motor vehicle collisions
> - Car vs. pedestrian collisions
> - Drownings and near-drownings
> - Penetrating injuries
> - Burns
> - Physical abuse

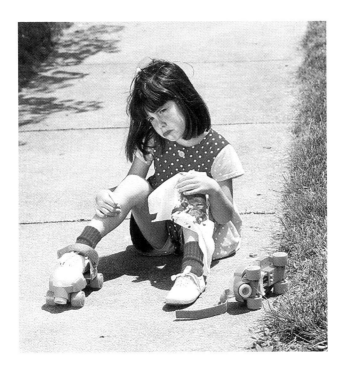

FIGURE 2-36 Falls are the most common cause of injury in young children.

Car vs. Pedestrian Injuries

Car versus child pedestrian injuries are more common in cities where children play close to the street. Car/pedestrian injuries are a particularly lethal form of trauma in children, as their short stature tends to push them down under the car. There are two phases of injury in car versus pedestrian accidents. The first group of injuries occur when the auto contacts the child. Because of the energy present, the child may be propelled away from the car or pushed down underneath the car. It is at this point that the second group of injuries occur as the child contacts the

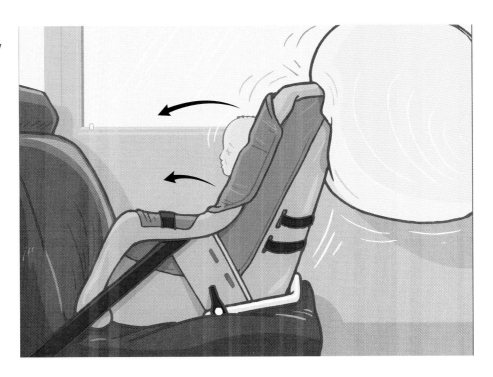

FIGURE 2-37 A deploying airbag can propel a child safety seat back into the vehicle's seat, seriously injuring the child secured in it.

ground or other objects. Head and spinal injuries often occur with the secondary impact. The best treatment for car versus child pedestrian accidents is prevention. This too can be a major area of emphasis for prehospital prevention programs.

Drownings and Near-Drownings

Drowning is the third leading cause of death in children between birth and 4 years of age, with approximately 2,000 deaths occurring in the United States annually. The term *drowning* is used to describe deaths that occur within 24 hours of the accident. *Near-drowning* refers to injuries where the child did not die or where the death occurred more than 24 hours after the injury. Many children who do not die from drowning suffer severe and irreversible brain injuries as a result of anoxia. Approximately 20 to 25 percent of near-drowning survivors exhibit severe neurological deficits. The outcomes are better when the water is cold, as the body's protective mechanisms protect against brain injury.

Again, as with the other injury processes, the best treatment is prevention. EMS systems, in conjunction with local building inspectors, can inspect pools for safety. A pool should be fenced off with a gate that closes automatically. Essential rescue equipment (pole, life saver) should be immediately available and the local emergency number posted. The best time for drowning prevention is late spring and early summer. Encourage parents to enroll their children in water safety classes as soon as possible.

Penetrating Injuries

Until 20 years ago, penetrating injuries in children were fairly uncommon. Since then, an increase in violent crime (although violent crime rates have both risen and fallen within that period) has resulted in an increasing number of children sustaining penetrating trauma. Stab wounds and firearm injuries account for approximately 10–15 percent of all pediatric trauma admissions. The risk of death increases with age. Children are usually innocent victims of crimes perpetrated against adults. However, children are sometimes the intended victims of gunfire and stabbings, as in the shootings that have taken place in schools.

It is important to remember that visual inspection of external injuries does not provide adequate evaluation of internal injuries. This is especially true with high-energy, high-velocity weapons that can cause massive internal injury with only minimal external trauma.

Paramedics can play a major role in preventing pediatric shootings. During public education and community service programs, it is prudent to talk about gun safety, including such measures as using trigger locks or locking weapons in places where children cannot reach them. You might emphasize the fact that children have an uncanny ability to find and gain access to weapons that adults think they have hidden and secured. As with many other pediatric emergencies, the best treatment is prevention.

Burns

Burn injuries are the leading cause of accidental death in the home for children under 14 years of age. Children can sustain both burn injuries and smoke inhalation in house fires. Unsupervised children with matches or cigarette lighters are responsible for many fires that result in pediatric injury.

Fire prevention programs are a major area of emphasis for fire departments. The importance of smoke detectors cannot be overemphasized. Citizens should be encouraged to change the batteries in their smoke detectors when the clock is moved backwards or forwards for daylight savings time. Many fire departments

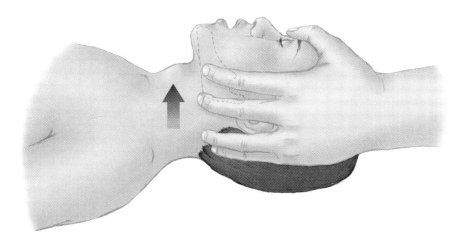

FIGURE 2-38 In the pediatric trauma victim, use the combination of jaw-thrust/spine stabilization maneuver to open the airway.

and EMS systems replace smoke detector batteries as a part of their fire prevention program. Part of the fire prevention program should be specifically directed at children. It is especially important to teach children how to exit their house in case fire erupts.

Physical Abuse

Unfortunately, children are at risk for physical abuse by adults and older children. Factors leading to child abuse are known to include social phenomena such as poverty, domestic disturbances, younger-aged parents, substance abuse, and community violence. Paramedics are often the first members of the health care team to come into contact with the abused child. It is very important to not accuse the parents or to confront a suspected abuser. Instead, document all pertinent findings, treatments, and interventions and report these to the proper authorities. (Child abuse is discussed in more detail later in this chapter.)

SPECIAL CONSIDERATIONS

As mentioned previously, children are not small adults. You should keep this in mind and modify treatment accordingly. Specific items to consider include the following:

Airway Control

Special considerations are related to characteristics of the child's airway. These include the following:

- Maintain in-line stabilization in neutral instead of the sniffing position to prevent possible pinching of the trachea (Figure 2-38).
- Administer 100% oxygen to all trauma patients.
- Maintain a patent airway with suctioning and the jaw-thrust maneuver.
- Be prepared to assist ineffective respirations. Remember that airway pressures can be high in children and it may be necessary to depress the pop-off valve to ventilate the child adequately.

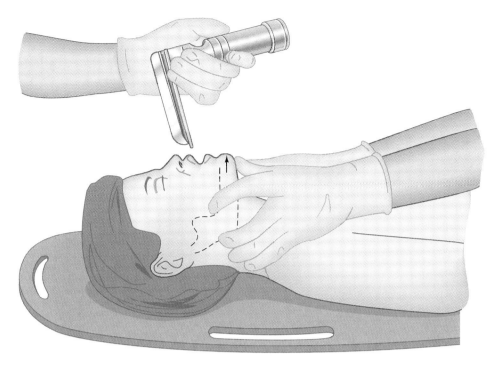

FIGURE 2-39   Simultaneous cervical spine immobilization and intubation in a pediatric patient.

- Intubate the child when the airway cannot be maintained, while simultaneously maintaining cervical spine stabilization (Figure 2-39).
- A gastric tube should be placed following intubation to decompress the stomach.
- Needle cricothyrotomy is rarely indicated for traumatic upper airway obstruction.

Immobilization

Use appropriate-sized pediatric immobilization equipment including:

- Rigid cervical collar
- Towel or blanket roll
- Child safety seat
- Pediatric immobilization device
- Vest-type device (KED)
- Short wooden backboard
- Straps and cravats
- Tape
- Padding

Keep infants, toddlers, and preschoolers supine with the cervical spine in a neutral in-line position by placing padding from the shoulders to the hips. (Review the discussion of pediatric immobilization earlier in this chapter.)

Fluid Management

Management of the airway and breathing takes priority over management of circulation, as circulatory compromise is less common in children than in adults. When obtaining vascular access, remember the following:

- If possible, insert a large-bore intravenous catheter into a peripheral vein.
- Do not delay transport to gain venous access.
- Intraosseous access in children less than 6 years of age is an alternative when a peripheral IV cannot be obtained.
- Administer an initial fluid bolus of 20 mL/kg of lactated Ringer's solution or normal saline
- Reassess the vital signs and re-bolus with another 20 mL/kg if there is no improvement.
- If improvement does not occur after the second bolus, there is likely to be a significant blood loss that may require surgical intervention. Rapid transport is essential.

Pediatric Analgesia and Sedation

An often overlooked aspect of prehospital pediatric care is pain control. Many pediatric injuries are painful and analgesics are indicated. These include burns, long bone fractures, dislocations, and others. Unless there is a contraindication, pediatric patients should receive analgesics. Commonly used analgesics include meperidene, morphine, and fentanyl. It is best to avoid using the synthetic analgesics (e.g., butorphanol [Stadol], nalbuphine [Nubain]) as their effects on children are unpredictable. Also, certain pediatric emergencies may benefit from sedation. These include such problems as penetrating eye injuries, prolonged rescue from entrapment in machinery, cardioversion, and other painful procedures. Always consult medical direction if you feel pediatric analgesia or sedation may be indicated.

Traumatic Brain Injury

Children, because of the relatively large size of their head and weak neck muscles, are at increased risk for traumatic brain injury. These injuries can be devastating and are often fatal. Early recognition and aggressive management can reduce both morbidity and mortality. Pediatric head injuries can be classified as follows:

- Mild – Glasgow coma score is 13–15
- Moderate – Glasgow coma score is 9–12
- Severe – Glasgow coma score is less than or equal to 8

Traumatic head injuries can cause intracranial bleeding or swelling. This ultimately results in an increase in intracranial pressure. The signs of increased intracranial pressure can be subtle. They include:

- Elevated blood pressure
- Bradycardia
- Rapid, deep respirations progressing to slow, deep respirations
- Bulging fontanelle in infants

Increased intracranial pressure will eventually lead to herniation of a portion of the brain through the foramen magnum. This is an ominous development that is often associated with irreversible injury. Signs and symptoms of herniation include:

- Asymmetrical pupils
- Decorticate posturing
- Decerebrate posturing

Specific management of traumatic head injuries in children is similar to that for adults. As a rule, follow these steps.

- Administer a high concentration of oxygen for mild to moderate head injuries.
- Intubate children with a Glasgow coma score of less than or equal to 8 (severe head injury) and ventilate at a normal rate with 100% oxygen.
- Consider using intravenous or tracheal lidocaine prior to intubation to blunt the rise in intracranial pressure that often occurs in association with this procedure.
- Consider rapid sequence intubation (RSI) for children with a Glasgow coma score of less than or equal to 8 who have too much muscle tone to allow endotracheal intubation.

Consider hyperventilation if there is a deterioration in the child's condition as evidenced by asymmetric pupils, active seizures, or neurological posturing. Children with traumatic head injuries do best at facilities that treat a great number of children and who have pediatric neurosurgeons on staff. Consider diverting to a pediatric trauma facility if a moderate or severe traumatic head injury is present.

SPECIFIC INJURIES

As previously mentioned, more pediatric patients die of trauma than of any other cause. Statistics reveal that nearly 50 percent of these deaths occur within the first hour of injury. The quick arrival of EMS at the scene can literally mean the difference between life and death for a child. Although management of trauma is basically the same for children as adults, anatomical and physiological differences cause pediatric patients to have different patterns of injury.

Head, Face, and Neck

The majority of children who sustain multiple trauma will suffer associated head and/or neck injuries. As previously mentioned, the larger relative mass of the head and lack of neck muscle strength provide for increased momentum in acceleration-deceleration injuries and a greater stress on the cervical spine. The fulcrum of cervical mobility in the younger child is at the C2–C3 level. As a result, nearly 60 to 70 percent of pediatric fractures occur in C1–C2.

Injuries to the head are the most common cause of death in pediatric trauma victims. School-age children tend to sustain head injuries from bicycle accidents, falls from trees, or auto-pedestrian accidents. Older children most commonly suffer head injuries from sporting events. Heads injuries in all age groups may result from abuse.

In treating head injuries, remember that diffuse injuries are common in children, while focal injuries are rare. Because the skull is softer and more compliant in children than in adults, brain injuries occur more readily in infants and young children. Because of open fontanelles and sutures, infants up to an average age of 16 months may be more tolerant to an increase in intracranial pressure and can have delayed signs. (Keep this fact in mind when taking the history of children in the 1-month to 2-year age range.)

Children also frequently injure their faces. The most common facial injuries are lacerations secondary to falls. Young children are very clumsy when they first start walking. A fall onto a sharp object, such as the corner of a coffee table, can result in a laceration. Older children sustain dental injuries in falls from bicycles, skateboard accidents, fights, and sports activities.

Spinal injuries in children are not as common as in adults. However, as noted earlier, a child's proportionally larger and heavier head makes the cervical spine vulnerable to injury. Any time a child sustains a severe head injury, always assume that a neck injury may also be present.

Chest and Abdomen

Most injuries to the chest and abdomen result from blunt trauma. As noted earlier, infants and young children lack the rigid rib cages of adults. Therefore, they suffer fewer rib fractures and more intrathoracic injuries. Likewise, their relatively undeveloped abdominal musculature affords minimal protection to the viscera.

Because of the high mortality associated with blunt trauma, children with significant blunt abdominal or chest trauma should be transported immediately to a pediatric trauma center with appropriate care provided en route.

Children tend to develop pulmonary contusions, sometimes massive, following blunt trauma to the chest.

Injuries to the Chest Chest injuries are the second most common cause of pediatric trauma deaths. Because of the compliance of the chest wall, severe intrathoracic injury can be present without signs of external injury. Pneumothorax and hemothorarax can occur in the pediatric patient, especially if the mechanism of injury was a motor vehicle collision. Tension pneumothorax can also occur in children. The condition is poorly tolerated by pediatric patients and a needle thoracostomy may be lifesaving. Tension pneumothorax presents with the following signs and symptoms:

- Diminished breath sounds over the affected lung
- Shift of the trachea to the opposite side
- A progressive decrease in ventilatory compliance

Keep in mind that children with cardiac tamponade may have no physical signs of tamponade other then hypotension. Also remember that flail chest is an uncommon injury in children. When noted without a significant mechanism of injury, suspect child abuse.

Injuries to the Abdomen Significant blunt trauma to the abdomen can result in injury to the spleen or liver. In fact, the spleen is the most commonly injured organ in children. Signs and symptoms of a splenic injury include tenderness in the left upper quadrant of the abdomen, abrasions on the abdomen, and hematoma of the abdominal wall. Symptoms of liver injury include right upper quadrant abdominal pain and/or right lower chest pain. Both splenic and hepatic injuries can cause life-threatening internal hemorrhage.

In treating blunt abdominal trauma, keep in mind the small size of the pediatric abdomen. Be certain to palpate only one quadrant at a time. In cases of both chest and abdominal trauma, treat for shock with positioning, fluids, and maintenance of body temperature.

Extremities

Extremity injuries in children are typically limited to fractures and lacerations. Children rarely sustain amputations and other serious extremity injuries. An exception includes farm children who may become entangled in agricultural equipment.

The most common injuries are fractures, usually resulting from falls (Figure 2-40). Because children have more flexible bones than adults, they tend to have incomplete fractures such as **bend fractures, buckle fractures,** and **greenstick fractures.**

✱ **bend fractures** fractures characterized by angulation and deformity in the bone without an obvious break.

✱ **buckle fractures** fractures characterized by a raised or bulging projection at the fracture site.

✱ **greenstick fractures** fractures characterized by an incomplete break in the bone.

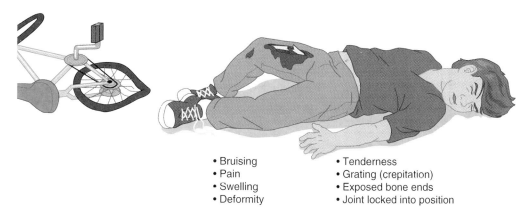

- Bruising
- Pain
- Swelling
- Deformity

- Tenderness
- Grating (crepitation)
- Exposed bone ends
- Joint locked into position

FIGURE 2-40   Signs and symptoms of a fracture in a child who has fallen off a bike.

In younger children, the bone growth plates have not yet closed. Some types of growth plate fractures can lead to permanent disability if not managed correctly.

Whenever indicated, perform splinting in order to decrease pain and prevent further injury and/or blood loss. In rare cases, the PSAG may be useful in unstable pelvic fractures with hypotension.

Burns

Burns are the second leading cause of death in children. They are the leading cause of accidental death in the home for children under 14. Burns may be chemical, thermal, or electrical. The most common type of burn injury encountered by EMS personnel is scalding. Children can scald themselves by pulling hot liquids off tables or stoves. In cases of abuse, they can be scalded by immersion in hot water.

Estimation of the burn surface area is slightly different for children than for adults (Figure 2-41). In adults, the "rule of nines" assigns 9 percent of the body surface area (BSA) to each of 11 body regions: the entire head and neck; the anterior chest; the anterior abdomen; the posterior chest; the lower back (posterior abdomen); the anterior surface of each lower extremity; the posterior surface of each lower extremity; and the entirety of each upper extremity. The remaining 1 percent is assigned to the genitalia.

In a child, the head accounts for a larger percentage of BSA while the legs make up a smaller percentage. So for children the rule of nines is modified to take away 8 percent from the lower extremities (2 percent from the front and 2 percent from the back of each leg) plus the 1 percent assigned to the adult genitalia. This 9 percent that is taken from the lower part of the body is reassigned to the head. So whereas the adult's entire head and neck are counted as 9 percent, in the child the anterior head and neck count as 9 percent and the posterior head and neck count as another 9 percent.

You can also use the child's palm as a guide (the "rule of palm"). The palm equals about 1 percent of the body surface area. You can calculate a burn area by estimating how many palm areas it equals. Usually, the rule of nines works best for more extensive burns and the rule of palm for less extensive ones.

Management considerations for pediatric burn patients include the following:

- Provide prompt management of the airway, as swelling can develop rapidly.
- If intubation is required, you may need to use an endotracheal tube up to two sizes smaller than normal.
- Thermally burned children are very susceptible to hypothermia. Be sure to maintain body heat.

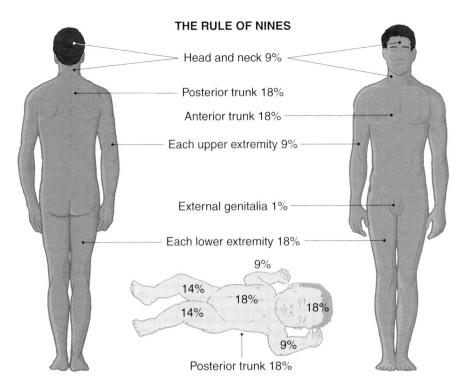

THE RULE OF NINES

Head and neck 9%

Posterior trunk 18%

Anterior trunk 18%

Each upper extremity 9%

External genitalia 1%

Each lower extremity 18%

9%

14%

18%

14%

18%

9%

Posterior trunk 18%

FIGURE 2-41   The rule of nines helps to estimate the extent of a burn in adults and children. Note the modifications for the child.

- When treating serious electrical burn patients, suspect musculoskeletal injuries and perform spinal immobilization.

SUDDEN INFANT DEATH SYNDROME (SIDS)

* **sudden infant death syndrome (SIDS)** illness of unknown etiology that occurs during the first year of life, with the peak at ages 2–4 months.

Sudden infant death syndrome (SIDS) is defined as the sudden death of an infant during the first year of life from an illness of unknown etiology. The incidence of SIDS in the United States is approximately 2 deaths per 1,000 births. SIDS is the leading cause of death between 2 weeks and 1 year of age. It is responsible for a significant number of deaths between 1 month and 6 months, with peak incidence occurring at 2–4 months.

SIDS occurs most frequently in the fall and winter months. It tends to be more common in males than in females. It is more prevalent in premature and low birthweight infants, in infants of young mothers, and in infants whose mothers did not receive prenatal care. Infants of mothers who used cocaine, methadone, or heroin during pregnancy are at greater risk. Occasionally, a mild upper respiratory infection will be reported prior to the death. SIDS is not caused by external suffocation from blankets or pillows. Neither is it related to allergies to cow's milk or regurgitation and aspiration of stomach contents. It is not thought to be hereditary.

Current theories vary about the etiology of SIDS. Some authorities feel it may result from an immature respiratory center in the brain that leads the child to simply stop breathing. Others think there may be an airway obstruction in the posterior pharynx as a result of pharyngeal relaxation during sleep, a hypermobile mandible, or an enlarged tongue. Studies strongly link SIDS to a prone sleeping position. Soft bedding, waterbed mattresses, smoking in the home, and/or an overheated environment are other potential associations. A small percentage of SIDS may be abuse related.

Although research into SIDS continues, the American Academy of Pediatrics suggests that infants be placed supine unless medical conditions prevent this. In addition, the academy urges parents or caregivers to avoid placing infants in overheated environments, overwrapping them with too many clothes or blankets, smoking before and after pregnancy, and filling the crib with soft bedding.

Assessment Infants suffering SIDS have similar physical findings. From an external standpoint, there is a normal state of nutrition and hydration. The skin may be mottled. There are often frothy, occasionally blood-tinged, fluids in and around the mouth and nostrils. Vomitus may be present. Occasionally, the infant may be in an unusual position as a result of muscle spasm or high activity at the time of death. Common findings noted at autopsy include intrathoracic petechiae (small hemorrhages) in 90 percent of cases. There is often associated pulmonary congestion and edema. Sometimes, stomach contents are found in the trachea. Microscopic examination of the trachea often reveals the presence of inflammatory changes.

Management The immediate needs of the family with a SIDS baby are many. Unless the infant is obviously dead, undertake active and aggressive care of the infant to assure the family that everything possible is being done. A first responder or other personnel should be assigned to assist the parents and to explain the procedures. At all points, use the baby's name.

After arrival at the hospital, direct management at the parents or caregivers, since nothing can be done for the child. Allow the family to see the dead child. Expect a normal grief reaction. Initially, there may be shock, disbelief, and denial. Other times, the parents or caregivers may express anger, rage, hostility, blame, or guilt. Often, there is a feeling of inadequacy as well as helplessness, confusion, and fear. The grief process is likely to last for years. SIDS has major long-term effects on family relations. It may also affect you, the on-scene paramedic. If so, do not be reluctant to request a Critical Incident Stress Debriefing.

In SIDS, active and aggressive care of the infant should continue until delivery to the emergency room unless the infant is obviously dead.

At all points in a SIDS case, use the baby's name when speaking with parents or caregivers.

CHILD ABUSE AND NEGLECT

A tragic truth is that some people cause physical and psychological harm to children, either through intentional abuse or through intentional or unintentional neglect. In fact, child abuse is the second leading cause of death in infants less than 6 months of age. An estimated 2,000 to 5,000 children die each year as a result of abuse or neglect.

There are several characteristics common to abused children. Often, the child is seen as "special" and different from others. Premature infants and twins stand a higher risk of abuse than other children. Many abused children are less than 5 years of age. Physically and mentally handicapped children as well as those with other special needs are at greater risk. So are uncommunicative (autistic) children. Boys are more often abused than girls. A child who is not what the parents wanted (e.g., the "wrong" gender) is at increased risk of abuse, too.

PERPETRATORS OF ABUSE OR NEGLECT

Abuse or neglect may be instigated by a parent, a legal guardian, or a foster parent. It can be carried out by a person, an institution, or an agency or program entrusted with custody. Abuse or neglect can also result from the actions of a caretaker, such as a baby-sitter or a "nanny."

The person who abuses or neglects a child can come from any geographic, religious, ethnic, racial, occupational, educational, or socioeconomic background. Despite their diversity, people who abuse children tend to share certain traits. The abuser is usually a parent or a full-time caregiver. When the mother spends the majority of the time with the child, she is the parent most frequently identified as the abuser. Most abusers were abused themselves as children.

Three conditions can alert you to the potential for abuse. They include:

- A parent or adult who seems capable of abuse—especially one who exhibits evasive or hostile behavior
- A child in one of the high-risk categories
- The presence of a crisis, particularly financial stress, marital or relationship stress, or physical illness in a parent or child

TYPES OF ABUSE

Child abuse can take several forms. These forms include:

- Psychological abuse
- Physical abuse
- Sexual abuse
- Neglect (either physical or emotional)

Abused children suffer every imaginable kind of mistreatment. They are battered with fists, belts, broom handles, hair brushes, baseball bats, electric cords, and any other objects that can be used as weapons (Figure 2-42). They are locked

FIGURE 2-42 An abused child. Note the marks on the legs associated with beatings with an electric wire. The burns on the buttocks are from submersion in hot water. (Courtesy of Scott and White Hospital and Clinic.)

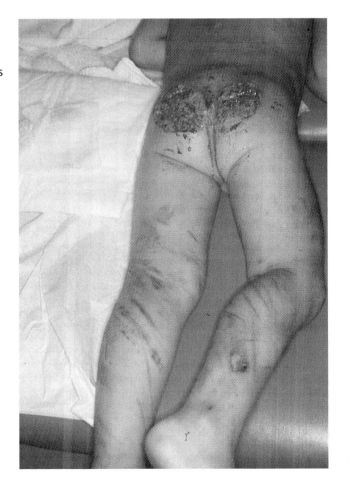

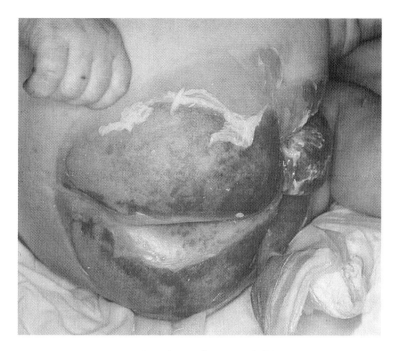

FIGURE 2-43   Burn injury from placing a child's buttocks in hot water as a punishment. (Courtesy of Scott and White Hospital and Clinic.)

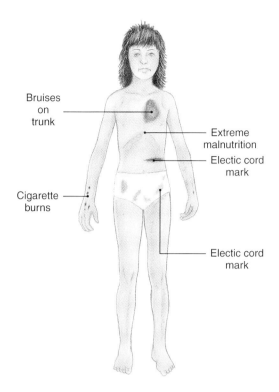

Bruises on trunk

Extreme malnutrition

Electic cord mark

Cigarette burns

Electic cord mark

FIGURE 2-44   The stigmata of child abuse.

in closets, denied food, or deprived of access to a toilet. They are intentionally burned or scalded with anything from hot water to cigarette butts to open flames (Figure 2-43). They are severely shaken, thrown into cribs, pushed down stairs, or shoved into walls. Some are shot, stabbed, or suffocated.

Sexual abuse ranges from adults exposing themselves to children to overt sexual acts to sexual torture. Sexual abuse can occur at any age, and the victims may be either male or female. Generally, the sexual abuser is someone the child knows and, perhaps, trusts. Stepchildren or adopted children face a greater risk for sexual abuse than biological children. Cases in which sexual abuse causes physical harm may get reported. Other cases, especially those with emotional and minor physical injury, may go undetected.

ASSESSMENT OF THE POTENTIALLY ABUSED OR NEGLECTED CHILD

Signs of abuse or neglect can be startling (Figure 2-44). As a guide, the following findings should trigger a high index of suspicion:

- Any obvious or suspected fractures in a child under 2 years of age
- Multiple injuries in various stages of healing, especially burns and bruises (Figure 2-45)
- More injuries than usually seen in children of the same age or size

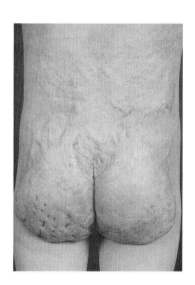

FIGURE 2-45   The effects of child abuse, both physical and mental, can last a lifetime. (Courtesy of Scott and White Hospital and Clinic.)

- Injuries scattered on many areas of the body
- Bruises or burns in patterns that suggest intentional infliction
- Increased intracranial pressure in an infant
- Suspected intra-abdominal trauma in a young child
- Any injury that does not fit with the description of the cause given

Information in the medical history may also raise the index of suspicion. Examples include:

- A history that does not match the nature or severity of the injury
- Vague parental accounts or accounts that change during the interview
- Accusations that the child injured himself intentionally
- Delay in seeking help
- Child dressed inappropriately for the situation
- Revealing comments by bystanders, especially siblings

Suspect child neglect if you spot any of the following conditions:

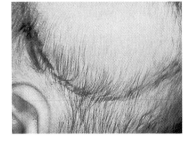

FIGURE 2-46 Child neglect from a lack of appropriate medical care.

- Extreme malnutrition
- Multiple insect bites
- Long-standing skin infections
- Extreme lack of cleanliness
- Verbal or social skills far below those you would expect for a child of similar age and background
- Lack of appropriate medical care (Figure 2-46)

MANAGEMENT OF THE POTENTIALLY ABUSED OR NEGLECTED CHILD

In cases of child abuse or neglect, the goals of management include appropriate treatment of injuries, protection of the child from further abuse, and notification of proper authorities. You should obtain as much information as possible, in a nonjudgmental manner. Document all findings or statements in the patient report. Don't "cross-examine" the parents—this job belongs to the police or other authorities. Try to be supportive toward the parents, especially if it helps you to transport the child to the hospital. Remember: Never leave transport to the alleged abuser.

Upon arrival at the emergency department, report your suspicions to the appropriate personnel. Complete the patient report and all available documentation at this time, since delay may inhibit accurate recall of data.

Child abuse and neglect are particularly stressful aspects of emergency medical services. You must recognize and deal with your feelings, perhaps taking them up at a Critical Incident Stress Debriefing.

Never leave transport of an abused child to an alleged abuser.

In many states, prehospital personnel are required by law to report suspected child abuse or neglect to the appropriate authorities.

RESOURCES FOR ABUSE AND NEGLECT

You can contact your local child protection agency for additional information on child abuse. Consider taking a course in the recognition of child abuse and neglect. These are often offered by children's hospitals. The Internet has several sites that provide up-to-date information on child abuse.

INFANTS AND CHILDREN WITH SPECIAL NEEDS

For most of human history, infants and children with devastating congenital conditions or diseases either died or remained confined to a hospital. In recent decades, however, medical technology has lowered infant mortality rates and allowed a greater number of children with special needs to live at home. (See more about home care in Chapter 6.) Some of these infants and children include:

- Premature babies
- Infants and children with lung disease, heart disease, or neurological disorders
- Infants and children with chronic diseases, such as cystic fibrosis, asthma, childhood cancers, cerebral palsy, and others
- Infants and children with altered functions from birth (Examples include cerebral palsy, spina bifida, and other congenital birth defects.)

In caring for these children, family members receive education relative to the special equipment required by the infant or child. Even so, they may feel a great deal of apprehension when care moves from the hospital to the home. As a result, they may summon EMS at the first indication of trouble. This is especially true in the initial weeks following discharge.

COMMON HOME-CARE DEVICES

Devices you might commonly find in the home include tracheostomy tubes, apnea monitors, home artificial ventilators, central intravenous lines, gastric feeding tubes, gastrostomy tubes, and shunts. In treating children with special needs, remember that the parents and caregivers are often very knowledgeable about their children and the devices that sustain their lives. Listen to them. They know their children better than anybody else.

Tracheostomy Tubes

Patients who are on prolonged home ventilators or who have chronic respiratory problems may have surgically placed tubes in the inferior trachea (Figure 2-47). A **tracheostomy** (trach) tube may be utilized as a temporary or a permanent device. Although there are various types of tubes, you might expect some common complications. They include:

* **tracheostomy** a surgical incision in the neck held open by a metal or plastic tube.

- Obstruction, usually by a mucous plug
- Site bleeding, either from the tube or around the tube
- An air leakage
- A dislodged tube
- Infection—a condition that will worsen an already impaired breathing ability

Management steps for a patient with a tracheostomy include:

- Maintaining an open airway
- Suctioning the tube, as needed
- Allowing the patient to remain in a position of comfort, if possible
- Administering oxygen in cases of respiratory distress

FIGURE 2-47 Tracheostomy tubes. Top: plastic tube. Bottom: metal tube with inner cannula.

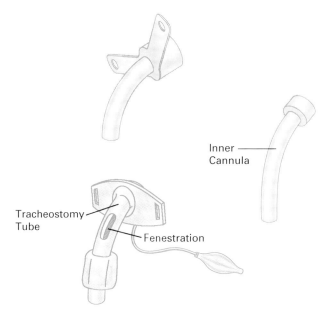

- Assisting ventilations in cases of respiratory failure/arrest by:
  – Intubating orally in the absence of an upper airway obstruction
  – Intubating via the **stoma** if there is an upper airway obstruction
- Transporting the patient to the hospital

Apnea Monitors

Apnea monitors are used to alert parents or caregivers to the cessation of breathing in an infant, especially a premature infant. Some types of monitors signal changes in heart rate, such as bradycardia or tachycardia. They operate via pads attached to the baby's chest and connected to the monitor by wires. If the device does not detect a breath within a specific time frame or if the infant's heart rate is too slow or too fast, an alarm will sound.

When an apnea monitor is placed in a home, the parents are typically instructed on what to do if the alarm sounds (stimulate the child, provide artificial respirations, and so on). If these fail, EMS may be summoned. Also, nervous parents who have just brought a baby home on an apnea monitor may panic the first couple of times the alarm sounds and call 911. Be patient and kind while instructing them on what to do when the alarm sounds.

Home Artificial Ventilators

Various configurations exist for home ventilators. Demand ventilators sense rate and quality of a patient's respiration as well as several other parameters, including pulse oximetry. They typically respond to pre-set limits. Other devices provide a constant PEEP (positive end-expiratory pressure) and a set oxygen concentration for the patient.

Two complications commonly result in EMS calls: (1) a device's mechanical failure and (2) shortages of energy during an electrical failure. Treatment typically includes:

- Maintaining an open airway
- Administering artificial ventilations via an appropriately sized BVM with oxygen
- Transporting the patient to a hospital until the home ventilator is working

✱ stoma a permanent surgical opening in the neck through which the patient breathes.

Most parents who have infants on apnea monitors have received training in pediatric CPR.

Central Intravenous Lines

Children who require long-term IV therapy will often have central lines placed into the superior vena cava near the heart. In cases where IV therapy is necessary for only several weeks, PIC (percutaneous intravenous catheter) lines may be placed in the arm and threaded into the superior vena cava. Otherwise the lines are placed through subclavian venipuncture. **Central IV lines** are commonly used to administer intravenous nutrition. antibiotics, or chemotherapy for cancer.

Possible complications for central IV lines include:

* Cracked line
* Infection, either at the site or at more distal aspects of the line
* Loss of patency—e.g., clotting
* Hemorrhage, which can be considerable
* Air embolism

✱ **central IV line** intravenous line placed into the superior vena cava for the administration of long-term fluid therapy.

Emergency medical care steps include control of any bleeding through direct pressure. If a large amount of air is in the line, try to withdraw it with a syringe. If this fails, clamp the line and transport. In cases of a cracked line, place a clamp between the crack and the patient. If the patient exhibits an altered mental status following the cracked line, position the child on the left side with head down. Transport the child to the hospital as quickly as possible.

Gastric Feeding Tubes and Gastrostomy Tubes

Children who are not capable of swallowing or eating receive nutrition through either a gastric feeding tube or a gastrostomy tube. (A gastric feeding tube is placed through the nostrils into the stomach. A gastrostomy tube is placed through the abdominal wall directly into the stomach.) These special devices are commonly used in disorders of the digestive system or in situations in which the developmental ability of the patient hinders feeding. Food consists of nutritious liquids.

Possible emergency complications include:

* Bleeding at the site
* Dislodged tube
* Respiratory distress, particularly if a tube feeding backs up into the esophagus and is aspirated into the trachea and lungs
* In the case of diabetics, altered mental status due to missed feedings

Emergency medical care involves supporting the ABCs, including possible suctioning and administration of supplemental oxygen. Patients should be transported to a definitive care facility, either in a sitting position or lying on the right side with the head elevated. The goal is to reduce the risk of aspiration, a serious condition.

Shunts

A **shunt** is a surgical connection that runs from the brain to the abdomen. It removes excess cerebrospinal fluid from the brain through drainage. A subcutaneous reservoir is usually palpable on one side of the patient's head. A pathological rise in intracranial pressure, secondary to a blocked shunt, is a primary complication. Shunt failure may also result when the shunt's connections separate, usually because of a child's growth.

✱ **shunt** surgical connection that runs from the brain to the abdomen for the purpose of draining excess cerebrospinal fluid, thus preventing increased intracranial pressure.

Cases of shunt failure present as altered mental status. The patient may exhibit drowsiness, respiratory distress, or the classic signs of pupil dysfunction or posturing. Be aware that an altered mental status may be caused by infection—a distinction to be made in a hospital setting.

Care steps involve maintenance of an open airway, administration of ventilations as needed, and immediate transport. Shunt failures require correction in the operating room, where the cerebrospinal fluid can be drained or, in rare cases, an infection identified and treated.

GENERAL ASSESSMENT AND MANAGEMENT PRACTICES

Remember that pediatric patients with special needs require the same assessment as other patients. Always evaluate the airway, breathing, and circulation. (Recall that in the initial assessment, "disability" refers to patient's neurological status—not to the child's special need.) If you discover life-threatening conditions in the initial assessment, begin appropriate interventions. Keep in mind that the child's special need is often an ongoing process. In most cases, you should concentrate on the acute problem.

During the assessment, ask pertinent questions of the patient, parent, or caregiver such as: "What unusual situation caused you to call for an ambulance?" As already mentioned, the parent or caregiver is usually very knowledgeable about the patient's condition.

In most cases, the physical examination is essentially the same as with other patients. It is important to explain everything that is being done, even if the patient does not seem to understand. Do not be distracted by the special equipment. Be aware of the help that the patient, parent, or caregiver may be able to provide in handling home-care devices.

In managing patients with special needs, try to keep several thoughts in mind.

- Avoid using the term "disability" (in reference to the child's special need). Instead, think of the patient's many abilities.
- Never assume that the patient cannot understand what you are saying.
- Involve the parents, caregivers, or the patient, if appropriate, in treatment. They manage the illness or congenital condition on a daily basis.
- Treat the patient with a special need with the same respect as any other patient.

SUMMARY

Pediatric emergencies can be stressful for both you and the adults responsible for the child's well-being. Most pediatric emergencies result from trauma, respiratory distress, ingestion of poisons, or febrile seizure activity. In addition, you must always be on the lookout for signs and symptoms of child abuse or neglect. The approach and management of pediatric emergencies must be modified for the age and size of the child. Certain skills generally considered routine, such as IV administration, become difficult in the pediatric patient because of size and other factors. It is important to remember that children are not "small adults." They have special considerations—both physical and emotional—that must be managed accordingly.

YOU MAKE THE CALL

Dispatch sends you to a residence in an affluent neighborhood. The call reports that "a child is hurt and bleeding." Upon arrival at the scene, the parents greet you and your crew with controlled anger. Apparently, the neighbors dialed 911 when they heard a child's loud cries coming from the house. The mother tells you that her 24-month-old son fell off the kitchen counter while trying to reach the cookie jar. "He's always climbing after something," she snaps. "I can't watch him 24 hours a day."

As you listen, the child remains strangely quiet. He avoids all eye contact and does not seek comfort from either his mother or father. You observe that a scalp laceration is bleeding profusely. You also observe a number of bruises and abrasions in various stages of healing on the patient's upper torso and arms.

1. What are your assessment priorities for this patient?
2. What interventions would you perform on scene and en route to the receiving hospital?
3. Describe possible transport considerations, including a potential refusal of transport by the angry parents.
4. What are the important factors in reporting this incident and documenting the call?

See Suggested Responses at the back of this book.

FURTHER READING

American Heart Association: "Guidelines 2000 for Cardiopulmonary Resuscitation and Emergency Cardiac Care." *Circulation*. 2000: 102 (supplement).

American Heart Association and American Academy of Pediatrics: *Textbook of Pediatric Advanced Life Support*. Dallas, TX. American Heart Association, 1998.

Beers, M.H., *et. al.: The Merck Manual of Diagnosis and Therapy*, 17th ed. Whitehouse Station, NJ. Merck Research Laboratories, 1999.

Eichelberger, M.R., *et. al.: Pediatric Emergencies*, 2nd ed. Upper Saddle River, NJ. Prentice-Hall, Inc., 1997.

Dickinson, E.T.: *Fire Service Emergency Care*. Upper Saddle River, NJ. Prentice-Hall, Inc., 1999.

Tunik, M.G., *et. al.: Teaching Resource for Prehospital Pediatrics*. New York, NY. Center for Pediatric Medicine, 1998.

ON THE WEB

Visit Brady's Paramedic Website at www.bradybooks.com/paramedic.

CHAPTER 3

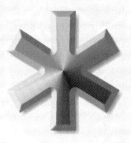

Geriatric Emergencies

Objectives

After reading this chapter, you should be able to:

1. Discuss the demographics demonstrating the increasing size of the elderly population in the United States. (pp. 140–141)
2. Assess the various living environments of elderly patients. (pp. 141–143.)
3. Discuss society's view of aging and the social, financial, and ethical issues facing the elderly. (pp. 140, 141–143, 145)
4. Describe the resources available to assist the elderly, and create strategies to refer at-risk patients to appropriate community services. (pp. 145–148)
5. Discuss common emotional and psychological reactions to aging, including causes and manifestations. (pp. 141–142, 148–149)
6. Apply the pathophysiology of multi-system failure to the assessment and management of medical conditions in the elderly patient. (p. 149)
7. Compare the pharmacokinetics of an elderly patient to that of a young patient, including drug distribution, metabolism, and excretion. (pp. 149–150)

Continued

8. Discuss the impact of polypharmacy, dosing errors, increased drug sensitivity, and medication non-compliance on assessment and management of the elderly patient (pp. 149–150)

9. Discuss the use and effects of commonly prescribed drugs for the elderly patient (pp. 149–150, 188–192)

10. Discuss the problem of mobility in the elderly, and develop strategies to prevent falls. (pp. 151–152)

11. Discuss age-related changes in sensations in the elderly, and describe the implications of these changes for communication and patient assessment. (pp. 152, 155–158)

12. Discuss the problems with continence and elimination in the elderly patient, and develop communication strategies to provide psychological support. (pp. 152–153)

13. Discuss factors that may complicate the assessment of the elderly patient. (pp. 148–149, 154–159)

14. Discuss the principles that should be employed when assessing and communicating with the elderly. (pp. 143, 152, 154–159)

15. Compare the assessment of a young patient with that of an elderly patient. (pp. 154–155, 159–166)

16. Discuss common complaints of elderly patients. (pp. 149, 167–188)

17. Discuss the normal and abnormal changes of age in relation to the:
    a. Pulmonary system. (pp. 160–162)
    b. Cardiovascular system. (pp. 161, 162–163)
    c. Nervous system. (pp. 161, 163–164)
    d. Endocrine system. (pp. 161, 164)
    e. Gastrointestinal system. (pp. 161, 164)
    f. Thermoregulatory system. (pp. 161, 165)
    g. Integumentary system. (pp. 161, 165)
    h. Musculoskeletal system. (pp. 161, 165)

18. Describe the incidence, morbidity/mortality, risk factors, prevention strategies, pathophysiology, assessment, need for intervention and transport, and management for elderly medical patients with:
    a. Pneumonia, chronic obstructive disease, and pulmonary embolism. (pp. 167–170)
    b. Myocardial infarction, heart failure, dysrhythmias, aneurysm, and hypertension. (pp. 170–175)
    c. Cerebral vascular disease, delirium, dementia, Alzheimer's disease, and Parkinson's disease. (pp. 175–179)
    d. Diabetes and thyroid diseases. (pp. 179–180)
    e. Gastrointestinal problems, GI hemorrhage, and bowel obstruction. (pp. 180–182)
    f. Skin diseases and pressure ulcers. (pp. 182–183)
    g. Osteoarthritis and osteoporosis. (pp. 183–185)
    h. Hypothermia and hyperthermia. (pp. 186–187)
    i. Toxicological problems, including drug toxicity, substance abuse, alcohol abuse, and drug abuse. (pp. 188–194)
    j. Psychological disorders, including depression and suicide. (pp. 194–196)

19. Describe the incidence, morbidity/mortality, risk factors, prevention strategies, pathophysiology, assessment, need for intervention and transport, and management of the elderly trauma patient with:
    a. Orthopedic injuries. (pp. 200–201)
    b. Burns. (pp. 201–202)
    c. Head injuries. (p. 202)

20. Given several pre-programmed simulated geriatric patients with various complaints, provide the appropriate assessment, management, and transport. (pp. 140–202)

CASE STUDY

"Turnpike Rescue, respond Priority One to 957 Homestead Road for a 79-year-old female with abdominal pain."

You've just arrived on duty when this call comes into the station. "The day is starting early," you say to a co-worker. Oh well, you think. It's a good chance to teach Andrew, the paramedic student intern assigned to your crew, about elderly patients. "Hey Andy," you call out. "What are the causes of abdominal pain in an elderly patient?"

Andy tells you that the pain could be related to any number of bowel complaints—from obstruction to simple constipation. He also mentions problems such as ulcers, urinary infections, and even trauma. He ends with a quip: "Probably isn't related to too many beers and a taco, huh?"

You've just pulled up to the house, so you let Andy's remark slide for now. A man standing in the doorway calls out: "Come quickly. I think my mother may be dying."

You and your partner allow Andy to conduct a complete scene survey. You concur with his decision that the scene is safe at the present time and enter what appears to be a well-kept home.

"Does your mother live alone?" you ask. The son, who identifies himself as Michae!, replies: "Yes, Mom lives alone. She's extremely independent. She drives everywhere, even at night. She does volunteer work and still likes to travel. This past summer, she took a cruise to the Bahamas all by herself." Michael then adds, "That's why I'm so worried. I stopped in to visit, and there was Mom still in bed, crying out in pain."

Upon entering the patient's bedroom, you see a well-nourished elderly woman, tossing and turning on her bed. "My stomach hurts so much," she sobs. Between cries of anguish, she manages to tell you that the pain woke her up early this morning. She has not gotten out of bed since. When you ask if she has fallen recently, she says "no."

You notice that Andy has instructed your partner to set up high flow O_2. You nod approval, and ask him to begin the initial survey. Meanwhile, you obtain a history from the son.

Michael explains that his mom, Mrs. Hildegaard, has been very healthy. She has hypertension, but is compliant with her medication of lisinopril-hydochlorthiazide. When you ask about allergies, Michael mentions aspirin. He knows of no changes in his mom's diet and her appetite has been good. In fact, she and his brother, Allen, went out to dinner last night. Michael explains that Mrs. Hildegaard was clinically depressed after the death of her husband

7 years ago, but "bounced back" after therapy. She's taken no antidepressants for more than five years.

After performing an initial assessment, Andy reports: "Airway is open and clear. Breathing is slightly fast at 22 per minute, but is interspersed with crying. Lungs are clear. Skin is cool, but dry. No overt bleeding. Pupils equal and reactive, with no neuro deficits noted." He then states the vital signs as BP 154/90, pulse 110 and irregular, respirations 22 and non-labored. Upon examination of the patient's abdomen, Andy found no evidence of guarding and no specific area of tenderness. Mrs. Hildegaard told him: "My stomach hurts all over, everywhere you touch."

Andy has started oxygen at 10 liters by nonrebreather mask, per protocols. Your partner has also established an IV line of normal saline and placed the patient on the cardiac monitor. The monitor shows atrial fibrillation with an average rate of 110 bpm.

The patient is packaged and transported to the emergency department. En route, you contact medical direction.

In the ED, the attending physician orders blood work, chest film, and an abdominal CT. Following an exploratory laparotomy, the physician admits Mrs. Hildegaard to the surgical intensive care unit. The diagnosis is an infarcted bowel. The patient's prognosis is poor.

Back at the station, you take time to address Andy's quip about the "beers and a taco." You say: "You probably know that as people age they often lose life-long support systems, like a job or a spouse. But did you realize that the elderly sometimes turn to alcohol to relieve the pain, just like people our own age?"

You then offer some pointers for providing quality EMS care to the elderly. "The most important thing to remember about the elderly patient is that while many changes occur as a result of aging, you must avoid jumping to conclusions. Give proper attention to assessment, and think about normal changes of aging versus changes as a result of disease. Provide prompt treatment as the elderly patient has less physiologic reserve than a younger patient. Once the elderly patient starts to deteriorate, the process is difficult to stop. Always remember that when complaints of abdominal pain are out of proportion to your exam, you should suspect a serious medical condition—in this case, bowel infarct."

As you walk away, you say: "So Andy, do you want to talk about what went right with this call and what we could have done better while we restock the ambulance?"

"You bet," he replies.

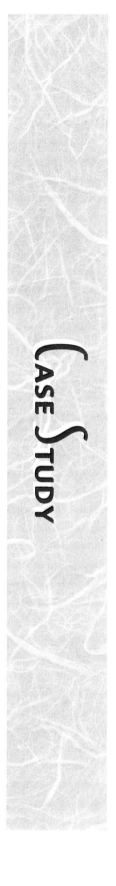

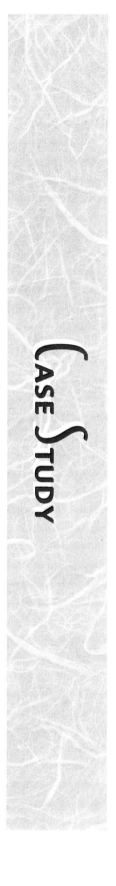
CASE STUDY

INTRODUCTION

Aging—the gradual decline of biological functions—varies widely from one individual to another. Most people reach their biological peak in the years before age 30. For practical purposes, however, the aging process does not affect their daily lives until later years. Many of the decrements commonly ascribed to aging are caused by other factors, such as lifestyle, diet, behavior, or environment. The aging process becomes even more complicated if we remember that age-related changes in organ functions also occur at different rates. For example, a person's kidneys may decline rapidly with age, while the heart remains strong or vice versa.

As people age, they actually become less alike, both physiologically and psychologically. Although some functional losses in old age are due to normal age-related changes, many others result from abnormal changes, particularly disease. In assessing and treating older patients, it is important to distinguish, when possible, normal age-related changes from abnormal changes. The purpose of this chapter is to present some of the most common physiological changes associated with aging and the implications of these changes to the quality of EMS care provided to the **elderly**—one of the fastest-growing segments of our population.

Many of the decrements commonly ascribed to aging are caused by other factors, such as lifestyle, diet, behavior, or environment.

✱ elderly a person age 65 or older.

EPIDEMIOLOGY AND DEMOGRAPHICS

The twentieth century—with its tremendous medical and technological advances—witnessed both a reduction in infant mortality rates and an increase in life expectancies. The cumulative effect was a population boom worldwide, with the greatest gains seen among people age 65 or older. During the 1900s, the population of the United States increased threefold, while the number of elderly increased tenfold. The growing number of elderly patients presents a challenge to all health-care services, including EMS, not only in terms of resources, but in the enormous impact that aging has upon our society.

POPULATION CHARACTERISTICS

America is getting older. Between 1960 and 1990, the number of elderly people in the United States nearly doubled. By late 1998, the total reached more than 34 million, with nearly 400,000 people ages 95 and older. As the 2000s opened, demographers talked about the "graying of America," a process in which the number of elderly people is pushing up the average age of the U.S. population as a whole. Reasons for this trend include:

- The mean survival rate of older persons is increasing.
- The birth rate is declining.
- There has been an absence of major wars and other catastrophes.
- Health care and standards of living have improved significantly since World War II.

In 2030, when the post-World War II baby boomers enter their 80s, more than 70 million people will be age 65 or older. By 2040, the elderly will represent roughly 20 percent of the population. In other words, one in five Americans will be age 65 or older.

Not only will the elderly population increase in size, its members will live longer, which in turn will swell the number of the **old-old**. By 2040, the number of people age 85 and over is expected to rise by 17 percent. Whether longer life spans mean longer years of active living or longer years of disease and disability is unknown.

✱ old-old an elderly person age 80 or older.

Gerontology—the study of the effects of aging on humans—is a relatively new science. (The Gerontological Society of America [GSA] was formed in 1945.) Gerontologists still do not fully understand the underlying causes of aging. However, most believe that some form of cellular damage or loss, particularly of nerve cells (neurons), is involved. The result is a general decline in the body's efficiency, such as a reduction in the size and function of most internal organs.

To treat age-related changes, physicians and other health care workers have increasingly specialized in the care of the elderly. This aspect of medicine, known as **geriatrics,** is essential in caring for our aging population.

The demographic changes will also affect your EMS career. Today nearly 36 percent of all EMS calls involve the elderly. The percentage is expected to grow. Therefore, you will need to be familiar with the fundamental principles of geriatrics, especially those related to advanced prehospital care. You will also need to be aware of the social issues that can affect the health and mental well-being of the elderly patients that you will be treating.

* **gerontology** scientific study of the effects of aging and of age-related diseases on humans.

* **geriatrics** the study and treatment of diseases of the aged.

SOCIETAL ISSUES

For a typical working person, the post-retirement years can be up to one-third of an average life span. The years include a series of transitions, such as reduced income, relocation, and loss of friends, family members, spouse, or partner.

After years of working and/or raising a family, an elderly person must not only find new roles to fulfill, but in many cases, must overcome the societal label of "old person." A lot of elderly people disprove **ageism**—and all the stereotypes it engenders—by living happy, productive, and active lives (Figure 3-1). Others, however, feel a sense of social isolation or uselessness. Physical and financial difficulties reinforce these feelings and help create an emotional context in which illnesses can occur. Therefore, successful medical treatment of elderly patients involves an understanding of the broader social situation in which they live.

* **ageism** discrimination against aged or elderly people.

Emotional, physical, and/or financial difficulties can help create a context in which illnesses can occur. Successful medical treatment of elderly patients involves an understanding of the broader social context in which they live.

Living Environments

The elderly live in both independent and dependent living environments. Many continue to live alone or with their partner well into their 80s or 90s. The "oldest" old are the most likely to live alone, and, in fact, nearly half of those age 85 and over live by themselves. The great majority of these people—

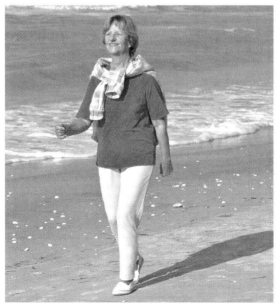

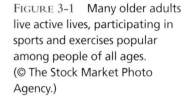

FIGURE 3-1 Many older adults live active lives, participating in sports and exercises popular among people of all ages. (© The Stock Market Photo Agency.)

an estimated 78 percent—are women. This is because married men tend to die before their wives, and widowed men tend to remarry more often than widowed women.

Poverty and Loneliness Elderly persons living alone represent one of the most impoverished and vulnerable parts of society. Death of a partner reduces income sharply, especially for women whose savings are depleted by long illnesses and/or who relied on their husband's retirement benefits. In the 1990s, roughly 45 percent of the elderly who lived alone tried to get by on less than $170 a week. Such low incomes force the elderly to choose between such basic necessities as food, shelter, or medicine.

In addition to poverty, many of the elderly who live alone, especially the old-old, have few or no living family members. Not surprisingly, more than 60 percent of those over age 75 report feelings of loneliness. Depression is also common, particularly among those who are both poor and alone.

Despite these difficulties, nearly 90 percent of the elderly who live alone choose to maintain their independence. Many fear any situation in which they would be treated as helpless human beings. Others do not want to burden family, friends, or even society with their problems. Some see their situation, including illness, as an inevitable part of aging and refuse to complain or ask for help. Keep this fact in mind whenever you question an elderly patient: The elderly often do not reveal problems beyond the chief complaint, either because they fear the loss of independence or because they consider the illnesses as "normal" for their age.

Social Support Of the elderly people who live alone and who cannot perform some everyday tasks, nearly 74 percent receive no form of assistance. To avoid the dangers of social isolation, doctors encourage the elderly to interact with other people. This helps them to build a network of social support—a critical factor to mental health and physical well-being (Figure 3-2). Interaction may be with family members, neighbors, and other elderly people at "senior centers." Levels of interaction can be gauged by questions such as, "Is there anyone you can call if you have trouble with your medications tonight?" "Can someone stay with you when you return from the hospital?"

Among the elderly who receive help, more than 43 percent rely on paid assistance. Another 54 percent use unpaid assistance, and 3 percent use both types of help. Those elderly that turn to dependent care arrangements may choose among a variety of options, including live-in nursing, **life-care communities, congregate care,** or **personal-care homes.** Approximately 5 percent of the elderly, live in nursing homes.

There are benefits and drawbacks to both independent and dependent living arrangements. Independence is an important concept. Older persons with the desire and ability should be allowed to remain in their homes. Keep in mind, however, that tight finances and limited mobility may prevent an independent elderly person from maintaining adequate nutrition and safety. As a result, elderly patients may be at increased risk of accidental hypothermia, carbon monoxide poisoning, or fires. They may also reduce their medications, or "half dose," to save money.

Many states have few or no restrictions on personal care aides or others who provide assistance in the home. The elderly can be at risk for criminal activities. Living in an adult community or nursing home removes some of the concerns of self-care. Tradeoffs include the loss, in varying degrees, of independence; exposure to illnesses found in an institutional setting; and a lack of contact with people of varying ages, particularly the young.

As a paramedic, you may be called on to assist elderly patients in any number of environments, both independent and dependent. These conditions will be

---

Elderly persons living alone represent one of the most impoverished and vulnerable parts of society.

The elderly often do not reveal problems behind the chief complaint, either because they fear the loss of independence or because they consider the illnesses as "normal" for their age.

* **life-care community** communities that provide apartments/homes for independent living and a range of services, including nursing care. Usually the elderly own their own homes.

* **congregate care** living arrangement in which the elderly live in, but do not own, individual apartments or rooms and receive select services.

* **personal-care home** living arrangement that includes room, board, and some supervision.

Keep in mind that tight finances and limited mobility may prevent an elderly person from maintaining adequate nutrition and safety.

The environment in which an elderly person lives will be part of your history and often will play a key role in your assessment of the patient's condition.

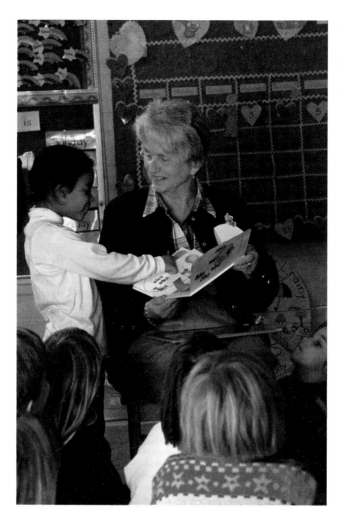

FIGURE 3-2 Many elderly people form social networks by joining a senior center or by taking part in volunteer programs. (© The Stock Market Photo Agency.)

a part of the patient's history and often will play a key role in your assessment of the elderly patient. For example, a deterioration in independence is not necessarily a function of aging. It may well be a sign of an untreated illness.

Whenever you treat elderly patients, remember that illness carries a special meaning for them. They are more aware than any other age group of the potential of death. They also realize that many "curable" injuries or diseases can lead to functional impairment and a reduction in self-sufficiency. An elderly patient may recover, but be unable to meet his or her own needs. An EMS call is almost always a stressful event for the elderly person. Communication and psychological support is of utmost importance in reducing patient anxiety and finding out the underlying causes of the medical condition that brought you to the patient's home.

Ethics

In the course of caring for elderly patients, ethical concerns frequently arise. You may be confronted with multiple decision makers, particularly in dependent living environments. You may also have a question about the patient's competency to give informed consent or refusal of treatment. Finally, you may be faced with **advance directives,** such as "living wills" and Do Not Resuscitate (DNR) Orders (Figure 3-3).

A deterioration in independence is not necessarily a function of aging. It may well be a sign of a heretofore untreated illness.

Remember at all times that illness carries a special—and often fearful—meaning for the elderly.

✳ **advance directive** legal document prepared when a person is alive, competent, and able to make informed decisions about health care. The document provides guidelines on treatment if the person is no longer capable of making decisions.

Department of Health

Nonhospital Order Not to Resuscitate (DNR order)

Person's Name (Print) _____

Date of Birth ____/____/____

Do not resuscitate the person named above.

Person's Signature_____

Date____/____/____

Physician's Signature_____

Print Name_____

License Number _____

Date____/____/____

It is the responsibility of the physician to determine, at least every 90 days, whether this order continues to be appropriate, and to indicate this by a note in the person's medical chart. The issuance of a new form is **NOT** required, and under the law this order should be considered valid unless it is known that it has been revoked. This order remains valid and must be followed, even if it has not been reviewed within the 90 day period.

FIGURE 3-3   An example of a Do Not Resuscitate order.

These situations may be confusing to emergency care providers. In cases of multiple decision makers, you should usually honor the wishes of the patient, if judged competent. If a caregiver opposes treatment, keep in mind the possibility of abuse. This also applies to institutionalized settings, such as nursing homes, where an elderly patient may have been subjected to neglect.

In matters of consent, follow the same general guidelines as you would with any other patient. (See Volume 1, Chapter 6.) However, remain aware of the high incidence of depression and suicide in the elderly. (The topic of suicide will be discussed in greater detail later in the chapter.) If you think a patient should be transported to the hospital, make every effort to get the person there.

Whenever you are presented with advance directives, you should follow state laws and local EMS system protocols. Some states have standard legal forms for DNR orders to prevent confusion. Cases in which you received an advance directive are truly life-and-death situations. If you have any doubt about what the directive says or its legality, begin treatment and contact medical direction. In all situations involving ethical decisions, document the reasons for your choice of action.

If you have any doubt about what an advance directive says or its legality, begin treatment and contact medical direction.

In all situations involving ethical decisions, document the reasons for your choice.

FINANCING AND RESOURCES FOR HEALTH CARE

Caring for an increasing number of elderly patients places a huge demand on traditional health-care resources, including EMS. Currently, social security pays a significant portion of monthly bills with medical support provided by three major publicly funded programs. They include:

- *Medicare.* This program basically operates as a two-part complementary system. Part A covers in-hospital care; Part B provides medical insurance to cover physicians, outpatient care, therapy, and durable medical equipment. About 95 percent of all people over age 65 are enrolled in Part A; nearly all of them are also enrolled in Part B, which is voluntary. Under Medicare, people may enroll in Health Maintenance Organizations (HMO) that accept Medicare benefits.

- *Medicaid.* Under Medicaid, the federal and state governments share responsibility for providing health care to the aged poor, the blind, the disabled, and low-income families with dependent children. Although Medicaid was created to help the poor, the high cost of medical care has brought large numbers of elderly people into the program. Today Medicaid provides the largest share of public funding for long-term care. It contributes approximately 45 percent of the financing for nursing home services.

- *Veterans Administration (VA).* The Veterans Administration offers health care to veterans with disabilities or service-related problems (Figure 3-4). It operates more than 170 hospitals and over 100 nursing homes. Services may be provided for free or on a sliding scale.

With the number of younger tax-paying workers shrinking, publicly funded medical programs face an uncertain future. A growing number of private insurers have started offering policies for long-term care during a person's older years. These policies, however, may be too expensive for many of the elderly, and younger people may not be willing to purchase them when premiums are low. Many experts worry that the booming elderly population projected for the 2030s and 2040s may have to rely increasingly on private savings, retirement plans, and state assistance in whatever form it exists.

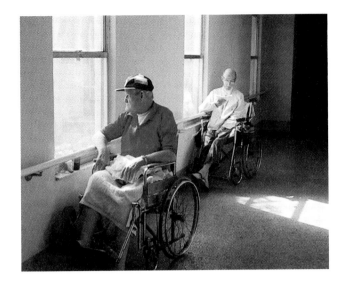

FIGURE 3-4 VA hospitals provide a variety of medical services, including nursing home facilities, to Americans who served in the nation's military.

Health-Care Alternatives

One of the biggest health care debates of the early 2000s centers around the question of preventing death at all costs. Most health-care dollars are spent during a person's last month of life with more than one-third of the expenditure occurring during the final 10 days. Governmental and independent agencies have advised that it might be better to spend money on preventing disease rather than preventing death.

In an effort to bring down the cost of acute medical care, hospitals have shifted patient care increasingly to the home. The emphasis on home care—with appropriate medical and nursing assistance—has become a recognized medical practice. (See Chapter 6.) This development has gone hand-in-hand with the hospice movement, which allows terminally ill patients to live the remainder of their lives outside a hospital. Both trends impact heavily on EMS personnel, who will be called upon to provide more complicated care for more patients, particularly the elderly, in an out-of-hospital setting.

Prevention and Self-Help

In treating the elderly, remember that the best intervention is prevention.

In treating the elderly, remember that the best intervention is prevention (Table 3-1). The goal of any health-care service, including EMS, should be to help keep people from becoming sick or injured in the first place. As previously mentioned, disease and disability in later life are often linked to unhealthy or unsafe behavior. As a paramedic, you can reduce morbidity among the elderly by taking part in community education programs and by cooperating with agencies or organizations that support the elderly. Some possible resources are described in the following sections.

Senior Centers Many communities have senior centers, which provide a social atmosphere for education, recreation, and entertainment. These centers also support health-care endeavors such as flu shots, blood pressure monitoring, and transport to clinics. Meals on Wheels—a program providing from 1 to 3 meals a day—may be part of a senior volunteer organization (Figure 3-5).

Religious Organizations Religious organizations commonly serve as a resource for the elderly. Some provide services, including dependent living environments, for their members. Others keep in touch with governmental agencies, provide food or clothing for the aged poor, and offer volunteer programs in which the elderly can make useful contributions, thus reducing their sense of isolation.

Table 3-1   PREVENTION STRATEGIES FOR THE OLDER PERSON

Issues	Strategies
Lifestyle	
Exercise:	Weight-bearing and cardiovascular exercise (walking) for 20–30 minutes at least three times a week
Nutrition:	Varies, but generally low fat, adequate fiber (complex carbohydrates), reduced sugar (simple carbohydrates), moderate protein; adequate calcium, especially for women*
Alcohol/tobacco:	Moderate alcohol, if any; abstinence from tobacco
Sleep:	Generally 7–8 hours a night
Accidents	Maintain good physical condition; add safety features to home (handrails, nonskid surfaces, lights, etc.); modify potentially dangerous driving practices (driving at night with impaired night vision, traveling in hazardous weather, etc.)
Medical Health	
Disease/Illness:	Routine screening for hearing, vision, blood pressure, hemoglobin, cholesterol, etc.; regular physical examinations; immunizations (tetanus booster, influenza vaccine, once-in-a-lifetime pneumococcal vaccine)
Pharmacological:	Regular review of prescriptive and over-the-counter medications, focusing on potential interactions and side effects
Dental:	Regular dental checkups and good oral hygiene (important for nutrition and general well-being)
Mental/emotional:	Observe for evidence of depression, disrupted sleep patterns, psychosocial stress; ensure effective support networks and availability of psychotherapy; compliance with prescribed antidepressants

*Vitamin supplements may be required, but should be taken only after other medications are reviewed and in correct dosages. Excessive doses of vitamin A or D, for example, can be toxic.

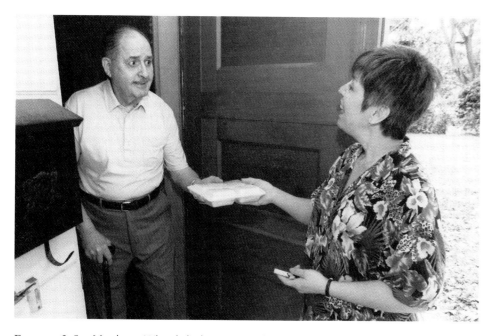

FIGURE 3-5   Meals on Wheels helps ensure that elderly people receive adequate nutrition by providing from 1–3 meals a day.

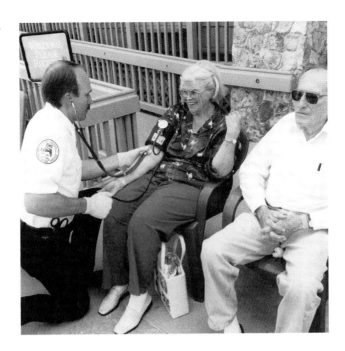

FIGURE 3-6 In some communities, paramedics offer free medical screening programs, such as blood pressure checks, to the elderly.

National and State Associations A number of associations serve as clearinghouses for information to aid the elderly. Some of these groups include the AARP, the Alzheimer's Association, and the Association for Senior Citizens. The AARP is one of the largest, most visible, and most politically connected non-profit organizations in the world today advocating for the elderly. These organizations provide significant advocacy for retired persons. They often have local chapters within a county or region and usually maintain web pages, where elderly patients can access information from their homes.

Governmental Agencies A wide range of services can be found through governmental agencies, such as the Department of Health. Many areas maintain an Office for the Aging, which refers the elderly to a wide range of community programs, including nutrition centers, senior citizen law projects, home-care services, senior citizen discount programs, transportation services, and more.

Familiarize yourself with agencies and organizations in your area that work with the elderly. They can be found through use of the Internet, the Department of Health, or special pages in the telephone book, usually at the front or in the Yellow Pages under the heading "Senior Citizens." You can either pass this information on to elderly patients, as needed, or work with one of these groups to initiate programs such as free blood pressure checks (Figure 3-6). You might also start a prevention program that helps the elderly to safeguard their environment against fires, theft, carbon monoxide poisoning, or extremes in temperature.

GENERAL PATHOPHYSIOLOGY, ASSESSMENT, AND MANAGEMENT

✳ **functional impairment** decreased ability to meet daily needs on an independent basis.

In treating elderly patients, it is important to recall several facts. First, medical disorders in the elderly often present as **functional impairment** and should be treated as an early warning of a possibly undetected medical problem. Second, signs and symptoms do not necessarily point to the underlying cause of the problem or illness. For example, while confusion often indicates a brain disease in younger patients, this may not be the case in an elderly patient. The confused patient may be suffering from a wide range of disorders, including drug toxicity, malnutrition, or accidental hypothermia.

A thorough evaluation must always be done to detect possible causes of an impairment. If identified early, an environmental- or disease-generated impairment can often be reversed. Your success depends upon a knowledge of age-related changes and the implications of these changes for patient assessment and management.

PATHOPHYSIOLOGY OF THE ELDERLY PATIENT

As mentioned, patients become less alike as they enter their elderly years, Even so, certain generalizations can be made about age-related changes and the disease process in the elderly.

Multiple-System Failure

There is no escaping the fact that the body becomes less efficient with age, increasing the likelihood of malfunction. The body is susceptible to all the disorders of young people, but its maintenance, defense, and repair processes are weaker. As a result, the elderly often suffer from more than one illness or disease at a time. On average, six medical disorders may coexist in an elderly person and perhaps even more in the old-old. Neither the patient nor the patient's doctor may be aware of all of these problems. Furthermore, disease in one organ system may result in the deterioration of other systems, compounding existing acute and/or chronic conditions.

Because of concomitant diseases (**comorbidity**) in the elderly, complaints may not be specific to any one disorder. Common complaints of the elderly include: fatigue and weakness, dizziness/vertigo/syncope, falls, headaches, insomnia, **dysphagia**, loss of appetite, inability to void, and/or constipation/diarrhea.

Elderly patients often accept medical problems as a part of aging and fail to monitor changes in their condition. In some cases, such as a silent myocardial infarction, pain may be diminished or absent. In others, an important complaint may seem trivial, such as constipation.

Although many medical problems in the young and middle-aged populations present with a standard set of signs and symptoms, the changes involved in aging lead to different presentations. In pneumonia, for example, the classic symptom of fever is often absent in the elderly. Chest pain and a cough are also less common. Finally, many cases of pneumonia among the elderly are due to aspiration, not infection. The presentation of pneumonia and other diseases commonly found in the elderly will be covered later in the chapter.

Pharmacology in the Elderly

The existence of multiple chronic diseases in the elderly leads to the use of multiple medications. Persons age 65 and older use one-third of all prescriptive drugs in the United States, taking an average of 4.5 medications per day. This does not include over-the-counter medications, vitamin supplements, or herbal remedies.

If medications are not correctly monitored, **polypharmacy** can lead to a number of problems among the elderly. In general, a person's sensitivity to drugs increases with age. When compared to younger patients, the elderly experience more adverse drug reactions, more drug-drug interactions, and more drug-disease interactions. Because of age-related pharmacokinetic changes such as a loss of body fluid and atrophy of organs, drugs concentrate more readily in the plasma and tissues of elderly patients. As a result, drug dosages often must be adjusted to prevent toxicity. (The problem of toxicity will be discussed in more detail later in the chapter.)

The elderly often suffer from more than one illness or disease at a time.

* **comorbidity** having more than one disease at a time.

* **dysphagia** inability to swallow or difficulty swallowing.

Content Review

COMMON COMPLAINTS IN THE ELDERLY

- Fatigue/weakness
- Dizziness/vertigo/syncope
- Falls
- Headaches
- Insomnia
- Dysphagia
- Loss of appetite
- Inability to void
- Constipation/diarrhea

The existence of multiple chronic disease in the elderly often leads to the use of multiple medications. Keep this in mind throughout the assessment.

* **polypharmacy** multiple drug therapy in which there is a concurrent use of a number of drugs.

In taking a medical history of an elderly patient, remember to ask if the patient is taking a prescribed medication as directed.

In taking a medical history of an elderly patient, remember to ask questions to determine if a patient is taking a prescribed medication as directed. Noncompliance with drug therapy, usually underadherence, is common among the elderly. Up to 40 percent do not take medications as prescribed. Of these individuals, 35 percent experience some type of medical problem. Factors that can decrease compliance in the elderly include:

- Limited income
- Memory loss due to decreased or diseased neural activity
- Limited mobility
- Sensory impairment (cannot hear/read/understand directions)
- Multiple or complicated drug therapies
- Fear of toxicity
- Child-proof containers (especially with arthritic patients)
- Duration of drug therapy (The longer the therapy, the less likely a patient will stick with it.)

Factors that can increase compliance among the elderly include:

- Good patient-physician communication
- Belief that a disease or illness is serious
- Drug calendars or reminder cards
- Compliance counseling
- Blister-pack packaging or other easy-to-open packaging (Figure 3-7)
- Multi-compartment pill boxes
- Transportation services to pharmacy
- Clear, simple directions written in large type
- Ability to read

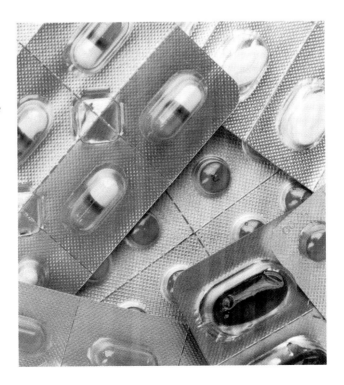

FIGURE 3-7 "Child-proof" pill vials are sometimes "elder-proof" as well. Blister-packs make it easier for elderly patients, especially those suffering from arthritis, to take their medicines, thus furthering compliance.

Problems with Mobility and Falls

Regular exercise and a good diet are two of the most effective preventive measures for ensuring mobility among the elderly. However, not all elderly take these measures. They may suffer from a severe medical problem, such as crippling arthritis. They may fear for their personal safety, either from accidental injury or intentional injury, such as robbery. Certain medications also may increase their lethargy. Whatever the cause, a lack of mobility can have detrimental physical and emotional effects. Some of these include:

- Poor nutrition
- Difficulty with elimination
- Poor skin integrity
- A greater predisposition for falls
- Loss of independence and/or confidence
- Depression from "feeling old"
- Isolation and lack of a social network

Falls present an especially serious problem for the elderly. Fall-related injuries represent the leading cause of accidental death among the elderly and the seventh highest cause of death overall. Only children and young adults have a higher incidence of falls. However, unlike the elderly, children and young adults rarely die from fall-related injuries.

Falls may be either intrinsic (related to the patient) or extrinsic (related to the environment). Intrinsic factors include a history of repeated falls, dizziness, a sense of weakness, impaired vision, an altered gait, CNS problems, decreased mental status, or use of certain medications. Extrinsic factors include environmental hazards such as slippery floors, a lack of handrails, or loose throw rugs (Table 3-2).

Table 3-2 MAKING A HOME SAFE FOR THE ELDERLY

Hazard	Intervention	Reason
Torn or slippery rugs	Repair or replace.	To prevent tripping or slipping
Chair without armrests	Install armrests.	To provide leverage in getting out of chair
Chair with low back	Replace with chair with high backs.	To support neck; prevent falling backward for patients who must rock to get out of a chair
Chair with wheels	Replace with chair with sturdy legs.	To prevent chair from sliding when elder is getting into or out of it
Obstructing furniture	Move items so that clutter is minimized and pathways are clear.	To help those with poor mobility and poor peripheral vision
Slippery bathtub	Install skid-resistant strips or mat.	To provide more stable footing
Dim lighting	Provide adequate lighting in all areas, perhaps with automatic timers.	To improve ability to see, especially in darkened rooms and at night
High cabinet shelves	Place frequently used items on lower shelves or in easy-to-reach places.	To eliminate unnecessary reaching or climbing
Missing handrails on stairways	Install handrail.	To allow elder to grab onto railing for support
High steps on stairways	Rebuild for a rise of less than 6 inches between steps or install a ramp.	To reduce the risk of tripping, falling, or overexertion (especially for cardiac or pulmonary patients)

In assessing an elderly patient who has fallen, remember that a fall often has multiple causes.

In assessing an elderly patient who has fallen, remember that a fall often has multiple causes. An over-medicated patient, for example, trips over a throw rug. A fall may also be a presenting sign of an acute illness, such as a myocardial infarction, or a sign that a chronic illness has worsened. Bear in mind the possibility of physical abuse, especially if the injury does not match the story.

Communication Difficulties

Most elderly patients suffer from some form of age-related sensory changes. Normal physiological changes may include impaired vision or blindness, impaired or loss of hearing, an altered sense of taste or smell, and/or a lower sensitivity to pain (touch). Any of these conditions can affect your ability to communicate with the patient. For communication strategies, see Table 3-3. (A discussion on the implications of sensory impairment on patient assessment appears later in the chapter.)

Problems with Continence and Elimination

The elderly often find it embarrassing to talk about problems with continence and elimination. They may feel stigmatized, isolated, and/or helpless. When confronted with these problems, DO NOT make a big deal out of them. Respect the patient's dignity, and assure the person that, in many cases, the problem is treatable.

✱ incontinence inability to retain urine or feces because of loss of sphincter control or cerebral or spinal lesions.

Incontinence The problem of **incontinence** can affect nearly any age group, but is most commonly associated with the elderly. Incontinence may be either urinary or fecal. An estimated 15 percent of the elderly who live at home experience some form of urinary incontinence. Nearly 30 percent of the hospitalized elderly and 50 percent of those living in nursing homes suffer from the same condition. Although fecal, or bowel, incontinence is less common, it seriously impairs activity and may lead to dependent care. Between 16–60 percent of the institutionalized elderly have some kind of fecal incontinence.

Incontinence can lead to a variety of conditions such as rashes, skin infections, skin breakdown (ulcers), urinary tract infections, sepsis, and falls or fractures. As mentioned, the condition takes a high emotional toll, on both the patient and the caregiver. Management of incontinence costs billions of dollars each year.

Table 3-3 AGE-RELATED SENSORY CHANGES AND IMPLICATIONS FOR COMMUNICATION

Sensory Change	Result	Communication Strategy
Clouding and thickening of lens in eye	Cataracts; poor vision, especially peripheral vision	Position yourself in front of patient where you can be seen; put hand on arm of blind patient to let patient know where you are; locate a patient's glasses, if necessary.
Shrinkage of structure in ear	Decreased hearing, especially ability to hear high frequency sounds; diminished sense of balance	Speak clearly; check hearing aids as necessary; write notes if necessary; allow the patient to put on the stethoscope, while you speak into it like a microphone.
Deterioration of teeth and gums	Patient needs dentures, but they may inflict pain on sensitive gums, so patient doesn't always wear them	If patient's speech is unintelligible, ask patient to put in dentures, if possible.
Lowered sensitivity to pain and altered sense of taste and smell	Patient underestimates the severity of the problem or is unable to provide a complete pertinent history	Probe for significant symptoms, asking questions aimed at functional impairment.

In general, effective continence requires several physical conditions. These include:

- An anatomically correct GI/GU tract
- Competent sphincter mechanism
- Adequate cognition and mobility

Although incontinence is not necessarily caused by aging, several factors predispose older patients to this condition. As mentioned, the elderly tend to have several medical disorders, each of which may require drug therapy. These disorders and/or the drugs used to treat them may compromise the integrity of either the urinary or bowel tracts. In addition, bladder capacity, urinary flow rate, and the ability to postpone voiding appear to decline with age. Certain diseases, such as diabetes and autonomic neuropathy, may also cause sphincter dysfunction. Diarrhea, or lack of physical sensation, may produce bowel incontinence as well.

Management of incontinence depends upon the cause, which cannot be easily diagnosed in the field. Some cases of incontinence can be managed surgically. In most cases, however, patients use some type of absorptive devices, such as leak-proof underwear or panty liners. Indwelling catheters are less common and may cause infections when used, particularly if not properly managed. Of critical importance is respect for the patient's modesty and dignity.

Elimination Difficulty with elimination can be a sign of a serious underlying condition (Table 3-4). It can also lead to other complications. Straining to eliminate may have serious effects on the cerebral, coronary, and peripheral arterial circulations. In elderly people with cerebrovascular disease or impaired baroreceptor reflexes, efforts to force a bowel movement can lead to a **transient ischemic attack (TIA)** or syncope. In the case of prolonged constipation, the elderly may experience colonic ulceration, intestinal obstruction, and urinary retention.

In assessing a patient with difficulty eliminating, remember to inquire about their medications. Any of the following drugs can cause constipation:

- Opioids
- Anticholinergics (e.g., antidepressants, antihistamines, muscle relaxants, antiparkinsonian drugs)
- Cation-containing agents (e.g., antacids, calcium supplements, iron supplements)
- Neurally active agents (e.g., opiates, anticonvulsants)
- Diuretics

In treating incontinence, remember to respect the patient's modesty and dignity.

Difficulty with elimination can be a sign of a serious underlying condition.

✱ transient ischemic attacks (TIA) reversible interruptions of blood flow to the brain; often seen as a precursor to a stroke.

Table 3-4 POSSIBLE CAUSES OF ELIMINATION PROBLEMS

Difficulty in Urination	Difficulty with Bowel Movements
Enlargement of the prostate in men	Diverticular disease
Urinary tract infection	Constipation*
Acute or chronic renal failure	Colorectal cancer

*Constipation may be related to dietary, medical, or surgical conditions. It could also be the result of a malignancy, intestinal obstruction, or hypothyroidism. Treat constipation as a serious medical problem.

ASSESSMENT CONSIDERATIONS

As with all patients, be sure to take appropriate BSI precautions when assessing an elderly patient. Because of the increased risk of tuberculosis in patients who are in nursing homes, consider wearing a HEPA or N-95 respirator. Remain alert to the environment, particularly the temperature of the surroundings and evidence of prescription medications.

In general, assessment of the elderly patient follows the same basic approach used with any patient. However, you need to keep in mind several factors that will improve the quality of your evaluation and make subsequent treatment more successful.

General Health Assessment

As already mentioned, you need to set a context for illness when assessing an elderly patient. When performing a general health assessment, take into account the patient's living situation, level of activity, network of social support, level of independence, medication history (both prescription and non-prescriptive), and sleep patterns.

Pay particularly close attention to the patient's nutrition. Elderly patients often have a decreased sense of smell and taste, which decrease their pleasure in eating. They also may be less aware of internal cues of hunger and thirst. Although caloric requirements generally decrease with age, an elderly patient may still suffer from malnutrition. Conditions that may complicate or discourage eating among the elderly include:

Content Review

FACTORS IN FORMING A GENERAL ASSESSMENT
- Living situation
- Level of activity
- Network of social support
- Level of independence
- Medication history
- Sleep patterns

- Breathing or respiratory problems
- Abdominal pain
- Nausea/vomiting, sometimes a drug-induced condition as with antibodies or aspirin
- Poor dental care
- Medical problems, such as hyperthyroidism, hypercalcemia, and chronic infections (e.g., cancer or tuberculosis)
- Medications (e.g., digoxin, vitamin A, fluoxetine)
- Alcohol or drug abuse
- Psychological disorders, including depression and **anorexia nervosa**
- Poverty
- Problems with shopping or cooking

✱ **anorexia nervosa** eating disorder marked by excessive fasting.

As with any person, nutrition greatly affects a patient's overall health. Because of reasons cited above, patients may suffer from a number of by-products of malnutrition, including vitamin deficiencies, dehydration, and hypoglycemia. Also remember that when a malnourished elderly person is fed, the food may produce yet other side effects, including electrolyte abnormalities, hyperglycemia, aspiration pneumonia, and a significant drop in blood pressure.

Content Review

BY-PRODUCTS OF MALNUTRITION
- Vitamin deficiencies
- Dehydration
- Hypoglycemia

Pathophysiology and Assessment

Assessment of the elderly reflects the pathophysiology of this age group. As already mentioned, the chief complaint of the elderly may seem trivial or vague at first. Also, the patient may fail to report important symptoms. Therefore, you should try to distinguish the patient's chief complaint from the patient's primary problem. A patient may report nausea, which is the chief complaint.

The primary problem, however, may be the rectal bleeding that the patient neglected to mention.

The presence of multiple diseases also complicates the assessment process. The presence of chronic problems may make it more difficult to assess an acute problem. It is easy to confuse symptoms from a chronic illness with those of an acute condition. When confronted with an elderly patient who has chest pain, for example, it is difficult to determine whether the presence of frequent premature ventricular contractions is acute or chronic. Lacking access to the patient's medical record, you should treat the patient on a "threat-to-life" basis.

Other complications stem from age-related changes in an elderly patient's response to illness and injury. Pain may be diminished, causing both you and the patient to underestimate the severity of the primary problem. In addition, the temperature-regulating mechanism may be altered or depressed. This can result in the absence of fever, or a minimal fever, even in the face of a severe infection. Alterations in the temperature-regulating mechanism, coupled with changes in the sweat glands, also makes the elderly more prone to environmental thermal problems.

Because of the complexity of factors that can affect assessment, you must probe for significant symptoms, and ultimately, the primary problem. Patience, respect, and kindness will elicit the answers needed for a pertinent medical history.

History

You should be prepared to spend more time obtaining histories from elderly patients. You may need to split the interview into sessions. For example, you might need to allow patients time to rest, if they become fatigued during the interview, or you might take a break to talk with caregivers.

When gathering the history, keep in mind the complications that arise from multiple diseases and multiple medications. Medications can be an especially important indicator of the patient's diseases. Therefore, you should find the patient's medications and take them to the hospital with the patient. Try to determine which of the medications, including over-the-counter medications, are currently being taken. In cases of multiple medications, there is an increased incidence of medication errors, drug interactions, and noncompliance.

Communication Challenges As previously mentioned, communications may be more difficult when dealing with the aged. **Cataracts** (Figure 3-8) and **glaucoma** can diminish sight. Blindness, often resulting from diabetes and stroke, is more common in the elderly. The level of anxiety increases when a patient is unable to see his or her surroundings clearly. As a result, you should talk calmly to the visually impaired patient. Yelling does not help. Instead, position yourself so the patient can see or touch you.

Age also affects hearing. Overall hearing decreases and patients may suffer from auditory disorders such as **tinnitus** or **Meniere's disease.** Diminished hearing or deafness can make it virtually impossible to obtain a history. In such cases, try to determine the history from a friend or family member. DO NOT shout at the patient. This will not help if the patient is deaf, and it may distort sounds and make it difficult for the patient who still has some hearing to understand you. Write notes if necessary. If the patient can lip-read, speak slowly and directly toward the patient. Whenever possible, verify the history with a reliable source. Also, because loss of hearing may result from other causes (such as a build up of earwax), confirm whether deafness is a pre-existing condition.

Patients may also have trouble with speech. They find it difficult to retrieve words. They will often speak slowly and exhibit changes in voice quality, which may be a normal age-related change. If a patient has forgotten to put in dentures, politely ask the person to do so.

Age-related alterations in the temperature-regulating mechanism, coupled with changes in the sweat glands, make the elderly more prone to environmental thermal problems.

Be prepared to spend more time obtaining a history from an elderly patient.

✱ **cataracts** medical condition in which the lens of the eye loses its clearness.

✱ **glaucoma** medical condition where the pressure within the eye increases.

✱ **tinnitus** subjective ringing or tingling sound in the ear.

✱ **Meniere's disease** a disease of the inner ear characterized by vertigo, nerve deafness, and a roar or buzzing in the ear.

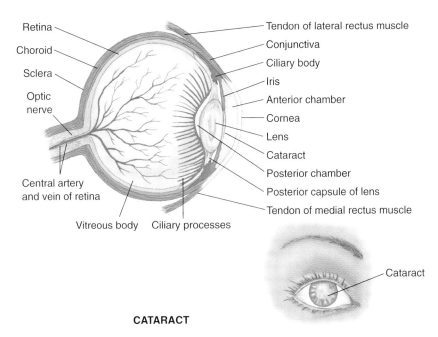

CATARACT

FIGURE 3-8   Cataracts, which cloud the lens, can diminish eyesight in the elderly.

To improve your skill at communicating with the elderly, keep these techniques in mind.

- Always introduce yourself.
- Speak slowly, distinctly, and respectfully.
- Speak to the patient first, rather than family members, caregivers, or bystanders.
- Speak face to face, at eye level with eye contact (Figure 3-9).
- Locate the patient's hearing aid or eyeglasses, if needed.
- Allow the patient to put on the stethoscope, while you speak into it like a microphone (Figure 3-10).
- Turn on the room lights.

FIGURE 3-9   If possible, talk *to* the elderly patient rather than talking about the patient to others.

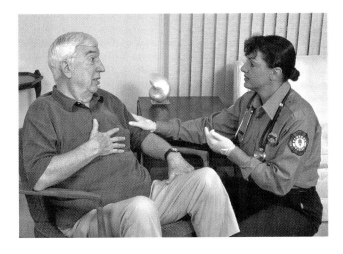

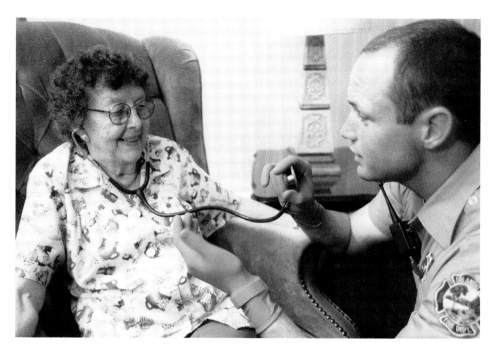

FIGURE 3-10   Allow the elderly patient with hearing difficulties to put on the stethoscope while you speak into it like a microphone.

- Display verbal and nonverbal signs of concern and empathy.
- Remain polite at all times.
- Preserve the patient's dignity.
- Always explain what you are doing and why.
- Use your power of observation to recognize anxiety—tempo of speech, eye contact, tone of voice—during the telling of the history.

Altered Mental Status and Confusion Remember that age sometimes diminishes mental status. The patient can be confused and unable to remember details. In addition, the noise of radios, ECG equipment, and strange voices may add to the confusion. Both senility and organic brain syndrome may manifest themselves similarly. Common symptoms include:

- Delirium
- Confusion
- Distractibility
- Restlessness
- Excitability
- Hostility

When confronted with a confused patient, try to determine whether the patient's mental status represents a significant change from normal. DO NOT assume that a confused, disoriented patient is "just senile," thus failing to assess for a serious underlying problem (Figure 3-11). Alcoholism, for example, is more common in the elderly than was once recognized. It can further complicate taking the history.

DO NOT assume that a confused, disoriented patient is "just senile," thus failing to assess for a serious underlying problem.

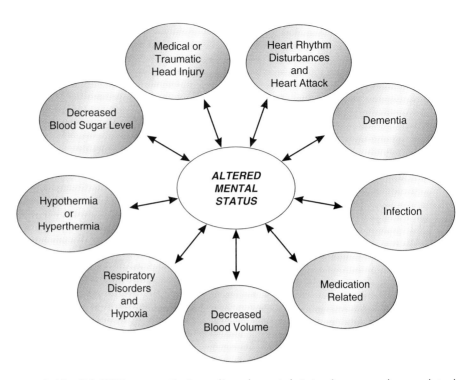

FIGURE 3-11 DO NOT assume that an altered mental status is a normal age-related change. A number of serious underlying problems may be responsible for changes in consciousness.

Treat depression as a warning sign of substance abuse and/or suicide ideation—both more common among the elderly than previously understood.

Another complication results from depression, which can be mistaken for many other disorders. It can often mimic senility and organic brain syndrome. Depression may also inhibit patient cooperation. The depressed patient may be malnourished, dehydrated, overdosed, contemplating suicide, or simply imagining physical ailments for attention. If you suspect depression, question the patient regarding drug ingestion or suicidal ideation. It is important to remember that suicide is now the fourth-leading cause of death among the elderly in the United States.

Concluding the History After obtaining the history, and if time allows, try to verify the patient's history with a credible source. This will often be less offensive to the patient if done out of his or her presence. While at the scene, it is important to observe the surroundings for indications of the patient's self-sufficiency. Look for evidence of drug or alcohol ingestion or for Medic-Alert or Vial-of-Life items. It is also important to spot signs of abuse or neglect, particularly in dependent living arrangements.

Physical Examination

Certain considerations must be kept in mind when examining the elderly patient. Remember that some patients are often easily fatigued and cannot tolerate a long examination. Also, because of the problems with temperature regulation, the patient may be wearing several layers of clothing, which can make examination difficult. Be sure to explain all actions clearly before initiating the examination, especially to patients with impaired vision. Be aware that the patient may minimize or deny symptoms because of a fear of becoming institutionalized or loss of self-sufficiency.

Try to distinguish signs of chronic disease from an acute problem. Peripheral pulses may be difficult to evaluate, because of peripheral vascular disease and arthritis. The elderly may also have non-pathological crackles (rales) upon lung auscultation. In addition, the elderly often exhibit an increase in mouth breathing and a loss of skin elasticity, which may be easily confused with dehydration. Dependent edema may be caused by inactivity, not congestive heart failure. Only experience and practice will allow you to distinguish acute from chronic physical findings.

Only experience and repeated practice will allow you to distinguish acute from chronic physical findings in the elderly patient.

MANAGEMENT CONSIDERATIONS

As you have read, people become less alike as they age. Therefore, each elderly patient presents a unique challenge in terms of assessment and management. You will need to tailor your management plan to fit a patient's illness, injury, and overall general health. Because of the potential for rapid deterioration among the elderly, you must quickly spot conditions requiring rapid transport. As with any other patient, your first concern is the ABCs. Remain alert at all times for changes in an elderly patient's neurological status, vital signs, and general cardiac status. (Management of specific disorders and the administration of medications to the elderly are covered in other sections of this chapter.)

In general, remember that transport to a hospital is often more stressful to the elderly than to any other age group except for the very young. Avoid lights and sirens in all but the most serious cases, such as when you suspect a pulmonary embolism or bowel infarction. A calm, smooth transport helps to reduce patient anxiety—and the resulting strain that anxiety places on an elderly patient's heart.

Provide emotional support at every phase of the call. Nearly any serious illness or injury in the elderly can provoke a sense of impending doom. Death is a very real possibility to this age group. To help reduce patient fears, keep these guidelines in mind.

- Encourage patients to express their feelings.
- DO NOT trivialize their fears.
- Acknowledge nonverbal messages.
- Avoid questions that are judgmental.
- Confirm what the patient says.
- Recall all you have learned about communicating with the elderly, thus avoiding communication breakdowns.
- Assure patients that you understand that they are adults on an equal footing with their care providers, including you.

SYSTEM PATHOPHYSIOLOGY IN THE ELDERLY

Although aging begins at the cellular level, it eventually affects virtually every system in the body (Figure 3-12). Age-related changes in the structure and function of organs increase the probability of disease, modify the threshold at which

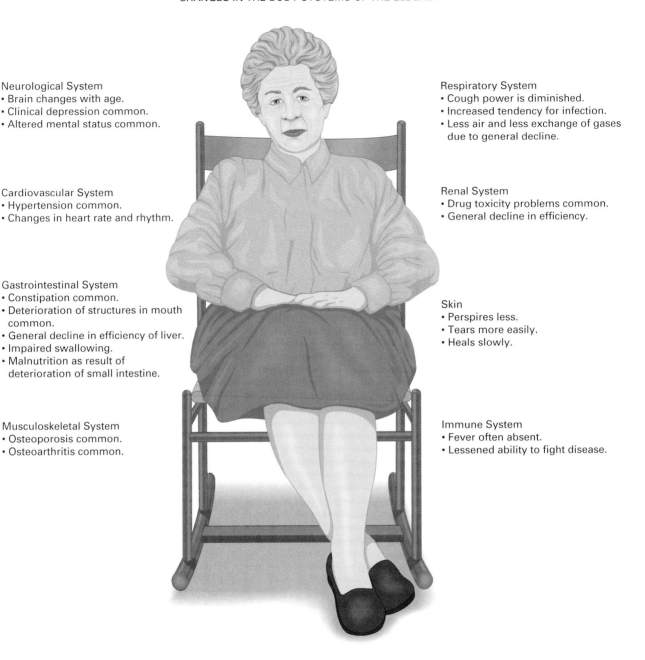

Neurological System
• Brain changes with age.
• Clinical depression common.
• Altered mental status common.

Cardiovascular System
• Hypertension common.
• Changes in heart rate and rhythm.

Gastrointestinal System
• Constipation common.
• Deterioration of structures in mouth common.
• General decline in efficiency of liver.
• Impaired swallowing.
• Malnutrition as result of deterioration of small intestine.

Musculoskeletal System
• Osteoporosis common.
• Osteoarthritis common.

Respiratory System
• Cough power is diminished.
• Increased tendency for infection.
• Less air and less exchange of gases due to general decline.

Renal System
• Drug toxicity problems common.
• General decline in efficiency.

Skin
• Perspires less.
• Tears more easily.
• Heals slowly.

Immune System
• Fever often absent.
• Lessened ability to fight disease.

FIGURE 3-12   Some changes in the body systems of the elderly.

signs and symptoms appear, and affect assessment and treatment of the elderly patient (Table 3-5). You should be familiar with normal systemic changes related to aging so that you can more easily identify the abnormal changes that may point to a serious underlying problem.

RESPIRATORY SYSTEM

The effects of aging on the respiratory system begin as early as age 30. Without regular exercise and/or training, the lungs start to lose their ability to defend

Table 3-5	COMMON AGE-RELATED SYSTEMIC CHANGES	
Body System	**Changes with Age**	**Clinical Importance**
Respiratory	Loss of strength and coordination in respiratory muscles Cough and gag reflex reduced	Increased likelihood of respiratory failure
Cardiovascular	Loss of elasticity and hardening of arteries Changes in heart rate, rhythm, efficiency	Hypertension common Greater likelihood of strokes, heart attacks Great likelihood of bleeding from minor trauma
Neurological	Brain tissue shrinks Loss of memory Clinical depression common Altered mental status common Impaired balance	Delay in appearance of symptoms with head injury Difficulty in patient assessment Increased likelihood of falls
Endocrine	Lowered estrogen production (women) Decline in insulin sensitivity Increase in insulin resistance	Increased likelihood of fractures (bone loss) and heart disease Diabetes mellitus common with greater possibility of hyperglycemia
Gastrointestinal	Diminished digestive functions	Constipation common Greater likelihood of malnutrition
Thermoregulatory	Reduced sweating Decreased shivering	Environmental emergencies more common
Integumentary (Skin)	Thins and becomes more fragile	More subject to tears and sores Bruising more common Heals more slowly
Musculoskeletal	Loss of bone strength (osteoporosis) Loss of joint flexibility and strength (osteoarthritis)	Greater likelihood of fractures Slower healing Increased likelihood of falls
Renal	Loss of kidney size and function	Increased problems with drug toxicity
Genitourinary	Loss of bladder function	Increased urination/incontinence Increased urinary tract infection
Immune	Diminished immune response	More susceptible to infections Impaired immune response to vaccines
Hematological	Decrease in blood volume and/or RBCs	Slower recuperation from illness/injury Greater risk of trauma-related complications

themselves and to carry out their prime function of ventilation. Age-related changes in the respiratory system include:

- Decreased chest wall compliance
- Loss of lung elasticity
- Increased air trapping due to collapse of the smaller airways
- Reduced strength and endurance of the respiratory muscles

Functionally, by the time we reach age 65, vital capacity may be reduced by as much as 50 percent. In addition, the maximum breathing capacity may decrease by as much as 60 percent, while the maximum oxygen uptake may decrease by as much as 70 percent. These changes ultimately result in decreased ventilation and progressive hypoxemia. Any presence of underlying pulmonary diseases, such as emphysema and chronic bronchitis, further reduces respiratory function.

In addition, there is a decrease in an effective cough reflex and the activity of the cilia—the small hairlike fibers that trap particles and infectious agents. The decline of these two defense mechanisms leave the lungs more susceptible to recurring infection.

Other factors that may affect pulmonary function in the elderly include:

* **Kyphosis**
* Chronic exposure to pollutants
* Long-term cigarette smoking

The management of respiratory distress in elderly patients is essentially the same as for all age groups. Position the patient for adequate breathing, usually upright or sitting. Teach breathing patterns that assist in exhalation, such as "pursed-lip breathing." (Tell patients to pretend they are blowing out a candle with each exhalation.) Use bronchodilators as needed, and provide high concentration supplemental oxygen.

At all points, remain attentive for possible complications, such as **anoxic hypoxemia**. Monitor ventilations closely as an elderly patient can become easily fatigued from any increase in the work of breathing. Remember that many elderly patients with respiratory disease have underlying cardiac disease. With this in mind, drugs such as theophylline and the beta agonists should be used with extreme caution. Monitor cardiovascular status, and administer IV fluids judiciously. DO NOT FLUID OVERLOAD. When infusing fluids, frequently reassess lung sounds to check for the pressure of pulmonary edema.

CARDIOVASCULAR SYSTEM

A number of variables unrelated to aging influence cardiovascular function. They include diet, smoking and alcohol use, education, socioeconomic status, and even personality traits. Of particular importance is the level of physical activity. Even though maximum exercise capacity and maximum oxygen consumption decline with age, a well-trained elderly person can match—or even exceed—the aerobic capacity of an unconditioned younger person.

This said, the cardiovascular system still experiences, in varying degrees, age-related deterioration. The wall of the left ventricle may thicken and enlarge (**hypertrophy**), often by as much as 25 percent. This is even more pronounced if there is associated hypertension. In addition, **fibrosis** develops in the heart and peripheral vascular system, resulting in hypertension, arteriosclerosis, and decreased cardiac function.

The aorta also becomes stiff and lengthens. This results from deposits of calcium and changes in the connective tissue. These changes predispose the aorta to partial tearing, resulting in dissection (thoracic) or aneurysm (abdominal).

As a person ages, the pattern of ventricular filling changes. Less blood enters the left ventricle during early diastole when the mitral valve is open. Therefore, filling and stretch (preload) depend on atrial contraction. Loss of the atrial kick (as will occur with atrial fibrillation) is not well tolerated in the elderly.

Over time, the conductive system of the heart degenerates, often causing dysrhythmias and varying degrees of heart block. Ultimately, the stroke volume declines and the heart rate slows, leading to decreased cardiac output. Because of

* **kyphosis** exaggeration of the normal posterior curvature of the spine.

* **anoxic hypoxemia** an oxygen deficiency due to disordered pulmonary mechanisms of oxygenation.

In treating respiratory disorders in the elderly patient, DO NOT FLUID OVERLOAD.

* **hypertrophy** an increase in the size or bulk of an organ.

* **fibrosis** the formation of fiber-like connective tissue, also called scar tissue in an organ.

this, the heart's ability to respond to stress diminishes. In such situations, expect exercise intolerance—an inability of the heart to meet an exercising muscle's need for oxygen.

To adequately manage complaints related to the cardiovascular system, ask the patient to stop all activity. This reduces the myocardial oxygen demand. DO NOT walk a patient with a cardiovascular complaint to your rig. Take the following basic steps per local protocols.

DO NOT walk a patient with a cardiovascular disorder to your rig.

- Provide high concentration supplemental oxygen.
- Start an IV for medication administration. Medications will vary with the complaint, but may include:
  —Antianginal agents
  —Aspirin
  —Diuretics
  —Antidysrhythmics
- Inquire about age-related dosages.
- Monitor vital signs and rhythm.
- Acquire a 12-lead ECG.
- Remain calm, professional, and empathetic. A heart-attack is one of the most fearful situations for the elderly.

NERVOUS SYSTEM

Unlike cells in other organ systems, cells in the central nervous system cannot reproduce. The brain can lose as much as 45 percent of its cells in certain areas of the cortex. Overall, there is an average 10 percent reduction in brain weight from age 20 to age 90. Keep in mind that reductions in brain weight and ventricular size are not well correlated with intelligence, and elderly people may still be capable of highly creative and productive thought. Once again, DO NOT assume that an elderly person possesses less cognitive skill than a younger person. Slight changes that may be expected include:

- Difficulty with recent memory
- Psychomotor slowing
- Forgetfulness
- Decreased reaction times

Although brain size may not have clinical implications in terms in intelligence, it does have implications for trauma. A reduction in brain size leaves room for increased bleeding following a blow to the head, making the elderly more prone to subdural hematomas. In cases of altered mental status, maintain a suspicion of trauma, especially when an accident has been reported.

Whenever you assess an elderly patient for mental status, determine a baseline. Presume your patient to have been mentally sharp unless proven otherwise. (Talk with partners, caregivers, family members, and so on.) Focus on the patient's perceptions, thinking processes, and communication. In questioning an elderly patient, provide an environment with minimal distractions. As already mentioned, ask clear and unhurried questions.

In assessing an elderly patient with altered mental status, presume the patient to have been mentally sharp unless proven otherwise.

In forming a patient plan, observe for weakness, chronic fatigue, changes in sleep patterns, and syncope or near syncope. If you suspect a stroke, think "brain attack" and assign the patient a priority status. (Additional material on strokes will appear later in the chapter.) Consider blood pressure control per local protocol—but remember that perfusion of the brain tissue depends upon an adequate BP. DO NOT plan to reduce the blood pressure to an average of 120/80 as cerebral blood flow may be diminished. Consider the causes of changes in mental status, keeping in mind the possibility of trauma. Apply oxygen, and monitor ventilations. Depending upon the situation, you may be called on to administer dextrose, thiamine, and naloxone.

ENDOCRINE SYSTEM

Early diagnosis of disorders in the endocrine system offers some of the greatest opportunities to prevent disabilities through appropriate hormonal therapy and/or lifestyle changes. Diabetes mellitus, for example, is extremely common among the elderly. However, normalization of glucose levels—through diet, exercise, and/or drug therapy—can reduce some of the devastating vascular and neurological complications.

In women, menopause—a normal age-related hormonal deficiency—can be similarly treated in a variety of ways, including hormone replacement therapy (HRT). By taking preventive measures, women can reduce and/or delay the incidence of heart disease, bone loss, and possibly Alzheimer's disease.

Thyroid disorders are "clinical masqueraders," especially in the elderly. Common signs and symptoms may be absent or diminished. When signs and symptoms are present, they may be attributed to aging or tied to other diseases, such as cardiovascular, GI, or neuromuscular disorders. However, it has been shown that thyroid disorders, especially hypothyroidism and thyroid nodules, increase with age. (For more on thyroid disorders, see "Metabolic and Endocrine Disorders" later in the chapter.)

With the exception of glucose disorders, most endocrine disorders cannot be easily determined in the field. Many endocrine emergencies will present as altered mental status, especially with insulin-related diseases. Monitor for cardiovascular effects of endocrine changes such as aortic aneurysm in a patient with **Marfan's Syndrome**—a disorder resulting in abnormal growth of distal tissues and a dilatation of the root of the aorta. Also remain alert to blood pressure swings in thyroid disorders such as hyperthyroidism and hypothyroidism.

GASTROINTESTINAL SYSTEM

Age affects the gastrointestinal system in various ways. The volume of saliva may decrease by as much as 33 percent, leading to complaints of dry mouth, nutritional deficiencies, and a predisposition to choking. Gastric secretions may decrease to as little as 20 percent of the quantity present in younger people. Esophageal and intestinal motility also decrease, making swallowing more difficult and delaying digestive processes. The production of hydrochloric acid also declines, further disrupting digestion and, in some adults, contributing to nutritional anemia. Gums atrophy and the number of taste buds decrease, reducing even further the desire to eat.

Other conditions may also develop. **Hiatal hernias** are not age-related per se, but can have serious consequences for the elderly. They may incarcerate, strangulate, or, in the most severe cases, result in massive GI hemorrhage. A diminished liver function, which is associated with aging, can delay or impede detoxification. A common drug toxicity problem for EMS personnel is the use of lidocaine for ventricular arrythmias. (See "Toxicological Emergencies" later in the chapter.) A diminished liver function can also reduce the production of clotting proteins, which in turn leads to bleeding abnormalities.

Complications in the gastrointestinal system can be life-threatening. Use shock protocols as necessary, and remember that not all fluid loss occurs outside the body.

Many endocrine emergencies encountered in the field present as altered mental status, especially with insulin-related disorders.

* **Marfan's Syndrome** hereditary condition of connective tissue, bones, muscles, ligaments, and skeletal structures characterized by irregular and unsteady gait, tall lean body type with long extremities, flat feet, stooped shoulders. The aorta is usually dilated and may become weakened enough to allow an aneurysm to develop.

* **hiatal hernia** protrusion of the stomach upward into the mediastinal cavity through the esophageal hiatus of the diaphragm.

A diminished liver function, which is associated with aging, can delay or impede detoxification. A common drug toxicity problem for EMS personnel is the use of lidocaine for ventricular arrythmias.

THERMOREGULATORY SYSTEM

The elderly and infants are highly susceptible to variations in environmental temperatures. This occurs in the elderly because of altered or impaired thermoregulatory mechanisms. Aging seems to reduce the effectiveness of sweating in cooling the body. Older persons tend to sweat at higher core temperatures and have less sweat output per gland than younger people. As people age, they also experience deterioration of the autonomic nervous system, including a decrease in shivering and lower resting peripheral blood flow. In addition, the elderly may have a diminished perception of the cold. Drugs and disease can further affect an elderly patient's response to temperature extremes, resulting in hyperthermia or accidental hypothermia.

Environmental emergencies are common causes of EMS calls, especially among the elderly living alone or in poverty. For more on these emergencies, see the discussion of heatstroke, hypothermia, and hyperthermia later in the chapter.

INTEGUMENTARY SYSTEM

As people age, the skin loses collagen, a connective tissue that gives elasticity and support to the skin. Without this support, the skin is subject to a greater number of injuries from bumping or tearing. The lack of support also makes it more difficult to start an IV, as the veins "roll away." Furthermore, the assessment of tenting skin becomes an inaccurate indicator of fluid status in the elderly. Without elasticity, the skin often will remain tented regardless of water balance.

As the skin thins, cells reproduce more slowly. Injury to skin is often more severe than in younger patients and healing time is increased. As a rule, the elderly are at a higher risk of secondary infection, skin tumors, drug-induced eruptions, and fungal or viral infections. Decades of exposure to the sun also makes the elderly vulnerable to melanoma and other sun-related carcinomas (e.g., basal cell carcinoma, squamous cell carcinoma).

MUSCULOSKELETAL SYSTEM

An aging person may lose as much as 2–3 inches of height from narrowing of the intervertebral discs and **osteoporosis.** Osteoporosis is the loss of mineral from the bone, resulting in softening of the bones. This is especially evident in the vertebral bodies, thus causing a change in posture. The posture of the aged individual often reveals an increase in the curvature of the thoracic spine, commonly called kyphosis, and slight flexion of the knee and hip joints. The demineralization of bone makes the patient much more susceptible to hip and other fractures. Some fractures may even occur from simple actions such as sneezing.

In addition to skeletal changes, a decrease in skeletal muscle weight commonly occurs with age—especially with sedentary individuals. To compensate, elderly women develop a narrow, short gait, while older men develop a wide gait. These changes make the elderly more susceptible to falls and, consequently, a possible loss of independence.

Because of the changes in the musculoskeletal system, simple trauma in the elderly can lead to complex injuries. In treating musculoskeletal disorders, supply supplemental oxygen, initiate an IV line, and consider pain control. Many extremity injuries should be splinted as found because of changes in the bone and joint structure of the elderly. To determine the cause of any injury, be sure to look beyond the obvious. Keep in mind the possibility of underlying medical conditions, drug complications, abuse or neglect, and ingestion of alcohol or drugs.

✱ **osteoporosis** softening of bone tissue due to the loss of essential minerals, principally calcium.

Many extremity injuries should be splinted as found because of changes in the bone and joint structure in the elderly.

RENAL SYSTEM

* nephrons the functional units
  of the kidneys.

Aging affects the renal system through a reduction in the number of functioning **nephrons,** which may be decreased by 30–40 percent. Renal blood flow may also be reduced by up to 45 percent, increasing the waste products in the blood and upsetting the fluid and electrolyte balance. Because the kidneys are responsible for the production of erythropoietin (which stimulates the production of red blood cells in the bone marrow) and renin (which stimulates vasoconstriction), a decrease in renal function may result in anemia or hypertension in the older patient.

Prehospital treatment of complaints involving the renal and urinary systems is directed toward adequate oxygenation, fluid status, monitoring output, and pain control. Pay attention to the airway as nausea and vomiting are complications of pain secondary to renal obstruction. Also monitor vital signs to detect changes in blood pressure and pulse.

GENITOURINARY SYSTEM

As people age, they experience a progressive loss of bladder sensation and tone. The bladder does not empty completely and consequently the patient may sense a frequent need to urinate. This urge increases the risk of falls, especially during the middle of the night when lighting is dim or the patient is sleepy. Furthermore, the lack of emptying increases the likelihood of urinary tract infection and perhaps sepsis. In the male, the prostate often becomes enlarged (benign prostatic hypertrophy), causing difficulty in urination or urinary retention. As already mentioned, the elderly also commonly develop, in varying degrees, problems with incontinence.

Treatment for a complaint in the genitourinary system is described in the preceding section on the renal system and in the earlier discussion of incontinence.

IMMUNE SYSTEM

* immune senescence diminished vigor of the immune response to the challenge and rechallenge by pathogens.

As a person ages, the function of T cells declines, making them less able to notify the immune system of invasion by antigens. A diminished immune response, sometimes called **immune senescence,** increases the susceptibility of the elderly to infections. It also increases the duration and severity of an infection.

Unless contraindicated, the elderly should receive vaccinations suggested by the Health Department. However, keep in mind that aging impairs the immune response to vaccines. The best prevention is adequate nutrition, infection control measures (e.g., washing hands), and exercise. Recognition and treatment of diseases such as diabetes mellitus, heart failure, thyroid disease, and occult malignancy also reduce the risk and severity of infections. As a paramedic, you should treat alterations in immune status as life threats and seek to prevent exposure of patients to infectious agents. DO NOT transmit an illness—even a mild cold—to an elderly patient.

DO NOT transmit an illness—even a mild cold—to an elderly patient.

HEMATOLOGY SYSTEM

The hematology system is affected by a failure of the renal system to stimulate the production of red blood cells. Nutritional abnormalities may also produce abnormal RBCs. Since there is less body water present in the elderly, blood volume similarly decreases. This makes it difficult for an elderly patient to recuperate from an illness or injury. Intervention must be started early in order to make a lasting difference.

In addition to providing supplemental oxygen, you should prepare for increases in bleeding time. Monitor the elderly patient closely as deterioration is difficult to stop.

COMMON MEDICAL PROBLEMS
IN THE ELDERLY

In general, the elderly suffer from the same kinds of medical emergencies as younger patients. However, illnesses may be more severe, complications more likely, and classic signs and symptoms absent or altered. In addition, the elderly are more likely to react adversely to stress and deteriorate much more quickly than young or middle-aged adults. The following are some of the medical disorders that you may encounter.

PULMONARY/RESPIRATORY DISORDERS

Respiratory emergencies are some of the most common reasons elderly persons summon EMS or seek emergency care. Most elderly patients with a respiratory disorder present with a chief complaint of dyspnea. However, coughing, congestion, and wheezing are also common chief complaints.

Many factors can trigger respiratory distress among the elderly (Figure 3-13). Descriptions of the most common ones follow.

Pneumonia

Pneumonia is an infection of the lung. It is usually caused by a bacterium or virus. However, aspiration pneumonia may also develop as a result of difficulty swallowing.

Pneumonia is a serious disease for the elderly. It is the fourth leading cause of death in people age 65 and older. Its incidence increases with age at a rate of 10 percent for each decade beyond age 20. It is found in up to 60 percent of the

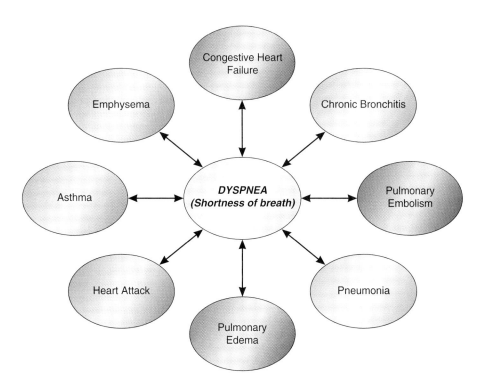

FIGURE 3-13 Dyspnea can be caused by a number of respiratory and cardiac problems in the elderly.

autopsies performed on the elderly. Reasons the elderly develop pneumonia more frequently than younger patients include:

- Decreased immune response
- Reduced pulmonary function
- Increased colonization of the pharynx by gram-negative bacteria
- Abnormal or ineffective cough reflex
- Decreased effectiveness of mucociliary cells of the upper respiratory system

The elderly who are at greatest risk for contracting pneumonia include frail adults and those with chronic, multiple diseases or compromised immunity. Institutionalized patients—either in hospitals or nursing homes—are especially vulnerable because of increased exposure to microorganisms and limited mobility. A patient in an institutional setting is up to 50 times more likely to contract pneumonia than an elderly patient receiving home care.

Common signs and symptoms of pneumonia include increasing dyspnea, congestion, fever, chills, tachypnea, sputum production, and altered mental status. Occasionally, abdominal pain may be the only symptom. Because of thermoregulatory changes, a fever may be absent in an elderly patient.

Prevention strategies include prophylactic treatment with antibiotics. Efforts should also be taken to reduce exposure to infectious patients and to promote patient mobility.

In treating an elderly patient with pneumonia, manage all life threats. Maintain adequate oxygenation. Transport the patient to the hospital for diagnosis, keeping in mind that patients with respiratory disease often have other underlying problems.

Chronic Obstructive Pulmonary Disease

Chronic obstructive pulmonary disease (COPD) is really a collection of diseases, characterized by chronic airflow obstruction with reversible and/or irreversible components. Although each COPD has its own distinct features, elderly patients commonly have two or more types at the same time. COPD usually refers to some combination of emphysema, chronic bronchitis, and, to a lesser degree, asthma. Pneumonia, as well as other respiratory disorders, can further complicate chronic obstructive pulmonary disease in the elderly.

In the United States, chronic obstructive pulmonary disease is among the ten leading causes of death. Its prevalence has been increasing over the past 20 years. Several factors combine to produce the damage of COPD. They include:

- Genetic disposition
- Exposure to environmental pollutants
- Existence of a childhood respiratory disease
- Cigarette smoking, a contributing factor in up to 80 percent of all cases of COPD

The physiology of COPD varies, but may include inflammation of the air passages with increased mucus production or actual destruction of the alveoli. The outcome is decreased airflow in the alveoli, resulting in reduced oxygen exchange. Usual signs and symptoms include:

- Cough
- Increased sputum production

- Dyspnea
- Accessory muscle use
- Pursed-lip breathing
- Tripod positioning
- Exercise intolerance
- Wheezing
- Pleuritic chest pain
- Tachypnea

COPD is progressive and debilitating (Figure 3-14). The patient can often keep the signs and symptoms under control until the body is stressed. When the condition becomes disabling, it is called exacerbation of COPD. This condition can lead rapidly to patient death as hypoxia and hypercapnia alter acid-base balance and deprive the tissues of the oxygen needed for efficient energy production.

The most effective prevention involves elimination of tobacco products and reduced exposure to cigarette smoke (in non-smokers). Recent legislation has sought to keep public places smoke free and to discourage cigarette smoking in the young. Once the disease is present, patients are taught to identify stresses that exacerbate the condition. Appropriate self care includes exercise, avoidance of infections, appropriate use of drugs, and, when necessary, calling EMS.

When confronted with an elderly patient with COPD, treatment is essentially the same as for all age groups. Supply supplemental oxygen and possibly drug therapy, usually for reducing dyspnea.

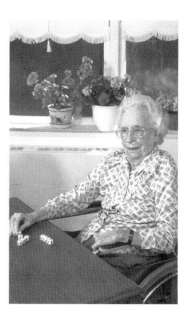

FIGURE 3-14   The COPD patient may use a nasal cannula with a home oxygen unit.

Pulmonary Embolism

Pulmonary embolism (PE) should always be considered as a possible cause of respiratory distress in the elderly. Although statistics for the elderly are unavailable, approximately 650,000 cases occur annually in the United States alone. Of this number, a pulmonary embolism is the primary cause of death in 100,000 people and a contributing factor in another 100,000 deaths. Nearly 11 percent of PE deaths take place in the first hour and 38 percent in the second hour.

Blood clots are the most frequent cause of pulmonary embolism. However, the condition may also be caused by fat, air, bone marrow, tumor cells, or foreign bodies. Risk factors for developing pulmonary embolism include:

- Deep venous thrombosis
- Prolonged immobility, common among the elderly
- Malignancy (tumors)
- Paralysis
- Fractures of the pelvis, hip, or leg
- Obesity
- Trauma to the leg vessels
- Major surgery
- Presence of a venous catheter
- Use of estrogen (in women)
- Atrial fibrillation

Pulmonary emboli usually originate in the deep veins of the thigh and calf. The condition should be suspected in any patient with the acute onset of dyspnea. Often, it is accompanied by pleuritic chest pain and right heart failure. If the pulmonary embolus is massive, you can expect severe dyspnea, cardiac dys-rhythmias, and, ultimately, cardiovascular collapse.

Definitive diagnosis of a pulmonary embolism takes place in a hospital setting. The goals of field treatment are to manage and minimize complications of the condition. General treatment considerations include delivery of high-flow oxygen via mask, maintaining oxygen levels above an SaO_2 of 90 percent. Establishment of an IV for possible administration of medications is appropriate, but vigorous fluid therapy should be avoided, if possible.

Prehospital pharmacological therapy for pulmonary embolism is limited. Upon advice from medical direction, you may administer small doses of morphine sulfate to reduce patient anxiety. After confirming the absence of GI bleeding, medical direction may also prescribe anticoagulants to prevent clot formation and/or to speed clot dissolution. If the administration of a vasopressor is indicated by low blood pressure, then dopamine may be prescribed. In such cases, remember to titrate the dopamine to a desirable blood pressure.

The risk of death from pulmonary embolism is greatest in the first few hours. As a result, rapid transport is essential. Position the patient in an upright position and avoid lifting the patient by the legs or knees, which may dislodge thrombi in the lower extremities. During transport, continue to monitor changes in skin color, pulse oximetry, and changes in breathing rate and rhythm. Your field assessment and interventions can save the patient's life and guide the hospital physician in a direction that will result in an accurate diagnosis and rapid treatment.

The risk of death from pulmonary embolism is greatest in the first few hours. As a result, rapid transport is essential.

Pulmonary Edema

Pulmonary edema is an effusion or escape of serous fluids into the alveoli and interstitial tissues of the lungs. Acute pulmonary edema can develop rapidly in the elderly. Although most commonly associated with acute myocardial infarction, it can also occur due to other factors including pulmonary infections, inhaled toxins, narcotic overdose, pulmonary embolism, and decreased atmospheric pressure.

Pulmonary edema causes severe dyspnea associated with congestion. Other signs and symptoms include rapid labored breathing, cough with blood-stained sputum, cyanosis, and cold extremities. Physical examination usually reveals the presence of moist crackles and accessory muscle use. Severe cases will exhibit rhonchi.

Treatment is directed toward altering the cause of the condition. The existence of pulmonary edema can be life-threatening and is often the symptom of a fatal cardiovascular disease.

The existence of pulmonary edema can be life-threatening and is often the symptom of a fatal cardiovascular disease.

Lung Cancer

North America has the highest incidence of lung cancer in the world. The incidence increases with age, with about 65 percent of all lung cancer deaths occurring among people age 65 and older. The leading cause of lung cancer is cigarette smoking.

Often, progressive dyspnea will be the first presentation of a cancerous lesion. Hemoptysis (bloody sputum), chronic cough, and weight loss are also common symptoms.

Treatment of lung cancer occurs in a hospital setting. However, you may be called to assist in the follow-up home care or, in terminal stages, a hospice. (See Chapter 6 for more information on this subject.)

CARDIOVASCULAR DISORDERS

The leading cause of death in the elderly is cardiovascular disease. Assessment and treatment of cardiovascular disease in the elderly patient is often complicated by non-age-related factors and disease processes in other organ systems. In conducting your history, determine the patient's level of cardiovascular fitness, changes in exercise tolerance, recent diet history, use of medications, and use of cigarettes and/or alcohol. Ask questions about breathing difficulty, especially at night, and evidence of palpitations, flutter, or skipped beats.

In performing the physical exam, look for hypertension and orthostatic hypotension (a decrease in blood pressure and an increase in heart rate when rising from a seated or supine position). Watch for dehydration or dependent edema. When taking an elderly patient's blood pressure, consider checking both arms. Routinely determine pulses in all the extremities. In auscultating the patient, remember that a bruit or noise in the neck, abdomen, or groin indicates a high probability of carotid, aortorenal, or peripheral vascular disease. Keep in mind, too, that heart sounds are generally softer in the elderly, probably because of a thickening of lung tissue between the heart and chest wall.

In evaluating the problem, recall the cardiovascular disorders commonly found in elderly patients. They include angina pectoris, myocardial infarction, heart failure, dysrhythmias, aortic dissection, aneurysm, hypertension, and syncope.

In auscultating a patient, remember that a bruit in the neck, abdomen, or groin indicates a high probability of carotid, aortorenal, or peripheral vascular disease.

Keep in mind that heart sounds are generally softer in the elderly, probably because of a thickening of lung tissues between the heart and chest wall.

Angina Pectoris

The likelihood of developing angina increases dramatically with age. This is especially true of women, who are estrogen protected until after menopause. Angina is usually triggered by physical activity, especially after a meal, and by exposure to very cold weather. Attacks vary in frequency, from several a day to occasional episodes separated by weeks or months.

Angina pectoris literally means "pain in the chest." However, the pain of angina is actually felt in only about 10–20 percent of elderly patients. The changes in sensory nerves, combined with the myocardial changes of aging, make dyspnea a more likely symptom of angina than pain.

Angina develops when narrowing of coronary vessels due to plaque or vasospasm lead to an inability to meet the oxygen demands of the heart muscle. The heart muscle usually responds by sending out pain signals, which represent a build-up of lactic acid. In an elderly patient, exercise intolerance is a key symptom of angina. In obtaining a history, you should ask the patient about sudden changes in routine. In addition, inquire about any increased stresses on the heart, such as anemia, infection, dysrhythmias, and thyroid changes.

General prevention strategies in the elderly are similar to those in young patients. Blood pressure control, combined with diet, exercise, and smoking modifications reduces the risk in all groups.

In an elderly patient, exercise intolerance is a key symptom of angina.

Myocardial Infarction

A myocardial infarction (MI) involves actual death of muscle tissue due to a partial or complete occlusion of one or more of the coronary arteries. The greatest number of patients hospitalized for acute myocardial infarction are older than 65. The elderly patient with myocardial infarction is less likely to present with classic symptoms such as chest pain than a younger counterpart. Atypical presentations that may be seen in the elderly include:

- Absence of pain
- Exercise intolerance
- Confusion/dizziness
- Syncope
- Dyspnea—common in patients over age 85
- Neck, dental, and/or epigastric pain
- Fatigue/weakness

The elderly patient with myocardial infarction is less likely to present with classic symptoms than a younger counterpart.

silent myocardial infarction a myocardial infarction that occurs without exhibiting obvious signs and symptoms.

The mortality rate associated with myocardial infarction and/or resulting complications doubles after age 70. Unlike younger patients, the elderly are more likely to suffer a **silent myocardial infarction.** They also tend to have larger myocardial infarctions. The majority of deaths that occur in the first few hours following a myocardial infarction are due to dysrhythmias.

A myocardial infarction is most commonly triggered by some form of physical exertion or a preexisting heart disease. Because of the high mortality associated with myocardial infarctions in the elderly, early detection and emergency management are critical.

Heart Failure

Heart failure takes place when cardiac output cannot meet the body's metabolic demands. The incidence rises exponentially after age 60. The condition is widespread among the elderly and is the most common diagnosis in hospitalized patients over age 65. The causes of heart failure fall in one of four categories: impairment to flow, inadequate cardiac filling, volume overload, and myocardial failure.

Typical age-related factors, such as prolonged myocardial contractions, make the elderly vulnerable to heart failure. Other factors that place them at risk include:

- Noncompliance with drug therapy
- Anemia
- Ischemia
- Thermoregulatory disorders (hypothermia/hyperthermia)
- Hypoxia
- Infection
- Use of non-steroidal anti-inflammatory drugs

Signs and symptoms of heart failure vary. In most patients, regardless of age, some form of edema exists. However, edema in the elderly can indicate a range of problems, including musculoskeletal injury. Assessment findings specific to the elderly include:

- Fatigue (left failure)
- **Two pillow orthopnea**
- Dyspnea on exertion
- Dry, hacking cough progressing to productive cough
- Dependent edema (right failure)
- **Nocturia**
- Anorexia, **hepatomegaly,** ascites

two-pillow orthopnea the number of pillows—in this case, two—needed to ease the difficulty of breathing while lying down; a significant factor in assessing the level of respiratory distress.

nocturia excessive urination during the night.

hepatomegaly enlarged liver.

Nonpharmacologic management of heart failure includes modifications in diet (e.g., less fat and cholesterol), exercise, and reduction in weight, if necessary. Pharmacologic management may include treatment with diuretics, vasodilators, antihypertensive agents, or inotropic agents. Check to see if the patient is already on any of these medications and if the patient is compliant with scheduled doses.

Dysrhythmias

Many cardiac dysrhythmias develop with age. Atrial fibrillation is the most common dysrhythmia encountered.

Dysrhythmias occur primarily as a result of degeneration of the patient's conductive system. Anything that decreases myocardial blood flood can produce a dysrhythmia. They may also be caused by electrolyte abnormalities.

To complicate matters further, the elderly do not tolerate extremes in heart rate as well as a younger person would. For example, a heart rate of 140 in an older patient may cause syncope, while a younger patient can often tolerate a heart rate greater than 180. In addition, dysrhythmias can lead to falls from cerebral hypoperfusion. They can also result in congestive heart failure (CHF) or a transient ischemic attack (TIA).

Treatment considerations depend upon the type of dysrhythmia. Patients may already have a pacemaker in place. In such cases, keep in mind that pacemakers have a low but significant rate of complications such as a failed battery, fibrosis around the catheter site, lead fracture, or electrode dislodgment. In a number of situations, drug therapy may be indicated. Whenever you discover a dysrhythmia, remember that an abnormal or disordered heart rhythm may be the only clinical finding in an elderly patient suffering acute myocardial infarction.

Aortic Dissection/Aneurysms

Aortic dissection is a degeneration of the wall of the aorta, either in the thoracic or abdominal cavity. It can result in an **aneurysm** or in a rupture of the vessel.

Approximately 80 percent of thoracic aneurysms are due to atherosclerosis combined with hypertension. The remaining cases occur secondary to other factors, including Marfan's Syndrome or blunt trauma to the chest. Patients with dissections will often present with tearing chest pain radiating through to the back or, if rupture occurs, cardiac arrest.

The distal portion of the aorta is the most common site for abdominal aneurysms. Approximately 1 in 250 people over age 50 die from a ruptured abdominal aneurysm. The aneurysm may appear as a pulsatile mass in a patient with a normal girth, but lack of an identifiable mass does not eliminate this condition. Patients may present with tearing abdominal pain or unexplained low back pain. Pulses in the legs are diminished or absent and the lower extremities feel cold to the touch. There may be sensory abnormalities such as numbness, tingling, or pain in the legs. The patient may fall when attempting to stand.

Treatment of an aneurysm depends on its size, location, and the severity of the condition. In the case of thoracic aortic dissection, continuous IV infusion and/or administration of drug therapy to lower the arterial pressure and to diminish the velocity of left ventricle contraction may be indicated. Rapid transport is essential, especially for the older patient who most commonly requires care and observation in an intensive care unit.

Hypertension

Hypertension appears to be a product of industrial society. In developed nations, such as the United States, the systolic and diastolic pressures have a tendency to rise until age 60. Systolic pressure may continue to rise after that time, but diastolic pressure stabilizes. Since this rise in blood pressure is not seen in less developed nations, experts believe that hypertension is not a normal age-related change.

Today more than 50 percent of Americans over age 65 have clinically diagnosed hypertension—defined as blood pressure greater than 140/90 mmHg. Prolonged elevated blood pressure will eventually damage the heart, brain, or kidneys. As a result of hypertension, elderly patients are at greater risk for heart failure, stroke, blindness, renal failure, coronary heart disease, and peripheral vascular disease. In men with blood pressure greater than 160/95 mmHg, the risk of mortality nearly doubles.

Content Review

POSSIBLE PACEMAKER COMPLICATIONS
- Failed battery
- Fibrosis around the catheter site
- Lead fracture
- Electrode dislodgment

Remember that an abnormal or disordered heart rhythm may be the only clinical finding in an elderly patient suffering acute myocardial infarction.

✱ **aortic dissection** a degeneration of the wall of the aorta.

✱ **aneurysm** abnormal dilation of a blood vessel, usually an artery, due to a congenital defect or a weakness in the wall of the vessel.

Most abdominal aortic aneurysms occur below the renal arteries.

✱ **epistaxis** nosebleed.

Hypertension increases with atherosclerosis, which is more common with the elderly than other age groups. Other contributing factors include obesity and diabetes. The condition can be prevented or controlled through diet (sodium reduction), exercise, cessation of smoking, and compliance with medications.

Hypertension is often a silent disease that produces no clinically obvious signs or symptoms. It may be associated with nonspecific complaints such as headache, tinnitus, **epistaxis,** slow tremors, or nausea and vomiting. An acute onset of high blood pressure without any kidney involvement is often a telltale indicator of thyroid disease.

Management of hypertension depends upon its severity and the existence of other conditions. For example, hypertension is often treated with beta-blockers—medications that are contraindicated in patients with chronic obstructive lung disease, asthma, or heart block greater than first degree. Diuretics, another common drug used in treating hypertension, should be prescribed with care for patients on digitalis. Keep in mind that centrally acting agents are more likely to produce negative side effects in the elderly. Unlike younger patients, the elderly may experience depression, forgetfulness, sleep problems, or vivid dreams and/or hallucinations.

Syncope

Syncope is a common presenting complaint among the elderly. The condition results when blood flow to the brain is temporarily interrupted or decreased. It is most often caused by problems with either the nervous system or the cardiovascular system. In general, syncope has a higher incidence of death in elderly patients than in younger individuals. The following are some of the common presentations that you may encounter:

✱ **varicosities** an abnormal dilation of a vein or group of veins.

✱ **autonomic dysfunction** an abnormality of the involuntary aspect of the nervous system.

✱ **valsalva maneuver** forced exhalation against a closed glottis, such as with coughing. This maneuver stimulates the parasympathetic nervous system via the vagus nerve, which in turn slows the heart rate.

✱ **Stokes-Adams syndrome** a series of symptoms resulting from heart block, most commonly syncope. The symptoms result from decreased blood flow to the brain caused by the sudden decrease in cardiac output.

✱ **sick sinus syndrome** a group of disorders characterized by dysfunction of the sinoatrial node in the heart.

- *Vasodepressor Syncope.* Vasodepressor syncope is the common faint. It may occur following emotional distress, pain, prolonged bed rest, mild blood loss, prolonged standing in warm, crowded rooms, anemia, or fever.

- *Orthostatic Syncope.* Orthostatic syncope occurs when a person rises from a seated or supine position. There are several possible causes. First, there may be a disproportion between blood volume and vascular capacity. That is, there is a pooling of blood in the legs, reducing blood flow to the brain. Causes of this include hypovolemia, venous **varicosities,** prolonged bed rest, and **autonomic dysfunction.** Many drugs, especially blood pressure medicines, can cause drug-induced orthostatic syncope due to the effects of the medications on the capacitance vessels.

- *Vasovagal Syncope.* Vasovagal syncope occurs as a result of a **valsalva maneuver,** which happens during defecation, coughing, or similar maneuvers. This effectively slows the heart rate and cardiac output, thus decreasing blood flow to the brain.

- *Cardiac Syncope.* Cardiac syncope results from transient reduction in cerebral blood flow due to a sudden decrease in cardiac output. It can result from several mechanisms. Syncope can be the primary symptom of silent myocardial infarction. In addition, many dysrhythmias can cause syncope. Dysrhythmias that have been shown to cause syncope include bradycardias, **Stokes-Adams syndrome,** heart block, tachydysrhythmia, and **sick sinus syndrome.**

- *Seizures.* Syncope may result from a seizure disorder or syncope (prolonged) may cause seizure activity. Syncope due to seizures tends to occur without warning. It is associated with muscular jerking or convulsions, incontinence, and tongue-biting. Postictal confusion may follow.

- *Transient Ischemic Attacks.* Transient ischemic attacks occur more frequently in the elderly. They may cause syncope.

NEUROLOGICAL DISORDERS

Elderly patients are at risk for several neurological emergencies. Often, the exact cause is not initially known and may require probing at the hospital.

Many of the neurological disorders that you will encounter in the field will exhibit an alteration in mental status. You may discover a range of underlying causes from stroke to degenerative brain disease. Some of the most common causes of altered mental status include:

- Cerebrovascular disease (stroke or transient ischemic attack)
- Myocardial infarction
- Seizures
- Medication-related problems (drug interactions, drug underdose, and drug overdose)
- Infection
- Fluid and electrolyte abnormalities (dehydration)
- Lack of nutrients (hypoglycemia)
- Temperature changes (hypothermia, hyperthermia)
- Structural changes (dementia, subdural hematoma)

As mentioned, it is often impossible in the field to distinguish the cause of an altered mental status. Even so, you should carry out a thorough assessment. Administer supplemental oxygen. As soon as practical, obtain a blood glucose level to exclude hypoglycemia as a possible cause. Overall, the approach to the elderly patient with altered mental status is the same as with any other patient presenting with similar symptoms.

As soon as practical, obtain a blood glucose level to exclude hypoglycemia as a possible cause of altered mental status in an elderly patient.

Cerebrovascular Disease (Stroke/Brain Attack)

Stroke is the third leading cause of death in the United States. Annually, about 500,000 people suffer strokes and about 150,000 die. Incidence of stroke and the likelihood of dying from a stroke increase with age. Occlusive stroke is statistically more common in the elderly and relatively uncommon in younger individuals. Older patients are at higher risk of stroke because of atherosclerosis, hypertension, immobility, limb paralysis, congestive heart failure, and atrial fibrillation. Transient ischemic attacks (TIAs) are also more common in older patients. More than one-third of patients suffering TIAs will develop a major, permanent stroke. As previously mentioned, TIAs are a frequent cause of syncope in the elderly.

Strokes usually fall in one of two major categories. **Brain ischemia**—injury to brain tissue caused by an inadequate supply of oxygen and nutrients—accounts for about 80 percent of all strokes. Brain hemorrhage, the second major category, may be either **subarachnoid hemorrhage** or **intracerebral hemorrhage**. These different patterns of bleeding have different presentations, causes, and treatments. However, together they account for a high percentage of all stroke deaths.

Because of the various kinds of strokes, signs and symptoms can present in many ways—altered mental status, coma, paralysis, slurred speech, a change in

✳ stroke injury to or death of brain tissue resulting from interruption of cerebral blood flow and oxygenation.

✳ brain ischemia injury to brain tissues caused by an inadequate supply of oxygen and nutrients.

✳ subarachnoid hemorrhage bleeding that occurs between the arachnoid and dura mater of the brain.

✳ intracerebral hemorrhage bleeding directly into the brain.

mood, and seizures. Stroke should be highly suspect in any elderly patient with a sudden change in mental status.

Whenever you suspect a stroke, it is essential that you complete the Glasgow Coma Scale for later comparison in the emergency department. Thrombolytic agents administered to a patient suffering an occlusive (ischemic) stroke can decrease the severity of damage if administered within 3 hours of onset. Rapid transport is essential for avoiding brain damage or limiting its extent. In the case of stroke, "time is brain tissue."

By far the most preferred treatment is prevention of strokes in the first place. Strategies include:

- Control of hypertension
- Treatment of cardiac disorders, including dysrhythmias and coronary artery disease
- Treatment of blood disorders, such as anemia and **polycythemia**
- Cessation of smoking
- Cessation of recreational drugs
- Moderate use of alcohol
- Regular exercise
- Good eating habits

Seizures

Seizures may be easily mistaken for stroke in the elderly. Also, a first-time seizure may occur due to damage from a previous stroke. Not all seizures experienced by the elderly are of the major motor type. Some are more subtle. Many causes of seizure activity in the elderly have been identified. Common causes include:

- Seizure disorder (epilepsy)
- Syncope
- Recent or past head trauma
- Mass lesion (tumor or bleed)
- Alcohol withdrawal
- Hypoglycemia
- Stroke

Often the cause of the seizure cannot be determined in the field. As a result, treat the condition as a life-threatening emergency and transport as quickly as possible to eliminate the possibility of stroke. If the patient has fallen during a seizure, check for evidence of trauma and treat accordingly.

Dizziness/Vertigo

Dizziness is a frightening experience and a frequent complaint of the elderly. The complaint of dizziness may actually mean that the patient has suffered syncope, pre-syncope, light-headedness, or true **vertigo**. Vertigo is a specific sensation of motion perceived by the patient as spinning or whirling. Many patients will report that they feel as though they are spinning. Vertigo is often accompanied with sweating, pallor, nausea, and vomiting. Meniere's disease can cause severe, **intractable** vertigo. It is often, however, associated with a constant "roaring" sound in the ears, as well as ear "pressure."

Table 3-6	DISTINGUISHING DEMENTIA AND DELIRIUM*
Dementia	**Delirium**
Chronic, slowly progressive development	Rapid in onset, fluctuating course
Irreversible disorder	May be reversed, especially if treated early
Greatly impairs memory	Greatly impairs attention
Global cognitive deficits	Focal cognitive deficits
Most commonly caused by Alzheimer's disease	Most commonly caused by systemic disease, drug toxicity, or metabolic changes
Does not require immediate treatment	Requires immediate treatment

*These are general characteristics that apply to most, but not all cases. For example, some forms of dementia, such as those caused by hypothyroidism, may be reversed.

Vertigo results from so many factors that it is often hard, even for the physician, to determine the actual cause. Any factor that impairs visual input, inner-ear function, peripheral sensory input, or the central nervous system can cause dizziness. In addition, alcohol and many prescription drugs can cause dizziness. So can hypoglycemia in its early stages. It is virtually impossible to distinguish dizziness, syncope, and pre-syncope in the prehospital setting.

Delirium, Dementia, Alzheimer's Disease

Approximately 15 percent of all Americans over age 65 have some degree of dementia or delirium. **Dementia** is a chronic global cognitive impairment, often progressive or irreversible. The best-known form of dementia is **Alzheimer's disease,** a condition that affects 4 million Americans. **Delirium** is a global mental impairment of sudden onset and self-limited duration. (For differences between dementia and delirium, see Table 3-6.)

Delirium Many conditions can cause delirium. The cause may be either organic brain disease or disorders that occur elsewhere in the body. Delirium in the elderly is a serious condition. According to some estimates, about 18 percent of hospitalized elderly patients with delirium die. Possible etiologies or causes include:

* Subdural hematoma
* Tumors and other mass lesions
* Drug-induced changes or alcohol intoxication
* CNS infections
* Electrolyte abnormalities
* Cardiac failure
* Fever
* Metabolic disorders, including hypoglycemia
* Chronic endocrine abnormalities, including hypothyroidism and hyperthyroidism
* Postconcussion syndrome

The presentation of delirium varies greatly and can change rapidly during assessment. Common signs and symptoms include the acute onset of anxiety, an inability to focus, disordered thinking, irritability, inappropriate behavior, fearfulness, excessive energy, or psychotic behavior such as hallucinations or paranoia. Aphasic

✱ **dementia** a deterioration of mental status that is usually associated with structural neurological disease. It is often progressive and irreversible.

✱ **Alzheimer's disease** a progressive, degenerative disease that attacks the brain and results in impaired memory, thinking, and behavior. It affects 4 million American adults.

✱ **delirium** an acute alteration in mental functioning that is often reversible.

or speaking errors and/or prominent slurring may be present. Normal patterns of eating and sleeping are almost always disrupted.

In distinguishing between delirium and dementia, err on the side of delirium. The condition is often caused by life-threatening, but reversible, conditions. Causes of delirium such as infections, drug toxicity, and electrolyte imbalances generally have a good prognosis if identified quickly and managed promptly.

Dementia   Dementia is more prevalent in the elderly than delirium. Over 50 percent of all nursing home patients have some form of dementia. It is usually due to an underlying neurological disease. This mental deterioration is often called "organic brain syndrome," **"senile dementia,"** or "senility." It is important to find out whether an alteration in mental status is acute or chronic. Causes of dementia include:

- Small strokes
- Atherosclerosis
- Age-related neurological changes
- Neurological diseases
- Certain hereditary diseases (e.g., Huntington's disease)
- Alzheimer's disease

Signs and symptoms of dementia include progressive disorientation, shortened attention span, **aphasia** or nonsense talking, and hallucinations. Dementia often hampers treatment through the patient's inability to communicate and exhausts caregivers. In moderate to severe cases, you will need to rely on the caregiver for information. (Remain alert to signs of abuse or neglect, which occurs in a disproportionate number of elderly suffering from dementia.)

Alzheimer's Disease   Alzheimer's disease is a particular type of dementia. It is a chronic degenerative disorder that attacks the brain and results in impaired memory, thinking, and behavior. It accounts for more than half of all forms of dementia in the elderly.

Alzheimer's disease generally occurs in stages, each with different signs and symptoms. These stages include:

- *Early Stage.* Characterized by loss of recent memory, inability to learn new material, mood swings, and personality changes. Patients may believe someone is plotting against them when they lose items or forget things. Aggression or hostility is common. Poor judgment is evident.
- *Intermediate Stage.* Characterized by a complete inability to learn new material; wandering, particularly at night; increased falls; loss of ability for self-care, including bathing and use of the toilet.
- *Terminal Stage.* Characterized by an inability to walk and regression to infant stage, including the loss of bowel and bladder function. Eventually the patient loses the ability to eat and swallow.

Families caring for an Alzheimer's patient at home also present signs of stress. Remember to treat both the Alzheimer patient and the family and/or caregivers with respect and compassion. Evaluate the needs of the family and make an appropriate report at your facility. There are support groups available to assist families.

In distinguishing between delirium and dementia, err on the side of delirium. The condition is often caused by life-threatening, but reversible, conditions.

* **senile dementia** general term used to describe an abnormal decline in mental functioning seen in the elderly; also called "organic brain syndrome" or "multi-infarct dementia."

* **aphasia** absence or impairment of the ability to communicate through speaking, writing, or signing as a result of brain dysfunction.

Remember to treat both the Alzheimer patient and family and/or caregivers with respect and compassion.

Parkinson's Disease

Parkinson's disease is a degenerative disorder characterized by changes in muscle response, including tremors, loss of facial expression, and gait disturbances. It mainly appears in people over age 50 and peaks at age 70. The disease affects about 1 million Americans, with 50,000 new cases diagnosed each year. It is the fourth most common neurodegenerative disease among the elderly.

The cause of primary Parkinson's disease remains unknown. However, it affects the basal ganglia in the brain, an area that deciphers messages going to muscles. Secondary Parkinson's disease is distinguished from primary Parkinson's disease by having a known cause. Some of the most common causes include:

- Viral encephalitis
- Atherosclerosis of cerebral vessels
- Reaction to certain drugs or toxins, such as antipsychotics or carbon monoxide
- Metabolic disorders, such as anoxia
- Tumors
- Head trauma
- Degenerative disorders, such as **Shy-Drager syndrome**

It is impossible in a field setting to distinguish primary and secondary Parkinson's disease. The most common initial sign of a Parkinson's disorder is a resting tremor combined with a **pill-rolling motion**. As the disease progresses, muscles become more rigid and movements become slower and/or more jerky. In some cases, patients may find their movements halted while carrying out some routine task. Their feet may feel "frozen to the ground." Gaits becomes shuffled with short steps and unexpected bursts of speed, often to avoid falling. Kyphotic deformity is a hallmark of the disease.

Patients with Parkinson's disease commonly develop mask-like faces devoid of all expression. They speak in slow, monotone voices. Difficulties in communication, coupled with a loss of mobility, often lead to anxiety and depression.

There is no known cure for Parkinson's disease, with the exception of drug-induced secondary Parkinson's disorders. Exercise may help maintain physical activity or teach the patient adaptive strategies. In calls involving a Parkinson's patient, observe for conditions that may have involved the EMS system, such as a fall or the inability to move. Manage treatable conditions and transport as needed.

METABOLIC AND ENDOCRINE DISORDERS

As previously mentioned, the endocrine system undergoes a number of age-related changes, which affect hormone levels. The most common endocrine disorders include diabetes mellitus and problems related to the thyroid gland. Of the two, you will more often treat diabetic-related emergencies, particularly hypoglycemia.

Diabetes Mellitus

An estimated 20 percent of older adults have diabetes mellitus, primarily Type II diabetes. Almost 40 percent have some type of glucose intolerance. Reasons that the elderly develop these disorders include:

- Poor diet
- Decreased physical activity
- Loss of lean body mass

✶ **Parkinson's disease** chronic, degenerative nervous disease characterized by tremors, muscular weakness and rigidity, and a loss of postural reflexes.

✶ **Shy-Drager syndrome** chronic orthostatic hypotension caused by a primary autonomic nervous system deficiency.

✶ **pill-rolling motion** an involuntary tremor, usually in one hand or sometimes in both, in which fingers move as if they were rolling a pill back and forth.

- Impaired insulin production
- Resistance by body cells to the actions of insulin

Diagnosis of Type II diabetes usually occurs during routine screening in a physical exam. In some cases, urine tests may register negative because of an increased renal glucose threshold in the elderly. The condition may present, in its early stages, with such vague constitutional symptoms as fatigue or weakness. Allowed to progress, diabetes can result in neuropathy and visual impairment. These manifestations often lead to more aggressive blood testing, which in most cases will reveal elevated glucose levels.

The treatment of diabetes involves diet, exercise, the use of sulfonylurea agents, and/or insulin. Many diabetics use self-monitoring devices to test glucose levels. Unfortunately, the cost of these devices and the accompanying test strips, sometimes discourages the elderly from using them. Elderly patients on insulin also risk hypoglycemia, especially if they accidentally take too much insulin or do not eat enough food following injection. The lack of good nutrition can be particularly troublesome to elderly diabetics. They often find it difficult to prepare meals, fail to enjoy food because of altered taste perceptions, have trouble chewing food, or are unable to purchase adequate and/or the correct food because of limited income.

Management of diabetic and hypoglycemic emergencies for the elderly are generally the same as for any other patient. DO NOT rule out alcohol as a complicating factor, especially in cases of hypoglycemia. In addition, remember that diabetes places the elderly at increased risk of other complications, including atherosclerosis, delayed healing, **retinopathy,** blindness, altered renal function, and severe peripheral vascular disease, leading to foot ulcers and even amputations.

DO NOT rule out alcohol as a complicating factor in cases of hypoglycemia.

* retinopathy any disorder of the retina.

Thyroid Disorders

With normal aging the thyroid gland undergoes moderate atrophy and changes in hormone production. An estimated 2 to 5 percent of people over age 65 experience hypothyroidism, a condition resulting from inadequate levels of thyroid hormones. It affects women in greater numbers than men, and the prevalence rises with age.

Less than 33 percent of the elderly present with typical signs and symptoms of hypothyroidism. When they do, their complaints are often attributed to aging. Common nonspecific complaints in the elderly include mental confusion, anorexia, falls, incontinence, and decreased mobility. Some patients also experience an increase in muscle or joint pain. Treatment involves thyroid hormone replacement.

Hyperthyroidism is less common among the elderly but may result from medication errors such as an overdose of thyroid hormone replacement. The typical symptom of heat intolerance is often present. Otherwise, hyperthyroidism presents atypically in the elderly. Common nonspecific features or complaints include atrial fibrillation, failure to thrive (weight loss and apathy combined), abdominal distress, diarrhea, exhaustion, and depression.

The diagnosis and treatment of thyroid disorders does not take place in the field. Elderly patients with known thyroid problems should be encouraged to go to the hospital for medical evaluation.

GASTROINTESTINAL DISORDERS

Gastrointestinal emergencies are common among the elderly. The most frequent emergency is gastrointestinal bleeding. However, older people will also describe a variety of other gastrointestinal complaints—nausea, poor appetite, diarrhea, and constipation, to name a few. Remember, that like other presenting complaints, these conditions may be symptomatic of more serious diseases. Bowel problems, for example, may point to cancer of the colon or other abdominal organs.

Regardless of the complaint, remember that prompt management of a GI emergency is essential for young and old alike. For the elderly, there is a significant risk of hemorrhage and shock. There is a tendency to take GI patients less seriously than those suffering moderate or severe external hemorrhage. This is a serious mistake. Patients with gastrointestinal complaints should be aggressively managed, especially the elderly. Keep in mind that older patients are far more intolerant of hypotension and anoxia than younger patients. Treatment should include:

- Airway management
- Support of breathing and circulation
- High-flow oxygen therapy
- IV fluid replacement with a crystalloid solution
- PASG placement, if indicated
- Rapid transport

Some of the most critical GI problems that you may encounter in the field will involve internal hemorrhage and bowel obstruction. You may also be called upon to treat **mesenteric infarct**—a serious and life-threatening condition in an elderly patient. The following will help you to recognize each of these gastrointestinal disorders.

GI Hemorrhage

Gastrointestinal bleeding falls into two general categories: upper GI bleed and lower GI bleed.

Upper GI Bleed This form of gastrointestinal bleeding includes:

- *Peptic Ulcer Disease.* Injury to the mucous lining of the upper part of the gastrointestinal tract due to stomach acids, digestive enzymes, and other agents, such as anti-inflammatory drugs.
- *Gastritis.* An inflammation of the lining of the stomach.
- *Esophageal Varices.* An abnormal dilation of veins in the lower esophagus; a common complication of cirrhosis of the liver.
- *Mallory-Weiss Tear.* A tear in the lower esophagus that is often caused by severe and prolonged retching.

Lower GI Bleed Conditions categorized as lower gastrointestinal bleeding include:

- *Diverticulosis.* The presence of small pouches on the colon that tend to develop with age; causes 70 percent of life-threatening lower GI bleeds.
- *Tumors.* Tumors of the colon can cause bleeding when the tumor erodes into blood vessels within the intestine or surrounding organs.
- *Ischemic Colitis.* An inflammation of the colon due to impaired or decreased blood supply.
- *Arterio-Venous Malformations.* An abnormal link between an artery and a vein.

Signs of significant gastrointestinal blood loss include the presence of "coffee ground" emesis; black tar-like stools (**melena**); obvious blood in the emesis or stool; orthostatic hypotension; pulse greater than 100 (unless on beta blockers); and

Patients with gastrointestinal complaints should be aggressively managed, especially the elderly.

✳ **mesenteric infarct** death of tissue in the peritoneal fold (mesentery) that encircles the small intestine; a life-threatening condition.

✳ **melena** a dark, tarry stool caused by the presence of "digested" free blood.

confusion. Gastrointestinal bleeding in the elderly may result in such complications as a recent increase in angina symptoms, congestive heart failure, weakness, or dyspnea.

Bowel Obstruction

Bowel obstruction in the elderly typically involves the small bowel. Causes include tumors, prior abdominal surgery, use of certain medications, and occasionally the presence of vertebral compression fractures. The patient will typically complain of diffuse abdominal pain, bloating, nausea, and vomiting. The abdomen may feel distended when palpated. Bowel sounds may be hypoactive or absent. If the obstruction has been present for a prolonged period of time, the patient may have fever, weakness, shock, and various electrolyte disturbances.

Mesenteric Infarct

Vessels arising from the superior or inferior mesenteric arteries generally serve the bowel. An infarct occurs when a portion of the bowel does not receive enough blood to survive. Certain age-related changes make the elderly more vulnerable to this condition. First, as a person ages, changes in the heart (such as atrial fibrillation) or the vessels (atherosclerosis) predispose the patient to a clot lodging in one of the branches serving the bowel. Second, changes in the bowel itself can promote swelling that effectively cuts off blood flow.

The primary symptom of a bowel infarct is pain out of proportion to the physical exam. Signs include:

- Bloody diarrhea, but usually not a massive hemorrhage
- Some tachycardia, although there may be a vagal effect masking the sign
- Abdominal distention

The patient is at great risk for shock as the dead bowel attracts interstitial and intravascular fluids, thus removing them from use. Necrotic products are released to the peritoneal cavity, leading to a massive infection. The prognosis is poor due, in part, to decreased physiologic reserves on the part of the older patient.

SKIN DISORDERS

Younger and older adults experience common skin disorders at about the same rates. However, age-related changes in the immune system make the elderly more prone to certain chronic skin diseases and infections. They are also more likely to develop **pressure ulcers** (bedsores) than any other age group.

Skin Diseases

Elderly patients commonly complain about **pruritus,** or itching. This condition can be caused by dermatitis (eczema) or environmental conditions, especially during winter (i.e., from hot dry air in the home and cold windy air outside). Keep in mind that generalized itching can also be a sign of systemic diseases, particularly liver and renal disorders. When itching is strong and unrelenting, suspect an underlying disease and encourage the patient to seek medical evaluation.

Slower healing and compromised tissue perfusion in the elderly makes them more susceptible to bacterial infection of wounds, appearing as cellutitis, impetigo, and, in the case of immunocompromised adults, staphylococcal scalded skin. The elderly also experience a higher incidence of fungal infections, partly because of decreases in the cutaneous immunologic response. In addition, they

---

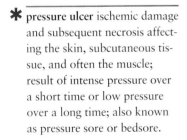

* **pressure ulcer** ischemic damage and subsequent necrosis affecting the skin, subcutaneous tissue, and often the muscle; result of intense pressure over a short time or low pressure over a long time; also known as pressure sore or bedsore.

* **pruritus** itching; often occurs as a symptom of some systemic change or illness.

Keep in mind that generalized itching can also be a sign of systemic diseases, particularly liver and renal disorders.

---

suffer higher rates of **herpes zoster** (shingles), which peaks between ages 50 and 70. Although these skin disorders occur in the young, their duration and severity increases markedly with age.

In treating skin disorders, remember that many conditions may be drug-induced. Beta-blockers, for example, can worsen psoriasis, which occurs in about 3 percent of elderly patients. Question patients about their medications, keeping in mind that certain prescription drugs (e.g., penicillins and sulfonamides) and some over-the-counter drugs can cause skin eruptions. Also ask about topical home remedies, such as alcohol or soaps, that may cause or worsen the disorder. Find out if the patient is compliant with prescribed topical treatments. Finally, remember that some drugs and topical medications commonly used to treat skin disorders in the young can worsen or cause other problems for the elderly. Antihistamines and corticosteroids are two to three times more likely to provoke adverse reactions in the elderly than in younger adults.

✱ **herpes zoster** an acute eruption caused by a reactivation of latent varicella virus (chicken pox) in the dorsal root ganglia; also known as shingles.

Antihistamines and corticosteroids are two to three times more likely to provoke adverse reactions in the elderly than in younger patients.

Pressure Ulcers (Decubitus Ulcers)

Most pressure ulcers occur in people over age 70. As many as 20 percent of patients enter the hospital with a pressure ulcer or develop one while hospitalized. The highest incidence occurs in nursing homes where up to 25 percent of patients may develop this condition.

Pressure ulcers typically develop from the waist down, usually over bony prominences, in bedridden patients. However, they can occur anywhere on the body and with the patient in any position. Pressure ulcers usually result from tissue hypoxia and affect the skin, subcutaneous tissues, and muscle. Factors that can increase the risk of this condition include:

- External compression of tissues (i.e., pressure)
- Altered sensory perception
- **Maceration,** caused by excessive moisture
- Decreased activity
- Decreased mobility
- Poor nutrition
- Friction or shear

✱ **maceration** process of softening a solid by soaking in a liquid.

To reduce the development of pressures ulcers or to alleviate their condition, you may take these steps.

- Assist the patient in changing position frequently, especially during extended transport, to reduce the length of time pressure is placed on any one point.
- Use a pull sheet to move the patient, reducing the likelihood of friction.
- Reduce the possibility of shearing by padding areas of skin prior to movement.
- Unless a life-treating condition is present, take time to clean and dry areas of excessive moisture, such as urinary or fecal incontinence and excessive perspiration.
- Clean ulcers with normal saline solution and cover with hydrocolloid or hydrogel dressings, if available. With severe ulcers, pack with loosely woven gauze moistened with normal saline.

MUSCULOSKELETAL DISORDERS

The skeleton, as you know, is a metabolically active organ. Its metabolic processes are influenced by a number of factors, including age, diet, exercise, and

osteoarthritis a degenerative joint disease, characterized by a loss of articular cartilage and hypertrophy of bone.

osteoporosis softening of bone tissue due to the loss of essential minerals, principally calcium.

Wear and tear is the most common factor leading to osteoarthritis.

hormone levels. The musculoskeletal system is also subject to disease. In fact, musculoskeletal diseases are the leading cause of functional impairment in the elderly. Although usually not fatal, musculoskeletal disorders often produce chronic disability, which in turn creates a context for illness. Two of the most widespread musculoskeletal disorders include **osteoarthritis** and **osteoporosis**.

Osteoarthritis

Osteoarthritis is the leading cause of disability among people age 65 and older. Many experts think the condition may not be one disease but several with similar presentations. While wear and tear as well as age-related changes such as loss of muscle mass predispose the elderly to osteoarthritis, other factors may play a role as well. Presumed contributing causes include:

- Obesity
- Primary disorders of the joint, such as inflammatory arthritis
- Trauma
- Congenital abnormalities, such as hip dysplasia

Osteoarthritis in the elderly presents initially as joint pain, worsened by exercise and improved by rest. As the disease progresses, pain may be accompanied by diminished mobility, joint deformity, and crepitus or grating sensations. Late signs include tenderness upon palpation or during passive motion.

The most effective treatment involves management before the disability develops or worsens. Prevention strategies include stretching exercises and activities that strengthen stress-absorbing ligaments (Figure 3-15). Immobilization, even for short periods, can accelerate the condition. Drug therapy is usually aimed at lessening pain and/or inflammation. Surgery—i.e., total joint replacement—is usually the last resort after more conservative methods have failed.

Osteoporosis

Osteoporosis affects an estimated 20 million Americans and is largely responsible for fractures of the hip, wrist, and vertebral bones following a fall or other injury. Risk factors include:

- *Age.* Peak bone mass for men and women occurs in their third and fourth decades of life and declines at varying rates thereafter. Decreased bone density generally becomes a treatment consideration at about age 50.
- *Gender.* The decline of estrogen production places women at a higher risk of developing osteoporosis than men. Women are more than twice as likely to have brittle bone, especially if they experience early menopause (before age 45) and do not take estrogen replacement therapy.
- *Race.* Whites and Asians are more likely to develop osteoporosis than African Americans and Latinos, who have higher bone mass at skeletal peak.
- *Body Weight.* Thin people, or people with low body weight, are at greater risk of osteoporosis than obese people. Increased skeletal weight is thought to promote bone density. However, weight-bearing exercise can have the same effect.
- *Family History.* Genetic factors—i.e., peak bone mass attainment—and a family history of fractures may predispose a person to osteoporosis.

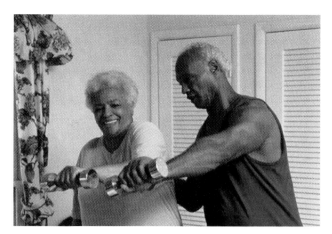

FIGURE 3-15 Regular stretching and weight-bearing exercises help prevent the development of osteoarthritis. (© The Stock Market Photo Agency.)

- *Miscellaneous.* Late menarche, nulliparity, and use of caffeine, alcohol, and cigarettes are all thought to be important determinants of bone mass.

Unless a bone density test is conducted, persons with osteoporosis are usually asymptotic until a fracture occurs. The precipitating event can be as slight as turning over in bed, carrying a package, or even a forceful sneeze. Management includes prevention of fractures through exercise and drug therapy, such as the administration of calcium, Vitamin D, estrogen, and other medications or minerals. Once the condition occurs, pain management also becomes a consideration.

RENAL DISORDERS

The most common renal diseases in the elderly include renal failure, **glomerulonephritis,** and renal blood clots. These problems may be traced to two age-related factors: (1) loss in kidney size and (2) changes in the walls of the renal arteries and in the arterioles serving the glomeruli. In general, the kidney loses approximately one-third of its weight between the ages of 30 and 80. Most of this loss occurs in the tissues that filter blood. When filtering tissue is gone, blood is shunted from the precapillary side directly to venules on the postcapillary side, thus bypassing any tissue still capable of filtering. The result is a reduction in kidney efficiency. This condition is complicated by changes in renal arteries, which promote the development of renal emboli and thrombi.

With renal changes, elderly patients are more likely to accumulate toxins and medications within the bloodstream. Occasionally, this will be obvious to the patient as he or she experiences a substantial decrease in urine output. More often, however, the elderly are prone to a type of renal failure in which urine output remains normal to high while the kidney remains ineffective in clearing wastes.

Processes that precipitate acute renal failure include hypotension, heart failure, major surgery, sepsis, angiographic procedures (the dye is nephrotoxic), and use of nephrotoxic antibiotics (i.e., gentamycin, tobramycin). Ongoing hypertension also figures in the development of chronic renal failure.

URINARY DISORDERS

Urinary tract infections (UTI) affect as much as 10 percent of the elderly population each year. Younger women generally suffer more UTIs than young men, but in the elderly the distribution is almost even. Most of these infections result from bacteria and easily lead to **urosepsis** due to reduced immune system function among the elderly.

✱ **glomerulonephritis** a form of nephritis, or inflammation of the kidneys; primarily involves the glomeruli, one of the capillary networks that are part of the renal corpuscles in the nephrons.

✱ **urosepsis** septicemia originating from the urinary tract.

A number of factors contribute to the high rate of UTIs among the elderly. They include:

- Bladder outlet obstruction from benign prostatic hyperplasia (in men)
- atrophic vaginitis (in women)
- Stroke
- Immobilization
- Use of indwelling bladder catheters
- Diabetes
- Upper urinary tract stone
- Dementia, with resulting poor hygiene

Signs or symptoms of a UTI range from cloudy, foul smelling urine to the typical complaints of bladder pain and frequent urination. Urosepsis presents as an acute process, including fever, chills, abdominal discomfort, and other signs of septic shock. The septicemia generally begins within 24–72 hours after catheterization or cystoscopy.

Treatment of urosepsis commonly includes placement of a large-bore IV catheter for administration of fluids and parenteral antibiotics. Diagnosis of urosepsis is based on history and other physical findings. Prompt transport is critical. The prognosis for elderly patients with urosepsis is poor, with a mortality rate of approximately 30 percent. Maintenance of fluid balance as well as adequate blood pressure is essential.

Prompt transport is critical for elderly patients with suspected urosepsis, as the condition has a mortality rate of approximately 30 percent.

* **heatstroke** life-threatening condition caused by a disturbance in temperature regulation; in the elderly, characterized by extreme fever and, in extreme cases, delirium or coma.

ENVIRONMENTAL EMERGENCIES

As previously mentioned, environmental extremes represent a great health risk for the elderly. Nearly 50 percent of all **heatstroke** deaths in the United States occur among people over age 50. The elderly are just as susceptible to low temperatures, suffering about 750,000 winter deaths annually, primarily from hypothermia and "winter risks" such as pneumonia and influenza. As you may already know from your EMT experience, thermoregulatory emergencies represent some of the most common EMS calls involving the elderly.

Hypothermia

A number of factors predispose the elderly to hypothermia. These include:

- Accidental exposure to cold
- CNS disorders, including head trauma, stroke, tumors, or subdural hematomas
- Endocrine disorders, including hypoglycemia and diabetes (Patients with diabetes are six times as likely to develop hypothermia as other patients.)
- Drugs that interfere with heat production, including alcohol, antidepressants, and tranquilizers
- Malnutrition or starvation
- Chronic illness
- Forced inactivity as a result of arthritis, dementia, falls, paralysis, or Parkinson's disease
- Low or fixed income, which discourages the use of home heating

- Inflammatory dermatitis
- A-V shunts, which increase heat loss

Signs and symptoms of hypothermia can be slow to develop. Many times, elderly patients with hypothermia lose their sensitivity to cold and fail to complain. As a result, hypothermia may be missed. Nonspecific complaints may suggest a metabolic disorder or stroke. Hypothermic patients may exhibit slow speech, confusion, and sleepiness. In the early stages, patients will exhibit hypertension and an increased heart rate. As hypothermia progresses, however, blood pressure drops and the heart rate slows, sometimes to a barely detectable level.

Remember that the elderly patient with hypothermia often does not shiver. Check the abdomen and back to see if the skin is cool to the touch. Expect subcutaneous tissues to be firm. If your unit has a low-temperature thermometer, check the patient's core temperature. (Regular thermometers often do not "shake down" far enough for an accurate reading.)

Remember that the elderly hypothermic patient often does not shiver.

As with other medical disorders, prevention is the preferred treatment. However, once elderly patients develop hypothermia, they become progressively impaired. Treat even mild cases of hypothermia, or suspected hypothermia, as a medical emergency. Focus on the rewarming techniques used with other patients and rapid transport. Maintain ongoing assessment to ensure that the hypothermia does not complicate existing medical problems or heretofore untreated disorders. Death most commonly results from cardiac arrest or ventricular fibrillation.

Treat even a mild case of hypothermia, or suspected hypothermia, as a medical emergency.

Hyperthermia (Heatstroke)

Age-related changes in sweat glands and increased incidence of heart disease place the elderly at risk of heat stress. They may develop heat cramps, heat exhaustion, or heatstroke. While the first two disorders rarely result in death, heatstroke is a serious medical emergency. Risk factors for severe hyperthermia include:

Heatstroke in the elderly is a serious medical emergency.

- Altered sensory output, which would normally warn a person of overheating
- Inadequate liquid intake
- Decreased functioning of the thermoregulatory center
- Commonly prescribed medications that inhibit sweating such as antihistamines and tricyclic antidepressants
- Low or fixed income, which may result in a lack of air conditioning or adequate ventilation
- Alcoholism
- Concomitant medical disorders
- Use of diuretics, which increase fluid loss

Like hypothermia, early heatstroke may present with nonspecific signs and symptoms, such as nausea, light-headedness, dizziness, or headache. High temperature is the most reliable indicator, but consider even a slight temperature elevation as symptomatic if coupled with an absence of sweating and neurological impairment. Severe hypotension also exists in many critical patients.

Prevention strategies include adequate fluid intake, reduced activity, shelter in an air conditioned environment, and use of light clothing. If hyperthermia develops, however, rapid treatment and transport are necessary.

TOXICOLOGICAL EMERGENCIES

As previously mentioned, aging alters pharmacokinetics and pharmacodynamics in the elderly. Functional changes in the kidneys, liver, and gastrointestinal system slow the absorption and elimination of many medications. In addition, the various compensatory mechanisms that help buffer against medication side effects are less effective in the elderly than in younger patients.

Approximately 30% of all hospital admissions are related to drug-related illnesses. About 50% of all drug-related deaths occur in people over age 60. Accidental overdoses may occur more frequently in the aged due to confusion, vision impairment, self-selection of medications, forgetfulness, and concurrent drug use. Intentional drug overdose also occurs in attempts at self-destruction. Another complicating factor is the abuse of alcohol among the elderly.

It is essential for the paramedic to be familiar with the range of side effects that can be caused by the polypharmacy of medications taken by geriatric patients. In assessing the geriatric patient, always take these steps:

- Obtain a full list of medications currently taken by the patient.
- Elicit any medications that are newly prescribed. (Some side effects appear within a few days of taking a new medication.)
- Obtain a good past medical history. Find out if your patient has a history of renal or hepatic depression.
- Know your medications, their routes of elimination, and their potential side effects.
- If possible, always take all medications to the hospital along with the patient.

A knowledge of pharmacology is important in all patients. However, it is critical in recognizing potential toxicological emergencies in the geriatric patient. Some of the drugs or substances that have been identified as commonly causing toxicity in the elderly are described in the following sections.

Lidocaine

Lidocaine is a class Ib cardiac antidysrhythmic recommended for the treatment of ventricular dysrhythmias in the acute setting, especially in acute myocardial infarction and in dysrhythmias that arise from cardiac surgery or catherization. Nearly 90% of the drug is metabolized in the liver and approximately 10% is excreted through the kidneys. Patients with hepatic impairment and decreased renal function should receive reduced doses of the medication to lessen the risk of the drug accumulating in their system and causing adverse reactions.

Lidocaine toxicity is characterized by vision disturbances (blurred or double vision), GI effects, tinnitus, trembling, breathing difficulties, dizziness/syncope, seizures and bradycardia dysrhythmics. Since the cardiac antidysrhythmics in general can cause a decrease in cardiac function and output, you should observe for shortness of breath, lightheadedness, loss of consciousness, fatigue, chest discomfort, and palpitations.

Betablockers

Betablockers are widely used to treat hypertension, angina pectoris, and cardiac dysrhythmias. Although fairly well tolerated in younger adults, elderly patients tend to be more susceptible to the side effects of these agents. In particular, central nervous system side effects—depression, lethargy, and sleep disorders—are more common in the elderly.

Because geriatric patients often have pre-existing cardiovascular problems that can cause decreased cardiac function and output, beta-blockers will limit the heart's ability to respond to postural changes, causing orthostatic hypotension. Beta blockers also limit the heart's ability to increase contractile force and cardiac output whenever a sympathetic response is necessary in situations such as exercise or hypovolemia. This can be detrimental to the trauma patient who is hemorrhaging and cannot mount the sympathetic response necessary to maintain perfusion of vital organs. Also remember that all beta-blockers can worsen heart failure in patients with poor left ventricular function. Beta-blockers decrease intraocular pressure and are often used to treat glaucoma in the elderly. Remember, even beta-blocker eye drops can cause systemic effects.

Treatment of beta-blocker overdose includes general supportive measures, the removal of gastric contents, cardio-respiratory support, fluids, and administration of nonadrenergic inotropic agents such as glucagon for hypotension. Excessive bradycardia can be treated with atropine.

Commonly prescribed beta-blockers include: propranolol hydrochloride (Inderal), nadolol, atenolol, sotalol, timolol, esmolol, metroprolol, penbutolol and labetalol.

Antihypertensives/Diuretics

Diuretics act on the kidneys to increase urine flow and the excretion of water and sodium. They are used primarily in the treatment of hypertension and congestive heart failure.

This group of medications includes hydrochlorthiazide (HCTZ), furosemide, ethacrynic acid, bumetanide, and torsemide. Of these drugs, furosemide is the most widely used diuretic in the elderly. The elimination half-life of furosemide is markedly prolonged in the patient with acute pulmonary edema and renal and hepatic failure. As a result, the geriatric patient is at risk for a drug build-up.

Because the elderly may be sensitive to adult dosages, a smaller dose is often prescribed and the patient usually takes a daily potassium supplement. Excessive urination caused by the drug may put the elderly at risk for postural hypotension, circulatory collapse, potassium depletion, and renal function impairment.

Angiotensin-Converting Enzyme (ACE) Inhibitors

ACE inhibitors are a relatively recent addition to the group of medications used in the treatment of hypertension and congestive heart failure. They are used either as a first-line treatment or when other more established drugs are contraindicated, poorly tolerated, or fail to produce the desired effect.

For the treatment of congestive heart failure, ACE inhibitors reduce renin-angiotensin-mediated vasoconstriction, which reduces the pressure against which the heart has to pump (afterload). Geriatric patients generally respond well to treatment with ACE inhibitors. However, these drugs can cause chronic hypotension in patients with severe heart failure who are also taking high-dose loop diuretics. ACE inhibitors can also cause plasma volume reduction and hypotension with prolonged vomiting and diarrhea, especially in the elderly. Some hemodialysis patients can experience anaphylactic reactions if treated with ACE inhibitors.

Other side effects of ACE inhibitors include dizziness or lightheadedness upon standing, presence of a rash, muscle cramps, swelling of the hands, face or eyes, cough (especially in women), headache, stomach upset, and fatigue. Catopril, in particular, can cause a loss of taste.

Specific examples of ACE inhibitors include captopril, enalapril, lisinopril, fosinopril, benazepril, quinapril, and ramipril.

Digitalis (Digoxin, Lanoxin)

Digoxin is the most widely used cardiac glycoside for the management of congestive heart failure, atrial fibrillation, atrial flutter, paroxysmal atrial tachycardia, and cardiogenic shock. The drug is unique in that it has a positive inotropic effect, but a negative chronotropic effect. In congestive heart failure, digoxin increases the strength of myocardial contractions (positive inotropic effect) with a resulting increase in cardiac output. Digoxin also slows conduction and increases the refractory period in cardiac conducting tissue, resulting in a reduced ventricular rate (negative chronotropic effect). This allows the ventricle to adequately fill with blood, also improving cardiac output.

In the patient with moderate-to-severe heart failure, digitalis is often combined with ACE inhibitors and diuretics. Remember that digoxin has a low therapeutic index. As a result, the dose must be adjusted for each patient.

Digoxin serum levels should be monitored carefully during therapy. The drug is excreted in the urine, with 50–70% of the dose as unchanged drug. The half-life ranges from 32–48 hours in patients with normal renal function. Because the elderly have reduced volume of distribution for digoxin and may have impaired renal or hepatic function, the dose should be reduced and individualized to minimize risk of toxicity. Digitalis-induced appetite loss is also a danger in frail elderly patients.

The most common adverse drug effect that occurs in elderly patients is digoxin toxicity. The primary reason is that digoxin has a low margin of safety and a narrow therapeutic index. The amount of the drug needed to produce beneficial or therapeutic effects is close to the toxic amount.

Digoxin toxicity in the elderly occur can result from accidental or intentional ingestion. For the renal-impaired elderly patient, any change in kidney function usually warrants an alteration in the dosing of digoxin. Failure to adjust the dose can lead to toxicity. Diuretics, which are often given to patients with congestive heart failure, cause the loss of large amounts of potassium in the urine. If potassium is not adequately replenished in the patient taking digoxin, toxicity will develop. Therefore, elderly patients on digoxin should be taking a daily potassium supplement such as potassium chloride (Micro-K, K-Tabs, Slow-K).

Signs and symptoms of digoxin toxicity include: visual disturbances, fatigue, weakness, nausea, loss of appetite, abdominal discomfort, dizziness, abnormal dreams, headache, and vomiting. Patients who are taking digoxin for the first time are instructed to call their physician if any of these symptoms occur.

Low potassium (hypokalemia) is also common with chronic digoxin toxicity due to concurrent diuretic therapy. Dysrhythmias commonly associated with digoxin toxicity include: sinoatrial exit block, SA arrest, second- or third-degree AV block, atrial fibrillation with a slow ventricular response, accelerated AV junctional rhythms, patterns of premature ventricular contractions (bigeminy and trigeminy), ventricular tachycardia, and atrial tachycardia with AV block.

Management of digoxin toxicity includes gastric lavage with activated charcoal, correction of confirmed hypokalemia with K^+ supplements, treatment of bradycardias with atropine or pacing, and treatment of rapid ventricular rhythms with lidocaine. Digoxin-specific FAB fragment antibodies (Digibind), an antidote for digoxin toxicity, is used in the treatment of potentially life-threatening situations.

Antipsychotics/Antidepressants

Psychotropic medications comprise a variety of agents that affect mood, behavior, and other aspects of mental function. The elderly often experience a high incidence of psychiatric disorders and may take any number of medications, including antidepressants, antianxiety agents, sedative-hypnotic agents, and antipsychotics.

Depression is the most common mental disorder in the elderly. Drug therapy may be prescribed to help resolve the feelings of sadness or hopelessness that result from the death of a spouse, divorce, declining health, and/or loss of independence. Commonly prescribed antidepressants include the serotonin reuptake inhibitors (SSRI) such as Prozac and Wellbutrin. The tricyclic antidepressants (Elavil and Tofranil) are less popular. Monamine oxidase inhibitors (Marplan and Nardil) are rarely used.

Antidepressant use in the elderly may result in side effects such as sedation, lethargy, and muscle weakness. Some antidepressants tend to produce anticholinergic effects, including dry mouth, constipation, urinary retention, and confusion. Newly prescribed tricyclic antidepressants can also cause orthostatic hypotension, which can be compounded if the geriatric patient is taking diuretics or other antihypertensive medications. Side effects such as sedation and confusion may also impair the patient's cognitive abilities and possibly endanger the elderly patient who lives alone.

Elderly patients with a history of manic depression may be treated with lithium carbonate. This drug stabilizes the mood swings associated with manic depression. Since lithium cannot be degraded by the body into an inactive form, the kidneys are the sole routes of elimination for this drug. If renal function is impaired, the drug may quickly accumulate to toxic levels, causing lithium toxicity. Symptoms include a metallic taste in the mouth, hand tremors, nausea, muscle weakness, and fatigue. As the levels of toxicity increase, blurred vision, lack of coordination, coma, and even death may occur.

Antipsychotic medications produce a number of minor side effects such as sedation and anticholinergic effects. Extrapyramidal side effects can also occur, including restlessness and involuntary muscle movements, particularly in the face, jaw, and extremities. Examples of these medications include Thorazine, Mellaril, Taractan, Navane and Haldol.

Sedative-hypnotic drugs are prescribed to relax the patient, allay anxiety, and promote sleep. Antianxiety medications, chemically similar to the sedative-hypnotics, are intended to decrease anxiety without producing sedation. These drugs are helpful in geriatric patients who suffer from insomnia and feelings of fear or apprehension.

Benzodiazepines are the most commonly prescribed sedative-hypnotic and anxiolytic drugs. These medications can produce drowsiness, sluggishness, and addiction if used over a long period of time. Examples of bendodiazipines include flurazepam (Dalmane), temazepam (Restoril), and triazolam (Halcion). Specific anti-anxiety agents include diazepam (Valium), lorazepam (Ativan), and chlordiazepoxide (Librium).

Field treatment for overdoses of these medications are aimed primarily at the ABCs, with special emphasis on airway management.

Medications for Parkinson's Disease

Parkinson's disease is a common disorder of the elderly and is caused by a breakdown of dopamine-secreting neurons located in the basal ganglia. This leads to an imbalance in other neurotransmitters, which eventually results in the parkinsonian motor symptoms of rigidity, bradykinesia, resting tremor, and postural instability.

Drug treatment is aimed at restoring the balance of neurotransmitters in the basal ganglia. The most commonly prescribed medications include carbidopa/levadopa (Sinemet), bromocriptine (Parlodel), benztropine mesylate (Cogentin), and amantadine (Symmetrel).

Toxicity of these drugs commonly presents as dyskinesia (the inability to execute voluntary movements) and psychological disturbances such as visual hallucinations and nightmares. When these medications are first taken, orthostatic hypotension may also occur.

Tsmar—a recently approved Parkinson's drug—is given in combination with Sinemet. It potentiates the effects of Sinemet and can cause liver failure. Toxicity in a patient on Tsmar will present as acute jaundice.

The goal of field management is aimed at decreasing the patient's anxiety and providing a supportive environment. Remember that patients with gross involuntary motor movements are a risk for aspiration and choking. Continued assessment of this patient is necessary.

Anti-Seizure Medications

Seizure disorders are not uncommon in elderly patients. In most cases, the cause of seizures is related to a previous central nervous system injury such as stroke or trauma, tumor, or degenerative brain disease. The selection of a specific anti-seizure medication depends on the type of seizure present in the patient.

The most common side effect of anti-seizure medications is sedation. Other side effects include GI distress, headache, dizziness, lack of coordination, and dermatological reactions (rashes). Recommended treatment involves airway management and supportive therapy.

Analgesics and Anti-Inflammatory Agents

Treatment of pain and inflammation for chronic conditions such as rheumatoid arthritis and osteoarthritis includes narcotics and non-narcotic analgesics and corticosteroids. The narcotic analgesics used to reduce pain in the elderly include codeine, meperidine (Demerol), morphine, oxycodone (Percodan), and propoxyphene (Darvon). Remember that these agents alter pain perception, rather than eliminating the condition. As they wear off, pain reappears, encouraging a patient to increase the frequency of dosage.

Adverse side effects of these drugs include sedation, mood changes, nausea, vomiting, and constipation. Orthostatic hypotension and respiratory depression may also occur. Over long periods of time, patients may develop drug tolerance and physical dependence on narcotic agents.

The nonsteroidal anti-inflammatory drugs (NSAIDs) and acetaminophen (Tylenol) are prescribed for mild to moderate pain. They are also the principle therapeutic agents for osteoarthritis and other inflammatory musculoskeletal considerations. The most common side effect of these agents is gastric irritation. Higher doses can cause renal and hepatic toxicity. Acetaminophen is particularly toxic to the liver when taken in high doses. Confusion and hearing problems (ringing or buzzing in the ears) and gastrointestinal hemorrhaging may occur with aspirin use.

Corticosteroids

Corticosteroids are powerful anti-inflammatory agents used to treat rheumatoid arthritis and other inflammatory conditions. Side effects from these agents include hypertension, peptic ulcer, aggravation of diabetes mellitus, glaucoma, increased risk of infection, and suppression of normally produced corticosteroids. Commonly prescribed corticosteroids include cortisone (Cortone), hydrocortisone (Hydrocortone), and prednisone (Deltasone).

Substance Abuse

Substance abuse is a widespread problem in the United States. It affects nearly all age groups, including the elderly. Up to 17 percent of Americans over age 60 are addicted to substances. That number is expected to rise as the baby boom generation swells the size of the elderly population.

In general, the factors that contribute to substance abuse among the elderly are different from those of younger people. They include:

- Age-related changes
- Loss of employment
- Loss of spouse or partner
- Multiple prescriptions
- Malnutrition
- Loneliness
- Moving from a long-loved house to an apartment

Like other age groups, the elderly may intentionally abuse substances, to escape pain or life itself. Other times, particularly in the case of prescription drugs, the abuse is accidental. Substance abuse in the elderly may involve drugs, alcohol, or both drugs and alcohol.

Drug Abuse

As previously mentioned, people age 65 and older have more illnesses, consume more drugs, and are more sensitive to adverse drug reactions than younger adults. The sheer number of medications taken by the elderly make them vulnerable to drug abuse. Of the 1.5 billion prescriptions written each year in the United States, more than one-third go to the elderly. People age 65 and older fill an average of 13 prescriptions per year. The elderly also use a disproportionate percentage of over-the-counter drugs.

Polypharmacy, coupled with impaired vision and/or memory, increase the likelihood of complications. The elderly might experience drug-drug interactions, drug-disease interactions, and drug-food interactions.

The elderly who become physically and/or psychological dependent upon drugs (or alcohol) are more likely to hide their dependence and less likely to seek help than other age groups. Common signs and symptoms of drug abuse include:

- Memory changes
- Drowsiness
- Decreased vision/hearing
- Orthostatic hypotension
- Poor dexterity
- Mood changes
- Falling
- Restlessness
- Weight loss

In cases of suspected drug abuse, carefully document your findings. Collect medications for identification at the hospital, where the patient can be evaluated and, if necessary, referred for substance abuse treatment.

✳ **substance abuse** misuse of chemically active agents such as alcohol, psychoactive chemicals, and therapeutic agents; typically results in clinically significant impairment or distress.

Alcohol Abuse

In a national survey, nearly 50 percent of the elderly reported abstinence from alcohol. However, the same survey found that 15 percent of the men and 12 percent of the women interviewed regularly drank in excess of the one-drink-a-day limit suggested by the National Institute on Alcohol Abuse and Alcoholism. Those percentages are expected to rise with the aging of the baby boom generation, which has generally used alcohol more frequently than their predecessors.

The use or abuse of alcohol places the elderly at high risk of toxicity. Physiological changes, such as organ dysfunction, makes older adults more susceptible to the effects of alcohol. Consumption of even moderate amounts of alcohol can interfere with drug therapy, often leading to dangerous consequences. Severe stress and a history of heavy and/or regular drinking predisposes a person to alcohol dependence or abuse in later life.

Unless a patient is openly intoxicated, discovery of alcohol abuse depends on a thorough history. Signs and symptoms of alcohol abuse in the elderly may be very subtle or confused with other conditions. Remember that even small amounts of alcohol can cause intoxication in an older person. If possible, question family, friends, or caregivers about the patient's drinking patterns. Pertinent findings include:

Unless an elderly patient is openly intoxicated, discovery of alcohol abuse often depends upon a thorough history.

- Mood swings, denial, and hostility (especially when questioned about drinking)
- Confusion
- History of falls
- Anorexia
- Insomnia
- Visible anxiety
- Nausea

Treatment follows many of the same steps as for any other patient with a pattern of abusive drinking. DO NOT judge the patient. Evaluate the need for fluid therapy, and keep in mind the possibility of withdrawal. Transport the patient to the hospital for evaluation and referral for treatment. Ideally, these patients will seek support from community organizations such as Alcoholics Anonymous (AA). Many communities have AA groups specifically for senior citizens.

BEHAVIORAL/PSYCHOLOGICAL DISORDERS

When behavioral or psychological problems develop later in life, they are often dismissed as normal age-related changes. This attitude denies an elderly person the opportunity to correct a treatable condition and/or overlooks an underlying physical disorder. Studies have shown that the elderly retain their basic personalities and their adaptive cognitive abilities. In other words, intellectual decline and/or regressive behavior are not normal age-related changes. Unless an organic brain disorder is involved, alterations in behavior should be considered symptomatic of a possible psychological problem.

It is important to keep in mind the emotionally stressful situations facing many elderly people—isolation, loneliness, loss of self-dependence, loss of strength, fear of the future, and more. The elderly also face a higher incidence of secondary depression as a result of neuroleptic medications such as Haldol and Thorazine. Some of the common classifications of psychological disorders related to age include:

- Organic brain syndrome
- Affective disorders (depression)

- Personality disorders (dependent personality)
- Dissociative disorders (paranoid schizophrenia)

As with other people, the emotional well-being of the elderly impacts upon their overall physical health. Therefore, it is important that you note evidence of altered behavior in any elderly patient that you assess and examine. Common signs and symptoms of a psychological disorder include lapses in memory, cognitive difficulty, changes in sleep patterns, fear of death, changes in sexual interest, thoughts of suicide, or withdrawal from society.

In general, management of psychological disorders in the elderly is the same as for other age groups. Two of the most common emotional disturbances that you may encounter in the elderly are depression and suicide.

Depression

Up to 15 percent of the non-institutionalized elderly experience depression. Within institutions, that figure rises to about 30 percent. The incidence of depression among the elderly is expected to rise in the early 2000s as the baby boomers—with their larger numbers and more prevalent depression at an earlier age—enter their 60s.

Some of the general signs and symptoms noted previously may indicate depression. Ask the patient about feelings of sadness or despair. Determine if he or she has suffered episodes of crying. Inquire about past psychological treatment and current stressful events, particularly the death of a loved one. Keep in mind that sensory changes—especially deafness and blindness—may make the patient vulnerable to depression. Serious acute diseases can have the same effect. If the patient recognizes the depression, ask about the duration and any prior bouts. Find out if the patient has been given any medications to treat the depression. If so, check compliance.

Some depressed patients may exhibit **hypochondriasis** (hypochondria). If this condition is a side effect of the depression, the patient will still show some degree of emotional pain and/or **dysphoria.** Although you may not be able to identify hypochondria in the field, remember that the condition is an illness and requires treatment by trained medical personnel.

In general, depressed patients should receive supportive care. Encourage them to talk, delicately raising questions about suicidal thoughts. The seriously depressed patient should be transported to the hospital. Treatment of depression usually entails psychotherapy and/or antidepressants.

Suicide

The highest suicide rates in the United States are among people over age 65, especially men. The elderly account for 20 percent of all suicides, but represent only 12 percent of the total population. Someone over age 65 completes suicide about every 90 minutes. Suicide is the third leading cause of death among the elderly, following falls and car accidents.

Depression is the leading cause for suicide among the elderly. As a group, the elderly are less likely to seek help than the young. They are also less likely to express their anger or sorrow, turning their feelings inward instead. Other stressors that put the elderly at risk of suicide include:

- Chronic illness
- Physical impairment
- Unrelieved pain
- Living in a youth-oriented society

* **hypochondriasis** an abnormal concern with one's health, with the false belief of suffering from some disease, despite medical assurances to the contrary; commonly known as hypochondria.

* **dysphoria** an exaggerated feeling of depression or unrest, characterized by a mood of general dissatisfaction, restlessness, discomfort, and unhappiness.

Remember that hypochondriasis is an illness, too.

- Family issues
- Financial problems
- Isolation and loneliness
- Substance abuse
- Low serotonin levels (Serotonin declines with age.)
- Bereavement
- Family history of suicide

Suicidal behavior is related to stress. As a paramedic, you should try to evaluate the stress from an elderly patient's point of view, keeping the preceding factors in mind. In cases of a seriously depressed patient, elicit behavior patterns from family, friends, or caregivers. Warning signs may include:

- Loss of interest in activities that were once enjoyable
- Curtailing social interaction, grooming, and self-care
- Breaking from medical or exercise regimens
- Grieving a personal loss ("I don't want to live without him/her.")
- Feeling useless ("Nobody would miss me.")
- Putting affairs in order, giving away things, finalizing a will
- Stock-piling medications or other lethal means of self-destruction, including firearms

Be particularly alert to suicide among the acutely ill. With more patients being returned home to care for themselves, there is a higher incidence of suicide among the terminally ill, especially cancer victims. A lack of post-acute hospital care can be interpreted as a lack of caring in general.

Prevention of suicide among the elderly involves intervention by all levels of society, from family to EMS to hospital workers. It is important to dispel the common myths about aging and age-related diseases. Recognition of warning signs and involvement of appropriate individuals and agencies is critical.

Your first priorities in the management of a suicidal elderly patient are to protect yourself and then to protect the patient from self-harm. To do this, you must gain access to the patient. This may require breaking into a house or room, particularly if the patient is unconscious or can be readily seen. Remember to summon law enforcement personnel as necessary. DO NOT RULE OUT FIREARMS AMONG THE ELDERLY.

DO NOT rule out firearms among the elderly.

If you reach the patient, emergency care has the highest priority secondary to crew safety. Conduct a brief interview with the patient, if possible, to determine the need for further action. DO NOT leave the suicidal patient alone. Administer medications with caution, keeping in mind polypharmacy and drug interactions in the elderly. (Consult with medical direction.) ALL SUICIDAL ELDERLY PATIENTS SHOULD BE TRANSPORTED TO THE HOSPITAL.

All suicidal elderly patients should be transported to the hospital.

TRAUMA IN THE ELDERLY PATIENT

Trauma is the leading cause of death among the elderly. Older patients who sustain moderate to severe injuries are more likely to die than their younger counterparts. Post-injury disability is also more common in the elderly than in the young.

CONTRIBUTING FACTORS

A number of factors contribute to the high incidence and severity of trauma among the elderly. Slower reflexes, arthritis, and diminished eyesight and hearing predispose the elderly to accidents, especially falls. The elderly, because of their physical state and vulnerability, are also at high risk from trauma caused by criminal assault. Purse-snatching, armed robbery, and assault occur all too frequently in the elderly population, especially among those living in urban areas.

Age-related factors that place the elderly at risk of severe injury and complications include:

- Osteoporosis and muscle weakness—increased likelihood of fractures
- Reduced cardiac reserve—decreased ability to compensate for blood loss
- Decreased respiratory function—increased likelihood of **acute respiratory distress syndrome (ARDS)**
- Impaired renal function—decreased ability to adapt to fluid shifts
- Decreased elasticity in the peripheral blood vessels—greater susceptibility to tearing

✱ **acute respiratory distress syndrome (ARDS)** respiratory insufficiency marked by progressive hypoxemia, due to severe inflammatory damage.

GENERAL ASSESSMENT

As with any other trauma patient, determine the mechanism of injury. Leading causes of trauma in the elderly include: falls, motor vehicle crashes, burns, assault or abuse, and underlying medical problems such as syncope.

In assessing elderly trauma patients, remember that blood pressure readings may be deceptive. Older patients typically have a higher blood pressure than younger patients. Although a blood pressure of 110/70 may be normal for a 30-year-old, it could represent a low blood pressure, and possibly shock, for an older patient. Elderly trauma patients also may not exhibit an elevated pulse—a common early sign of hypoperfusion. This may be because of a chronic heart disease or the use of medications to treat hypertension or a myocardial infarction. Fractures may also be obscured or concealed because of a diminished sense of pain among the elderly. One of the best indicators of shock in the elderly is an altered mental status or changes in consciousness during assessment. Elderly trauma patients who exhibit confusion or agitation are candidates for rapid transport.

In assessing elderly trauma patients, remember that blood pressure and pulse readings can be deceptive indicators of hypoperfusion.

Observing for Abuse/Neglect

Make sure you observe the scene for signs of abuse and neglect. Abuse of the elderly is as big a problem in our society as child abuse and neglect. **Geriatric abuse** is defined as a syndrome in which an elderly person has received serious physical or psychological injury from family members or other caregivers. Abuse of the elderly knows no socioeconomic bounds. It often occurs when an older person is no longer able to be totally independent, and the family has difficulty upholding their commitment to care for the patient. It can also occur in nursing homes and other health care facilities. The profile for the potential geriatric abuser may often show a great deal of life stress. In many cases, there is sleep deprivation, marital discord, financial problems, and work-related problems. As the abuser's life gets in further disarray, and as the patient further deteriorates, abuse may be the outcome.

Signs and symptoms of geriatric abuse and neglect are often obvious (Figure 3-16). Unexplained trauma is usually the primary presentation. The average abused patient is older than 80 and has multiple medical problems, such

✱ **geriatric abuse** a syndrome in which an elderly person is physically or psychologically injured by another person.

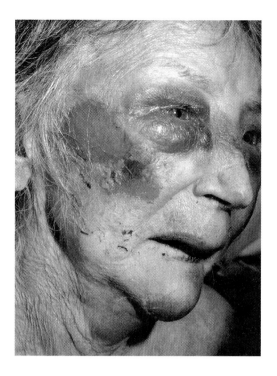

FIGURE 3-16 When you encounter evidence of serious head injury, maintain a suspicion of geriatric abuse until proven otherwise.

as cancer, congestive heart failure, heart disease, and incontinence. Senile dementia is often present. In these cases, it can be hard to determine whether the dementia is chronic or acute, especially if there is an increased likelihood of head trauma from abuse.

Whenever you suspect geriatric abuse, obtain a complete patient and family history. Pay particular attention to inconsistencies. *DO NOT confront the family.* Instead, report your suspicions to the emergency department and the appropriate governmental authority. Many states have very strong laws protecting the elderly from abuse or neglect. In fact, many states consider it a criminal offense *not* to report suspected geriatric abuse. These states also offer legal immunity to those who report geriatric abuse, as long as the report is made in good faith.

Many states have laws that require prehospital personnel to report suspected cases of geriatric abuse and/or neglect.

GENERAL MANAGEMENT

The priorities of care for the elderly trauma patient are similar to those for any trauma patient. However, you must keep in mind age-related systemic changes and the presence of chronic diseases. This is especially true of the cardiovascular, respiratory, and renal systems.

Cardiovascular Considerations

Recent or past myocardial infarctions may contribute to the risk of dysrhythmia or congestive heart failure in the trauma patient. In addition, there may be a decreased response of the heart, in adjusting heart rate and stroke volume, to hypovolemia. An elderly trauma patient may require higher than usual arterial pressures for perfusion of vital organs, due to increased peripheral vascular resistance and hypertension. Care must be taken in intravenous fluid administration because of decreased myocardial reserves. Hypotension, hypovolemia, and hypervolemia are poorly tolerated in the elderly patient.

Respiratory Considerations

In managing the airway and ventilation in an elderly trauma patient, you must consider the physical changes that may affect treatment. Check for dentures and determine whether they should be removed. Keep in mind that age-related changes can decrease chest wall movement and vital capacity. Age also reduces the tolerance of all organs for anoxia. Remember, too, that chronic obstructive pulmonary disease is widespread among the elderly.

Make necessary adjustments in treatment to provide adequate oxygenation and appropriate CO_2 removal. It is important to remember that use of 50 percent nitrous oxide (Nitronox) for elderly patients may result in more respiratory depression than would occur in younger patients. Positive pressure ventilation should also be used cautiously. There is an increased danger of resultant alkalosis and rupture of emphysematous bullae, making the elderly more vulnerable to pneumothorax.

Renal Considerations

The decreased ability of the kidneys to maintain normal acid/base balance, and to compensate for fluid changes, can further complicate the management of the elderly trauma patient. Any preexisting renal disease can decrease the kidney's ability to compensate. The decrease in renal function, along with a decreased cardiac reserve, places the elderly injured patient at risk for fluid overload and pulmonary edema. Remember, too, that renal changes allow toxins and medications to accumulate more readily in the elderly.

Transport Considerations

You may have to modify the positioning, immobilization, and packaging of the elderly trauma patient before transport. Be attentive to physical deformities such as arthritis, spinal abnormalities, or frozen limbs that may cause pain or special care (Figure 3-17a-c). Recall the frailty of an elderly person's skin and avoid creating skin tears or pressure sores. Keep in mind that trauma places an elderly person at increased risk of hypothermia. Ensure that the patient is kept warm at all times.

Keep in mind that trauma places an elderly person at increased risk of hypothermia. Ensure that the patient is kept warm at all times.

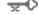

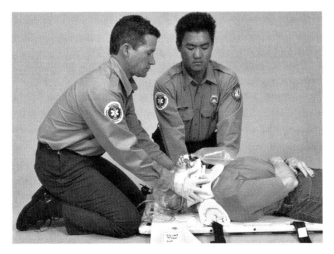

FIGURE 3-17a In an elderly patient with curvature of the spine, place padding behind the neck when immobilizing a patient to a long spine board.

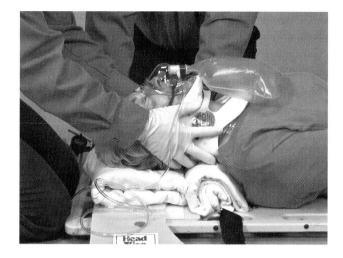

FIGURE 3-17b Additional padding, such as rolled blankets or towels behind the head, may be needed to keep the head in a neutral, in-line position.

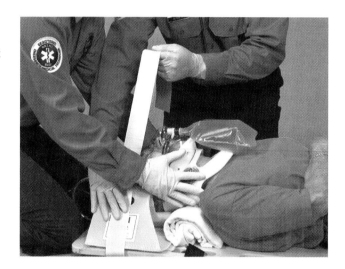

FIGURE 3-17c Secure the patient's head with a head immobilizer device. To prevent spinal damage, maintain manual stabilization until the head is secured.

SPECIFIC INJURIES

The elderly can be subject to a variety of injuries, just like any other age group. The three most common categories of injuries among the elderly include orthopedic injuries, burns, and injuries of the head and spine.

Orthopedic Injuries

As previously mentioned, the elderly suffer the greatest mortality and greatest incidence of disability from falls. Approximately 33 percent of falls in the elderly result in at least one fractured bone. The most common fall-related fracture is a fracture of the hip or pelvis (Figure 3-18). Osteoporosis and general frailty contribute to this. The older patient who has fallen should be assumed to have a hip fracture until proven otherwise. Signs and symptoms of a hip fracture include tenderness over the affected joint and shortening and external rotation of the leg. The patient is unable to bear weight on the affected leg. Those patients who live alone may not be able to get to a phone to summon help. Because of this, they may remain on the floor for a prolonged period of time. This can lead to hypothermia, hyperthermia, and/or dehydration.

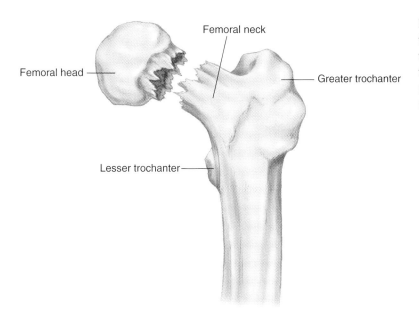

Femoral head

Femoral neck

Greater trochanter

Lesser trochanter

FIGURE 3-18 Subcapital femoral neck fracture. Patients with a displaced femoral neck fracture present with groin pain and a shortened externally rotated leg.

Falls also result in a variety of other stress fractures in the elderly, including fractures of the proximal humerus, distal radius, proximal tibia, and thoracic and lumbar bodies. Falls may also lead to soft-tissue injuries and hot water burns, if the incident occurred in a tub or hot shower.

In treating orthopedic injuries, remember to ask questions aimed at detecting an underlying medical condition. Ask if the patient recalls "blacking out." Remain alert for evidence of potential cardiac emergencies. Package and transport the patient per the general guidelines mentioned earlier.

Burns

People age 60 and older are more likely to suffer death from burns than any other age group except neonates and infants. Several factors help explain the high mortality rate among elderly burn victims. They include:

- Reaction time slows as people age, so the elderly often stay in contact with thermal sources longer than their younger counterparts.
- Pre-existing diseases place the elderly at risk of medical complications, particularly pulmonary and cardiac problems.
- Age-related skin changes (thinning) result in deeper burns and slower healing time.
- Immunological and metabolic changes increase the risk of infection.
- Reductions in physiologic function and the reduced reserve of several organ systems make the elderly more vulnerable to major systemic stress.

Management of elderly burn patients follows the same general procedures as other patients. However, remember that the elderly are at increased risk of shock. Administration of fluids are important to prevent renal tubular damage. Assess hydration in the initial hours after a burn injury by blood pressure, pulse, and urine output (at least 1–2 mL/kg per hour).

In the case of the elderly, complications from a burn may manifest themselves in the days and weeks following the incident. For serious burns to heal, the body may use up to 20,000 calories a day. Elderly patients, with altered metabolisms and complications such as diabetes, may not be able to meet this demand, increasing the chances for infection and systemic failure. Part of your job may be to prepare the family for such a delayed response and to provide necessary psychological support.

Head and Spinal Injuries

As a group, the elderly experience more head injuries, even from relatively minor trauma than their younger counterparts. A major factor is the difference in proportion between the brain and the skull. As mentioned earlier, the brain decreases in size and weight with age. The skull, however, remains constant in size, allowing the brain more room to move, thus increasing the likelihood of brain injury. Because of this, signs of brain injury may develop more slowly in the elderly, sometimes over days and weeks. In fact, the patient may often have forgotten the offending injury.

The cervical spine is also more susceptible to injury due to osteoporosis and spondylosis. **Spondylosis** is a degeneration of the vertebral body. The elderly often have a significant degree of this disease. In addition, arthritic changes can gradually compress the nerve rootlets or spinal cord. Thus, injury to the spine in the elderly makes the patient much more susceptible to spinal cord injury. In fact, sudden neck movement, even without fracture, may cause spinal-cord injury. This can occur with less than normal pain, due to the absence of fracture. Therefore, it is important to provide older patients with suspected spinal injuries, especially those involved in motor vehicle accidents, with immediate manual cervical spinal stabilization at the time of initial assessment.

✱ **spondylosis** a degeneration of the vertebral body.

Summary

The practice of EMS in the 21st century means treating a growing elderly population. The "Graying of America" has resulted in a greater number of people age 65 and older, many of whom will be in home settings. When treating elderly patients, keep in mind the anatomical, physiological, and emotional changes that occur with age. However, never jump to conclusions based solely on age. Weigh normal age-related changes against abnormal changes—i.e., those resulting from a medical condition or trauma. Recall that elderly patients are much more susceptible to medication side effects and toxicity than younger patients. They also are more susceptible to trauma and environmental stressors. Abuse of the elderly occurs, and you should bear this in mind whenever injuries do not match the history. Any suspected abuse or neglect of an elderly patient should be reported to the emergency department and/or the appropriate governmental authorities.

You Make the Call

Just after 3 A.M., a call comes in to the station to assist an elderly man who has fallen. His wife requests lifting assistance because she is disabled. She reports: "I have arthritis and cannot possibly help him back into bed."

You arrive at a small, one-family home just off a major thoroughfare. A small, severely arthritic woman in a wheelchair greets you: "He's inside. The nerve of him. He won't even answer me—just makes fun of me by repeating everything I say and slurring his words. I'll bet he's been drinking and didn't want me to know. As if I couldn't tell by his behavior! We've been married for 47 years, and he still takes care of me. But not tonight!"

The home is clean and well cared for—not a speck of dust or a single cobweb to be seen. The woman's husband is lying on his side on the carpeted floor next to the bed. He is awake, drooling, and repeating words in a thick speech.

1. What general impression do you have of this patient?
2. Do you suspect that this is an acute or chronic problem? Explain.

During the initial assessment, the patient is V on AVPU. Pupils are deviated left. You ensure that all spinal precautions are taken. Then you check hand grasp—the left is strong, the right absent. The airway is open, but needs suctioning of saliva. Respirations are present and unlabored. You note strong, but irregular distal pulses.

You apply oxygen and determine that the patient, Mr. Jones, is a high priority due to the field diagnosis of a stroke. His airway will need close management and definitive treatment.

3. Aside from the patient's presentation and response to your interventions, what other information must be included in your hospital report?
4. What support do you provide for Mrs. Jones?

See Suggested Responses at the back of this book.

FURTHER READING

Abi-Hanna, P. and R. Gleckman: "Acute Abdominal Pain: A Medical Emergency in Older Patients," *Geriatrics* 52(7), July 1997 (pp. 72–74).

Abrams, W.B., *et. al.*, eds.: *The Merck Manual of Geriatrics*, 2nd ed. Whitehouse Station, NJ. Merck Research Laboratories. 1995.

Ball, R.: "Geriatric Assessment: Considerations of the Over 65 Patient," *Journal of Emergency Medical Services*, March, 1997 (pp. 96–102).

Bledsoe, B., Papa, F., and D. Clayden: *Prehospital Emergency Pharmacology*, 5th ed. Upper Saddle River, NJ. Brady/Prentice-Hall. 2001.

Ciccone, C.D.: "Geriatric Pharmacology," in *Geriatric Physical Therapy*. St. Louis, MO. Mosby-Year Book, Inc., 1993.

"Drug Therapy in the Elderly," in Beers, M.H., *et. al.*, eds.: *The Merck Manual of Diagnosis and Therapy*, 17th ed. Whitehouse Station, NJ. Merck Research Laboratories. 1999.

Duban, S.: "The Hospitalized Nursing Home Patient," *American Journal of Nursing*, January, 1998 (p. 35).

Emmett, K.R.: "Non-specific and Atypical Presentations of Diseases in the Older Patient," *Geriatrics* 53(2), February 1998 (pp. 50–60).

"Geriatric Considerations," in Harwood-Nuss, A.L., *et. al.*, eds.: *Clinical Practice of Emergency Medicine*, 2nd ed. Philadelphia, PA. Lippincott-Raven, 1996.

"Geriatric Trauma" and "Abuse in the Elderly and Impaired," in Tintinalli, J.E., *et. al.*, eds., *Emergency Medicine: A Comprehensive Study Guide*, 5th ed. New York, NY. McGraw-Hill, 1999.

Hamm, R.: "If You Could Feel What I Feel: Learning to Care for the Elderly," *JEMS*, October 1993 (pp. 57–60).

Potter, M.: "Pulmonary Embolism: A Lung Attack," *Emergency*, April 1998 (pp 33–37).

Schneider, S.M.: "Altered Mental Status in the Elderly: Current Assessment and Management Strategies for a Complex Clinical Syndrome," *Emergency Medicine Reports* 17(5), March 4, 1996 (pp. 43–52).

ON THE WEB

Visit Brady's Paramedic Website at www.bradybooks.com/paramedic.

CHAPTER 4

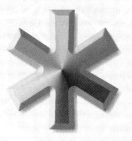

Abuse and Assault

Objectives

After reading this chapter, you should be able to:*

1. Discuss the incidence of abuse and assault. (p. 206)
2. Describe the categories of abuse. (pp. 206–217)
3. Discuss examples of spouse, elder, child, and sexual abuse. (pp. 206–220)
4. Describe the characteristics associated with the profile of a typical spouse, elder, or child abuser and the typical assailant of sexual abuse. (pp. 208–209, 211–212, 213, 218)
5. Identify the profile of the "at-risk" spouse, elder, and child. (pp. 207–208, 209, 211, 212, 213)
6. Discuss the assessment and management of the abused patient. (pp. 209–210, 211, 214–217)
7. Discuss the legal aspects associated with abuse situations. (pp. 206, 210, 217, 219–220)
8. Identify community resources that are able to assist victims of abuse and assault. (pp. 209, 211, 217)
9. Discuss the documentation necessary when caring for abused and assaulted patients. (pp. 210, 217, 219–220)

For more information on objectives relating to child and elder abuse, see Chapters 1 and 3.

CASE STUDY

You are awakened during the middle of the night to respond to an unknown emergency. You arrive to find a police officer on the scene with a 36-year-old woman who was found at the side of the road partially clothed. She is crying and nearly incoherent. You learn from scattered comments, and remarks by the police officer, that a male assailant abducted the patient at gunpoint and sexually assaulted her. He then threw the patient from a moving vehicle and fled the scene. A passing motorist spotted the woman curled up along the roadside and used a cell phone to summon police.

Because you have a female partner, you decide that she might be more appropriate to maintain contact with this patient. As you return to the ambulance to retrieve equipment, your partner begins an initial assessment. She looks for immediate life threats, while exhibiting a compassionate and consoling attitude just as any EMS professional should do. During the physical exam, she uses a blanket to protect the patient's privacy. Any clothing removed during the assessment is placed in a paper bag and given to the police officer as evidence.

Due to the mechanism of injury, you and your partner decide to apply spinal immobilization. You find extensive abrasions when you log-roll the patient, but do not detect any life-threatening injuries. Because your partner has

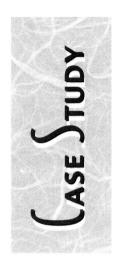

noted blood around the patient's perineum, she places a dressing over the patient's genitals.

Vital signs are good, so you begin transport to a hospital designated as a rape crisis center. En route, you notify the receiving hospital so that it can prepare for your arrival. The staff readies a private room for the patient and summons a social worker, a nurse with specialized training as a Sexual Assault Nurse Examiner (SANE), and a detective.

After you transfer the patient, you complete your patient report, giving special attention to the narrative. Both you and your partner realize that you might be called to testify in court sometime in the future.

INTRODUCTION

Because of underreporting, it is difficult to provide accurate statistics on the incidence of abuse and assault in the United States today. That makes available figures even more overwhelming in their seriousness. To grasp the magnitude of the problem, consider these facts.

- Nearly three million children suffer abuse each year and more than 1,000 die annually.
- Between two to four million women each year are battered by their partners or spouses.
- Elder abuse occurs at an incidence of between 700,000 to 1.1 million annually.

Abuse and assaults transcend gender, race, age, and socio-economic status.

Abuse and assaults transcend gender, race, age, and socio-economic status. The effects are serious and long-lasting. Victims may die as a result of their injuries or have long-term healthcare problems. No victim ever forgets his or her pain. Even after the physical wounds have healed, the emotional injuries never completely fade.

Unfortunately, the pattern of abuse and assault forms a cycle that is difficult to break. Parents who harm each other are more likely to abuse their children. Children who suffer abuse have a greater likelihood of becoming abusers themselves. At some point in their lives, they may abuse their dates, their partners, their children, their elders, or others.

The EMS system is involved with many cases of abuse. Although law enforcement is not always present, you have a responsibility to identify victims of abuse and initiate some kind of action. In many areas, laws require healthcare personnel to report actual or suspected incidences of abuse. Early detection is critical to breaking the cycle of abuse through social services support and alterations in behavior.

Early detection is critical to breaking the cycle of abuse through social services support and alterations in behavior.

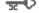

PARTNER ABUSE

partner abuse physical or emotional violence from a man or woman towards a domestic partner.

The potential for **partner abuse** has existed for as long as couples have interacted. It results when a man or woman subjects a domestic partner to some form of physical or psychological violence. The victim may be a husband or wife, someone who shares a residence, or simply a boyfriend or girlfriend.

The most widespread and best known form of abuse involves the abuse of women by men. However, battery is not limited to women. Men can be—and are—abused by women. They suffer the same feelings of guilt, humiliation, and a loss of control. A battered man feels trapped just like a battered woman, but is often even less likely to report the abuse, either out of a sense of shame or a lack of resources for support, or both.

Battery also affects same-sex couples. Abusive relationships between men or between women follow the same patterns and the same conditioning as those seen in heterosexual relationships. What can be said of women battered by men can generally be said of most battery situations, regardless of the gender of the victim or the abuser.

REASONS FOR NOT REPORTING ABUSE

Victims of partner abuse hesitate or fail to report the problem for a number of reasons. Fear presents one of the biggest obstacles to taking action. Most battered partners fear reprisals, either to themselves or to their children. They also fear being humiliated for their powerlessness or inability to stop the violence, especially if the battered partner is a male.

Reporting abuse is usually the last resort. Many partners hope the abusive behavior will simply just end. This hope is fueled when the abuser promises to change—a common reaction after a violent episode. The abused partner may also be in denial—claiming that the situation is less serious than it is or rationalizing that the violence is somehow justified. Some abused women, for example, believe they are the cause of the abusive behavior or that the abuse is part of the marriage and should be endured to preserve the family.

Finally, many victims of abuse lack the knowledge or financial means to seek help. They may not know where to turn or who to trust. They may also lack the money to seek counseling, intervention, or a safe place to live. A partner who lacks job training and/or who must support dependent children may find the prospect of starting life anew more frightening than the abuse. Unfortunately, an abusive situation rarely ceases without some kind of separation or intervention. Escalation of violence is common, with injuries becoming more severe. Over time, abuse becomes more frequent, often occurring without provocation, and more inclusive. If children were not initially involved, they may become victims as the episodes escalate.

> **Content Review**
>
> ## REASONS FOR NOT REPORTING ABUSE
> - Fear of reprisal
> - Fear of humiliation
> - Denial
> - Lack of knowledge
> - Lack of financial resources

IDENTIFICATION OF PARTNER ABUSE

Partner abuse can fall into several categories. The most obvious form is physical abuse, which involves the application of force in ways too numerous to list here. In addition to direct personal injury, physical abuse may exacerbate existing medical conditions, such as hypertension, diabetes, or asthma. These conditions can also be affected by verbal abuse, which consists of words chosen to control or harm a person. Verbal abuse may leave no physical mark, but it damages a person's self-esteem and can lead to depression, substance abuse, or other self-destructive behavior.

Sexual abuse, which is a form of physical abuse, can also occur between partners. It involves forced sexual contact and includes marital or date rape. (For more on sexual abuse and assault, see material later in the chapter.)

In identifying an abusive family situation, keep in mind the ten generic risk factors identified in "Domestic Violence: Cracking the Code of Silence," a source cited in the DOT's National Standard Curriculum. These factors, based on research of battered women, include:

1. Male is unemployed.
2. Male uses illegal drugs at least once a year.

In addition to direct personal injury, physical abuse may exacerbate existing medical conditions, such as hypertension, diabetes, or asthma.

3. Partners have different religious backgrounds.
4. Family income is below the poverty level.
5. Partners are unmarried.
6. Either partner is violent toward children at home.
7. Male did not graduate from high school.
8. Male is unemployed or has a blue-collar job.
9. Male is between 18 and 30 years old.
10. Male saw his father hit his mother.

CHARACTERISTICS OF PARTNER ABUSERS

As already indicated, partner abuse occurs in all demographic groups. However, abuse is more common in lower socio-economic levels in which wage earners have trouble paying bills, holding down jobs, or keeping pace with technological changes that make their job skills outdated or obsolete.

A history of family violence makes a person more likely to repeat the pattern as an adult. Typically the abuser does not like being out of control, but at the same time feels powerless to change. The situation is made worse if both parties do not know how to back down from a conflict. Lacking any alternative, one or both of the partners may turn to physical and/or verbal violence (Figure 4-1). In some cases, abusers will think they are demonstrating discipline rather than violent behavior.

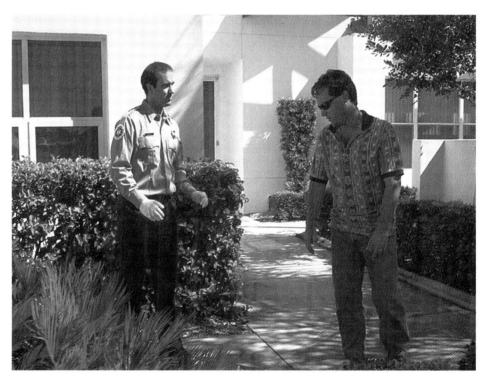

FIGURE 4-1 When called to the scene of domestic violence, you may encounter hostility from the person responsible for the abuse. Remain calm when you speak to the person and do not enter his or her personal space. Remain alert to changes in emotional status, and be prepared to summon law enforcement officials as necessary.

Abusers usually exhibit overly aggressive personalities—an outgrowth of low self-esteem. They often feel insecure and jealous, flying into sudden and unpredictable rages. Use of alcohol or drugs increases the likelihood that the abuser will lose control and may not even clearly remember his or her actions.

In the aftermath of an abusive incident, the abuser often feels a sense of remorse and shame. The person may seek to relieve his or her guilt by promising to change or even seeking help. For a time, the abuser may appear charming or loving, convincing an abused partner to think that perhaps the pattern has finally been broken. All too often, however, the cycle of violence repeats itself in just a few days, weeks, or months.

CHARACTERISTICS OF ABUSED PARTNERS

It may be difficult to identify the abused partner. As mentioned, the primary risk factor for abuse is a history of violence between parents, a factor that will not be immediately known to you or other EMS providers. However, studies have revealed that abused partners share certain common characteristics. They include:

- *Pregnancy:* Forty-five percent of women suffer some form of battery during pregnancy.
- *Substance abuse:* Abused partners often seek the numbing effect of alcohol and/or drugs.
- *Emotional disorders:* Abused partners frequently exhibit depression, evasiveness, anxiety, or suicidal behavior.

As mentioned earlier, the victim may seek to protect his or her attacker, either by delaying care and/or by providing alternative explanations for injuries. Remain alert to subtle signs that the patient is being less than honest. Many victims, for example, avoid eye contact, exhibit nervous behavior, and/or watch the abuser, if present. The victim may also provide verbal clues, saying such things as "we've been having some problems lately" or "I always seem to be causing some kind of trouble."

APPROACHING THE BATTERED PATIENT

In assessing the battered patient, direct questioning usually works best. Convey an awareness that the person's partner may have caused the harm or created conditions that led to the injury and/or the emotional trauma. Once the subject of abuse has been introduced, exhibit a willingness to discuss it. Remember to avoid both judgmental questions such as "Why don't you leave?" or judgmental statements such as "How awful!"

Throughout the assessment, listen carefully to the patient. Indicate your attention by saying, "I hear what you are telling me." Often victims of abuse feel a sense of relief when someone else knows about the situation. This can be the first step toward seeking help.

When speaking with abused patients, encourage them to regain control over their lives. Do this by helping them to identify what they want for themselves and, in many cases, for their children. Also, be prepared to share your knowledge of community resources, such as shelters and counseling services, that may offer help. Find out about the support services, both for the victim and the abuser, that are available in your area.

In assessing the battered patient, direct questioning usually works best.

Do not leave the scene of suspected abuse without advising the patient to take all necessary precautions.

Finally, do not leave the scene without advising the patient to take all necessary precautions. Rehearse the quickest way to leave the home. Find out where the patient will go and/or who the patient will call. If the patient drives, suggest carrying the keys to the vehicle at all times. Remind the patient that it is a crime to beat another person and that, depending upon the type of injury, assault is either a misdemeanor or a felony.

Keep in mind that in cases of partner abuse, the abuser may be reported and taken into custody by the police. However, the person may soon be released on his or her own recognizance, sometimes within a matter of hours. The patient may already know this and be reluctant to take any action. If the patient does not know this, it is your duty to inform him or her of this possibility and to tell the person about available protection programs.

ELDER ABUSE

As noted in Chapter 3, elder abuse is a widespread medical and social problem caused by many factors. They include:

- Increased life expectancies
- Increased dependency on others, as a result of longevity
- Decreased productivity in later years
- Physical and mental impairments, especially among the "old old"
- Limited resources for long-term care of the elderly
- Economic factors, such as strained family finances
- Stress on middle-age caretakers responsible for two generations— children and parents

The problem of elder abuse is expected to grow along with the size of the elderly population, which will increase dramatically within the next 20–30 years as baby boomers turn age 65 and older. It is your responsibility to be aware of this situation and to remain alert to signs of elder abuse (Figure 4-2).

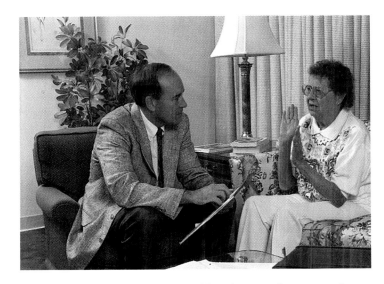

FIGURE 4-2 You are obligated to report suspected elder abuse to the appropriate authorities. In the case of institutional elder abuse, your actions may result in an investigation by an outside agency who will question the patient more closely.

IDENTIFICATION OF ELDER ABUSE

There are basically two types of elder abuse—domestic and institutional. **Domestic elder abuse** takes place when an elder is being cared for in a home-based setting, usually by relatives. **Institutional elder abuse** occurs when an elder is being cared for by a person with a legal or contractual responsibility to provide care, such as paid caregivers, nursing home staff, or other professionals. Both types of abuse can be either acts of commission (acts of physical, sexual, or emotional violence) or acts of omission (neglect).

In some cases, signs of elder abuse are subtle, such as theft of the victim's belongings or loss of freedom. Other signs, such as wounds, untreated decubitus ulcers, or poor hygiene, are more obvious. For additional information on the signs of elder abuse, see Chapter 3.

✳ **domestic elder abuse** physical or emotional violence or neglect when an elder is being cared for in a home-based setting.

✳ **institutional elder abuse** physical or emotional violence or neglect when an elder is being cared for by a person paid to provide care.

THEORIES ABOUT DOMESTIC ELDER ABUSE

There are four main theories about causes of domestic elder abuse. Commonly, caregivers feel stressed and overburdened. They are ill-equipped to provide care or simply lack the knowledge to do the job correctly. Another cause of elder abuse is their physical and/or mental impairment. Elders in poor health are more likely to be abused than elders in good health. This situation results, in part, from their inability to report the abuse. Yet another cause of elder abuse is family history, or the cycle of violence mentioned earlier. Finally, elder abuse increases proportionately with the personal problems of the caregivers. Abusers of the elderly tend to have more difficulties, either financial or emotional, than non-abusers.

CHARACTERISTICS OF ABUSED ELDERS

Like partner abuse, elder abuse cuts across all demographic groups. As a result, it is difficult to outline an accurate profile of the abused elder. The most common cases involve elderly women abused by their sons. However, this pattern is skewed by the fact that women live longer than men. Elder abuse most frequently occurs among people who are dependent upon others for their care, especially among those elders who are mentally or physically challenged. In such cases, elders may be repeatedly abused by relatives who believe the elder will not or cannot ask for help.

In cases of neglect, abused elders most commonly live alone. They may be mentally competent, but fear asking for help because relatives have complained about providing care or have threatened to place them in a nursing home. Like abused partners, they may be reluctant to give information about their abusers for fear of retaliation.

CHARACTERISTICS OF ELDER ABUSERS

It is also difficult to profile the people who are most likely to abuse elders. According to the National Aging Resource Center on Elder Abuse, the percentages in Table 4-1 reflect the reported perpetrators of elder abuse in domestic settings. As you can see, the most typical abusers are adult children, who are either overstressed by care of the elder or who were abused themselves.

As with partner abusers, there are several characteristics commonly found in abusers of the elderly. Often, the perpetrators exhibit alcoholic behavior, drug addiction, or some mental impairment. The abuser may also be dependent upon the income or assistance of the elder—a situation that can cause resentment, anger, and, in some cases, violence.

For more on the management of elder abuse, see Chapter 3.

Table 4-1	PERPETRATORS OF DOMESTIC ELDER ABUSE
Group	**Percentage**
Adult children	32.5
Grandchildren	4.2
Spouse	14.4
Sibling	2.5
Other relatives	12.5
Friend/neighbor	7.5
All others	18.2
Unknown	2.0

CHILD ABUSE

 child abuse physical or emotional violence or neglect towards a person from infancy to eighteen years of age.

Child abuse can occur from infancy to age 18 and can be inflicted by any number of caregivers.

As pointed out in Chapters 1 and 2, child abuse is one of the most difficult circumstances that you will face as a paramedic. **Child abuse** may range from physical or emotional impairment to neglect of a child's most basic needs (Figure 4-3). It can occur from infancy to age 18 and can be inflicted by any number of caregivers—parents, foster parents, step-parents, babysitters, siblings, step-siblings, or other relatives or friends charged with a child's care.

Although you may be familiar with some of the following information from your training or from earlier chapters in this book, it bears repeating. The damage done to a child can last a lifetime and, as stressed, perpetuate a cycle of violence in generations to come.

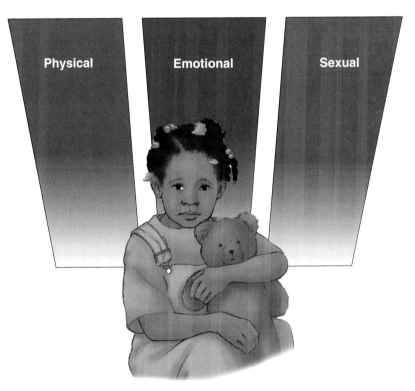

FIGURE 4-3   Child abuse comes in many forms. Be alert and report any concerns you may have regarding abuse or neglect.

CHARACTERISTICS OF CHILD ABUSERS

As with other types of abusers, you cannot relate child abuse to social class, income, or education. However, certain patterns do emerge, most notably a history of abuse within their own families. Most child abusers were physically or emotionally abused as children. They often would prefer to use other forms of discipline, but under stress they regress to the earliest and most familiar patterns. Once resorting to physical discipline, the punishments become more severe and more frequent.

In cases of reported physical abuse, perpetrators tend to be men. However, the statistics for men and women even out when neglect is taken into account. As indicated earlier, potential child abusers can include a wide variety of caregivers. In most cases, however, one or both parents are the most likely abusers. Frequent behavioral traits include:

- Use or abuse of drugs and/or alcohol
- Immaturity and preoccupation with self
- Lack of obvious feeling for the child, rarely looking at or touching the child
- Seemingly unconcerned about the child's injury, treatment, or prognosis
- Openly critical of the child, with little indication of guilt or remorse for involvement in the child's condition
- Little identification with the child's pain, whether it be physical or emotional

Any one of these signs should raise suspicion in your mind of possible child abuse. The infant or child will provide other clues, even before you begin your physical examination.

CHARACTERISTICS OF ABUSED CHILDREN

A child's behavior is one of the most important indicators of abuse. Some behavior is age-related. For example, abused children under age six usually appear excessively passive, while abused children over age six seem aggressive. Other behavioral clues include:

A child's behavior is one of the most important indicators of abuse.

- Crying, often hopelessly, during treatment or not crying at all
- Avoiding the parents or showing little concern for their absence
- Unusually wary or fearful of physical contact
- Apprehensive and/or constantly on the alert for danger
- Prone to sudden behavioral changes
- Absence of nearly all emotions
- Neediness, constantly requesting favors, food, or things

In general, use your instincts and knowledge of age-appropriate behavior (see Chapters 1 and 2) to guide your first impression of the child. If the child's behavior is atypical, maintain an index of suspicion throughout your assessment.

Use your instincts and knowledge of age-appropriate behavior to guide your first impression of a child whom you suspect may have been abused.

IDENTIFICATION OF THE ABUSED CHILD

As you know, children very commonly get injured and not all injured children are abused. If a child volunteers the story of his or her injury without hesitation and if it matches the story told by the parent and the symptoms of injury,

Table 4-2	COLOR OF BRUISES AND THEIR AGE*
Age	**Skin Appearance**
0 to 2 days	tender and swollen, red
0 to 5 days	blue, purple
5 to 7 days	green
7 to 10 days	yellow
10 or more days	brown
2 or more weeks	cleared

*Adapted from Richardson, A.C., "Cutaneous Manifestations of Abuse" in Reece, R.M. *Child Abuse: Medical Diagnosis and Management.*

Soft-tissue injuries are common indicators of abuse, especially multiple bruises in different places on the body, in different stages of healing, and/or with distinctive shapes.

child abuse is very unlikely. However, in cases in which the behavior of a caregiver and/or child has raised an index of suspicion, you may face a challenge in distinguishing between an intentional injury and an authentic accident. Conditions commonly mistaken for abuse are car seat burns, staphylococcal scalded skin syndrome, chicken pox (cigarette burns), and hematological disorders that can cause bruising. In assessing a child, look for common patterns of physical abuse, evidence of emotional abuse, and/or environmental clues of neglect.

Physical Examination

In most cases, signs of physical mistreatment of a child should be the easiest type of abuse for you to recognize. Soft tissue injuries are the most common indicators, especially multiple bruises in different planes of the body, in different stages of healing, and with distinctive shapes (Table 4-2 and Figure 4-4). Other common warning signs include defensive wounds on the hands and forearms and symmetrical injuries such as bites or burns. Any of these conditions carry a high index of suspicion of abuse.

Burns and Scalds As Figure 4-5 indicates, abusive burns often have distinctive patterns that indicate the implement or source used to injure the child. The burns tend to be in certain common locations—the soles of the feet, palms of the hands, back, or buttocks. They may or may not be found in conjunction with other injuries.

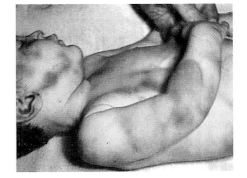

FIGURE 4-4   Severe multiple bruises can lead to death.

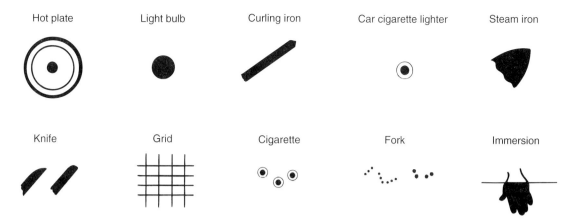

Hot plate	Light bulb	Curling iron	Car cigarette lighter	Steam iron

Knife	Grid	Cigarette	Fork	Immersion

FIGURE 4-5   You can often recognize the source of intentional burns by their shape and/or pattern.

Because children have thinner skin than adults (other than elders), they also tend to scald more easily. The temperature of hot water in most residences is about 140°F, which can scald an adult in only about five seconds. (Bath water for children should be kept below 120°F.) When children accidentally get into water that is too hot, you can expect to see "splash" burns—marks created by spattering water as children try to escape. Intentional scalding, however, is characterized by the conspicuous lack of splash burns. Such "dipping injuries" are a common form of child abuse.

Intentional scalding is characterized by the conspicuous lack of splash burns.

Fractures   Fractures constitute the second most common form of child abuse. Sites of fractures include the skull, nose, facial structures, and upper extremities (Figure 4-6). Twisting and jerking fractures result from grabbing a child by an extremity, while neck injuries occur from shaking a child. Because children have soft, pliable ribs, they rarely experience accidental fractures to this region. As a result, you should maintain a high index of suspicion of abuse whenever you encounter a child with fractured ribs.

Because children have soft, pliable ribs, they rarely experience accidental fractures to this region.

Head Injuries   Over time, injuries from abuse tend to progress from the extremities and trunk to the head. Head injuries commonly found in abused children include scalp wounds, skull fractures, subdural or subgaleal hematomas, and repeated contusions.

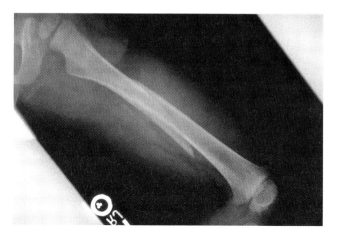

FIGURE 4-6   Evidence of child abuse—X-ray of a spiral femur fracture.

Injuries to the head claim the largest number of lives among abused children. They also account for most of the long-term disability associated with child abuse.

Shaken Baby Syndrome Shaken baby syndrome frequently occurs when a parent or caregiver becomes frustrated with a crying infant and all other attempts to quiet the baby have failed. It happens when a person picks up the infant and shakes the baby vigorously. The movement can cause permanent brain damage such as subdural hematomas or diffuse swelling. It may also result in injuries to the neck and spine or retinal hemorrhages, which in turn can lead to blindness. If the infant is shaken hard enough or repeatedly, the baby may die from the injuries.

Abdominal Injuries Although abdominal injuries represent a small proportion of the injuries suffered by abused children, they are usually very serious. Blunt force can result in trauma to the liver, spleen, or mesentery. You should look for pain, swelling, and vomiting, as well as hemodynamic compromise from these injuries.

Signs of Neglect

Some forms of child abuse are less obvious than physical injuries. Abuse may result from neglect. Caregivers simply do not provide children with adequate food, clothing, shelter, or medical care.

As a paramedic, you may be in a unique position to observe and report neglect. Unlike many other healthcare or public-safety workers, EMS personnel get an opportunity to see the child's home environment for themselves. Unhealthy or unclean conditions are clear evidence of a caregiver's inability to provide for a child's safety or well-being.

In examining a child, keep in mind the following common signs of neglect:

- Malnutrition (Neglected children are often underweight, sometimes by up to 30 percent.)
- Severe diaper rash
- Diarrhea and/or dehydration
- Hair loss
- Untreated medical conditions
- Inappropriate, dirty, or torn clothing
- Tired and listless attitudes
- Near constant demands for physical contact or attention

Signs of Emotional Abuse

Emotional abuse is often the hardest form of abuse to identify. It may take any one of the following six forms:

1. Parents or caregivers simply ignore the child, showing indifference to the child's needs and failing to provide any stimulation.
2. Parents or caregivers reject, humiliate, or criticize the child.
3. The child may be isolated and deprived of normal human contact or nurturing.
4. A child may be terrorized or bullied through verbal assaults and threats, creating feelings of fear and anxiety.

5. A parent or caregiver may encourage destructive or antisocial behavior.

6. The child may be over-pressured by unrealistic expectations of success.

RECORDING AND REPORTING CHILD ABUSE

As with all other forms of abuse, you have a responsibility to report suspected cases of child abuse. In some instances, you might have a chance to provide early intervention. An abusive adult may actively seek help or may send out signals for help. For example, a potential abuser may make several calls within a 24-hour period. The person may also summon help for inconsequential symptoms or demonstrate an inability to handle an impeding crisis. These are warning signs and should be duly noted.

When confronted with an actual case of child abuse, try to conduct the examination with another colleague present. You must keep your personal reactions to yourself and record only your objective observations. Assumptions must not be included in your report. The final document should be objective, legible, and written with the knowledge that it may be used in a future court or child custody case. At all times, put the child's interest first, treating him or her with utmost kindness and gentleness. (For more on your EMS and legal responsibilities, see material later in the chapter.)

As with all other forms of abuse, you have a responsibility to report suspected cases of child abuse.

When confronted with a case of child abuse, try to conduct the examination with another colleague present.

SEXUAL ASSAULT

Anyone can be a victim of sexual violence. Statistics from the National Victims Center and the U.S. Department of Justice reveal that males and females of all backgrounds, from infancy to old age, have reported crimes involving forced or unwanted sexual contact. According to the Bureau of Justice Statistics, over 260,000 rapes and nearly 100,000 sexual assaults are reported each year. However, these figures reflect only a small percentage of cases, with an estimated 63–74 percent of all incidents going unreported.

Although the legal definitions vary from state to state, courts generally interpret **sexual assault** as unwanted sexual contact, whether it be genital, oral, rectal, or manual. **Rape** is usually defined as penile penetration of the genitalia or rectum (however slight) without consent of the victim. Both forms of sexual violence are prosecuted as crimes, with rape constituting a felony offense. As a result, your actions at the scene and the report that you file will in all likelihood impact on the outcome of a trial.

✱ **sexual assault** unwanted oral, genital, rectal, or manual sexual contact.

✱ **rape** penile penetration of the genitalia or rectum without the consent of the victim.

CHARACTERISTICS OF VICTIMS OF SEXUAL ASSAULT/RAPE

It is difficult to profile a victim of sexual assault or rape because of the variety of victims. However, statistics reveal certain patterns. The group most likely to be victimized is made up of adolescent females younger than age 18. Nearly two-thirds of all rapes and sexual assaults take place between the hours of 6 P.M. and 6 A.M. at the victim's home or at the home of a friend, relative, or acquaintance. A woman is raped, on average, every two minutes in the United States and is four times as likely to be raped by someone she knows than by a stranger.

Particularly alarming is the number of children who suffer some form of sexual abuse. According to the Department of Justice, one in two rape victims are

The legal definition of rape varies from state to state. You should review the appropriate laws in your state pertaining to rape and sexual assault.

under age 18; one in six are under age 12. Other government figures show that approximately one-third of all juvenile victims of sexual abuse are children younger than 6 years of age. Typically, contact involves a male assailant and a female victim, but not always. The contact can range from exposure to fondling to penetration. Although sexual abuse can occur in families of all descriptions, children raised in families where there is domestic violence are eight times more likely to be sexually molested within that family.

Sexual assault and rape carry serious consequences. Victims may be physically injured during the assault or even killed. They commonly suffer internal injuries, particularly if multiple assailants are involved in the attack. Rape can result in infections, sexually transmitted diseases, and unwanted pregnancies. The psychological damage is deep and long-lasting. Shame, anger, and a lack of trust may persist for years—or even a lifetime.

Children, in particular, find it difficult to speak about molestation. It is likely that they know the person and fear reprisal or, in some instances, even seek to protect the individual. In many cases, the assailants physically explore the child without intercourse or force the child to touch or fondle them. Victims, especially very young children, may be confused about the situation or, lacking physical evidence of abuse, fear that nobody will believe them. Symptoms of sexual abuse, regardless of its form, may include:

- Nightmares
- Restlessness
- Withdrawal tendencies
- Hostility
- Phobias related to the offender
- Regressive behavior, such as bed wetting
- Truancy
- Promiscuity, in older children and teens
- Drug and alcohol abuse

CHARACTERISTICS OF SEXUAL ASSAILANTS

Like the victims of sexual assaults, the assailants can come from almost any background. However, the violent victimizers of children are substantially more likely than the victimizers of adults to have been physically or sexually abused as children. Many assailants, particularly adolescents and abusive adults, think domination is part of any relationship. Such thinking can lead to date rape or marital rape. In a significant percentage of all cases, the assailants are under the influence of alcohol or drugs. Nearly 30 percent of all rapists use weapons, underscoring the fact that sexual assaults are violent crimes.

In cases of date rape, the assailant may have drugged the unknowing victim with flunitrazepam (Rohypnol), known by the street names of "roofie," "roche," "rib," or "rope." The victim may exhibit extreme intoxication without a corresponding strong smell of alcohol or may have drug-induced amnesia (a common effect), making questioning difficult or impossible. More often than not, the alleged assailant in such cases lives on a college campus, the location of most EMS calls involving what is known as the "date rape drug."

EMS RESPONSIBILITIES

Your response to a call involving a sexual assault is in many ways similar to your response to any abusive situation. In both instances, your primary responsibil-

In calls involving abuse or assault, your primary responsibility is safety—both your own and that of the patient.

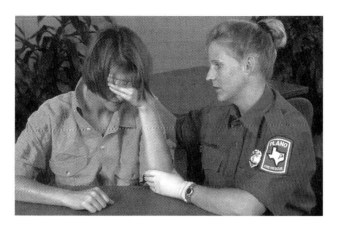

FIGURE 4-7 If possible, a same-sex paramedic or EMT should maintain contact with the victim of rape or an alleged sexual assault, accompanying the patient to the hospital.

ity is safety—both your own and that of the patient. You should never enter a scene if your safety is compromised, and you should leave the scene as soon as you feel unsafe.

You can expect victims of assault or abuse to feel unsafe as a result of the violence they have suffered. One of your primary responsibilities is to provide a safe environment for an already traumatized patient. Sometimes you can provide safety merely by your official presence. Other times, you may have to move the patient to the ambulance where you can lock the doors or move to a different location entirely. In still other instances, you may have to summon additional personnel. (For more on crime scene management, see Chapter 12.)

You are also responsible for providing proper psychosocial care for the victims of abuse and assault. Privacy is a major consideration. In many cases, a same-sex paramedic—you or a colleague—should maintain contact with the victim (Figure 4-7). Although you may need to expose the victim during assessment, you should cover the patient and remove him or her from public view as soon as possible.

When talking with the patient, use open-ended questions to reestablish a sense of control. You might say, for example, "Would you like to sit on a seat or ride on the stretcher?" Or you might ask, "Is there someone you would like us to call?" As mentioned in earlier sections, remain non-judgmental throughout treatment, avoiding subjective comments both of the patient and the assailant. In a reassuring voice, encourage the patient to report the rape, explaining the importance of preserving evidence.

Medical treatment of victims of abuse and assault is essentially the same as with other patients. However, you should always remember the origins of the patient's injuries and provide appropriate emotional support. Keep in mind that the patient has been harmed by another human being, in many cases a person that they know intimately.

In many cases, a same-sex paramedic—you or a colleague—should maintain contact with the victim of an alleged sexual assault.

When talking with a victim of sexual assault, use open-ended questions to help the patient regain a sense of self-control.

LEGAL CONSIDERATIONS

As noted throughout this chapter, abuse and assault constitute crimes. Although their nature and extent of the crime often depends upon local laws, you have a responsibility to report suspected cases to the appropriate law enforcement officials. Because the assailants may be detained only a short time, you also have an obligation to find out about the victim and witness protection programs available in your area.

Specialized resources include both private and state or federally funded programs. Make a point of learning about hospital units for the victims of sexual assault, public and private shelters for battered persons, and state agencies responsible for youths and their families. Also acquaint yourself with nurses trained as Sexual Assault Nurse Examiners (SANE). They have completed programs allowing them to perform the physical exam for sexual assaults. They have detailed information on the protection of evidence, something that you must keep in mind throughout the call.

As you have read, your actions can affect the prosecution of a crime. Clothing should only be removed from a patient when necessary for assessment and treatment. All items should then be turned over to the proper authorities.

In the case of rape, patients should not urinate, defecate, douche, bathe, eat, drink, or smoke. Some jurisdictions have specific rules for evidence protection, such as using paper bags to collect evidence or placing bags over the patient's hands to preserve trace evidence. Remember that any evidence that you collect must remain in your custody until you can give it directly to a law enforcement official to preserve the **chain of evidence.**

As indicated, it is important that you carefully and objectively document all your findings. You may end up defending your words in a court of law. Regardless of the emotions evoked by the call, you must remain a professional at all times.

Finally, you should study the local laws and protocols regarding cases of abuse and assault. All 50 states require healthcare workers to report suspected cases of child abuse. Some states require EMS personnel to report even a suspicion of abuse or assault. Some states allow minors to seek medical care for sexual assault without parental consent. The Joint Commission of Accreditation of Healthcare Organizations (JCAHO) mandates that hospital personnel screen incoming patients for abuse. Regardless of where you live, take time to learn the rules and regulations that affect your practice, both for your sake and for the sake of your patients.

* **chain of evidence** legally retaining items of evidence and accounting for their whereabouts at all times to prevent loss or tampering.

Your actions in the case of alleged sexual assaults can affect the prosecution of a crime. Protect the evidence.

Regardless of the emotions evoked by a call involving abuse or assault, you must remain professional at all times.

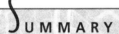

$\int$ UMMARY

The incidence of abuse is widespread today, and you will encounter many cases during your paramedic career. You should learn the hallmarks of partner abuse, elder abuse, child abuse, and sexual assaults. You should also learn to recognize significant physical and emotional assessment findings as well as characteristics of the victims and assailants. Proper treatment of victims of abuse and assault includes knowing the legal requirements of your area, protecting evidence, and properly documenting your findings and actions.

Y OU MAKE THE CALL

Y ou and your partner respond to a police request to evaluate an injured child. You find several police officers on the scene of a domestic disturbance. The patient is a three-year-old boy found sitting quietly on the couch. The boy's parents are present and being questioned by the police officers.

You find the patient dressed in underwear with no other clothing during wintertime. He has obvious and different colored bruises to both his upper arms and his back. During your exam, the boy is silent, not answering your questions or looking towards either of his parents.

1. What do you suspect is taking place?
2. What physical evidence do you have to support this suspicion?
3. What emotional evidence do you have to support this suspicion?
4. What other clues lead you to believe that abuse might be taking place?
5. What are your priorities in this case?

See Suggested Responses at the back of this book.

FURTHER READING

American Nurses Associations: *Culturally Competent Assessment for Family Violence.* Washington, DC. American Nurses Publishing, 1998.

Federal Bureau of Investigation: *Uniform Crime Statistics.* Washington, DC. FBI, 1996.

Garnett, Co.: "Health Seminar Series Examines Domestic Violence," *The WIH Record*, April 12, 1994, pp. 1, 4.

Hamberger, L.K. and C. Renzetti: *Domestic Partner Abuse.* New York, NY. Springer Publishing. 1996.

Hobbs, C.J. and J.M. Wynne: *Physical Signs of Child Abuse: A Color Atlas.* London. W.B. Saunders. 1996.

Kaplan, S.J.: *Family Violence: A Clinical and Legal Guide.* Washington, DC. American Psychiatric Press. 1996.

McCurdy, D., *et. al.*: *Current Trends in Child Abuse Reporting and Fatalities.* Chicago, IL. Committee to Prevent Child Abuse, 1994.

Monteleone, J.A.: *Recognition of Child Abuse for the Mandated Reporter.* St. Louis, MO. Mosby-Year Book, Inc. 1994.

Presidential Task Force on Violence and the Family: *Report of the American Psychological Association Presidential Task Force on Violence and the Family.* Washington, DC. Government Printing Office, 1996.

Reece, R.M.: *Child Abuse: Medical Diagnosis and Management.* Philadelphia, PA. Lea & Febiger. 1994.

U.S. Department of Justice: *National Crime Victimization Survey.* Washington, DC. Bureau of Justice Statistics, 1996.

U.S. Department of Justice: *Violence Against Women.* Washington, DC. Bureau of Justice Statistics, 1994.

ON THE WEB

Visit Brady's Paramedic Website at www.bradybooks.com/paramedic.

CHAPTER 5

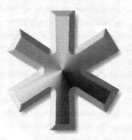

The Challenged Patient

Objectives

After reading this chapter, you should be able to:

1. Describe the various etiologies and types of hearing impairments. (pp. 225–226)
2. Recognize the patient with a hearing impairment. (p. 226)
3. Anticipate accommodations that may be needed in order to properly manage the patient with a hearing impairment. (p. 227)
4. Describe the various etiologies and types, recognize patients with, and anticipate accommodations that may be needed in order to properly

manage each of the following conditions:
   a. visual impairments (pp. 227–228)
   b. speech impairments (pp. 228–230)
   c. obesity (pp. 230–231)
   d. paraplegia/quadriplegia (pp. 231–232)
   e. mental illness (p. 232)
   f. developmentally disabled (pp. 232–233, 234)
   g. Down syndrome (pp. 233–234)
   h. emotional impairment (p. 232)

Continued

CASE STUDY

You sit down for the first meal on your shift at Medic 211. Just as you take out something to eat, you are dispatched to a private residence for a fall victim. You and your partner look at each other, throw your food back into your lunch bags, and hit the road.

En route to the call, you learn that a 72-year-old woman has fallen out of her wheelchair and is unable to get back up. Dispatch tells you that the door is locked, but the woman has hidden a spare key under a fake rock in the garden near the front door.

Fifteen minutes later, you and your partner gain access to the house. You find a woman lying on her side on the bedroom floor, her wheelchair off to the side behind her. You notice what appears to be a brace on the woman's right leg.

When you introduce yourself, the patient tells you her name is Mrs. Bonnie Wade. "I was trying to put a dress up in my closet," explains Mrs. Wade, "when I lost my balance and fell."

Upon further questioning, Mrs. Wade indicates that she is widowed and lives alone. Although she can ambulate for short periods of time, she is, for the most part, wheelchair bound. Mrs. Wade denies losing consciousness and says

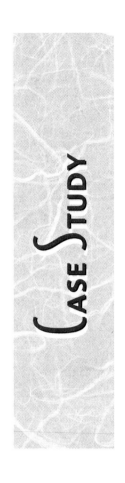
she feels no neck or back pain and no tingling in her extremities. When asked about pain, she replies, "My left hip and shoulder hurt real bad. I fell so hard that I almost dropped the mobile phone. I carry it all the time just in case I ever need help."

During your neurological exam, you find that the patient is unable to move her right leg. Mrs. Wade responds, "Oh that, I had polio when I was young—long before the vaccination they give to kids today." She also tells you that her left arm is weak from post-polio syndrome.

Your partner goes to the ambulance to get the scoop stretcher. Meanwhile, you put the patient's left arm in a cravat sling. You then explain how the scoop stretcher works and assure Mrs. Wade that it is the safest and most comfortable way to get her off the floor. When Mrs. Wade asks whether her leg brace will be in the way, you tell her that you'd like to keep it in place until a doctor evaluates her.

Once you have packaged the patient in the scoop stretcher, you carefully place her on the ambulance stretcher. Mrs. Wade tells you that the sling has relieved some of the pain in her arm, but asks you to take the bumps slowly due to pain in her leg. You place her in the back of the ambulance and begin transport to Memorial Hospital.

INTRODUCTION

Throughout your EMS career, you can expect to encounter a number of patients who live with a variety of impairments or special challenges. Many will have met these challenges so successfully that you may not notice them right away. For example, people with hearing impairments might lip read so well that you may not initially realize they cannot hear. People with more obvious challenges, such as paralysis, may have accepted their impairments and built active and rewarding lives. A patient with a history of polio, for example, may have lived with the problem so long that he or she neglects to tell you about it right away. Instead the patient talks about a more immediate problem—the reason for summoning EMS.

The one thing that challenged patients share is their variety. They might have any number of physical, mental, or emotional impairments. They might have contracted a pathological illness that necessitates a special living or working arrangement. They might be suffering from a terminal illness or a communicable disease. They may come from a cultural or financial situation that dictates medical practices contrary to those of the EMS community. The key to treating the "challenged" patient is to understand and recognize the special condition or situation and to make any accommodations that may be needed for proper patient care.

PHYSICAL CHALLENGES

A number of physical impairments—conditions that limit the use of one or more parts of the body—can affect patient assessment and/or treatment. These impairments may be the result of accidents, birth injuries, chronic illnesses, aging, and more. Impairments can limit the ability of a patient to hear, see, speak, or move. Patients will react to their impairments in different ways—from acceptance, to denial, to anger, to shame. It is important that you quickly recognize the impairment and exhibit knowledge and sensitivity to assure the patient that you understand his or her special needs.

HEARING IMPAIRMENTS

Hearing impairments involve a decrease or loss in the ability to distinguish or hear sounds, particularly those involving speech. An inability to hear is commonly described as **deafness.** A person may be completely deaf or partially deaf. Deafness may be in one ear or both ears. The condition may be present at birth or may occur later in life as a result of an accident, illness, or aging.

Types of Hearing Impairments

There are basically two types of deafness—**conductive deafness** and **sensorineural deafness.** Many forms of conductive deafness may be treated and cured, especially if caught early. Sensorineural deafness, on the other hand, is often incurable.

Conductive Deafness Conductive deafness results from any condition that prevents sound waves from being transmitted from the external ear to the middle or inner ear. The condition can be either temporary or permanent.

If an infant or child does not respond to verbal stimulation or questions, rule out the possibility of conductive deafness when performing your assessment of disability. Congenital malformation of the ear is a possible, but rare cause of conductive deafness in the neonate. A more common cause of conductive deafness in children is **otitis media,** an infection of the middle ear. This condition often arises from various childhood illnesses, particularly those involving the upper respiratory tract. To prevent hearing loss, children under age six who experience recurrent otitis media may need to take daily prophylactic antibiotics or have tympanostomy (myringotomy) tubes placed.

In addition to infection, a number of other conditions can result in a temporary loss of hearing. Anyone can experience conductive deafness during an airline flight, where changes in air pressure can affect hearing. A deep-water dive can have a similar effect. Impacted **cerumen,** or earwax, is yet another common and easily treatable cause of conductive deafness.

Other causes might be the temporary blockage of the ear canal by various irritants such as dust, hair spray, insects, or water ("swimmer's ear"). Patient attempts to clean the canal with cotton applicators may disrupt the ear's natural cleaning process and push the debris deeper into the ear, which sets the stage for bacterial infections and conductive deafness.

Obstructions can also be caused by hematomas, which may result from blunt trauma to the ear. Force to the mandible, such as a fractured jaw, can also produce a temporary loss of hearing and may in fact result in fragments of bone displaced to the ear canal. Although these conditions cannot be treated in the field, they should be taken into account when a trauma patient appears not to respond to, or "hear," your questions.

Sensorineural Deafness Sensorineural deafness arises from the inability of nerve impulses to reach the auditory center of the brain because of damage either to the inner ear or to the brain itself. It is usually a permanent condition.

In the case of infants and children, sensorineural deafness often results from congenital defects or birth injuries. Preterm infants are particularly at risk for sensorineural deafness, especially those with severe asphyxia or recurrent apnea in the neonatal period. Ototoxic drugs, such as furosemide (Lasix) and gentamycin,

It is important that you quickly recognize the impairment and exhibit the knowledge and sensitivity to assure the patient that you understand his or her special needs.

✱ **deafness** the inability to hear.

✱ **conductive deafness** deafness caused when there is a blocking of the transmission of the sound waves through the external ear canal to the middle or inner ear.

✱ **sensorineural deafness** deafness caused by the inability of nerve impulses to reach the auditory center of the brain because of nerve damage either to the inner ear or to the brain.

✱ **otitis media** middle ear infection.

✱ **cerumen** ear wax.

can also cause sensorineural deafness if administered to infants in neonatal intensive care units. Finally, many children who develop this type of hearing loss have mothers who contracted rubella (German measles) or cytomegalovirus (CMV), during the first three months of pregnancy.

Diseases, such as bacterial meningitis, or viral illnesses, such as **labrynthitis** (inner ear infection), can lead to sensorineural deafness at any age. Taking high does of ototoxic drugs such as aspirin can also cause sensorineural deafness in both children and adults. A common symptom of aspirin toxicity is "ringing in the ears" (tinnitus). Other causes of sensorineural deafness include tumors of the brain or middle ear, concussion, severe blows to the ear, and repeated loud noises such as chain saws, heavy machinery, gun fire, rock music, or sudden blasts of sound.

Conditions associated with aging can also lead to permanent hearing loss. **Presbycusis** is a progressive sensorineural hearing loss that begins after age 20, but is usually significant only in people over age 65. More common in men than women, this type of hearing loss affects high-frequency sounds first, then low-frequency sounds. Eventually, human voices becomes harder to detect, especially if background noise is present. Elderly people with this condition will often tell others not to "mumble" or will ask them to speak louder.

✱ **labrynthitis** inner ear infection that causes vertigo, nausea, and an unsteady gait.

✱ **presbycusis** progressive hearing loss that occurs with aging.

Recognition of Deafness

As mentioned, it is important to detect deafness early in your assessment. A partially deaf person may ask questions repeatedly, misunderstand answers to questions, or respond inappropriately. Such reactions can easily be mistaken for head injury, leading to misdirected treatment.

The most obvious sign of deafness is a hearing aid (Figure 5-1). Unfortunately, hearing aids do not work for all types of deafness. Also, many people do not wear hearing aids, even when they have been prescribed. In addition, deaf people may have poor diction due to partial hearing loss or hearing loss later in life. They might use their hands to gesture or use sign language. As noted, deaf people may ask you to speak louder or they may speak excessively loud themselves. Finally, deaf people will commonly face you so that they can read your lips.

A partially deaf person may ask questions repeatedly, misunderstand answers to questions, or respond inappropriately. Such reactions can easily be mistaken for head injury, leading to misdirected treatment.

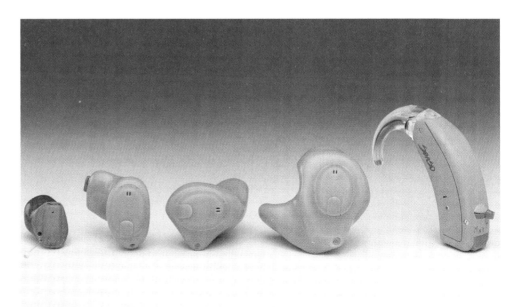

FIGURE 5-1   Hearing aids come in various shapes and sizes.

Accommodations for Deaf Patients

When managing a patient with a hearing impairment, you can do several things to ease communication. Begin by identifying yourself and making sure the patient knows that you are speaking to him or her. Get the patient's attention by moving so you can be seen or by gently touching the person, if appropriate. By addressing deaf patients face to face, you give them the opportunity to read your lips and interpret your expression.

When talking with a deaf patient, speak slowly in a normal voice. Never yell or use exaggerated gestures. These techniques often distort your facial and body language, making you seem angry or threatening. Keep in mind that nearly 80 percent of hearing loss is related to high-pitched sounds. As a result, you might use a low-pitched voice to speak directly into the patient's ear. Whatever you do, make sure that background noise is reduced as much as possible, turning off the TV, radio, or other sources of sound.

If you are called to a deaf patient's home during the night, you may need to help find or adjust a hearing aid. If you cannot locate the device, you might put a stethoscope on the patient and try speaking into it. Alternatively, you might make use of an "amplified" listener—e.g., an ear microphone.

Don't forget one of the most simple and effective means of communication—use of pen and paper. As long as you don't need to move quickly, you can write out notes for the patient to read and wait for the person to respond in the same way. You can also use a pen and paper to draw pictures to illustrate basic needs or procedures. This approach can ease a patient's anxiety, reducing the fear of miscommunication or lack of control over his or her treatment.

Finally, many people with hearing impairments know sign language, usually American Sign Language (ASL). If this is the case, try to utilize an interpreter, often a family member or even a neighbor. Make sure that you document the name of the person who did the interpreting and the information received. Also, notify the receiving hospital of the need to have an interpreter on hand if the person is unable to accompany you.

> *By addressing deaf patients face to face, you give them the opportunity to read your lips and interpret your expression.*
>

> *If you use an interpreter, make sure that you document the name of the person who did the interpreting and the information received.*
>

VISUAL IMPAIRMENTS

When caring for the patient with a visual impairment, it is important to note if the impairment is a permanent disability or if it is a new symptom as a result of the illness or injury for which you were called. It is necessary to understand the causes of blindness before this determination can be made.

Etiologies

Visual impairments can result from a number of causes. Possible etiologies include injury, disease, congenital conditions, infection (such as cytomegalovirus [CMV]), and degeneration of the retina, optic nerve, or nerve pathways. A description of each of the etiologies follows.

Injury A previous injury to the eye can cause a permanent vision loss. An injury to the orbit usually includes injury to the tissue around the orbit as well as to the eye itself. This can cause muscle and nerve damage that may lead to permanent loss of eyesight. Penetrating injuries can result in **enucleation,** which is removal of the eyeball. Chemical and thermal burns to the eye can result in damage to the cornea and can also lead to permanent vision loss if not treated quickly. A temporary loss of vision can result from an injury, such as the chemical burn that may occur with the deployment of an airbag, or from a corneal abrasion. Once treated, these injuries rarely lead to permanent loss of vision.

> **Content Review**
>
> **CAUSES OF VISUAL IMPAIRMENTS**
> - Injury
> - Disease
> - Congenital conditions
> - Infection
> - Degeneration of the retina, optic nerve, or nerve pathways

* **enucleation** removal of the eyeball after trauma or illness.

Disease Visual impairments may also be caused by a disease of the eye, or as a secondary result of the primary disease process. **Glaucoma,** for example, is a group of eye diseases that results in increased intraocular pressure on the optic nerve. If not treated, glaucoma leads to loss of peripheral vision and blindness.

The are two different types of glaucoma, primary and secondary. The cause of primary glaucoma remains unknown. However, secondary glaucoma results from other eye diseases. The incidence of glaucoma is higher in blacks than in whites. A black person between the ages of 45 and 65 is 15 times more likely to have glaucoma than a white person in the same age group.

Diabetic retinopathy is another disease-related visual impairment. It results from diabetes mellitus, which causes disorders in the blood vessels that lead to the retina. Small hemorrhages in these blood vessels leads to a slow loss of vision and possible blindness.

Congenital and Degenerative Disorders A congenital disorder that causes visual disturbances is cerebral palsy. Premature birth can lead to blindness in the neonate. Degeneration of the eyeball, optic nerve, or nerve pathways is most commonly caused by aging and can slowly lead to loss of vision. Cytomegalovirus (CMV), an opportunistic infection often seen in AIDS patients, can lead to blindness by causing retinitis—an inflammation of the retina.

Recognizing and Accommodating Visual Impairments

Many visually impaired people live independent, active lives (Figure 5-2). Depending upon the degree of impairment and a person's adjustment to the loss of vision, you may or may not recognize the condition right away. In cases of obvious blindness, identify yourself as you approach the patient so that the person knows you are there. Also, describe everything you are doing as you do it.

Many blind people have tools to assist them in their activities of daily living. The most obvious is a seeing eye dog. When approaching a person with a seeing eye dog, DO NOT pet the dog or disturb it while the dog is in its harness. For the dog, the harness means that it is working. Ask permission from the patient to touch the dog. Never grab the leash, the harness, or the patient's arm without asking permission. Doing this may place the dog or the owner in danger.

Accommodation must be made for transporting the guide dog with the patient. Circumstances and local protocols will dictate whether you transport the dog in the ambulance with the patient or have the dog transported in another vehicle.

If your patient does not have a guide dog, inquire about other tools that the person may want brought to the hospital. If the patient is ambulatory, have the person take your arm for guidance rather than taking the patient's arm.

SPEECH IMPAIRMENTS

When performing an assessment, you may come across a patient who is awake, alert, and oriented, but cannot communicate with you due to a speech impairment. Possible miscommunication can hinder both the treatment you administer and the information that you provide to the receiving facility.

Types of Speech Impairments

You may encounter four types of speech impairments—language disorders, articulation disorders, voice production disorders, and fluency disorders. A discussion of each disorder follows.

Language Disorders A language disorder is an impaired ability to understand the spoken or written word. In children, language disorders result from a num-

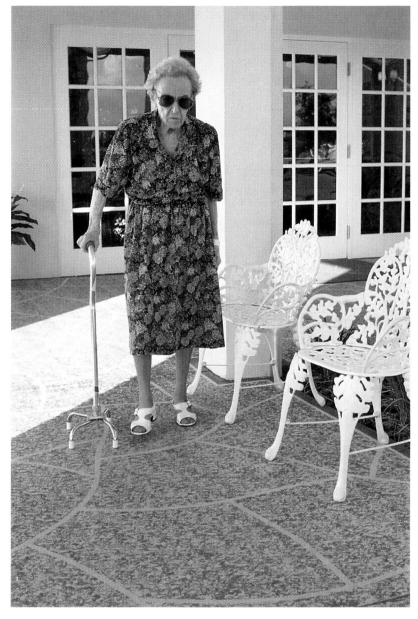

FIGURE 5-2   Individuals who are visually impaired can still maintain active, independent lives.

ber of causes such as congenital learning disorders, cerebral palsy, or hearing impairments. A child who receives inadequate language stimulation in the first year of life may also experience delayed speaking ability.

In an adult patient, language disorders may result from a variety of illnesses or injuries. The person may have experienced a stroke, aneurysm, head injury, brain tumor, hearing loss, or some kind of emotional trauma. The loss of ability to communicate in speech, writing, or signs is known as **aphasia**. Aphasia can manifest itself in the following ways:

- **Sensory aphasia**—a person can no longer understand the spoken word. Patients with sensory aphasia will not respond to your questions because they cannot understand what you are saying.

✳ **aphasia** occurs when the individual suffers a brain injury due to stroke or head injury and no longer has the ability to speak or read.

✳ **sensory aphasia** occurs when the patient cannot understand the spoken word.

✱ motor aphasia occurs when the patient cannot speak but can understand what is said.

Patients with motor aphasia will understand what you say. It is important to allow such patients to express their responses however they can.

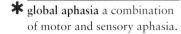

✱ global aphasia a combination of motor and sensory aphasia.

- **Motor aphasia**—a person can no longer use the symbols of speech. Patients with motor aphasia, also known as expressive aphasia, will understand what you say, but cannot clearly articulate a response. They may respond to your questions slowly, use the wrong words, or act out answers. It is important to allow such patients to express their responses in whatever way they can.
- **Global aphasia**—occurs when a person has both sensory and motor aphasia. These patients can neither understand nor respond to your questions. A brain tumor in Broca's region can cause this condition.

Articulation Disorders Articulation disorders, also known as dysarthria, affect the way a person's speech is heard by others. These disorders occur when sounds are produced or put together incorrectly or in a way that makes it difficult to understand the spoken word. Articulation disorders may start at an early age, when the child learns to say words incorrectly or when a hearing impairment is involved. This type of disorder can also occur in both children and adults when neural damage causes a disturbance in the nerve pathways leading from the brain to the larynx, mouth, or lips.

When speaking with someone who has an articulation disorder, you will notice that they pronounce their words incorrectly or that their speech is slurred. They may leave certain sounds out of a word because they are too difficult for them to pronounce. Again, it is important for you to listen carefully and let the person complete a response.

Voice Production Disorders When a patient has a voice production disorder, the quality of the person's voice is affected. This can be caused by trauma due to overuse of the vocal cords or infection. Cancer of the larynx can also cause a speech failure by impeding air from passing through the vocal cords. A patient with a production disorder will exhibit hoarseness, harshness, an inappropriate pitch, or abnormal nasal resonance.

Fluency Disorders Fluency disorders present as stuttering. Although the cause of stuttering is not fully understood, the condition is found more often in men than in women. Stuttering occurs when sounds or syllables are repeated and the patient cannot put words together fluidly. When speaking with patients who stutter, do not interrupt or finish their answers out of frustration. Let patients complete what they have to say, and do not correct how they say it.

Accommodations for Speech Impairments

When speaking to a patient with a speech impairment, try to form questions that require short, direct answers.

When speaking to a patient with a speech impairment, never assume that the person lacks intelligence. It will be difficult, if not impossible, to complete a thorough interview if you have insulted the patient. Do not to rush the patient or predict an answer. Try to form questions that require short, direct answers. Prepare to spend extra time during your interview.

When asking questions, look directly at the patient. If you cannot understand what the person has said, politely ask him or her to repeat it. Never pretend to understand when you don't. You might miss valuable information about the patient's chief complaint—the reason for the call. If all else fails, give the patient an opportunity to write responses to your questions.

OBESITY

Over 40 percent of people in the United States are considered obese, while many more are heavier than their ideal body weight. An obese patient can make a difficult job even more difficult for an EMS provider. Besides the obvious difficulty of lifting and moving the obese patient, excess weight can exacerbate the complaint for which you were called. Obesity can also lead to a number of serious medical conditions, including hypertension, heart disease, strokes, diabetes, and joint and muscle problems.

Etiologies

People require a certain amount of body fat in order to metabolize vitamins and minerals. Obesity occurs when a person has an abnormal amount of body fat and a weight 20 to 30 percent heavier than is normal for people of the same age, gender, and height.

Obesity occurs for a number of reasons. In many cases, it happens when a person's caloric intake is higher than the amount of calories required to meet his or her energy needs. In such cases, diet, exercise, and life style choices play a role in the person's condition. Genetic factors may also predispose a patient toward obesity. In rare cases, an obese patient may have a low basal metabolic rate, which causes the body to burn calories at a slower rate. In such cases, the condition may be produced by an illness, particularly hypothyroidism.

Accommodations for Obese Patients

Regardless of the cause of your patient's obesity, your primary responsibility is to provide thorough and professional medical care. Conduct an extensive medical history, keeping in mind the chronic medical conditions commonly associated with obesity.

Obese patients often mistakenly blame signs and symptoms of an untreated illness on their weight. For example, they may quickly dismiss shortness of breath by saying "When you're as heavy as me, you can't expect to walk up a flight of stairs without some extra breathing." Don't accept such an answer. The shortness of breath may be caused by congestive heart failure. Obtain a complete history of the symptoms and the activities the person was doing when they appeared. While the patient usually experiences shortness of breath when climbing stairs, this time the condition may have started while sitting down or may have been more severe than usual.

When doing your patient assessment, you may also have to make accommodations for the person's weight. For example, if the patient's adipose tissue presents an obstruction, you may need to place ECG monitoring electrodes on the arms and thighs instead of on the chest. You may also need to auscultate lung sounds anteriorly on a patient who is too obese to lean forward. In assessing an obese patient, flexibility is the key. Keep in mind that no two patients and no two environments will be just alike.

Positioning an obese patient for transport may prove especially difficult, as many EMS transportation devices are not designed or rated for high weights. Always be sure you have enough lifting assistance for the circumstances. Never compromise your health or safety during the transport process. Another EMS crew or the fire department may be necessary to move your patient safely. Finally, remember to let the emergency department know that extra lifting assistance and special stretchers will be needed upon your arrival.

PARALYSIS

Always expect the unexpected in EMS. During your career, you may respond to a call and find that your patient is paralyzed from a previous traumatic or medical event. You will have to treat the chief complaint while taking into account the accommodations that must be made when treating a patient who cannot move some or all of his or her extremities.

If the adipose tissue on an obese patient presents an obstruction, you may need to place ECG monitoring electrodes on the arms and thighs instead of on the chest.

When transporting an extremely obese patient, summon adequate assistance. Try not to draw excess attention to the patient in order to protect the person from further embarrassment.

Be prepared to be extremely innovative when determining how to transport a morbidly obese patient who will not fit the ambulance stretcher.

A paralyzed patient may be paraplegic or quadriplegic. A paraplegic patient has been paralyzed from the waist down, while a quadriplegic patient has paralysis of all four extremities. In addition, spinal cord injuries in the area of C3 to C5 and above may also paralyze the patient's respiratory muscles and compromise the ability to breathe.

If your patient depends on a home ventilator, it is important to maintain a patent airway and to keep the ventilator functioning. Also, a paralyzed patient may have been breathing through a tracheostomy for some time. Therefore, you should keep suction nearby in case the person experiences an airway obstruction. You may also need to use a bag-valve-mask to transport the patient to the ambulance if the ventilator does not transport easily. If your ambulance is equipped, use the ventilator with an onboard power supply to save the ventilator's batteries. This is an already anxious time for your patient, so you may need to spend some extra time reassuring the person before making any changes in the life-support system.

If the patient has suffered a recent spinal cord injury, halo traction may still be intact. Be sure to stabilize the traction before transport. The patient can probably tell you how to assist with the halo traction; if not, a call to the patient's physician may be necessary.

While performing your physical assessment, you may come across a **colostomy**. This device is necessary when the patient does not have normal bowel function due to paralysis of the muscles needed for proper elimination. Be sure to take any other assisting devices, such as canes or wheelchairs, so the patient can get around once out of your care. (For more on acute interventions for physically disabled and other chronic care patients, see Chapter 6.)

If a patient still has halo traction intact, be sure to stabilize the traction before transport.

---

* colostomy a surgical diversion of the large intestine through an opening in the skin where the fecal matter is collected in a pouch; may be temporary or permanent.

MENTAL CHALLENGES AND EMOTIONAL IMPAIRMENTS

Mental and emotional illnesses present a special challenge to the EMS provider. They may range from the psychoses caused by complex biochemical brain diseases, such as bipolar disorder (manic depression), to the personality disorders related to personality development, to a traumatic experience. Emotional impairments can include such conditions as hysteria, compulsive behavior, or anxiety. For a detailed discussion on the etiologies, assessment, management and treatment of these patients, see Chapter 12 in Volume 3 of *Paramedic Care: Principles and Practice*.

DEVELOPMENTAL DISABILITIES

People with developmental disabilities are those individuals with impaired or insufficient development of the brain who are unable to learn at the usual rate. In recent years, a large number of people with developmental disabilities have been mainstreamed into the day-to-day activities of life. They hold jobs and live in residential settings, either on their own, with their families, or in group homes.

Developmental disabilities can result from a variety of reasons. They can be genetic, such as in Down syndrome, or they can be the product of brain injury caused by some hypoxic or traumatic event. Such injuries can take place before birth, during birth, or anytime thereafter.

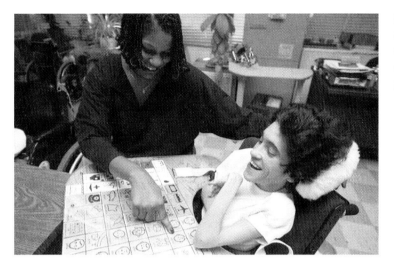

FIGURE 5-3 Developmentally disabled people may have trouble communicating, but can often still understand what you say.

ACCOMMODATIONS FOR DEVELOPMENTAL DISABILITIES

Unless a patient has Down syndrome, it may be difficult to recognize someone with a developmental disability unless the person lives in a group home or other special residential setting. The disability may only become obvious when you start your interview, and even then the person may be able to provide adequate information (Figure 5-3). Remember that a person with a developmental disability can recognize body language, tone, and disrespect just like anyone else. Treat them as you would any other patient, listening to their answers, particularly if you suspect physical or emotional abuse. As mentioned in previous chapters, this group has a higher than average chance of being abused, particularly by someone they know.

If a patient has a severe cognitive disability, you may need to rely on others to obtain the chief complain and history. In this case, plan to spend a little extra time on your physical assessment because the patient may not be able to tell you what is wrong. Also, many children or young people with learning disabilities have been taught to be wary of strangers who may seek to touch them. You will have to establish a basis of trust with the patient, perhaps by making it clear that you are a member of the medical community or by asking for the support of a person the patient does trust. Also, some people with developmental disabilities have been judged "stupid" or "bad" for behavior that results in an accident and they may try to cover up the events that led up to the call.

At all times, keep in mind that a person with a developmental disability may not understand what is happening. The ambulance, special equipment, and even your uniform may confuse or scare them. In cases of severe disabilities, it will be important to keep the primary caregiver with you at all times, even in the back of the ambulance. Talk to disabled patients in terms they will understand and demonstrate what you are doing, as much as possible, on yourself or your partner.

Remember that a person with a developmental disability can recognize body language, tone, and disrespect just like anyone else. Treat them as you would any other patient.

DOWN SYNDROME

Until the mid-1900s, people with Down syndrome lived largely out of public view and tended to die at an early age. Today, however, Down syndrome people attend special schools, hold paid jobs, and, because of improved medical care, can live long lives.

Down syndrome is named after J. Langdon Down, the British physician who studied and identified the condition. It results from an extra chromosome, usually on chromosome 21 or 22. Instead of 46 chromosomes, a person with Down syndrome has 47.

Although the cause is unknown, the chromosomal abnormality increases with the age of the mother, especially after age 40. It also occurs at a higher rate in parents with a chromosomal abnormality, such as the translocation of chromosome 21 to chromosome 14. In such cases, the parent, usually the mother, is phenotypically normal, but has 45 chromosomes. Theoretically the chance is one in three that the mother will have a Down syndrome child.

Typically Down syndrome presents with easily recognized physical features. They include:

- Eyes sloped up at the outer corners
- Folds of skin on either side of the nose that cover the inner corner of the eye
- Small face and features
- Large and protruding tongue
- Flattening on the back of the head
- Short and broad hands

Patients with Down syndrome are often loving and trusting. Be sure to treat them with respect and patience.

In addition to mild to moderate developmental disability, Down syndrome patients may have other physical ailments, such as heart defects, intestinal defects, and chronic lung problems. Down syndrome people are also at risk of developing cataracts, blindness, and Alzheimer's disease at an early age.

When assessing the Down syndrome patient, consider the level of their developmental delay and follow the general guidelines mentioned earlier. Transport to the hospital should be uneventful, especially if the care giver accompanies you.

FETAL ALCOHOL SYNDROME

Fetal Alcohol Syndrome (FAS) is sometimes confused with Down syndrome because of similar facial characteristics. Unlike Down syndrome, FAS is a preventable disorder, caused by excessive alcohol consumption during pregnancy. Children who suffer FAS have characteristic features, including:

- Small head with multiple facial abnormalities
- Small eyes with short slits
- Wide, flat nose bridge
- Lack of a groove between the nose and lip
- Small jaw

FAS patients often exhibit delayed physical growth, mental disabilities, and hyperactivity. Again, follow the preceding general guidelines when treating children with FAS.

PATHOLOGICAL CHALLENGES

As you will learn in Chapter 6, "Acute Interventions for the Chronic-Care Patient," you will encounter a number of challenged patients with chronic conditions. It is important for you to be aware of most common of these conditions, since chronic-care patients require higher-than-average interventions and transport.

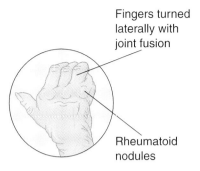

Fingers turned laterally with joint fusion

Rheumatoid nodules

FIGURE 5-4   Rheumatoid arthritis causes joints to become painful and deformed.

ARTHRITIS

The three most common types of arthritis include:

- Juvenile rheumatoid arthritis (JRA)—a connective tissue disorder that strikes before age 16
- Rheumatoid arthritis—an autoimmune disorder
- Osteoarthritis—a degenerative joint disease, the most common arthritis seen in elderly patients

All forms of arthritis cause painful swelling and irritation of the joints, making everyday tasks sometimes impossible. Arthritis patients commonly have joint stiffness and limited range of motion. Sometimes the smaller joints of the hands and feet become deformed (Figure 5-4). In addition, children with JRA may suffer complications involving the spleen or liver.

Treatment for arthritis includes aspirin, non-steroidal antiinflammatory drugs (NSAIDS), and/or corticosteroids. It is important for you to recognize the side effects of these medications because you may have been called upon to treat a medication side effect rather than the disease. NSAIDS can cause stomach upset and vomiting, with or without bloody emesis. Corticosteroids, such as prednisone, can cause hyperglycemia, bloody emesis, and decreased immunity. You should also take note of all the patient's medications so that you do not administer a medication that can interact with the ones already taken by the patient.

When transporting arthritis patients, keep in mind their high level of discomfort. Use pillows to elevate affected extremities. The most comfortable patient position might not be the best position to start an IV, but try to make the patient as comfortable as possible. Special padding techniques may be required due to the patient's arthritis.

Most cases of arthritis encountered in emergency medicine are due to osteoarthritis.

When transporting arthritis patients, keep in mind their high level of discomfort.

CANCER

Entire books have been written on the subject of cancer. It is impossible to list all that a health care provider needs to know about cancer in a small part of a single chapter. In fact, "cancer" is really many different diseases, each with its own characteristics. However, there are some basic points that a paramedic should keep in mind when treating the patient with cancer.

Cancer is caused by the abnormal growth of cells in normal tissue. The primary site of origin of the cancer cells determines the type of cancer that the patient has. If the cancer starts in epithelial tissue, it is called a carcinoma. If the cancer forms in connective tissue, it is called a sarcoma. It may be difficult for you to recognize a cancer patient because the disease often has few obvious signs and symptoms. Rather, the treatments for the disease take on telltale signs, such as anorexia leading to weight loss or alopecia (hair loss). Tattoos may be left on the skin by

FIGURE 5-5 Take every effort to protect cancer patients from infection. Keep a mask on yourself and the patient during transport and during transfer at the hospital.

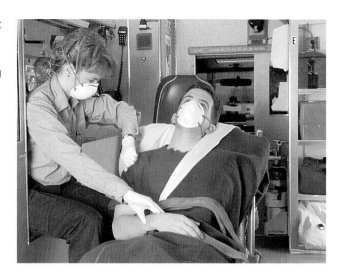

* **neutropenic** a condition that results from an abnormally low neutrophil count in the blood (less than 2000/mm^3).

If a person has recently undergone chemotherapy, assume that the patient is neutropenic. For this reason, keep a mask on the patient during transport and during transfer at the emergency department.

radiation oncologists to mark positioning of radiation therapy equipment. In addition, physical changes, such as loss of a breast (mastectomy), may be obvious.

Management of the cancer patient can present a special challenge to the paramedic. Many patients undergoing chemotherapy treatments become **neutropenic.** This is a condition in which chemotherapy creates a dangerously low level of neutrophils—the white blood cells responsible for the destruction of bacteria and other infectious organisms. Frequently during chemotherapy, the neutrophils are destroyed along with the cancer cells, severely increasing the patient's risk for infection.

If patients have recently undergone chemotherapy, assume that they are neutropenic. Decrease their exposure to infection as much as possible. Remember that once infected, a neutropenic patient can quickly go into septic shock, sometimes in a matter of hours. For this reason, keep a mask on a patient both during transport and during transfer at the emergency department (Figure 5-5).

In treating cancer patients, also keep in mind that their veins may have become scarred and difficult to access due to frequent IV starts, blood draws, and caustic chemotherapy transfusions. Cancer patients may also have an implanted infusion port, found just below the skin, with the catheter inserted into the subclavian vein or brachial artery. This port is accessed for infusion of chemotherapy drugs or IV fluids using sterile technique.

You need special training to use these ports and should not attempt to access them unless you have such training. Local protocols usually dictate whether an EMS provider may access one of these devices. The patient may request that you do not start a peripheral IV if their port can be accessed at the hospital. In such cases, you need to consider if your IV is a life-saving necessity that cannot wait or if the patient can indeed wait for access at the emergency department.

Cancer patients may also have a peripheral access device such as a Groshong catheter or Hickman catheter, which have access ports that extend outside the skin. In this situation, it may simply be a matter of flushing the line and then hooking up your IV fluids to this external catheter. Whatever you decide to do, involve the patient in the decision-making process whenever possible. Cancer patients lose much control over their lives during treatment, so it is important for them to maintain as much control over their EMS care as possible.

CEREBRAL PALSY

Cerebral palsy is a group of a disorders caused by damage to the cerebrum *in utero* or by trauma during birth. Prenatal exposure of the mother to German measles can cause cerebral palsy, along with any event that leads to hypoxia in the fetus. Premature birth or brain damage from a difficult delivery can also lead to cerebral palsy. Other causes include encephalitis, meningitis, or head injury from a fall or the abuse of an infant.

Patients with cerebral palsy have difficulty controlling motor functions, causing spasticity of the muscles. This condition may affect a single limb or the entire body. About two thirds of cerebral palsy patients have a below normal intellectual capacity and about half experience seizures. Conversely, a full third of CP patients have normal intelligence and a few are highly gifted.

There are three main types of cerebral palsy—spastic paralysis, athetosis, and ataxia. Spastic paralysis, which is the most common form of cerebral palsy, forces the muscles into a state of permanent stiffness and contracture. When both legs are affected, the knees turn inward, causing the characteristic "scissor gait." Athetosis causes an involuntary writhing movement, usually affecting arms, feet, hands, and legs. If the patient's face is affected, the person may demonstrate drooling or grimacing. Ataxic cerebral palsy is the rarest form of the disease and causes problems with coordination of gait and balance.

In treating patients with cerebral palsy, keep this fact in mind: Many people with atheotoid and diplegic cerebral palsy are highly intelligent. Do not automatically assume that a person with cerebral palsy cannot communicate with you. Also, as you might expect, many cerebral palsy patients rely on special devices to help them with their mobility. Diplegic patients, for example, may be dependent on wheelchairs.

When transporting cerebral palsy patients, make accommodations to prevent further injury. If they experience severe contractions, the patients may not rest comfortably on a stretcher. Use pillows and extra blankets to pad extremities that are not in proper alignment. Have suction available if a patient drools. If a patient has difficulty communicating, make sure that the care giver helps in your assessment. Be alert for cerebral palsy patients who sign. If you do not know sign language, find someone who does and alert the emergency department.

CYSTIC FIBROSIS (MUCOVISCIDOSIS)

Cystic fibrosis (CF) is an inherited disorder that involves the exocrine (mucus producing) glands, primarily in the lungs and the digestive system. Thick mucus forms in the lungs, causing bronchial obstruction and atelectasis, or collapse of the alveoli. In addition, the thick mucus causes blockages in the small ducts of the pancreas, leading to a decrease in the pancreatic enzymes needed for digestion. This results in malnutrition, even for patients on healthy diets.

Obtaining a complete medical history is important to the recognition of a CF patient. A unique characteristic of CF is the high concentration of chloride in the sweat, leading to the use of a diagnostic test known as the "sweat test." A CF patient may also complain of frequent lung infections, clay-colored stools, or clubbing of the fingers or toes.

Recent medical advances have extended the lives of CF patients so that some live well into their thirties. However, because of a poor prognosis, most of the CF patients that you see will be children and adolescents. In treating these patients, remember that they have been chronically ill for their entire life. The last thing they may want is another trip to the hospital. For this reason, transport can be difficult for both the patient and family members. To allay their fears, keep in mind the developmental stage of your patient. A child with cystic fibrosis is still a child. So recall everything you have learned about the treatment of pediatric patients.

Because of the high probability of respiratory distress in a CF patient, some form of oxygen therapy may be necessary. You may need to have a family member or care giver hold blow by oxygen, rather than use a mask, if that is all the patient will

Many people with atheotoid and diplegic cerebral palsy are highly intelligent. Do not automatically assume that they cannot communicate with you.

✱ **muscoviscidosis** cystic fibrosis of the pancreas resulting in abnormally viscous mucoid secretion from the pancreas.

In treating patients with cystic fibrosis, remember that they have been chronically ill for their entire lives. The last thing they may want is another trip to the hospital.

tolerate. Suctioning may be necessary to help the patient clear the thick secretions from the airway. CF patients may be taking antibiotics to prevent infection and using inhalers or Mucomyst to thin their secretions. Make sure that you take along all medications so that the hospital staff can continue with the patient's regimen.

MULTIPLE SCLEROSIS

Multiple sclerosis (MS) is a disorder of the central nervous system that usually strikes between the ages of 20 and 40, affecting women more than men. The exact cause of MS is unknown, but it is considered to be an autoimmune disorder. Characteristically, repeated inflammation of the myelin sheath surrounding the nerves leads to scar tissue, which in turn blocks nerve impulses to the affected area.

The onset of MS is slow. It starts with a slight change in the strength of a muscle and a numbness or tingling in the affected muscle. For example, a patient may start to drop things, blaming it on clumsiness. Doctors encourage MS patients to lead as normal a life as possible, but they become increasingly tired. Their gait may become unsteady, and their speech may slur. MS patients may also develop eye problems, such as double vision due to weakness of the eye muscles or eye pain due to neuritis of the optic nerve.

The initial signs of MS are usually temporary. However, they return and become more frequent and long lasting. As the symptoms progress, they become more permanent, leading to a weak extremity or paralysis. Over time, some patients may become bedridden and lose control of bladder function. Eventually an MS patient may develop a lung or urinary infection, which may lead to death. As with other chronically ill patients, people with MS may experience mood swings and seek medical attention for their feelings.

Transport of an MS patient to the hospital may require supportive care, such as oxygen therapy. Make sure the patient is comfortable and help position the person as necessary. Do not expect patients with MS to walk to the ambulance. Even if normally ambulatory, they may be in a more weakened state than usual. Again, be sure to bring assistive devices, such as a wheelchair or cane so that the patient can maintain as much independence as possible (Figure 5-6).

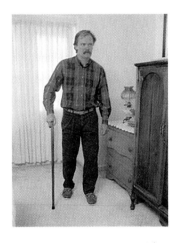

FIGURE 5-6 Patients with multiple sclerosis and muscular dystrophy may use a cane to aid in ambulation. Be sure to take such devices with you on the ambulance.

MUSCULAR DYSTROPHY

Muscular dystrophy (MD) is a group of hereditary disorders characterized by progressive weakness and wasting of muscle tissue. It is a genetic disorder, leading to gradual degeneration of muscle fibers. The most common form of MD is Duchenne muscular dystrophy, which typically affects boys between the ages of 3 and 6. It leads to progressive muscle weakness in the legs and pelvis and to paralysis by age 12. Ultimately, the disease affects the respiratory muscles and heart, causing death at an early age. The other various MD disorders are classified by the age of the patient at onset of symptoms and by the muscles affected.

Since MD is a hereditary disease, you should obtain a complete family history. You should also note the particular muscle groups that the patient cannot move. Again, since MD patients are primarily children; choose age-appropriate language. Respiratory support, such as oxygen, may be needed, especially in the later stages of the disease.

POLIOMYELITIS

Poliomyelitis is a communicable disease that affects the gray matter of the brain and the spinal cord. Although it is highly contagious, immunization has made outbreaks of polio extremely rare in developed nations. However, it is important to know about the disease since many people born before development of the polio vaccination in the 1950s were affected by the disease.

Typically, the polio virus enters the body through the gastrointestinal tract. It circulates through the digestive tract and then enters the blood stream. There, it is carried to the central nervous system where the virus enters the nerve cells and alters them. In cases of paralytic poliomyelitis, patients experience asymmetrical muscle weakness that leads to permanent paralysis.

Although most patients recover from the disease itself, they are left with permanent paralysis of the affected muscles. You may recognize a polio victim by the use of assistive devices for ambulation or by the reduced size of the affected limb due to muscle atrophy. Some patients may have experienced paralysis of the respiratory muscles, requiring assisted ventilation. Patients on long-term ventilators will typically have tracheotomies.

Along with polio, you should know about a related disorder called post-polio syndrome. Post-polio syndrome affects those patients who suffered severely from polio more than 30 years ago. Although the cause of post-polio syndrome remains unknown, researchers think the condition results from the stress of long-term weakness in the affected nerves. Patients with this condition quickly tire, especially after exercise, and develop an intolerance for cold in their extremities.

Many patients with polio or post-polio syndrome try to maintain their independence. They may insist on walking to the ambulance, but should not be encouraged to do so. The idea of hospitalization will frustrate them, since many polio survivors have memories of spending months or even years in hospitals as children. Unlike other chronically ill patients, most do not require frequent trips to the hospital. Therefore, this may be their first time in the back of an ambulance. Try to alleviate their anxiety as much as possible.

PREVIOUS HEAD INJURIES

A patient with a previous head injury may not be easily recognized. You may not notice anything different about the patient until the person starts to speak. A patient with a head injury may display similar symptoms to that of a stroke, without the hemiparesis, or paralysis to one side of the body. The presenting symptoms will be related to the area of the brain that has been injured. The patient may have aphasia, slurred speech, loss of vision or hearing, or may develop a learning disability. Such patients may also exhibit short-term memory loss and may not even have any recollection of their original injury.

Obtaining a medical history from these patients is very important, especially if you are responding to a traumatic event. Note any new symptoms the patient may be having or the recurrence of old ones. Conduct the physical assessment slowly. If the patient cannot speak, look for obvious physical signs of trauma or for facial expressions of pain. Transport considerations will depend upon the condition for which you were called. However, information about the previous head injury should be an important part of the patient's transfer.

SPINA BIFIDA

Spina bifida is a congenital abnormality that falls under the category of neural tube defects. It presents when there is a defect in the closure of the backbone and the spinal canal. In spina bifida occulta, the patient exhibits few outward signs of the deformity. In spina bifida cystica, the failure of the closure allows the spinal cord and covering membranes to protrude from the back, causing an obvious deformity.

Symptoms depend upon which part of the spinal cord is protruding through the back. The patient may have paralysis of both lower extremities and lack of bowel or bladder control. A large percentage of children born with spina bifida have hydrocephalus, which results from the accumulation of fluid in the brain. Permanent disabilities cannot be assessed until the defect is surgically corrected.

If the patient has hydrocephalus, a shunt will need to be inserted to help drain off the excess fluid.

When treating spina bifida patients, keep several things in mind. Recent research has shown that between 18 to 73 percent of children and adolescents with spina bifida have latex allergies. For safety, assume that all patients with spina bifida have this problem. In transporting a spina bifida patient, be sure to take along any devices that aid the patient. If you are called to treat an infant, safe transport to the hospital should be done in a car seat, unless contraindicated.

For safety, assume that all patients with spina bifida have a latex allergy.

MYASTHENIA GRAVIS

Myasthenia gravis is an autoimmune disease characterized by chronic weakness of voluntary muscles and progressive fatigue. The condition results from a problem with the neurotransmitters, which causes a blocking of nerve signals to the muscles. It occurs most frequently in women between the ages of 20 and 50.

A patient with myasthenia gravis may complain of a complete lack of energy, especially in the evening. The disease commonly involves muscles in the face. You may note eyelid drooping or difficulty in chewing or swallowing. The patient may also complain of double vision.

In severe cases of myasthenia gravis, a patient may experience paralysis of the respiratory muscles, leading to respiratory arrest. These patients may need assisted ventilations en route to the emergency facility. For less severe patients, accommodations will vary based upon presentation.

As a health care provider, you are ethically required to take care of all patients in the same manner, regardless of their race, religion, gender, ethnic background, and living situation.

OTHER CHALLENGES

In addition to the challenges described in the preceding sections, you can expect to meet a whole range of special situations that will affect the quality of the patient service that you provide. The following are some of the special situations or conditions that you will encounter, if you have not already done so.

CULTURALLY DIVERSE PATIENTS

Many ethnic groups believe in and practice varying forms of folk medicine. You should respect these beliefs and remember that some folk remedies may interact with traditional medical therapies. If you work in an area populated by a specific ethnic group, learn more about the group's folk medicine beliefs and practices.

As a health care provider, you are ethically required to take care of all patients in the same manner, regardless of their race, religion, gender, ethnic background, or living situation. What may make it difficult for you to treat culturally different patients may not be the differences per se, but your inability to understand them. Do not consider this a reason for refusing treatment. Rather, consider it a learning experience that will prepare you for a similar situation on another run. With United States society becoming more diverse, instead of less diverse, tolerance of cultural differences will become an important part of your career (Figure 5-7).

FIGURE 5-7 United States society is becoming diverse, with the largest number of immigrants coming from Asia and Latin America.

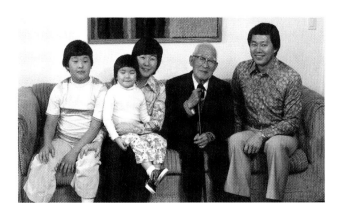

```
┌─────────────────────────────────────────────────────────────────────┐
│              REFUSAL OF TREATMENT AND TRANSPORTATION                   │
│                                                                       │
│  I, THE UNDERSIGNED HAVE BEEN ADVISED THAT MEDICAL ASSISTANCE ON MY   │
│  BEHALF IS NECESSARY AND THAT REFUSAL OF SAID ASSISTANCE AND          │
│  TRANSPORTATION MAY RESULT IN DEATH, OR IMPERIL MY HEALTH.            │
│  NEVERTHELESS, I REFUSE TO ACCEPT TREATMENT OR TRANSPORT AND ASSUME   │
│  ALL RISKS AND CONSEQUENCES OF MY DECISION AND RELEASE GOLD CROSS     │
│  AMBULANCE COMPANY AND ITS EMPLOYEES FROM ANY LIABILITY ARISING FROM  │
│  MY REFUSAL.                                                          │
│                                                                       │
│                                        _____  │
│                                             SIGNATURE OF PATIENT       │
│  _____                                        │
│         WITNESSED BY                                                   │
│                                        _____  │
│                                              DATE SIGNED               │
└─────────────────────────────────────────────────────────────────────┘
```

FIGURE 5-8   If a patient refuses care because of cultural or religious beliefs, be sure to have the person sign a Refusal of Treatment and Transportation form.

From time to time, you may encounter a patient who will make a decision about medical care with which you do not agree. For example, Christian Scientists do not believe in human intervention in sickness through the use of drugs or other therapies. You cannot force these patients to accept an IV or take nitroglycerin if they are having chest pain. Remember, the patient who has decision-making abilities has a right to self-determination. You should, however, obtain a signed document indicating informed refusal of consent (Figure 5-8).

Accommodation of a culturally diverse population will require patience and, in some cases, ingenuity. If your patient does not speak English, communication may be a problem. You may need to rely on a family member to act as an interpreter or on a translator device, such as telephone language line for non-English speaking people. In such cases, be sure to notify the receiving facility of the need for an interpreter.

TERMINALLY ILL PATIENTS

Caring for a terminally ill patient can be an emotional challenge. Many times, the patient will choose to die at home, but at the last minute the family compromises those wishes by calling for an ambulance. In other cases, the patient may call for an ambulance so that a newly developed condition can be treated or a medication adjusted. For more on caring for the terminally ill, either at home or in a hospice situation, see Chapter 6.

PATIENTS WITH COMMUNICABLE DISEASES

When treating people with communicable diseases, you should withhold all personal judgment. Although you will have to take BSI precautions just as you would with any patient, keep in mind the heightened sensitivity of a person with a communicable disease. Most of these patients are familiar with the health care setting and understand why you must take certain protective measures. However, you should still explain that you take these measures with other patients that

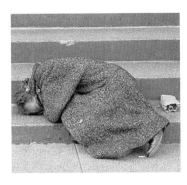

FIGURE 5-9 Homeless people sometimes refuse care, thinking they cannot afford to pay the medical bills. Become familiar with public hospitals and clinics that provide services to the needy.

Treat the patient, not the financial condition the patient is in.

have a similar disease. Also, you do not need to take additional precautions that are not required by departmental policy. The patient will generally spot these extra measures, feeling guilt, shame, or anger.

For more information on the etiologies and treatment of communicable diseases, see Chapter 11 in Volume 3 of *Paramedic Care: Principles & Practice.*

PATIENTS WITH FINANCIAL CHALLENGES

One of the exciting parts of a career in EMS is the opportunity to meet people of all backgrounds. You have the chance to get out into the street and see how people live, work, and play. This allows you to help and educate people who may not otherwise have access to health care. For example, you may get sent to a street corner where a homeless man has fallen and needs medical attention, but cannot afford to pay the medical bills. It is your job to help the patient understand that he can receive health care regardless of his financial situation (Figure 5-9).

Become familiar with public hospitals and clinics that provide services to people without money or adequate insurance coverage. Calm a patient's fears by discussing this or other information. In providing care, always keep this guideline in mind: Treat the patient, not the financial condition the patient is in.

SUMMARY

It is important to be aware of the pathophysiology of diseases that you may encounter throughout your career. You should also know the characteristics of impairments that are commonly found in the medical setting. They may be the primary reason that your patient seeks help, or they may not be the reason your patient called at all. Whatever the circumstances, it is important to learn the various etiologies of these impairments and illnesses in order to treat your patient with the knowledge and respect that each of your patients deserves every day.

YOU MAKE THE CALL

You and your partner are called out to the home of a 56-year-old female with a chief complaint of fever. You arrive on the scene to find the door unlocked and a woman calling to you to come to a back bedroom.

She stops you at the door of her bedroom and asks both you and your partner to put on a mask. She tells you that she is undergoing treatment for breast cancer and that the doctor told her that she shouldn't be around people who are sick because she has an increased risk of infection. She has a scarf around her head and you notice a wig on her bedside table.

She tells you that she has a fever of 102°F and her heart is beating very fast, and this is scaring her. She has had a decrease in appetite and some vomiting. The doctor told her that she should go to the hospital, but she lives alone and didn't have a ride so she called EMS.

Your partner has a cold, so he agrees to drive to the hospital. In the back of the ambulance you apply the monitor to your patient when she tells you she has had a recent mastectomy. The short transport to the hospital is uneventful. You arrive at the hospital and transfer patient care to the ER nurse.

1. Why did the patient's doctor tell her that she has an increased risk of infection from communicable diseases?
2. What signs indicate that this patient has cancer?
3. Is it necessary for all three of you to wear a mask? Explain.
4. Will you start a peripheral IV on this patient? Explain.
5. What information will you include in your patient report so the emergency department is prepared for this patient?

See Suggested Responses at the back of this book.

FURTHER READING

Barry, P.: *Mental Health & Mental Illness*. Philadelphia, PA: Lippincott, 1998.

Early Identification of Hearing Impairment in Infants and Young Children, Program and Abstracts. National Institutes of Health, 1993.

Phipps, W., et al.: *Medical-Surgical Nursing: Concepts and Clinical Practice*, 6th edition. St. Louis, MO: Mosby-Year Book, 1999.

ON THE WEB

Visit Brady's Paramedic Website at www.bradybooks.com/paramedic.

CHAPTER 6

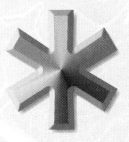

Acute Interventions for the Chronic-Care Patient

Objectives

After reading this chapter, you should be able to:

1. Compare and contrast the primary objectives of the paramedic and the home care provider. (pp. 249, 255–256)

2. Identify the importance of home health care medicine as it relates to emergency medical services. (pp. 247–250)

3. Differentiate between the role of the paramedic and the role of the home care provider. (pp. 249–250, 255–256)

4. Compare and contrast the primary objectives of acute care, home care, and hospice care. (pp. 248, 255–256, 283)

5. Discuss aspects of home care that enhance the quality of patient care and aspects that have the potential

to become detrimental. (pp. 247–248, 250–254)

6. List pathologies and complications in home care patients that commonly result in ALS intervention. (pp. 249–254, 263–283)

7. Compare the cost, mortality, and quality of care for a given patient in the hospital versus the home care setting. (pp. 247–248)

8. Discuss the significance of palliative care programs as related to a patient in a home health care or hospice setting. (pp. 255, 283–285)

9. Define hospice care, comfort care, and DNR/DNAR as they relate to local

Continued

practice, law, and policy. (pp. 262, 283–285)

10. List and describe the characteristics of typical home care devices related to airway maintenance, artificial and alveolar ventilation, vascular access, drug administration, and the GI/GU tract. (pp. 253–255, 263, 267–280)

11. Discuss the complications of assessing each of the devices described above. (pp. 270–271, 273–274, 275–276, 277–278, 279–280)

12. Describe indications, contraindications, and techniques for urinary catheter insertion in the male and female patient in an out-of-hospital setting. (pp. 276–277)

13. Identify failure of GI/GU, ventilatory, vascular access, and drain devices found in the home care setting. (pp. 275–276, 277–278, 279–280, 280–281)

14. Discuss the relationship between local home care treatment protocols/SOPs and local EMS Protocols/SOPs. (pp. 255–256)

15. Discuss differences in the ability of individuals to accept and cope with their own impending death. (p. 285)

16. List the stages of the grief process and relate them to an individual in hospice care. (p. 285)

17. Discuss the rights of the terminally ill patient. (pp. 283–285)

18. Summarize the types of home health care available in your area and the services provided. (pp. 248, 255)

19. Given a series of home care scenarios, determine which patients should receive follow-up home care and which should be transported to an emergency care facility. (pp. 249–285)

20. Given a series of scenarios, demonstrate interaction and support with the family members/support persons for a patient who has died. (pp. 283–285)

CASE STUDY

Pridemark 2 has just ordered a take-out dinner when dispatch reports an "elderly male, short of breath." With a shrug, the crew members cancel dinner and head to the address provided by the dispatcher. Upon arrival, they find the door slightly ajar and can see the patient sitting on the couch. As they pass through the vestibule, they notice several bottles of oxygen on the floor. They observe that their patient is on a nasal cannula. He is having obvious moderate dyspnea and is using some accessory muscles.

The patient speaks in four- to five-word sentences. He tells the crew that his name is Clarence Casey. Mr. Casey indicates that he is 74 years old. He complains that it has become increasingly difficult for him to breathe. He has used his puffers multiple times without relief. Although Mr. Casey says he has no chest pain, he feels like his breathing has become "heavier."

While the EMT puts together a nebulizer, the paramedic auscultates lung sounds. She notes diminished breathing in all fields with inspiratory and expiratory wheezes. She also observes a prolonged expiratory phase with pursing of lips. The patient is not tripoding and has a respiratory rate of 30 breaths per minute. Use of a pulse oximeter indicates a reading of 86% on 4 liters oxygen. The patient's skin is warm, dry, and pale.

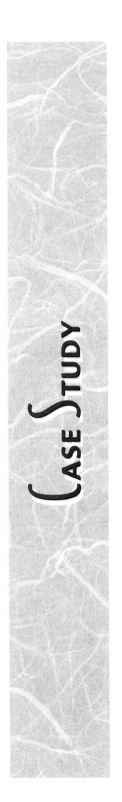

Upon questioning, Mr. Casey tells the crew that he has a history of emphysema, bronchitis, hypertension, glaucoma, and smoked a pack of cigarettes each day for sixty years. His medications include a Proventil inhaler, a Serevent inhaler, eye drops, and Cardura. He has no allergies. He usually uses oxygen only when walking around the house or doing light chores, such as washing dishes. He lives alone and has home care one day a week. Due to his end-stage COPD, Mr. Casey has authorized a valid prehospital Do Not Resuscitate (DNR) order with his physician, which he shows to the EMS crew.

The paramedic administers nebulized albuterol (2.5mg/2mL) at 8 liters per minute. She also leaves the patient's nasal cannula at 4 liters per minute. She encourages the patient to take deep breaths. Vital signs indicate a blood pressure of 162/94 and a pulse rate of 110 sinus tachycardia.

Upon moving Mr. Casey to the cot, his dyspnea increases and he becomes more anxious. Reassessment in the ambulance shows his respiratory rate has increased to 36 and there has been no subjective change in his wheezing. The patient now only speaks in one- to two-word sentences even though his oxygen saturation has increased to 90%. Mr. Casey appears to be growing tired from the work of breathing. The EMT establishes an IV and draws blood, while the paramedic contemplates intubating the patient. The prehospital DNR precludes intubation, so the paramedic is forced to continue pharmacological interventions only.

En route to the hospital, the paramedic administers a second albuterol treatment and continues to encourage Mr. Casey to take deep breaths. Through gentle reassurances, she succeeds in calming him down. Over the next five minutes, the patient's respiratory rate drops to 30, his wheezes become louder, and tidal volume increases. The patient appears less anxious and the SaO_2 rises slowly to 93%.

Upon arrival at the hospital, the crew administers a third albuterol treatment. The respiratory rate is now 28 breaths per minute, and the patient can again speak in four- to five-word sentences. In the emergency department, the admitting physician gives the patient 125 mg of Solu-Medrol and one more treatment of albuterol. The patient also receives blood tests, chest X-rays, arterial blood gas, and a 12-lead ECG. He is released five hours later with a diagnosis of exacerbation of COPD—the acute condition that Mr. Casey treats in a home-care setting.

The crew, meanwhile, carefully documents the run and drops off their chart. Luckily, they get a chance to eat dinner before the next call arrives.

INTRODUCTION

One of the major trends in modern health care involves the shifting of patients out of the hospital and back into their homes as soon as possible. The result has been a huge increase in home health care needs and services. In 1963, approximately 1,100 health care agencies existed in the United States. Today, more than 20,000 agencies employ over 665,000 caregivers—nurses, home health aides, physical therapists, occupational therapists, and other health care professionals. Experts predict the trend toward home health care to increase in the future. As a result, more and more patients will receive treatment, even of terminal illnesses, in an out-of-hospital setting.

EPIDEMIOLOGY OF HOME CARE

A number of factors have promoted the growth of home care in recent years. They include:

- Enactment of Medicare in 1965 (Table 6-1)
- The advent of health maintenance organizations (HMOs)
- Improved medical technology
- Studies showing improved recovery rates and lower costs with home care.

Supporters of home health care offer several arguments in its favor. First, they point out that patients often recover faster in the familiar environment of their homes than in the hospital. They also emphasize differences in the cost of home care vs. hospital care (Table 6-2). With total health expenditures expected to rise by an estimated 7.5 percent in the first decade of the 2000s, the savings promised by home health care continues to speed the dismissal of patients from hospitals and nursing homes.

The primary driving force in home health care is cost-containment.

The shift to home care has important implications for ALS providers. As patients assume greater responsibility for their own treatment and recovery, the likelihood of ALS intervention for the chronic-care patient increases. Calls may come from the patient, the patient's family, or a home health care provider.

Table 6-1	MEDICARE FUNDING OF HOME CARE FOR SELECTED YEARS, 1967–1997		
Year	Fee-for-ServiceOutlays (in millions)	Clients (in thousands)	Number of Visits (in thousands)
1967	$ 46	N.A.	N.A.
1980	$ 662	957	22,428
1985	$ 1,773	1,589	39,742
1990*	$ 3,860	1,940	69,532
1991	$ 5,566	2,223	99,183
1992	$ 7,724	2,523	132,494
1993	$10,198	2,868	168,029
1994	$13,269	3,175	220,495
1995	$15,976	3,457	266,261
1996	$17,266	3,583	283,936
1997**	$17,241	3,370	269,919

*Most of the growth from 1990-1996 resulted from court decisions and legislative actions that expanded Medicare benefits.

**Reductions in 1997 reflect new per-beneficiary limits designed to curb Medicare expenditures. As of 1999, Medicare and Medicaid still provided funds for nearly two-thirds of all home care, with the remainder paid for by out-of-pocket payments and private insurance.

Source: HCFA, Office of the Actuary and Bureau of Data Management and Strategy; reported on the National Association for Home Care web site, August 1999.

Table 6-2	SELECT MEDICAL CHARGES, 1995–1997		
Charge	1995	1996	1997
Hospital charges per day	$1,909	$2,071	$2,121
Skilled nursing facility charges per day	401	443	454
Home health care charges per visit	84	86	88

Source: Based on figures provided on the National Administration for Home Care web site, August 1999.

As a paramedic, you should become familiar with the basic functions of many of the common home care devices and, just as important, recognize the underlying need for them.

In home care settings, you can expect to encounter a sometimes dizzying array of devices, machines, and equipment designed to provide anything from supportive to life-sustaining care. As a paramedic, you should become familiar with the basic functions of the common home care devices and, just as important, recognize the underlying need for them. The failure or malfunction of this type of equipment has the potential to become a life-threatening or life-altering event. New technologies and machines are being developed constantly. It is your responsibility to stay informed of these changes and the assessment complications that may be involved with the use of each device.

PATIENTS RECEIVING HOME CARE

In 1992, the National Center for Health Statistics conducted its first annual National Home and Hospice Care Survey (NHHCS). The survey grew out of the proliferation of home care agencies throughout the United States. The results gave health care professionals their first in-depth look at the home health care population. Key findings from the survey included the following two points:

- Almost 75 percent of home care patients were age 65 or older.
- Of the elderly home care patients, almost two-thirds were female.

Today some eight million patients—both acute and chronic—receive formal health care treatment from paid providers. Millions of others receive unpaid assistance from family members or other volunteers. On average, these informal caregivers give up to four hours assistance per day, seven days a week.

Patients require home care for a variety of reasons (Table 6-3). Some simply don't need to recover from an injury or illness in a hospital or a rehabilitation facility. Their home care is transitory and their condition usually improves. Other patients have chronic conditions that require varying degrees of home assistance in order to live relatively normal lives. These patients usually adjust to their illness or disability, but never completely recover. Yet other patients have terminal illnesses that may or may not involve complicated supportive measures. Their condition is expected to worsen, and the patient may in fact be waiting to die.

All these situations require sensitivity to the special needs of the patient and consideration of the people involved in the patient's care. Strong emotions may emerge during the call. A previously manageable condition may have suddenly become unmanageable or more complicated. Unlike in a hospital, the patient or home care provider cannot push a button and summon immediate help. Instead, they often summon you, the ALS provider.

	Table 6-3	SELECT DIAGNOSES OF DISCHARGED HOME CARE PATIENTS, 1995–1996

Diagnosis Upon Hospital Admission	Number of Home Care Patients
Diseases of the circulatory system	1,776,900
Heart Disease	999,100
Injuries and poisonings	974,400
Neoplasms	948,200
Malignant neoplasms*	923,200
Diseases of the respiratory system	639,200
Diseases of the musculoskeletal system and connective tissue	629,200
Endocrine, nutritional, metabolic, and immunity disorders	456,200
Diabetes mellitus	333,400
Diseases of the digestive system	314,100
Diseases of the nervous system and sensory organs	271,700
Essential hypertension	260,700
Diseases of the skin and subcutaneous tissue	190,100
Diseases of the genitourinary system	181,300
Infectious and parasitic diseases	166,400
Mental disorders	138,800
Diseases of the blood and blood-clotting organs	130,500

*Does not include malignant neoplasms of the trachea, bronchus, lung, breast, and prostate, which accounted for the primary diagnoses of an estimated 237,200 discharged home care patients.

Source: National Center of Health Statistics; adapted from data on the National Association for Home Care web site, August 1999.

ALS RESPONSE TO HOME CARE PATIENTS

A number of situations may involve you in the treatment of a home care patient—equipment failure, unexpected complications, absence of a caregiver, need for transport, inability of the patient or caregiver to operate a device, and more. As already mentioned, you might also be called upon to provide emotional support or intervention. Taking responsibility for an illness or an ill family member can be a stressful and overwhelming experience. Some people may be ill-equipped to deal with complicated directions, mechanical problems, or the stress of long-term care. Do not minimize their frustrations or allow these frustrations to interfere with your care.

Your primary role as an ALS provider is to identify and treat any life-threatening problems. An important source of information is the home care provider—whether it be a nurse, nurse's aid, family member, or friend. Remember that this person usually knows the patient better than anyone else. The provider will often spot subtle changes in the patient's condition that may seem insignificant to the outsider. In assessing the patient, it is crucial that you listen carefully to what this person says (Figure 6-1).

Home care providers are often health care professionals, but be sensitive in questioning their training or background. You must obtain certain information to care for your patient, and the home care provider may be the only source you have for critical items such as the patient's baseline mental status. If you meet resistance,

Content Review

COMMON REASONS FOR ALS INTERVENTION
- Equipment failure
- Unexpected complications
- Absence of a caregiver
- Need for transport
- Inability to operate a device

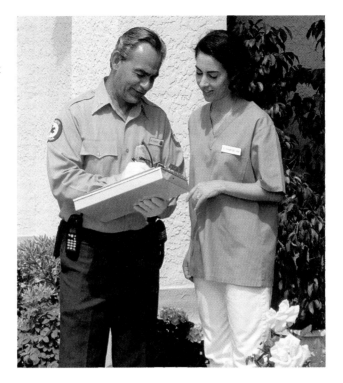

FIGURE 6-1 The home health care provider usually knows the patient better than anyone else and will often spot subtle changes in the patient's condition.

either from the home care provider's lack of training or a misunderstanding of your needs, try rephrasing your question or using less technical language. You may also find evidence of neglect or improper patient care by the home care provider. Correct any immediate life-threats that you find, and document your findings in your patient report. You should also report the situation to your supervisors for corrective action. However, do not confront the home care worker yourself.

At all times, keep in mind the presence of the patient. Involve him or her in the questioning process. If the caregiver mentions a change or reaction, you might say: "Did you notice this change, too?" "How do you think you reacted?" Your role is to perform as complete and accurate an assessment as possible.

Typical Responses

Many of the medical problems that you will encounter in a home care setting are the same as the ones that you will encounter elsewhere in the field. However, you must always keep in mind that the home care patient is in a more fragile state to begin with. A member of the medical community has already decided that the person needs extra help. A home care patient is more likely to decompensate and go into crisis more quickly than the general population. As a result, you need to monitor the home care patient carefully and be ready to intervene at all times. Some of the typical responses involve airway complications, respiratory failure, cardiac decompensation, alterations in peripheral circulation, altered mental status, GI/GU crises, infections and/or septic complications, and equipment malfunction. (For more specific information on examples of home care problems requiring acute intervention, see later sections of the chapter.)

Airway Complications The airway is always your paramount concern, and the home care patient is no exception. In the absence of documentation proving the patient's request to withhold intubation and mechanical ventilation, you should protect the airway at all costs. However, even if the patient has a valid Do Not Re-

A home care patient is more likely to decompensate and go into crisis more quickly than the general population.

suscitate (DNR) order, remember that, in certain situations, you still can use basic airway techniques and suctioning to protect the airway.

Airway compromise can be the result of many different etiologies. Problems that you might encounter include inadequate pulmonary toilet, inadequate alveolar ventilation, and inadequate alveolar oxygenation. (For more on airway problems, see material later in the chapter.)

Respiratory Failure As you will read later in the chapter, any number of respiratory problems can be treated in a home care setting. Some of the most common conditions that will lead to respiratory failure or acute crisis include:

- Emphysema
- Bronchitis
- Asthma
- Cystic fibrosis
- Congestive heart failure
- Pulmonary embolus
- Sleep apnea
- **Guillain-Barré syndrome**
- **Myasthenia gravis**

Cardiac Decompensation Regardless of the setting, cardiac decompensation is a true medical emergency that can lead to life-threatening shock. This condition requires aggressive identification and treatment. Home care patients who have borderline cardiac output may be placed at risk if their cardiac demand increases from stress or illness and their system cannot compensate. Some other common causes of cardiac decompensation include:

- Congestive heart failure
- Acute myocardial infarction (MI) (Home care patients are at higher risk.)
- Cardiac **hypertrophy**
- Calcification or degeneration of the heart's conductive system
- Heart transplant
- Sepsis

Alterations in Peripheral Circulation You already know that the heart circulates blood throughout the body. However, in the case of home care patients, remember that bodily movement also aids in circulation. If a patient has limited mobility, expect the entire circulatory system to be less effective and weaker. As muscle tone declines, so does the flow of blood. When circulation slows, movement becomes more difficult, thus creating a vicious cycle that leads to poorer circulation overall.

Keep in mind that alterations in peripheral circulation can complicate or worsen the course of treatment for a home care patient. Slowed circulation may result in delayed healing, increased risk of infections, or even **gangrene**. Diabetes, a problem that affects some 16 million Americans, commonly results in poor circulation, especially to the extremities. These patients are at high risk of unhealed wounds or ulcers, particularly on the feet.

Altered Mental Status A common ALS response to a home care patient involves some kind of subtle or obvious change in mental status. In the home care patient, always suspect an exacerbation of their condition as well as other causes. Never forget that these patients are at higher risk than the general population of

✳ **Guillain–Barré syndrome** acute viral infection that triggers the production of autoantibodies, which damage the myelin sheath covering the peripheral nerves; causes rapid, progressive loss of motor function, ranging from muscle weakness to full-body paralysis.

✳ **Myasthenia gravis** disease characterized by episodic muscle weakness triggered by an autoimmune attack of the acetylcholine receptors.

Regardless of the setting, cardiac decompensation is a true medical emergency that can lead to life-threatening shock.
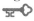

✳ **hypertrophy** an increase in the size or bulk of an organ or structure; caused by growth rather than by a tumor.

If a patient has limited mobility, expect the entire circulatory system to be less effective and weaker.

✳ **gangrene** death of tissue or bone, usually from an insufficient blood supply.

developing new medical problems. Some common causes of altered mental status include:

- Hypoxia (from any number of respiratory or airway problems)
- Hypotension (from any number of cardiac problems or shock)
- Sepsis
- Altered electrolytes or blood chemistries (common in dialysis patients)
- Hypoglycemia (diabetes)
- Alzheimer's disease
- Cancerous tumor or brain lesions
- Overdose
- Stroke (brain attack)

GI/GU Crises EMS personnel find themselves involved in a number of calls involving home care patients with gastrointestinal or genitourinary problems. The problem often revolves around a misplaced or removed catheter, such as a Foley or a percutaneous endoscopic gastrostomy (PEG) tube. This may not seem like an emergency to you, but the inability to eat or urinate for a period of time can easily compromise an already weakened patient. In addition, home interventions such as peritoneal dialysis can alter fluid balances or electrolytes, creating a subtle but life-threatening problem.

You should always maintain a high index of suspicion for infection in a home care patient with a decreased immune response.

Infections and Septic Complications You should always maintain a high index of suspicion for infection in a home care patient with a decreased immune response, either from poor general health or a specific disease. Be particularly alert to infections in patients with indwelling devices such as gastrostomy tubes, peripherally-inserted central catheter (PICC) lines, Foley catheters, or colostomies. Also remember that patients with limited lung function or tracheotomies cannot clear their airway easily, putting them at a higher risk of lung infections.

Patients who have decreased **sensorium** from a variety of conditions may have wounds and ulcers that they are unaware of, especially if they have been bedridden or inactive for long periods of time. Surgically implanted drains or wound closures may become infected without the patient realizing it. A bedbound patient may also develop decubitus wounds, or bedsores (Figure 6-2). If these problems are not identified or treated, they can progress from a generalized infection to gangrene and sepsis.

In identifying infections, look for the following general signs:

- Redness and/or swelling, especially at the insertion site of an indwelling device
- Purulent discharge at the insertion site
- Warm skin at the insertion site
- Fever

Infection at the cellular level is called **cellulitis** and is not life-threatening. When an infection spreads systemically, however, it can lead to sepsis—a serious medical emergency. This may cause a patient's immune system to fail, resulting in septic shock. Signs and symptoms of sepsis include:

- Redness at an insertion site
- Fever
- Altered mental status
- Poor skin color or **turgor**

* **sensorium** sensory apparatus of the body as a whole; also that portion of the brain that functions as a center of sensations.

* **cellulitis** inflammation of cellular or connective tissue.

* **turgor** ability of the skin to return to normal appearance after being subjected to pressure.

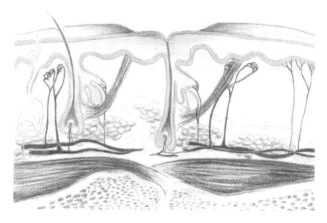

FIG. 6-2A **Stage 1** Inflammation or redness of the skin that does not return to normal after 15 minutes of removal of pressure. Edema is present. It involves the epidermis. Skin may or may not be broken.

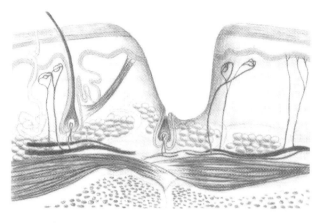

FIG. 6-2b **Stage 2** Skin blister or shallow skin ulcer. Involves the epidermis. Looks like a shallow crater. Area is red, warm, and may or may not have drainage.

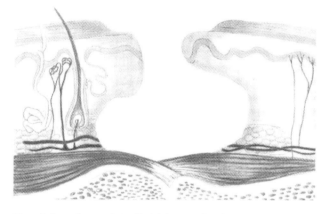

FIG. 6-2c **Stage 3** Full-thickness skin loss exposing subcutaneous tissue, may extend into the next layer. Edema, inflammation, and necrosis present. Drainage present, which may or may not have an odor.

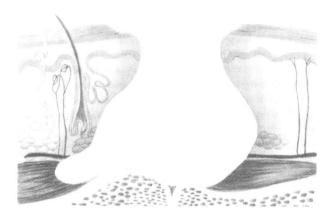

FIGURE 6-2d **Stage 4** Full-thickness ulcer. Muscle and/or bone can be seen. Infection and necrosis is present. Drainage present, which may or may not have an odor.

FIGURE 6-2 Pressure sores are classified by the depth of tissue destruction.

- Signs of shock
- Vomiting
- Diarrhea

Keep in mind that home care patients may already be receiving treatment for a generalized infection that has in fact worsened or spread. Inquire if a pattern of deterioration has been seen by the caregiver or home care provider. In cases of septic shock, ALS treatment is mainly supportive. Provide fluid for hypotension and necessary airway and oxygen support.

Equipment Malfunction Home care equipment has the normal limitations of any machine. The power may go out and stop the machine from functioning. The machine may break and/or need maintenance. Some machines, if inoperative, can create a life threat to a patient. Common examples include home ventilators, oxygen delivery systems, apnea monitors, and home dialysis machines.

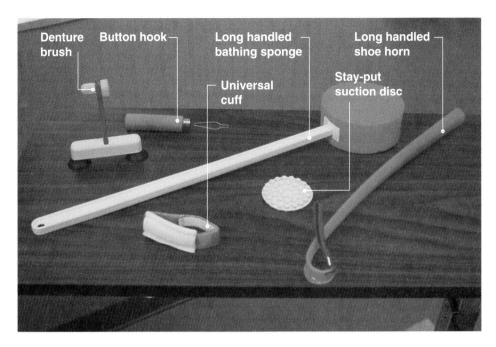

FIGURE 6-3 EMS personnel must become familiar with the common medical devices that they may encounter when providing interventions for the chronic-care patient.

In cases of equipment malfunction, you may be called upon to take the place of a device (such as a ventilator) or to treat problems that have arisen as a result of the malfunction. Even the malfunction of a glucometer for a diabetic can be a difficult situation for some patients to handle, especially if they suspect hypoglycemia. Your job is to assess the problem and take the appropriate actions.

Other Medical Disorders and Home Care Patients As already mentioned, you can expect to find a wide variety of problems treated in the home care setting. They can range from an infant on an apnea monitor to progressive dementia in a family member to psychosocial support of the family of a home care patient. Some other conditions that may be treated at home include:

- Brain or spinal trauma
- Arthritis
- Psychological disorders
- Cancer
- Hepatitis
- AIDS
- Transplants (including patients awaiting transplants)

Commonly Found Medical Devices

As previously mentioned, home care patients use a vast number of devices (Figure 6-3). They range from the simplicity of a nasal cannula to the complexity of a home ventilator. If you encounter an unfamiliar device—which may happen at some time in your career—don't panic. Find out what it's used for, and you will then have an idea on how to proceed. Don't be afraid to look foolish by asking questions. You won't. You will be foolish, and endanger the patient, if you pretend to understand a device, but don't. Some commonly used devices include:

- Glucometers
- IV infusions and in-dwelling IV sites
- Nebulized and aerosolized medication administrators
- Shunts, fistulas, and venous grafts
- Oxygen concentrators, oxygen tanks, and liquid oxygen systems
- Oxygen masks and nebulizers
- Tracheotomies and home ventilators
- G-tubes, colostomies, and urostomies
- Surgical drains
- Apnea monitors, cardiac monitors, and pulse oximeters
- Wheelchairs, canes, and walkers

Spend some time at the hospital talking with health care personnel about new devices being introduced for the home care setting. Study or make copies of the brochures that come with these devices. You might also talk with manufacturers or vendors, the people who commonly deliver equipment to home care patients.

Intervention by a Home Health Care Practitioner or Physician

Most calls involving home care patients will require acute intervention in problems such as inadequate respiratory support, acute respiratory events, acute cardiac events, acute sepsis, or GI/GU crises. Keep in mind, however, that you may not be the first person to provide intervention. If home care patients have a good relationship with their home health care practitioner or physician, they may contact this person first. In fact, they may be required to do so in order to receive reimbursement for medical services.

On any call involving a home care patient, be sure to ask whether a patient has called another health care professional. If so, find out what instructions or medications have been issued. Also inquire about written orders from the physician or the physician-approved health care plan. Health care agencies resubmit these plans to physicians at least every 62 days. So check the date to see when the plan was last revised.

In some cases, you may be called to a home care setting in which a home health practitioner or physician must intervene—i.e., the scope of treatment is beyond your training. In such cases, your role will be mainly supportive. Examples of such conditions include:

- Chemotherapy
- Pain management
- **Hospice** care

Remain especially alert to home care patients receiving medications for pain management. They are at risk for pharmacological side effects and possible overdose. The patient may also be taking non-prescription drugs that could interact with prescribed medications. Substance abuse, especially in critically ill patients, is also a possibility.

Hospice patients have unique psychological needs due to the terminal nature of their illness. Although they and their families will have been counseled about

You will be foolish, and endanger the patient, if you pretend to understand a device, but don't.

On any call involving a home care patient, be sure to ask whether a patient has called another health care professional.

* **hospice** program of palliative care and support services that addresses the physical, social, economic, and spiritual needs of terminally ill patients and their families.

Table 6-4	PREPARING THE HOME FOR PATIENT CARE
Room	**Strategies**
Bathroom	• Purchase a shower chair and/or tub seat.
	• Install grab bars.
	• Install a raised toilet seat.
	• Hang mirrors, shelves, racks at wheelchair level.
	• Set water temperature at a safe level (no higher than 120°F/48.8°C).
Kitchen	• Install easy-to-reach stove dials, counter tops, and storage areas.
	• Provide an easy-to-reach fire extinguisher.
	• Keep floors dry and non-slippery.
Living Room	• Arrange furniture for free access.
	• Provide sturdy seating at a suitable height.
Bedroom	• Install a telephone next to the bed.
	• Obtain a hospital-type bed.
	• Keep a night-light or flashlight near the bed.
	• Keep a bedpan or commode chair within patient reach.
General	• Install smoke alarms.
	• Provide adequate heating and air conditioning.
	• Provide good lighting.
	• Remove all hazards to mobility—throw rugs, electrical wires, etc.
	• Install wheelchair ramps into house and over doorsills.
	• Secure all banisters and railings.
	• Provide a mobile phone.

the disease process, emotional support is still part of your job. If a call involves a hospice patient, the situation will almost always require intervention by specially trained health care professionals. Find out the names of these people as quickly as possible and determine the advisability of consultation versus rapid transport. (For more on hospice care, see the closing sections of this chapter.)

Injury Control and Prevention

As has been mentioned in earlier chapters, the most effective intervention is prevention. Care of the patient begins even before he or she returns to the home. Some or all of the steps listed in Table 6-4 and Table 6-5 should be taken, depending upon the patient's condition. You should also keep in mind a matrix, or strategy, for injury prevention developed by William Haddon in 1972. His ten steps to injury prevention are essential to all aspects of emergency medicine. The steps include:

1. Prevent the creation of hazard to begin with.
2. Reduce the amount of the hazard brought into existence.
3. Prevent the release of the hazard that already exists.
4. Modify the rate of distribution of the hazard from the source.

Table 6-5 INJURY CONTROL AND PREVENTION

Organize for out-of-hospital care	• Find out about the patient's condition—length of time for recovery, possible impairments or limitations, prospects for recovery, prescribed treatment plan, frequency of check-ups, and possible side effects of medications.
	• Determine available health care agencies, including home-to-hospital transportation services.
	• Prepare the home for patient care (Table 6-4).
	• Rent or purchase appropriate equipment and learn how it operates.
	• Arrange for help—Meals on Wheels, visiting nurses, adult day care, and so on.
Provide proper bed care	• Apply restraints—safety vests, safety belts, limb holders, or mitts—as necessary.
	• Assist in elimination (and safe depose of wastes).
	• Encourage exercise.
	• Look for bedsores or other infections.
Prepare for emergencies	• Establish a patient baseline.
	• Learn the danger signs for the patient's particular condition.
	• Keep a list of emergency numbers at each phone (or program mobile or cell phones).
	• Notify fire and rescue squads of the patient's condition or special needs.
	• Obtain necessary Medic Alert identification.
	• Obtain a Vial of Life and post a decal on the refrigerator door.

5. Separate the hazard and that which is to be protected in both time and space.
6. Separate the hazard and that which is to be protected by a barrier.
7. Modify the basic qualities of the hazard.
8. Make that which is to be protected more resistant to the hazard.
9. Counter the damage already done by the hazard.
10. Stabilize, repair, and rehabilitate the object of the damage.

These ten steps can be used to protect paramedics from the hazards they encounter in the workplace or to protect patients from injuries at home. The steps can be seen in such simple areas as BSI precautions (barrier protection), the use of side rails to prevent falls, or the use of home rehabilitation to stabilize or repair a patient's injuries.

GENERAL SYSTEM PATHOPHYSIOLOGY, ASSESSMENT, AND MANAGEMENT

Assessment and management of home care patients can be challenging. You can gain confidence by becoming familiar with the pathophysiology of the diseases most commonly found in home care settings. You must also keep in mind the emotional needs of both the home care patient and the caregivers or family members affected by the patient's condition. Some caregivers love what they do and treat the patient's condition as part of their daily lives. Other households feel constant, unremitting stress, and possibly resentment toward the patient's condition.

Getting a feel for the emotional context of a patient's care should be a part of any call. However, in the case of home care patients, you must exhibit extra sensitivity. The way in which you interact with the patient and family can greatly affect the ease and efficiency with which you assess the patient and gather information. Developing a consistent, comprehensive approach to patient assessment and treatment can be your best strategy for dealing with these sometimes complicated responses. The one thing home care calls have in common is their diversity. Be prepared to draw on all your EMS skills and to think quickly as you figure out the most effective management plan.

The one thing home care calls have in common is their diversity.

ASSESSMENT

Assessment of the home care patient follows the same basic steps as any other patient—scene size-up, initial assessment, focused history and physical examination, ongoing assessment, and continued management. However, you will need to modify your mind set for the home care patient—i.e., observe for conditions that you might not ordinarily look for in the general population. This section highlights some of the points you should keep in mind or emphasize when assessing the home care patient. (For more on assessment, see Volume 2 of *Paramedic Care: Principles & Practices*. For information on assessment-based management, see Chapter 7 in this volume.)

Scene Size Up

As with any call, your assessment of the scene begins before you get out of your vehicle. In the case of home care patients, note any special equipment you may observe upon entering the home. This will alert you to any possible chronic problems that the patient might have. As you approach the scene, keep the following questions in mind:

- Is there a wheelchair ramp next to the front steps?
- Is there oxygen equipment in view?
- Is there a trail of oxygen tubing that leads into the patient's bedroom?
- Are there infection control supplies on the counter?
- Is there a sharps container present? (This means there are sharps too!)
- Is the patient in a hospital bed?

Introduce yourself to any other medical personnel on the scene—nurse, aide, hospice worker, and so on. By making personal contact, you will help create a health care team that can pool resources and share information. It is a serious mistake to arrive on the scene with a "take-over" mentality that all but eliminates the home care provider from the assessment process.

It is a serious mistake to arrive on the scene with a "take-over" mentality that all but eliminates the home care provider from the assessment process.

Scene Safety After you have identified the scene as a home care situation, remain alert for special hazards that might be present. As mentioned earlier, emotions often run high in a home care situation. Evaluate whether any of the people present have a threatening attitude that could be directed toward you. If at any time you don't feel comfortable, withdraw and seek assistance, either from the police or additional personnel. Ask someone to put any pets in another room and have all sources of sound (TV, radio, etc.) turned off so that you can work in a quiet, focused environment. As in any patient's home, look for weapons that the patient might use for self-defense—firearms, knives, or chemical sprays.

Other special hazards that you may face in a home care situation include infectious wastes, medical supplies such as needles, and potentially dangerous equipment. You would hope that all home care providers are meticulous with the safe disposal of sharps. However, don't take it for granted. You cannot help any patients if you are on disability because you contracted hepatitis or AIDS from a needle stick. Look around carefully.

In responding to any home care situation, keep in mind the following guidelines.

- Any patient with limited movement may be contaminated with feces, urine, or **emesis.**
- Any bed-bound patient may have weeping wounds, bleeding, or decubitus ulcers (bedsores).
- Sharps may be present.
- Collection bags for urine or feces sometimes leak.
- Tracheostomy patients clear mucus by coughing, which can spray.
- Any electrical machine has the potential for electric shock.
- A hospital bed, wheelchair, or walker could be contaminated with body fluid.
- Contaminated medical devices, such as a nebulizer, may be left around unprotected.
- Oxygen in the presence of flame has the potential for fire or explosion.
- Equipment may be in the way and cause you to fall—or it may be unstable and fall on you.
- Medical wastes may not be properly contained or discarded.

Don't minimize the impact of any of these hazards. You can always be contaminated by any patient, but treatment of the home care patient has the potential for a broader range of exposures. Be sure to remove any medical waste you generate so the patient does not return to an unsafe environment. If at all possible, you should also remove any medical waste that is already there for the same reason. Always use BSI precautions and be careful!

Patient Milieu Another important part of the scene size-up involves an evaluation of the patient's environment. Is the house clean or filthy? Is there nutritious food available? Are the sanitary facilities clean? Is the house heated and/or air conditioned? Is there adequate electricity? Is there insect or vermin infestation? The answers to such questions obviously have an impact upon the patient's health and his or her ability to recover.

Also note the condition of the patient's specific medical devices. For example, is the nasal cannula clean? Is the wheelchair in good working order? Is the ventilator well situated for safety and effectiveness? Again, these observations provide important clues to the quality of the home care received by the patient and the ability or willingness of the patient to comply with a prescribed treatment regimen.

* emesis vomitus.

Be sure to remove any medical wastes that you generate so the patient does not return to an unsafe environment.

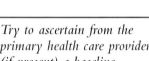

If the patient is living in a hazardous or unhealthy environment, you have an obligation to notify the proper agency to ensure that the person receives the necessary help.

Try to ascertain from the primary health care provider (if present) a baseline presentation for the patient.

Remember that you not only have a responsibility to treat the patient, but to act as an advocate. If a patient is living in a hazardous or unhealthy environment, you have an obligation to notify the proper agency to ensure that the person receives the necessary help. Often hospital social services will be of assistance. The patient's home care agency or the police might also intervene, depending upon the situation.

Remain alert to signs of abuse and/or neglect. In many states, you are required by law to report signs of child or elder abuse. (See Chapters 2, 3, and 4.) Know the laws that pertain to the practice of EMS in your state. Home care patients, whether old or young, may be helpless to improve their situation. It is the responsibility of all health care workers to look out for their safety and well being.

Initial Assessment, Focused History, Physical Exam

At this point in your assessment, you may already have a good base of information without actually having seen the patient! As you approach the patient, begin your initial assessment by observing general appearance, skin color and quality, quality of respiration, and level of distress. Also note any medical equipment that the patient may be currently using.

As you continue to assess the patient for the ABCs, try to ascertain from the primary care provider (if present) a baseline presentation for the patient. Were you called just because his or her condition has gotten worse? Or, are you here for a new problem? For some home care patients, respiratory distress may be a chronic condition. For example, a COPD patient might always have difficulty breathing. Your first impulse may be to reach for your airway supplies only to find that this is the patient's norm and that you were called to treat an unrelated problem. You must be flexible in your judgments and listen carefully to the report provided by the caregiver or family member who summoned EMS.

As with any patient, treat it as you see it! Once you have established the patient's baseline, assess for changes from the norm. Airway and breathing are always your first concern, followed by circulation. If there are any serious threats to the ABCs, you must treat them. If you are unable to stabilize the patient, complete your rapid assessment and transport immediately. In such cases, your detailed and ongoing assessments will be performed en route to the hospital, if possible.

In non-critical patients, you might take the opportunity to compare vital signs to the bedside records, if they are kept. The focus of your exam should be on the chief complaint and how it might relate to the patient's chronic condition. Be meticulous in your exam, especially with the home care patient. As stated earlier, home care patients are more susceptible to complications than most other patients and can deteriorate rapidly—i.e., a non-critical patient can quickly become a critical patient.

In examining a home care patient, be sure to inspect, palpate, and auscultate all potential problem areas. In bed-bound patients, look for decubiti (pressure sores or bed sores) on parts of the body subjected to constant pressure or friction. As mentioned, decubiti pose a significant danger to the patient through infection or sepsis and may require surgical debridement.

Mental Status If your patient has a preexisting altered mental status such as dementia or Alzheimer's disease, you must have a good understanding of his or her normal mentation before transport. This information is vital to the physician evaluating and treating the patient at the receiving facility. As stressed in Chapter 3, depression can mimic senility and senility can mimic organic brain syndrome. Dementia can also be a sign or symptom of a number of other serious medical problems, such as hypoglycemia and AIDS.

In general, assessment of mental status follows the same general procedure as with other patients. However, you must tailor your questions to the home care

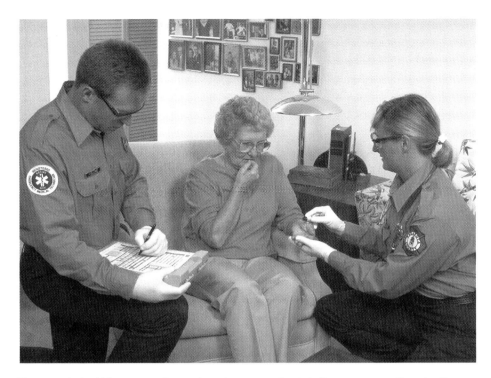

FIGURE 6-4   When assessing a chronic-care patient, tailor your questions to the home-care setting. Remember that the stress in many home-care settings, or fear of removal from the home, can increase patient confusion.

setting (Figure 6-4). For example, a person who does not work may be oriented but not know the date or even the day of the week. Also keep in mind the high level of stress in many home care situations and the effect this may have on patient confusion.

To avoid insulting the patient with what may appear to be childlike questions, preface your assessment by saying, "Since I don't know your condition very well, I need to ask you some very basic questions." If patients understand that you are following a systematic assessment, they usually cooperate in what, for them, is often a tedious process.

If a patient cannot or will not answer questions, rely on family members or health care providers to explain why the patient's current mental status is a departure from the norm. For example, belligerent behavior might be normal for a home care patient. If this is the case, find out what is different this time than other times. Perhaps, as pointed out earlier, nothing may be different—the family member or caregiver has just reached the breaking point and is in need of outside assistance.

Remember that home care patients, especially older or terminal patients, are fearful of being removed from the home environment. This can trigger depression, which in turn worsens a preexisting altered mental status. The key in such cases is tactful questioning combined with your own powers of observation. Pay particular attention to body language and interactions between household members. Note any evidence that the altered mental condition may have been triggered or worsened by a treatable cause and present this information as part of your focused history.

Other Considerations In preparing your history, take into account any long-term medical problems—i.e., the conditions that necessitated home care—and the specific events that led to the current crisis. Use the home health history and written orders from the physician, if available. As mentioned, talk to the health care provider and to the patient. What changes, if any, have taken place in the patient's life in the recent past? Has patient treatment and/or compliance changed? Are medical devices operating correctly?

Keep in mind that eating habits, fluid intake, and minor illnesses or injuries can have a dramatic effect on a seriously ill home-bound patient. Have a high index of suspicion for any new conditions that the patient may be developing. For example, evidence of dementia in an AIDS patient is a serious sign. Correlate this with your physical exam and use this information in developing your treatment plan.

In the case of home care patients, you may more commonly encounter Do Not Resuscitate (DNR) orders, Do Not Attempt Resuscitation (DNAR) orders, living wills, and so on. Ascertain whether these documents are in place before beginning any life-saving treatments. If that information is unavailable, act in the best interests of the patient. Also, keep in mind, that a DNR or DNAR doesn't mean that you have to withhold *all* treatment. For example, if a CHF patient with crackles and shortness of breath has a DNR, you may still be able to start a line, give nitroglycerin, administer an IV diuretic, and/or transport the patient to the hospital. However, you must read the specific instructions contained within the advance directives and consult with medical control.

Advance directives are designed to prevent useless treatment and invasion to the body when natural death or dying occurs. However, many people who have advance directives can be treated in crisis situations and recover. You must use your judgment on a case-by-case basis to determine what qualifies as a resuscitative or life-sustaining measure. (Additional material on advance directives appears later in the chapter.)

TRANSPORT AND MANAGEMENT TREATMENT PLAN

Transport and/or treatment of a home care patient often involves replacing home health treatment modalities with ALS modalities. Airway and ventilatory support should be straightforward, as EMS providers are usually equipped and trained in the use of most necessary supplies. Some home care interventions, such as Foley catheters, can simply be brought along with the patient. Other interventions, such as percutaneous endoscopic gastrostomy (PEG) tubes, must be flushed and capped, which you may not be trained or equipped to do. In this case, the home care provider should assist you.

In some instances, you may be forced to take the support mechanism on your ambulance if you cannot find a suitable replacement. Certain infusion pumps or other devices may be essential to the patient's well-being and you must bring them along. You should critically assess the risks of discontinuing the home care intervention versus transporting the mechanism. Seek advice from your base physician if you are unfamiliar with the intervention and if the home health provider is unable to help.

When taking a home care patient to a receiving facility, be sure to notify family members and caregivers, if they are not present. Before leaving the scene, secure the home, making sure that doors and windows are locked. In all likelihood, you will need to notify the patient's physician and/or the appropriate health care agency, if you have not already done so.

Document your findings and all care steps carefully. Your run report will become part of the home care patient's record and may in fact suggest modifications in the treatment plan. If the patient is not already using a home care agency, provide names of services in your community or refer the person to the proper social service agency. You might also mention non-medical attendant care such as housekeeping services and Meals-on-Wheels. As mentioned earlier, if you suspect the need for intervention in patient care, report your suspicions to the appropriate agency.

You should critically assess the risks of discontinuing the home health care intervention versus transporting the mechanism.

SPECIFIC ACUTE HOME HEALTH SITUATIONS

Content Review

COMMON ACUTE HOME CARE SITUATIONS
- Respiratory disorders
- Cardiac problems
- Use of VADs
- GI/GU disorders
- Acute infections

Although you will undoubtedly intervene in a wide variety of home care situations during your EMS career, you can expect to encounter certain conditions more commonly than others. The chronic-care patients that will most likely require acute ALS intervention include those with respiratory disorders, cardiac problems, vascular access devices (VADs), GI/GU disorders, and acute infections. You may also be called upon to intervene in the home care of mothers and their newborn infants and to provide assistance in hospice settings. A discussion of each of these situations will help you to prepare for your increasing involvement in the home health care system of the 2000s.

RESPIRATORY DISORDERS

Content Review

COMMON HOME RESPIRATORY EQUIPMENT
- Oxygen equipment
- Portable suctioning machines
- Aerosol equipment and nebulizers
- Incentive spirometers
- Home ventilators
- Tracheostomy tubes and collars

Respiratory disorders account for more than 630,000 of the hospital patients discharged for home care each year. Nearly 37 percent of patients with simple pneumonia and pleurisy and more than 50 percent of patients with chronic obstructive pulmonary disease (COPD) often receive home care within one day of their discharge from the hospital.

Some of the most common home care devices used to treat respiratory disorders include oxygen equipment, portable suctioning machines, aerosol equipment and nebulizers, incentive spirometers, various home ventilators, and tracheostomy tubes and collars. In order to provide intervention with these devices, you need to review pertinent respiratory anatomy and physiology as it relates to home oxygen and respiratory therapy. (See Volume 3, Chapter 1, "Pulmonology.") You also need to review the pathophysiology of the disorders that most frequently require home respiratory support.

Select respiratory disorders and the medical therapy used to treat them are discussed in the following sections. As you read this material, keep in mind earlier comments on the increased risk of airway infections and respiratory compromise in the home care patient.

Chronic Diseases Requiring Home Respiratory Support

Many home care patients have a lung capacity that is minimally able to meet their normal requirements. Sometimes even simple activities, such as climbing stairs, can severely stress their system. Unlike patients with normal lung capacities, they simply do not have the ability for any increased workload. Even walking from one room to another may require use of oxygen equipment. The following is a review of some of the conditions you may find in the respiratory compromised patient.

Many home care patients have a lung capacity that is minimally able to meet their normal requirements.

COPD As you know, COPD is a triad of diseases—emphysema, chronic bronchitis, and asthma. Some patients may have one, two, or all three disorders. All three are outflow obstructive diseases, impeding the exhalation of air from the lungs. This causes an increase in carbon dioxide and a decrease in oxygenation.

COPD patients work harder to breathe than healthy people. When that work becomes too much, they tire quickly. If home equipment fails for any reason, they often panic, worsening their situation. As with any COPD patient, direct your treatment toward increasing oxygen flow. Be prepared to take over their breathing as soon as patients can no longer move enough oxygen to sustain themselves.

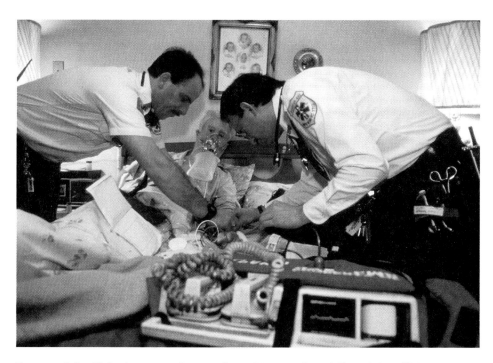

FIGURE 6-5   If the home equipment for a COPD patient fails or is insufficient, you may have to replace it with equipment from the ALS unit.

In some cases, this may mean fixing or replacing home respiratory equipment and/or transport to the hospital (Figure 6-5).

In treating the COPD patient, keep in mind the following disease-specific information.

Bronchitis and Emphysema   These two diseases go hand-in-hand. Most often they result from smoking, but can have other causes as well. Bronchitis involves the chronic overproduction of mucus, which narrows bronchial passages and restricts air flow. Emphysema typically leads to a stiffening and enlargement of the alveoli. This loss of elasticity and compliance requires higher pressures in the lungs to facilitate gas exchanges at the alveolar level. Usually these patients are thin (because breathing takes up a large portion of their daily caloric intake) and barrel chested (due to the retention of air in the lungs as a result of outflow obstruction).

In cases of acute exacerbation, these patients have a difficult time compensating. They may exhibit wheezing with diminished lung sounds, use of accessory muscles, retractions, tripod positioning, and the inability to speak in full sentences. Home treatments that you may see include oxygen, nebulized or aerosol medications, and possibly a ventilator utilizing **PEEP, CPAP,** or **BiPAP.** PEEP is provided through an endotracheal tube, while CPAP and BiPAP are provided through a tightly fitted mask.

When providing intervention, don't forget that home care patients usually have a high dosing regimen, which may make them less responsive to their medications. Always provide these patients with high flow oxygen. Medications that may be helpful include:

* Nebulized beta-2 specific agonist bronchodilators, such as albuterol or metaproterenol
* IV or oral corticosteroids, such as methylprednisolone (Solu-Medtrol)
* Nebulized anticholinergics (ipratropium)

✳ PEEP positive end expiratory pressure.

✳ CPAP continuous positive airway pressure.

✳ BiPAP bilevel positive airway pressure.

When providing intervention, don't forget that home care patients usually have a high dosing regimen, which may make them less responsive to their medications.

Asthma   Asthma, sometimes referred to as reactive airway disease, can be seen with any age patient. A crisis often occurs when some reactant causes an acute constriction of the bronchial passages. Home care patients with asthma can usually handle these episodes on their own. If the episode becomes severe, however, you may be called by a caregiver or parent. (Asthma in children can be especially stressful for the family, so be sure to review its treatment in Chapter 2 of this volume.)

With asthmatic patients, look for wheezing with diminished lung sounds, use of accessory muscles, and the inability to speak in full sentences. Head bobbing in children is an ominous sign of impending respiratory failure.

Home treatments you may see include oxygen, oral medications, and a variety of nebulizers and/or inhalers. In providing support, always administer high flow oxygen. Medications that may be helpful include the same ones used to treat bronchitis and emphysema. You may also consider an epinephrine IV or SQ. However, use this medication with caution when treating the elderly or very weak patients.

Long-term care of asthma involves the avoidance or elimination of reactants that can trigger the problem. Try to gather as much information as possible about the cause of the attack so that the physician and patient can take action to avoid future episodes.

Congestive Heart Failure (CHF)   CHF often presents as a respiratory problem. For more information on this condition, see "Cardiac Problems" in Volume 3, Chapter 2, "Cardiology."

Cystic Fibrosis (CF)   Cystic fibrosis is a genetic disorder usually identified during childhood, sometimes in the late teenage years. It is characterized by chronic and copious overproduction of mucus, inflammation of the small airways and hyperinflation of the alveoli, chronic infections, and erosion of the pulmonary blood vessels secondary to infection. CF is an **exocrine** disease that causes other systemic problems, such as GI disturbances, pancreatic disorders, and glucose intolerance.

> ✱ **exocrine** disorder involving external secretions.

Treatment of CF typically involves frequent postural drainage of mucus and chest percussion. Some patients may use mechanical vibrators to facilitate the percussions. They usually take medications aimed at mucus reduction and control of bacterial infection.

CF can be regarded as a terminal disease. Few patients live to the age of 40. Take this fact into account when treating the patient. At all times, remain sensitive to the emotional state of both the patient and any members of the family who may be present.

> *In the later stages, most CF patients will be colonized with respiratory system pathogens such as* Pseudomonas aerugionosa.
>
>

You may be summoned to help a CF patient for a variety of reasons. The vigorous coughing associated with the disease can result in **hemoptysis** and pneumothorax. Severe or fatal pulmonary hemorrhage can occur at any time. Patients can also suffer **cor pulmonale,** or right ventricular hypertrophy secondary to pulmonary hypertension.

> ✱ **hemoptysis** expectoration of blood arising from the oral cavity, larynx, trachea, bronchi, or lungs; characterized by sudden coughing with production of salty sputum with frothy bright red blood.

In treating a CF patient, ascertain the stage of the disease and inquire about any standing medical orders. Also find out if the patient or family has initiated any advance directives. Your treatment will flow from this information and your own assessment. There is no specific in-field treatment for acute problems stemming from CF. As a general rule, you will provide respiratory support, ventilation, and intubation, if indicated. Be sure to counsel the family or summon the proper counselor to do so, especially if the patient is in the terminal stage of the disease.

> ✱ **cor pulmonale** congestive heart failure secondary to pulmonary hypertension.

Bronchopulmonary Dysplasia (BPD)   This disease primarily affects infants of low birth weight. It is characterized by an ongoing need for mechanical ventilation in newborns who have been treated for respiratory distress of any cause. These infants may simply fail to wean from mandatory ventilation or from O_2. They are also at increased risk of lower respiratory tract infections, especially

> *In treating a CF patient, ascertain the stage of the disease and inquire about any standing orders.*
>
>

* Intermittent Mandatory Ventilation (IMV) respirator setting
where a patient-triggered
breath does not result in assistance by the machine.

*Keep in mind that pulmonary
congestion and edema may
develop in infants with BPD
if excessive fluids have been
administered.*

* demyelenation destruction or
removal of the myelin sheath
of nerve tissue; found in
Guillain–Barré syndrome.

viral infections, and may require immediate hospitalization if signs of respiratory infection or increased distress develop.

Home care providers will have been advised to wean infants to lower **Intermittent Mandatory Ventilation (IMV)** settings. However, if the process occurs too quickly, the infant may be at risk of becoming hypoxemic. Arterial oxygenation should be maintained at or above 88 to 90 percent saturation and should be monitored continuously with a pulse oximeter.

Keep in mind that pulmonary congestion and edema may develop in BPD infants if excessive fluids have been administered. Question caregivers about fluid intake, which may need to be restricted to about 120 mL/kg per day. Inquire, too, about the use of diuretic therapy, which is sometimes prescribed to these patients.

Even after an infant is weaned from a ventilator, supplemental oxygen may still be required for weeks or even months. In such cases, it is usually delivered by nasal cannula.

Remember that BPD is a serious condition in infants. Reduced lung compliance and increased airway resistance may persist for several years. The best treatment is adequate ventilatory support and prompt transport to the nearest neonatal unit.

Neuromuscular Degenerative Diseases As a group, these diseases affect respiratory action through degeneration of the muscles used for breathing. Patients who suffer from neuromuscular degeneration may at some point require respiratory support. Other problems, particularly an inability to ambulate, will have a huge impact on the patient's life.

Many patients with neuromuscular degenerative diseases will be cared for by family members. However, if the condition worsens, professional home care providers may be involved and ALS may be summoned. In cases of respiratory compromise, there is little that you can do other than provide airway and respiratory support and transport. Expect to see all manner of respiratory home care devices, including oxygen and ventilators.

In treating and transporting these patients, keep in mind the following information on the leading neuromuscular degenerative diseases.

Muscular Dystrophy This genetically inherited disorder causes a defect in the intracellular metabolism of muscle cells. The condition leads to degeneration and atrophy of muscles, which are eventually replaced by fatty and connective tissue. There is no cure as yet, and treatment is multidisciplinary because of the many muscle systems involved. These patients have difficulty moving and may need assistance with daily tasks. ALS involvement would almost certainly be for respiratory failure or accidental injuries, usually related to falls.

Poliomyelitis Poliomyelitis is an infectious disease rarely seen today because of effective vaccines. When it does occur, the disease causes destruction of motor neurons, leading to muscular atrophy, muscle weakness, and paralysis. Patients have difficulty ambulating. However, unless respiratory muscles are involved, there may be no systemic effects. Children who contract the disease may suffer permanent crippling or deformity. But once the disease is resolved, further degeneration will cease.

It has been shown that after polio patients recover normal functioning they sometimes experience a **demyelenation** of affected neurons and a return of the disability. This condition is known as post polio syndrome. Its pathophysiology is unknown.

Guillain–Barré Syndrome This syndrome is thought to be an autoimmune response to a viral (rarely bacterial) infection. It is usually preceded by a febrile episode with a respiratory and/or GI infection. The disease is characterized by muscle weakness leading to paralysis caused by nerve demyelenation. It usually starts in the distal extremities and progresses proximally.

Progression of this disorder may take several days. Once it reaches the patient's trunk, respiratory involvement becomes an obvious concern. One way to differentiate Guillain–Barré from a spinal injury is the increased motor involvement. In other words, motor deficits are greater than sensory deficits. As a rule, there is no cognitive or CNS involvement with the disease. With supportive ventilatory care, the patient can be expected to recover.

Myasthenia Gravis Myasthenia gravis is a rare disease that affects the neuronal junction. Due to the breakdown in acetylcholine receptors, nerve impulses are dampened. This disease is characterized by muscle weakness and can be more apparent in muscles proximal to the body than distally.

There is no cure for this disorder, and treatment is aimed at relieving symptoms. If the disease progresses to the diaphragm or intercostal muscles, respiratory compromise can result. Sometimes patients may have an acute exacerbation of the disease brought on by infection or stress. In such cases, intubation or artificial ventilation may be required. These episodes are most commonly preceded by difficulty swallowing or breathing.

Sleep Apnea Sleep apnea is a complex condition not yet fully understood by experts. It is characterized by long pauses in the respiratory cycle that can be caused by a relaxation of the pharynx or lack of respiratory drive. It can result in hypertension, cardiac arrhythmias, and chronic fatigue.

As a general rule, the muscles of the airway become more relaxed as the mind falls deeper and deeper into sleep. This is what leads to snoring and, in some cases, blockage of the airway. With sleep apnea, decreased oxygen levels cause a partial awakening of the patient. Breathing then resumes and the patient returns to sleep, often with no memory of the incident. Repeated over and over, such interruptions destroy normal sleep patterns and the patient spends much of the sleeping period in a hypoxic state.

People with sleep apnea often suffer alterations in their blood pressure and stroke volume. They lose the normal effect of declining blood pressure as they sleep and their pulse oximetry may fall to 80 percent or less. In patients who have ingested alcohol, the reading can fall to 50 percent.

Treatment of sleep apnea may include surgical alteration of the airway, medications, prescribed loss of weight, avoidance of any CNS depressant or alcohol, or use of a CPAP ventilator.

Patients Awaiting Lung Transplants Patients receive lung transplants for a variety of cardiopulmonary diseases. Single-lung transplants are performed for pulmonary fibrosis, COPD, or reversible hypertension or cardiac disease. Double-lung transplants are performed for cystic fibrosis, COPD, or **bronchiectasis.** Patients may also receive heart-lung transplants for primary pulmonary hypertension or various congenital diseases. Remember that patients awaiting organ transplants are in the end-stages of their diseases and traditional therapies are unlikely to be effective.

✱ **bronchiectasis** chronic dilation of a bronchus or bronchi, with a secondary infection typically involving the lower portion of the lung.

Medical Therapy Found in the Home Setting

The treatment of chronic respiratory disorders in the home setting requires a wide range of devices. The following are some of the most common types of medical therapy that you can expect to encounter.

Home Oxygen Therapy Oxygen therapy has many advantages for the home care patient. First, it is relatively simple to manage. Second, most patients tolerate it easily. Third, oxygen therapy can add much to the quality of a patient's life. Studies have shown that long-term oxygen use raises the life expectancy of COPD patients considerably. It also prevents hypoxic states that may result in permanent cognitive damage or degeneration.

Table 6-6 COMMON TECHNICAL PROBLEMS WITH OXYGEN SYSTEMS

Problem	Possible Cause	Corrective Action
Oxygen not flowing freely	Faulty tubing	Check for obstruction or replace tubing.
	Dirty or plugged humidifier	Remove from oxygen supply, clean, and refill with sterile water or replace with prefilled bottle.
Buzzer goes off on oxygen concentrator	Unit unplugged	Check plug.
	Power failure	Check fuses, circuit breaker, or, in cases of power outages, use backup oxygen tank until power is restored. (Or call EMS, as necessary.)
Oxygen tank empties too quickly or hisses	Leak in tank	Open all windows, extinguish all flames, and summon help, from the fire department, EMS, and/or supplier.

A medical equipment supplier usually delivers, sets up, and educates patients on the home oxygen delivery systems that they will use. In most cases, the systems include:

- A source of oxygen—e.g., concentrator, cylinder, or liquid oxygen reservoir
- Regulator-flow meter
- Nasal cannula, face mask, tracheostomy collar, oxygen tubing (large-bore for face tents or tracheostomy collars)
- Humidifier
- Sterile water for respiratory therapy (Make sure it is sterile!)

Very few problems arise from the systems themselves. When they do occur, patients or home care providers can usually correct the situation on their own (Table 6-6). However, you may be called upon to provide oxygen while a home system is repaired or to transport the patient to the hospital until the system is replaced. You may also be summoned if a condition unexpectedly worsens and the home oxygen system proves insufficient.

When you arrive at the scene, review the physician's prescription for the type of therapy and the source of the oxygen supply. As already noted, the three sources include:

- *Oxygen concentrators.* These systems supply the lowest concentrations of home oxygen. They extract oxygen from room air and add to the flow received by the patient. Home concentrators usually provide no more than six liters of oxygen per minute.
- *Oxygen cylinders.* Cylinders or tanks are used by patients who may require more than six liters/minute or for some reason cannot have a concentrator. Cylinders involve the same technology that you use on your own portable oxygen systems.
- *Liquid oxygen.* Patients who require constant oxygen may have a liquid oxygen system. This allows much more oxygen to be stored in the home. Patients will use this system as a reservoir to fill portable tanks that they make take outside the home.

Although these systems are relatively safe, any high pressure tank or liquid system has the potential for explosion. In a polite manner, ensure that the patient and home care provider adheres to these safety tips:

- Alert the local fire department to the presence of oxygen in the home.
- Keep a fire extinguisher on hand.
- If a fire does start, turn the oxygen off immediately and leave the house.
- Don't smoke—and do not allow others to smoke—near the oxygen system. (No open flames or smoking within ten feet of oxygen.)
- Do not use electrical equipment near oxygen administration.
- Store the oxygen tank in an approved, upright position.
- Keep a tank or reservoir away from direct sunlight or heat.
- Ground all oxygen cylinders.

In terms of the oxygen therapy itself, keep these guidelines in mind:

- Ensure the ability of the patient/home care provider to administer oxygen.
- Make sure the patient knows what to do in case of a power failure.
- Evaluate sterile conditions, especially disinfection of reusable equipment.
- As with any patient with chronic respiratory problems, remain alert to signs and symptoms of hypoxemia.

Artificial Airways/Tracheostomies Patients who have long-term upper airway problems often have a tracheostomy. A **tracheostomy** is a small surgical opening that a surgeon makes from the anterior neck into the trachea. The tracheostomy may be temporary or permanent. The technique is used on any patient who requires artificial ventilation for a long period of time. (Endotracheal or nasal intubation can only be used on a short-term basis. Pressure on the tracheal tissues, from the inflated cuff, can cause necrosis.) Tracheostomies may also be used on patients who have had damage to their larynx, epiglottis, or upper airway structures from surgery or trauma. They may also be performed on patients who have cancer of the larynx or neck.

The tracheostomy consists of the surgical opening (stoma), an outer cannula, and an inner cannula. The outer cannula keeps the stoma open and is held in place by twill tape or Velcro around the neck. The inner cannula is similar to a mini ET tube and slides down into the trachea a few inches. Due to the small size of the airway, the inner cannula usually has a low pressure cuff at the end to hold it in place and provide a good seal. In the case of infants, there is no inner cannula because of the small size of infant airways. Also, the airways of infants are more pliable than older patients and more susceptible to blockage.

Tracheostomy patients who have had a larygectomy may have some ability for speech, and some may have an air connection to the oropharynx or nasopharynx. Keep this in mind if you need to ventilate a person with a tracheostomy. It may be necessary to block off the nose and mouth to prevent air from escaping upwardly instead of being pushed into the lungs.

Those patients who are unable to speak will use an artificial larynx. This device looks like a small flashlight. It creates an electronic vibration, which the patient manipulates by pressing the device up against the neck and by changing the shape of his or her mouth (much as you do when you speak). If the patient does not have an artificial larynx, you will need to resort to writing or signing for communication. Remember that an inability to communicate can create a lot of stress and frustration for the patient. Try to be part of the solution, not part of the problem.

Routine care of the tracheostomy includes:

- Keeping the stoma clean and dry
- Periodic changing of the outer cannula
- Changing and cleaning the inner cannula from every few weeks to every few months, depending on the patient
- For ventilator patients, routine changing of the ventilator hose connections
- Frequent suctioning, due to increased secretions

Use sterile technique when changing or adjusting tracheostomy tubes to avoid colonizing the site with flora from your own skin.

It is important to remember that a tracheostomy eliminates a large part of the normal air-filtering process. The trapping of bacteria in the nasopharynx and oropharynx no longer occurs. Neither does the humidification and heating of air by the nasal passages. This means that bacteria have a more direct route to the lungs, and the air received in the lungs is drier and cooler than normal. Therefore, people with a tracheostomy have a higher incidence of lung infections, mucus production, and irritation. Since they have less control over their airway, it is also more difficult for them to clear blocked airways.

If a patient is not currently using a tracheostomy, it may be closed with a Trach-button. This device simply plugs up the opening until it is needed again.

Common Complications The most common problems faced by tracheostomy patients include blockage of the airway by mucus and a dislodged cannula. The patient can usually clear the obstructing mucus by coughing. (Be careful—the mucus can fly out of the stoma for quite a distance.) Sometimes suctioning, either by the patient or by the caregiver, will suffice. Cannulas can become dislodged by patient movement, or, in the case of children, by their growth. In assessing a child with a cannula problem, find out when it was last changed. Maybe the child is ready for the next size. Children can also have their stoma blocked by foreign objects that enter by accident or are put there by a sibling. Other complications include infection of the stoma, drying of the tracheal mucus leading to crusting or bleeding, and tracheal erosion from an over-inflated cuff (causing necrosis).

In assessing a child with a cannula problem, find out when it was last changed. Maybe the child is ready for the next size.

Management If EMS has been called, it means that neither the patient nor the caregiver has been able to solve the problem. If the tracheostomy patient is on a ventilator, you must rapidly determine if the problem is with the ventilator or with the airway itself. If the problem is simply a loose fitting or disconnected tube, fix it. If the problem is not immediately apparent, do not waste time trying to troubleshoot the machine—unless you are qualified to do so. Your bag-valve device will connect directly to where the ventilator tubing connects. Remove the tubing, connect the bag-valve device to the trach connector, and ventilate (Figure 6-6).

If the problem is not immediately apparent, do not waste time troubleshooting the machine.

If the problem is with the patient's airway, you will need to clear it. If the patient is hypoxic, always hyperventilate before suctioning. Be sure to evaluate any postural or positional considerations. If the patient is slumped over, straighten him or her up. Remember to ensure that ventilations are directed downward into the lungs, not upward into the mouth. (Ask the home care provider if there is a connection from the trachea to the upper airway.)

The tracheostomy stoma will close fairly quickly if a tube is not promptly replaced.

If you are unable to ventilate, clearing the airway is your first priority. Visualize as much of the airway as possible and check for obstructions. If none are visible, introduce a suction catheter and suction while withdrawing—no more than 10–15 seconds for an adult, 5 seconds for a child. Again, always hyperventilate before and after suctioning.

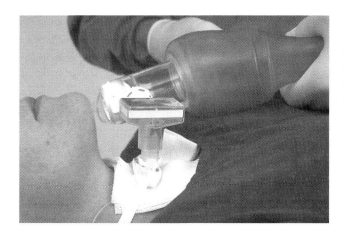

FIGURE 6-6 Artificial ventilation can be accomplished in the patient with a tracheostomy tube by attaching the bag-valve device directly to the tube.

If it appears that the inner cannula is blocked or dislodged, you may remove it. If cuffed, you must first deflate the cuff. Connect a 10 cc syringe to the cuff valve and withdraw the air. If a syringe is unavailable, you can cut off the valve and the air will escape. You can then remove the inner cannula, hyperventilate, and continue to suction as needed.

If necessary, you may intubate the stoma. The inner cannula must always be removed first. Use an appropriate sized tube to pass through the outer cannula, and advance so the ET cuff (if a cuffed tube is used) is 1-2 cm inside the trachea. Inflate the cuff and verify placement by auscultating the epigastrum and both lungs. Add an end tidal CO_2 device to the end of the tube. Pulse oximetry should also be used to monitor patient oxygenation.

Once the airway is secure, you may proceed with the rest of your assessment. It is inappropriate to proceed until you have protected the airway.

Home Ventilation Although you will see positive pressure ventilators with most home care patients, you may also encounter negative pressure ventilators. Both devices are used to ventilate patients for a wide variety of diseases and conditions.

Some of the most common reasons patients may be on a ventilator include:

- Decreased respiratory drive
  —spinal cord injury
- Ventilatory muscle weakness
  —muscular dystrophy
  —poliomyelitis
  —myasthenia gravis
  —Guillian–Barré syndrome
- Obstructive Pulmonary Disorders
  —COPD
  —sleep apnea
  —cystic fibrosis
  —bronchopulmonary dysplasia
- Other Disorders
  —pediatric sleep apnea
  —chest wall deformities

Ventilators provide ventilation in several different ways. They also have a number of operating controls and options, depending upon the manufacturer. Volume-cycled ventilation, for example, has long been the standard type of ventilatory support for all forms of severe respiratory failure. All modern ventilators can provide this feature as well as several other modes that vary in ventilatory waveform, method of terminating the machine-aided cycle, and so on.

Positive-Pressure Ventilators According to current practice, positive-pressure ventilation (PPV) is the recommended form of support for acute respiratory disorders. A positive pressure ventilator pushes air into the lungs, either through a face mask, nasal mask, or tracheostomy. Features of this type of ventilator include variations in tidal volume, respiratory rate, flow rate, and pressure. Optional connectors will be available for oxygen and a humidifier.

There are too many types of positive-pressure ventilators to list here. However, any home care provider should be familiar with a patient's particular machine—including the small ventilators that attach to a mobile patient's wheelchair.

Negative Pressure Ventilators Ventilators that apply negative pressure to the chest—tank, cuirass, or poncho-wrap—require a rigid structure to support the vacuum department. When they expand, they pull on the chest, causing it to expand and allowing air to flow into the lungs. This mimics the normal breathing process.

The iron lung is one of the best known examples of negative pressure ventilators. However, some home care patients may also be fitted with a poncho-wrap—a suit that it is sealed at all openings. Patients most commonly use this device at night.

PEEP, CPAP, and BiPAP These three ventilator options add pressure at various times in the respiratory cycle. They may be used by full-time or part-time ventilator patients. Keep in mind that there is a danger of pneumothorax because of the increased pulmonary pressure. Take this into account during your assessment of PEEP.

PEEP PEEP, or positive end expiratory pressure, is used to keep alveoli from collapsing. It works by providing a little back pressure at the end of expiration. This option can be used for newborns—usually premature—who have insufficient surfactant to keep the alveoli inflated or in adults who have surfactant washout from acute pulmonary edema, **ARDS,** or drowning.

PEEP also has a use in treating COPD. However, due to stiffening and degeneration of the alveoli in emphysema, patients require higher diffusion pressures for gas exchange. If you ever see COPD patients pursing their lips as they exhale, they are providing their own PEEP. By blowing against a slight resistance, they will keep their alveoli open. A COPD patient who is getting worse may deteriorate to the point where he or she needs occasional assistance from a ventilator with PEEP.

CPAP CPAP, or continuous positive airway pressure, is used to keep pharyngeal structures from collapsing at the end of a breath. This option is often prescribed for sleep apnea patients who need help in keeping their airways open. Most of these patients will use nasal CPAP—a mask that encompasses the nose (Figure 6-7). In these cases, patients must learn to keep their mouths closed for the mask to work correctly. Otherwise the pressure will be lost. The idea behind mask CPAP or nasal CPAP is the same as PEEP, except that CPAP is provided by mask, while PEEP is provided by endotracheal tube.

BiPAP BiPAP, or bilevel positive airway pressure, provides two levels of pressure—one on inspiration and one on exhalation. This option is used for patients who require more or higher levels of pressure than CPAP. Although the settings on the patient's home ventilator may be useful to the ED or to follow-up patient care, they are not essential to your assessment. Try to gather this information at the scene, but don't let it delay your management of any serious airway or breathing problems.

As you may already have inferred, a home care patient with a chronic respiratory problem might eventually progress from home oxygen, to occasional ventilator support (PEEP, CPAP, BiPAP), to full ventilator dependency. Knowing each stage of the illness and how it relates to the various ventilatory options will give you a more complete understanding of the patient's clinical progress.

* ARDS acute respiratory distress syndrome.

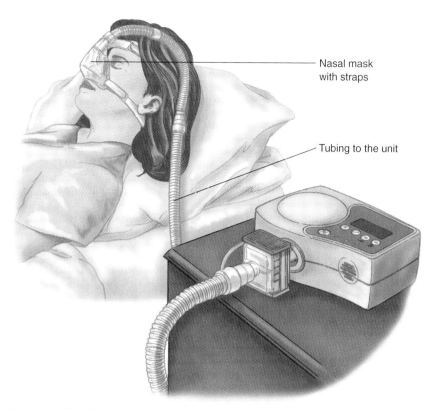

Nasal mask
with straps

Tubing to the unit

FIGURE 6-7 Sleep apnea patients will often use continuous positive pressure airway pressure—CPAP—to keep their airways open.

General Assessment Considerations Assessment of the respiratory patient should focus on the patient's entire respiratory apparatus. Any deficit found in the system must be rapidly identified and managed.

As you approach the patient, look at the effort required to breathe. Observe for head bobbing, retractions, respiratory rate, tripod posturing, pursed lips, cyanosis, and depth of respiration. Listen for sounds of wheezing or rales. Note any devices or medications that the patient is currently using.

Immediately assess the patient's mental status by talking to him or her as you approach. Patients will indicate understanding with their eyes even if they are unable to speak due to dyspnea. Note the number of words that they can speak without stopping for a breath. Rapidly confirm the patient's baseline respiratory effort and mental status from the home care worker, if present.

Next, auscultate the lungs to identify the type of problem that the patient may be having and to determine tidal volume. Look at the patient's chest to spot any irregularities, retractions, or abdominal breathing. You can use pulse oximetry as an adjunct to your assessment, but don't rely on it alone. If the patient has poor peripheral circulation, it may not give an accurate reading.

Finally, complete your assessment by considering the full range of problems that might have caused the patient's current complaint. Whenever assessing a home care patient, you must remain vigilant for complications other than the chronic medical condition being treated at home. An asthma patient, for example, might be having a myocardial infarction (MI).

General Management Considerations As always, your first considerations when intervening in the care of a chronically ill patient center on the ABCs. In the absence of documentation or a valid prehospital DNR, you must maintain a patent airway or improve on the airway that is already in place. This may be as simple as suctioning secretions from an airway device, such as a tracheostomy tube. You should also assess the placement of airway devices that you did not insert. It is easy for a device to become dislodged, obstructing the airway or failing to ensure patency. You may be forced to remove home airway devices and replace them with your own interventions, such as endotracheal tubes.

Ventilatory problems are traditionally easy to fix in the prehospital environment. If a home ventilator fails, you should begin manual positive pressure ventilation immediately. The failure may be easy to remedy, such as in the case of unplugged power cords or a temporary loss of electricity. If you are familiar with the ventilator, you can adjust the settings to restore or improve ventilations. However, if you are unfamiliar with the ventilator, play it safe and support ventilations with your own equipment.

As with ventilation, oxygenation problems are also generally easy for EMS providers to fix. First, assess the patency of the patient's home oxygen delivery system. The power may be off, the tubing damaged, or the oxygen supply depleted. You can adjust the flow rate of an intact home oxygen delivery system or replace it with your own system.

Whatever interventions you choose, you will have to make arrangements for the devices to be transported with you to the hospital. Flexibility is the key to transporting home care patients. You should reassure the patient that you will properly care for their needs, as they will be physically as well as psychologically dependent upon their home care systems.

VASCULAR ACCESS DEVICES

Vascular access devices (VADs) are used to provide any parenteral treatment on a long-term basis. The type of device and treatment depends upon the disease process involved. Patients may have chemotherapy, hemodialysis, peritoneal dialysis, Total Parenteral Nutrition (TPN) feedings, or antibiotic therapy provided through a VAD.

Types of VADs

There are approximately 500,000 long-term therapy catheters inserted each year. Some of the most common VADs that you can expect to find in the home are described in the following sections. Consult your local protocols and procedures for accessing VADs.

Hickman, Broviac, and Groshong Catheters These catheters may be single, double, or triple lumen and can be inserted into any central vein in the trunk of the body. The subclavian vein is the most common anatomical insertion site, as it is usually easy to locate and secure.

Although these catheters have slight differences, each has an external port that looks like a typical intravenous port. The external hub of the catheter is sutured to the skin and has a cuff that promotes fibrous in-growth. This growth helps anchor the catheter to the body and prevents infection from traveling down the catheter. The highest risk of infection or accidental removal of the catheter is during the first two weeks after insertion. Care of these devices consists of keeping the site clean and dry and the administration of anticoagulant therapy to prevent clot formations.

Peripherally Inserted Central Catheters Peripherally inserted central catheters, or PICC lines, are inserted into a peripheral vein, such as the median cubital vein in the antecubital fossa. These veins are easily accessible and allow a physician to thread a catheter from the insertion site into central venous circulation. PICC lines

If you are having problems ventilating patients with their home health equipment, remove it and use equipment from the EMS unit.

If a home ventilator fails, you should begin manual positive pressure ventilation immediately.

VADs will often be routed through a subcutaneous tunnel to protect the site of venous puncture.

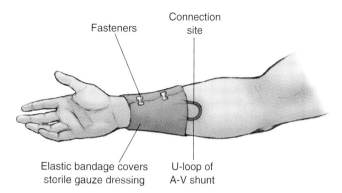

FIGURE 6-8 An A-V shunt is a loop connecting an artery and a vein, usually in the distal arm, where the dialysis apparatus draws and returns blood. It is used in home-care patients requiring dialysis.

Fasteners

Connection site

Elastic bandage covers sterile gauze dressing

U-loop of A-V shunt

are inserted under fluoroscopy by radiology rather than in an operating room. As a result, the procedure has relatively low complication rate.

Surgically Implanted Medication Delivery Systems Surgically implanted devices, such as the Port-A-Cath or Medi-Port, are similar to Hickman-style catheters. However, the infusion port is implanted completely below the skin. These devices are disc-shaped and have a diaphragm that requires a specially shaped needle, such as the Huber needle, to access. They are typically found in the upper chest and can be felt through the skin.

Never access a surgically implanted port unless local protocols allow you to do so. If such protocols exist, only properly trained personnel with proper equipment should complete the procedure. A regular intravenous catheter or needle will permanently damage an implanted port. Surgically implanted medication delivery devices should only be accessed using sterile technique.

Never access a surgically implanted port unless local protocols allow you to do so and only if you have the training and equipment to complete the procedure.

Dialysis Shunts Dialysis shunts are used for patients undergoing hemodialysis to filter their blood. An A-V shunt is a loop connecting an artery and a vein, usually in the distal arm, where the dialysis apparatus draws out and returns blood (Figure 6-8). A fistula connects an artery and a vein, creating an artificially large blood vessel for access. It is also usually found in the upper extremity.

Both shunts and fistulas are created surgically and are very delicate. As a result, you should avoid vascular access and application of blood pressure cuffs in the extremity where they are located. Some jurisdictions allow shunt access by paramedics during life-threatening emergencies. You will be able to see the shunt in the extremity, and you should be able to auscultate a bruit over the area. Failure to auscultate a bruit over the shunt area may indicate an obstruction, either a thrombus that has formed or an embolus that has lodged there.

Avoid obtaining vascular access and blood pressure in the extremity where a shunt is located.

Anticoagulant Therapy

Patients with vascular access devices will be on some type of anticoagulant therapy. The most commonly found anticoagulants will be those used to flush the device to prevent clot formation. Some patients may be on systemic anticoagulants as well. Because VADs are artificial, the body's natural clotting mechanism must be suppressed in order to ensure that the devices function properly. As a result, these patients will be much more prone to bleeding disorders. The most common sites for hemorrhage are GI bleeding, strokes, and extremity bruising.

VAD Complications

In treating patients with VADs, keep in mind possible complications. The most common complications result from various types of obstructions. A thrombus may form at the catheter site, or an embolus may lodge there after formation

It is prudent to have an orientation session on VADs used by the home health agencies in your area. Following this, an assortment of specialized needles and supplies should be carried.

elsewhere in the body. Inactivity increases the risk for clot formation. Other obstructive problems include catheter kinking or catheter tip embolus.

With central venous access devices, you should always be aware of the potential for an air embolus. The devices provide a clear pathway for air to enter central circulation. Signs and symptoms of an air embolus include:

- Headache
- Shortness of breath with clear lungs
- Hypoxia
- Chest pain
- Other indications of myocardial ischemia
- Altered mental status

Of course, any device implanted in the body has a risk of infection or hemorrhage. Look for redness, swelling, tenderness, localized heat, or discharge for a potentially infected catheter site. Because these catheters provide a channel into the central circulation, patients may quickly become septic, especially if they are weakened or immunosuppressed.

CARDIAC CONDITIONS

Many chronic-care patients receive treatment for a wide variety of cardiac conditions. You may be called to intervene in the following situations:

- Post MI recovery
- Post cardiac surgery
- Heart transplant
- CHF
- Hypertension
- Implanted pacemaker
- Atherosclerosis
- Congenital malformation (pediatric)

Home care for the cardiac patient can consist of oxygen, monitoring devices, and regular visits by a home health care provider. You can expect to find a variety of medications associated with the specific cardiac problem, bedside cardiac monitors (for adults and children), diagnostic devices such as a halter monitor, and possibly a defibrillator. For a review of the assessment, treatment, and management of cardiac problems, see Volume 3, Chapter 2.

GI/GU CRISIS

Patients with various long-term devices to support gastrointestinal or genitourinary functions may need ALS intervention. Your response may be directly related to a problem with the GI or GU device, or you may simply need to be aware of the device and support during transport.

Urinary Tract Devices

There are various medical devices designed to support patients with urinary tract dysfunction. External devices, such as Texas catheters (also called condom catheters), attach to the male external genitalia to collect urine (Figure 6-9). Because these devices are not inserted into the urethra, they reduce the risk of in-

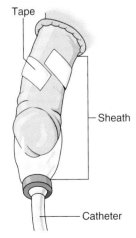

Tape

Sheath

Catheter

FIGURE 6-9 An external urinary tract device.

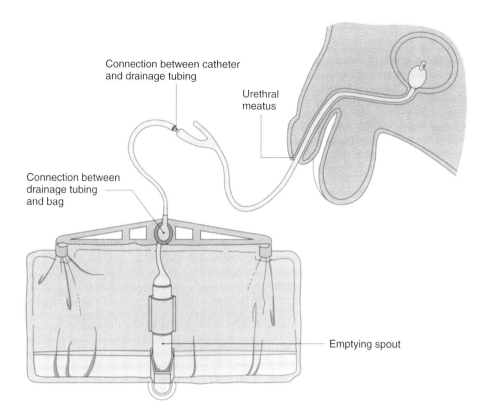

Connection between catheter
and drainage tubing

Urethral
meatus

Connection between
drainage tubing
and bag

Emptying spout

FIGURE 6-10   An internal urinary catheter with balloon. Note sites where bacteria can enter.

fection. However, they do not collect urine in a sterile manner, nor are they adequate for long-term use.

Internal catheters, such as Foley or indwelling catheters, are the most commonly used devices for urinary tract dysfunction. They are long catheters with a balloon tip that is inserted through the urethra into the urinary bladder. The balloon is then inflated with saline to keep the device in place (Figure 6-10). Internal catheters are well-tolerated for long-term use and are frequently found in hospitals, skilled nursing facilities, or home-care situations.

Suprapubic catheters are similar in purpose to internal catheters. However, they are inserted directly through the abdominal wall into the urinary bladder. Suprapubic catheters may be used instead of indwelling catheters in the event of surgery or other problems with the genitalia or bladder.

Urostomies are a surgical diversion of the urinary tract to a stoma, or hole, in the abdominal wall. A collection device will be attached to the stoma outside the body to collect urine. Urostomies are used when the bladder is unable to effectively collect urine.

* **urostomy** surgical diversion of the urinary tract to a stoma, or hole, in the abdominal wall.

Urinary Device Complications

Most complications related to urinary tract support devices result from infection or device malfunctions. Infection is a very common problem with urinary tract devices because the area is rich with pathogens and because the catheter provides a pathway directly into the body. Remain alert to foul-smelling urine or altered urine color, such as "tea" colored, cloudy, or blood-tinged urine. Also look for signs and symptoms of systemic infection, or urosepsis, as urinary infections can

FIGURE 6-11 A nasogastric feeding tube.

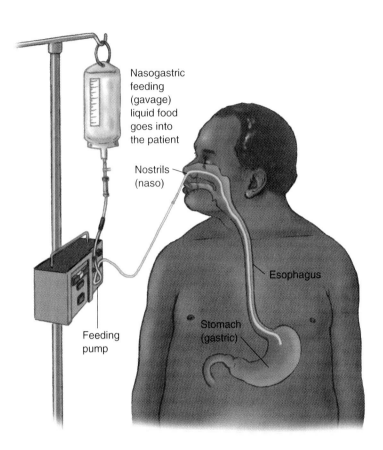

Nasogastric feeding (gavage) liquid food goes into the patient

Nostrils (naso)

Esophagus

Stomach (gastric)

Feeding pump

quickly spread in the immunocompromised patient. Suprapubic catheters or urostomies may also have infections at the abdominal wall site. You should note redness, swelling, heat, discharge, or loss of skin integrity.

Device malfunctions typically include accidental displacement of the device, obstruction, balloon ruptures in devices that use a balloon as an anchor, or leaking collection devices. Changes in the patient's anatomy, such as a shortened urinary tract or tissue necrosis can also cause malfunctions. Ensure that the collection device is empty and record the amount of urine output. Look for kinks or other obstructions in the device, and make sure that the collection bag is placed below the patient.

Gastrointestinal Tract Devices

You can expect to encounter a wide variety of devices to support the gastrointestinal tract. Nasogastric (NG) tubes are commonly seen by EMS personnel, as they are often used to decompress gastric contents in the prehospital environment (Figure 6-11). NG tubes may also be used to lavage the GI system in various situations, such as GI bleeding or substance ingestion. NG tubes are not usually long-term devices, as they cause discomfort and may lead to tissue necrosis in the nasal passages if left intact for an extended period.

Feeding tubes are more substantial than NG tubes and come to rest in either the duodenum or jejunum. Often they are weighted to help them pass through the pyloric sphincter and have a steel filament to facilitate insertion. Feeding tubes are used for supplemental nutrition when a person cannot swallow due to dysphagia, paralysis, or unconsciousness.

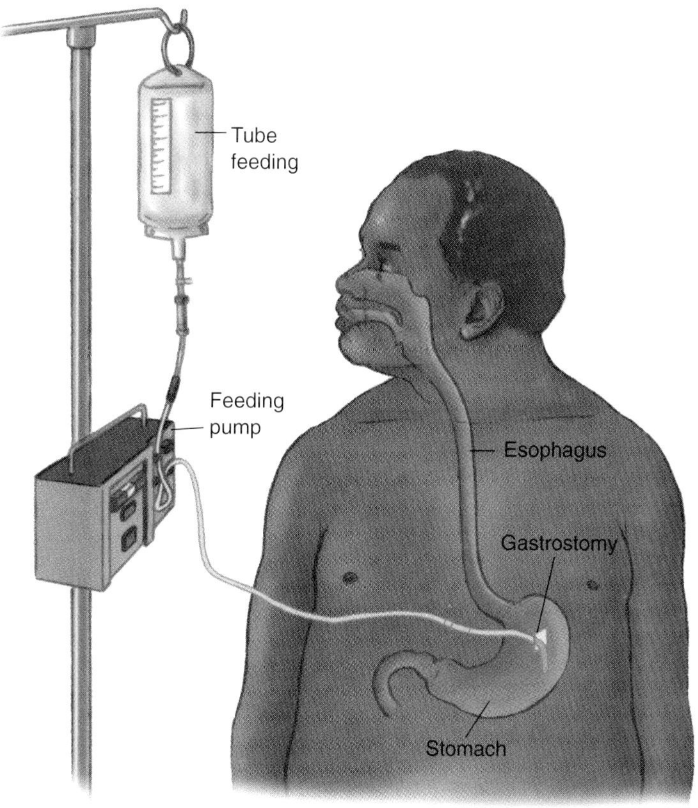

FIGURE 6-12   A gastrostomy feeding tube.

For longer-term supplemental nutrition, a gastric tube may be inserted through the abdominal wall into the small intestine (Figure 6-12). Indications for a gastrostomy tube include Alzheimer's disease, neurological deficits from strokes or head trauma, or mental retardation. Gastrostomy tubes come in many forms, such as percutaneous endoscopic gastrostomy (PEG) tubes, surgical gastrostomy tubes, and Jejunal tubes, to name a few. These tubes have different means of insertion (surgical vs. endoscopic), location (stomach vs. duodenum), and function (feeding vs. aspiration prevention).

A **colostomy** is used to bypass part of the large intestine and allow feces to be collected outside the body in a collection bag, either on a temporary or permanent basis. Indications for a colostomy include cancer of the bowel or rectum, diverticulitis, Crohn's disease, or trauma. A surgical connection of the bowel to an ostomy created in the skin results in diversion of feces into the collection bag (Figure 6-13).

✱ colostomy opening of a portion of the colon through the abdominal wall, allowing feces to be collected outside the body.

Gastrointestinal Tract Device Complications

Complications from GI tract devices include tube misplacement, obstruction, or infection. Because misplaced tubes can obstruct the airway or GI system, you should always ensure device patency if you have doubts about placement of the tube. First, have the patient speak to you. If he or she cannot speak, the tube may be in the airway and need to be removed. Second, to assure patency of an NG tube, used a 60 mL syringe to insert air into the stomach. Use your stethoscope to listen over the epigastrum for air movement within the stomach. A low-pitched, rumbling should be heard. You may also note stomach contents spontaneously moving up the tube or they may be aspirated with a 60 cc syringe. In such cases, patients may be repositioned to return patency, or the device may be reinserted.

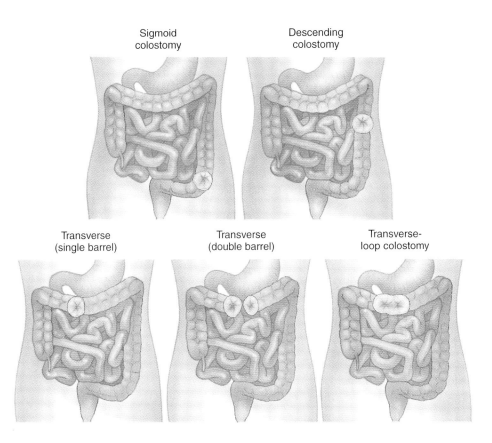

Sigmoid colostomy   Descending colostomy

Transverse (single barrel)   Transverse (double barrel)   Transverse-loop colostomy

FIGURE 6-13   Examples of colostomy stoma locations.

A displaced gastrostomy or jeuojenostomy tube must be replaced as soon as possible after dislodgement. Some services train paramedics in G-tube changes and insertions.

Tubes are also prone to obstructions. Colostomies may become clogged or otherwise obstructed. Feeding tubes can become clogged due to the thick consistency of supplemental feedings or pill fragments. As a result, the tubes may require irrigation with water. In addition, the thick consistency of food may cause bowel obstructions or constipation.

As might be expected, ostomies can become infected (or lose skin integrity from pressure). Look for signs and symptoms of skin or systemic infection. In addition, remember that digestive enzymes may leak from various ostomies and begin to digest the skin and abdominal contents.

Psychosocial Implications

Many patients with GI or GU support devices lead active and otherwise normal lives. These patients may be understandably self-conscious about their conditions and many experience embarrassment, avoidance, anger, or discomfort when questioned. You should be sensitive to the patient's emotions during your patient assessment and treatment.

ACUTE INFECTIONS

After physicians or hospital personnel treat open wounds, they typically release patients to home care. These wounds may be surgical wounds or loss of skin integrity for other reasons. In such instances, you may see dressings covering wounds to protect against infection, absorb drainage, or immobilize the wound area. Gauze packing may also be inserted in infected spaces to absorb drainage.

Drains may sometimes be inserted in a wound site to remove blood, serum bile, or pus from the area. Drains are typically soft rubber tubes that have one end in the wound and the other end attached to a bag or suction device. Common drains include the Penrose drain, which is a simple rubber tube, and the Jackson-Pratt drain, which includes a suction bulb.

Wounds are typically closed with sutures, wires, staples, or cyanoacrylate adhesives. The type of closure used depends upon the wound and the preferences of the physician closing it. Sutures are the most common device used to secure a wound, but staples and adhesives are becoming more widespread due to their ease of use. Wires are typically used to secure musculoskeletal structures, such as ribs or the sternum after a sternotomy.

In assessing wounds, always be aware of the potential for improper wound healing. As already mentioned, home care patients are at increased risk of infection. The immunological response and rate of wound healing expected in the general population is compromised in the home care patient by poor peripheral perfusion, a sedentary existence, the presence of percutaneous and implanted medical devices, the existences of chronic diseases, and more.

An infected superficial wound may quickly lead to major infections or sepsis in the immunocompromised or weakened patient. Keep in mind that the chronically ill or homebound patient, particularly the elderly, often have a decreased ability to perceive pain or to perform self-care. Pay particular attention to signs of infection in wounds found in home care patients. If you inspect a wound, be sure to use sterile technique and redress the wound. For more on the treatment of bedsores and shear, see Chapter 3.

Pay particular attention to signs of infection in wounds found in home care patients.

MATERNAL AND NEWBORN CARE

Today, many women who deliver their babies in a hospital will be discharged in 24 hours or less. This trend, fueled by rising health care costs, greatly shortens the transition time from hospital to home. Some parents may not yet be emotionally prepared to care for a new baby, especially first-time parents. Rapid discharge may also leave a mother or newborn with an unrecognized problem or complication stemming from delivery. As a result, you the ALS provider might be summoned to the home and called on to utilize the neonatology and pediatrics skills that you learned in Volume 3, Chapter 14, and in Chapters 1 and 2 of this volume.

Common Maternal Complications

For the mother, post partum bleeding and embolus (especially after Cesarean) are the most common complications. Management of an embolus would the same as with any patient with a similar complaint. Post partum bleeding can be a serious condition. Management steps include:

- Massage of uterus, if not already contracted
- Administration of fluids to correct hypotension
- Administration of certain medications, such as Pitocin (if ordered)
- Rapid transport to the hospital, if necessary

Mothers may also experience **post partum depression.** In such cases, women may have difficulty caring for both themselves and their newborn. In extreme cases, babies have been neglected or even harmed.

When entering the home, be sensitive to the needs of the parents. First-time mothers and/or fathers may be inexperienced in childrearing and may call EMS for what a more experienced parent might regard as normal. It is important that you always take any parent's concerns seriously, and if no medical support is needed, provide emotional reassurance. If you suspect neglect or abuse of the newborn, take actions recommended in Chapters 1, 2, and 4.

＊ **post partum depression** the "let down" feeling experienced during the period following birth occurring in 70-80% of mothers.

Common Infant/Child Complications

As pointed out in Chapter 1, newborns must rapidly adapt to a new environment and may well not have reached a state where they can thrive on their own. Newborns must be positioned properly to breathe, their noses must be clear (newborns are nose breathers), and they must be kept warm because of immature thermoregulation. Newborns also have immature immune systems and can develop rapid, life-threatening infections or septicemia.

Infants with recognized problems may already be receiving home care. They may have cardiac or respiratory abnormalities or other congenital defects. Premature or low birth weight babies—as well as babies with any number of respiratory disorders—are at risk for sleep apnea. Such babies may wear apnea monitors around their chest so that an alarm sounds at any pause in their breathing pattern. Some infants may also be on pulse oximetry. If you are summoned because of an alarm and find a normal breathing pattern, still encourage the parents or caregivers to have the baby examined as soon as possible.

As noted, newborns may also be discharged from the hospital with an undetected cardiac or respiratory condition. Signs and symptoms of cardiac or respiratory insufficiency include:

- Cyanosis
- Bradycardia (< 100 b/m)
- Crackles
- Respiratory distress

In such cases, resuscitation should be initiated immediately. Management should be towards respiratory support with BVM or intubation, as necessary. If any newborn has a heart rate < 80 b/m despite 30 seconds or more of oxygenation, start CPR. Preserve warmth and obtain a record from the parents of feeding intake since birth. If the infant has not been feeding or has been vomiting with diarrhea, it may be dehydrated. In this case, a fluid bolus of 20 mL/kg is indicated. If a peripheral IV cannot be obtained in two attempts or two minutes, obtain access via the intraosseus route. If blood sugar is below 80 mg/dl administer $D_{25}W$ (some experts suggest $D_{10}W$) at a dosage of 0.5 mg/kg.

For a newborn with infection or septicemia, look for fever, tachycardia, and irritability. If septicemia progresses to septic shock, you should initiate resuscitation as previously described.

Children who have serious, long-term health problems are usually cared for by their parents at home—with or without the help of a home care professional. Commonly found medical therapies for children who are home care patients include:

- Mechanical ventilators
- IV medications or nutrition
- Oxygen therapy
- Tracheostomies
- Feeding tubes
- Pulse oximeters
- Apnea monitors

Education of the parents or caregivers by doctors and nurses forms a critical component in their ability to deal with a crisis. Some people adapt well to the task and can deal with their child's chronic problems in a professional manner. Others, however, may become panicked or, either through misunderstanding or

Parents of children with special needs are often highly educated regarding their child's problem. Always listen to them even when their attitude may appear condescending.

Table 6-7	PERCENT OF HOSPICE PATIENTS BY AGE
Age	**Percent**
Under 45 years	8.1
45-54 years	7.9
55-64 years	14.8
65-69 years	8.7
70-74 years	15.6
75-79 years	14.5
80-84 years	12.3
85 years and older	16.4

Source: National Center for Health Statistics

denial, have little comprehension of the situation. As with any difficult call, maintain a professional demeanor at all times.

When dealing with children, remember to keep the parents or caregivers informed of your assessment and treatment plans. Children quickly pick up on a person's emotions. As a result, it is part of your job to act in a supportive and controlled manner. Calming a child could make a huge difference in the long-term effects of the current episode.

HOSPICE AND COMFORT CARE

Today more than 2,250 hospices—and hundreds of volunteer agencies—provide support for the terminally ill and their families. Initially philanthropic, these programs are now covered by Medicare. Some states—such as Florida, Michigan, Kentucky, and New York—also include them under Medicaid. Most programs are home-based, with Medicare and Medicaid stipulating that at least 80 percent of an agency's care be provided to patients in their homes.

Up to 450,000 patients a year receive services from hospices funded by Medicare or Medicaid. (Thousands more receive help from private or volunteer agencies.) Although the majority of Medicare patients are age 70 and older (Table 6-7), children receive benefits, too. Reimbursement is extended to those patients with a life expectancy of six months or less.

The goal of hospices is to provide palliative or comfort care rather than curative care (Table 6-8). This is a very different role than most other branches of the health care profession, including EMS. For an ALS team, care is usually geared toward aggressive and life-saving treatment. A hospice team, on the other hand, seeks to relieve symptoms, manage pain, and give patients control over the end of their lives. It is important to remember that these patients have, for the most part, exhausted or declined curative resources.

The goal of hospice care is to provide palliative or comfort care rather than curative care.

ALS Intervention

Involvement in a hospice situation can be a difficult and stressful call. In most cases, family members, caregivers, and health care workers have been instructed to call a hospice rather than EMS. However, you may be summoned for intervention, particularly in situations involving transport. You should always keep in mind that the hospice patient is in an end-stage disease and has already expressed wishes to withhold resuscitation. However, even a valid DNR order should not prevent you from performing palliative and/or comfort care.

Table 6-8 NATIONAL HOSPICE STANDARDS

The following are the National Hospice Organization Standards of a Hospice Program of Care, published by the National Hospice Association.

- Appropriate therapy is the goal of hospice care.
- Palliative care is the most appropriate form of care when cure is no longer possible.
- The goal of palliative care is the prevention of distress from chronic signs and symptoms.
- Admission to a hospice program of care depends upon patient and family needs.
- Hospice care consists of a blending of professional and nonprofessional services.
- Hospice care considers all aspects of the lives of patients and their families as valid areas of therapeutic concern.
- Hospice care is respectful of all patient and family belief systems and will employ resources to meet the personal philosophic, moral, and religious needs of patients and their families.
- Hospice care provides continuity of care.
- A hospice care program considers the patient and the family together as the unit of care.
- The patient's family is considered to be a central part of the hospice care team.
- Hospice care programs seek to identify, coordinate, and supervise persons who can give care to patients who do not have a family member available to take on the responsibility of giving care.
- Hospice care for the family continues into the bereavement period.
- Care is available 24 hours a day, 7 days a week.
- Hospice care is provided by an interdisciplinary team.
- Hospice programs will have structured and informal means of providing support to staff.
- Hospice programs will be in compliance with the standards of the National Hospice Organization and the applicable laws and regulations governing the organization and delivery of care to patients and families.
- The services of the hospice program are coordinated under a central administration.
- The optimal control of distressful symptoms is an essential part of a hospice care program requiring medical, nursing, and other services of the interdisciplinary team.
- The hospice care team will have a medical director on staff, physicians on staff, and a working relationship with the physicians.
- On the basis of patient's needs and preferences as determining factors in the setting and location for care, a hospice program provides inpatient care and care in the home setting.
- Education, training, and evaluation of hospice services is an on-going activity of a hospice care program.
- Accurate and current records are kept on all patients.

Common diseases that you can expect to see in hospice include:

- Congestive heart failure (CHF)
- Cystic fibrosis
- COPD
- AIDS (Figure 6-14)
- Alzheimer's
- Cancer

Terminally ill patients may take up to 3,000 milligrams of morphine a day with few side effects other than constipation.

In some instances, particularly with cancer, you may also be confronted with patients on high dosages of pain medications. In cases of cancer, for example, morphine is the drug of choice. It is important for you to know that patients, who often take doses of up to 3,000 milligrams a day, will have few side effects other than constipation. They will have grown used to the drug and normal side effects will not be seen. Other drugs that may be administered include Percocet, Oxycontin, or a Duragesic patch. Some patients may also have a portable pump that provides

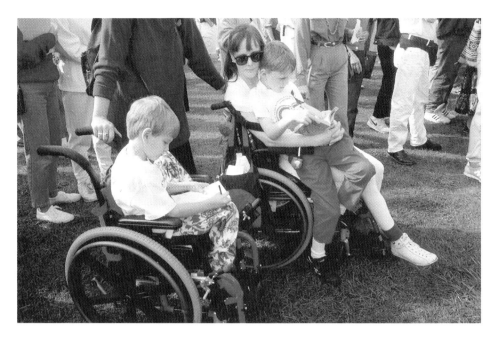

FIGURE 6-14   The incidence of AIDS and HIV infection in children is increasing worldwide. These children may be among the patients that you may encounter in a hospice setting.

a continuous infusion of medication through a PICC line. The pumps can be small and hidden by clothing.

In a hospice, you need to establish communication with the home health care worker as quickly as possible. Your inclination may be to intubate, start a line, or administer medications. However, as noted, palliative care supersedes curative care. A hospice worker, when faced with the end-stage of a disease, may do nothing in accordance with the patient's wishes. Therefore, it is vital that you gain a clear understanding of these wishes, whether through a family member or a written document. If you are called to the house, it is your responsibility to respect the wishes of the patient and the ideals of hospice care.

In a hospice situation, family members might panic at a patient's imminent death and appropriate care might involve support for the family rather than resuscitation of the patient. Local protocols may also vary in respect to DNRs, DNARs, living wills, and durable power of attorney documents. Be sure that you are familiar with these legal statements and their implications for care of the terminally ill. (See Volume 1, Chapter 6, "Medical/Legal Aspects of Prehospital Care.")

Terminally ill patients who are not involved in a hospice present a potentially gray area. Remember that while hospice prepares families for the impending death of their loved ones, families without hospice may be ill-prepared for the end-stages of life. Don't assume that all terminal patients are under hospice care. A simple question to determine the presence of hospice may alter your course of treatment and approach to the family.

Regardless of whether a patient is in hospice or not, keep in mind the stages of the grief process—denial, anger, depression, bargaining, and acceptance. Remember that both the patient and the family will go through these stages, and, in the case of the terminally ill, the patient may have reached acceptance well ahead of those who remain behind.

If you are called to the house of a terminally ill patient, it is your responsibility to respect the wishes of the patient and the ideals of hospice care.

Caring for a hospice patient can be a challenge for paramedics as they must act within the scope of the patient's wishes.

Content Review

STAGES OF DEATH AND GRIEF
- Denial
- Anger
- Depression
- Bargaining
- Acceptance

SUMMARY

The shift toward home health care is one of the most important trends of the 2000s and will have a great impact on the ALS profession. You can expect in your career to provide acute intervention for a growing number of chronic-care patients of all ages and in all stages of the disease process. These calls will challenge you to use all of your assessment skills in developing an effective management plan, which in many cases will be based on input from an extended team of home health care workers.

YOU MAKE THE CALL

Pridemark Paramedic 4 receives a call to assist a patient who has fallen out of a wheelchair. En route to the scene, dispatch informs the crew that the patient is a 32-year-old female with possible head injuries. A home health care worker is with the patient.

Upon arrival, the crew finds the patient supine on the floor, A/O ×3, with a relatively minor amount of blood caked into her hair over the left temple. The health care worker introduces herself as the nursing assistant who regularly visits the patient. When she arrived for her normal visit about 20 minutes earlier, she knocked on the door and heard the patient call out for help. She then opened the door with a key and found the patient on the floor.

While the EMT assesses the patient, the paramedic interviews the home care worker for a complete history and baseline presentation. During this time, the fire department arrives with three firefighters to assist per local protocol. The Pridemark crew notes that the patient's apartment is messy and dirty.

The home care worker explains that the patient has a left-sided neurological deficit from a right-sided head injury caused by a motor vehicle accident when the patient was 18 years old. The patient does have sensation on her left side, but movement is limited. Her left arm is normally contracted, and she has a left-sided facial droop. The home care worker shows the paramedic where the patient keeps her medications, but does not know what they are. Examination of the bottles reveals that the patient takes Tegretol, glucophage, and Zoloft.

Firefighters offer further history as they know the patient from past runs. They explain that the patient smokes heavily, uses marijuana, and can be hostile at times.

Members of the Pridemark crew meet to share what they have learned. The EMT reports that the patient fell out of her wheelchair last night—approximately 14 hours before the crew's arrival. She apparently lost her balance and was not dizzy, weak, or sick. She complains of being cold and demands a cigarette. There is blood on the left side of her temple, but the wound cannot be visualized due to matted hair. The patient denies loss of consciousness and does not want to go to the hospital. Blood pressure is 110/84, pulse is 72 normal and regular, and respirations are normal and non-labored. Skin is cool, dry, and normal in color. The patient's eyes are equal and reactive. The abdomen is soft and non-tender. No other injuries are noted.

The EMT reports that the patient is lying in a pool of urine. The home care worker states that the patient is normally incontinent. However, she seems quieter than usual.

Although the patient has no neck or back pain, c-spine stabilization is taken. The paramedic talks to the patient and attempts to get her consent for treatment and transport. After explaining that she could have a possible c-spine injury, the patient changes her mind and gives her approval. Although c-spine clearance is allowed in the local protocol, the paramedic feels that due to the patient's baseline neurological deficits, more caution is required.

The crew applies a rigid cervical collar. They then log roll the patient onto a long spine board and secure her in place. En route to the hospital, the crew conducts a secondary assessment with no new findings. Upon further questioning, the patient vehemently denies a history of diabetes or seizures, despite medications to the contrary. She repeatedly states, "I am normal!" She also denies allergies. A blood glucose test is not done due to the patient's strong emotional response to the procedure.

At the emergency department, the crew give a full report and transfers care of the patient to the hospital staff. The patient is later released from the hospital with a butterfly bandage for a one-inch head laceration and returned home by wheelchair van.

1. What does the condition of the apartment tell you?
2. Why is it important to immediately interview the home care worker?
3. What are some of the causes of urinary incontinence?
4. How can you rule out spinal injury to this patient?
5. Why do you think the patient denies a history of diabetes and seizures if she takes Tegretol and glucophage?
6. Why is it acceptable to defer the glucose test when patient medications indicate a possible blood sugar problem?
7. Was there any need for an IV?
8. Should the patient have been placed on oxygen?

See Suggested Responses at the back of this book.

FURTHER READING

Balinsky, W.: *Home Care: Current Problems and Future Solutions.* San Francisco, CA. Jossey-Bass Publishers, 1994.

Schmidt, C.A.: "EMS on the Acute Interventions for Chronic-Care Patients," JEMS, December 1999, pp. 68-76.

Spratt, S.J., *et. al.,* eds.: *Home Health Care: Principles and Practices.* Delray Beach, FL. GR/St. Lucie Press, 1997.

Illustrated Guide to Home Health Care. Springhouse, PA. Springhouse Corporation, 1995.

ON THE WEB

Visit Brady's Paramedic Website at www.bradybooks.com/paramedic.

CHAPTER 7

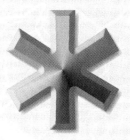

Assessment-Based Management

Objectives

After reading this chapter, you should be able to:

1. Explain how effective assessment is critical to clinical decision making. (pp. 292–294)
2. Explain how the paramedic's attitude and uncooperative patients affect assessment and decision making. (pp. 294–296)
3. Explain strategies to prevent labeling, tunnel vision, and decrease environmental distractions. (pp. 293–297)
4. Describe how personnel considerations and staffing configurations

affect assessment and decision making. (pp. 296–297)
5. Synthesize and apply concepts of scene management and choreography to simulated emergency calls. (p. 297)
6. Explain the roles of the team leader and the patient care person. (p. 297)
7. List and explain the rationale for bringing the essential care items to the patient. (pp. 297-298)

Continued

8. When given a simulated call, list the appropriate equipment to be taken to the patient. (p. 298)
9. Explain the general approach to the emergency patient. (pp. 298–302)
10. Explain the general approach, patient assessment differentials, and management priorities for patients with various types of emergencies that may be experienced in prehospital care. (pp. 304, 305–314)
11. Describe how to effectively communicate patient information face to face, over the telephone, by radio, and in writing. (pp. 302–304)
12. Given various preprogrammed and moulaged patients, provide the appropriate scene size-up, initial assessment, focused assessment, and detailed assessment, then provide the appropriate care, ongoing assessments, and patient transport. (pp. 291–314)

CASE STUDY

It's after midnight. In fact, a glance at the clock on the station wall tells me it's 3:05 on Sunday morning. I sigh with relief, thinking the worst is probably over for the weekend. Just then, the bell rings, signaling another call. Dispatch reports a single-vehicle crash on Moonglow Road, just outside of town. The caller has given no additional information.

I'm thinking: I wish the caller had provided more information. It's a single-vehicle crash, but we don't know how bad it is or how many patients there might be. The injuries could be minor or severe. Maybe the driver had a medical condition that caused the crash. My partner and I agree that we have to keep an open mind. No tunnel vision. We need to be prepared for anything. While my partner drives to the scene, I'm making a mental list of all the possible medical conditions and injuries that could be involved, and I'm mentally reviewing equipment that we'll need, including airway and ventilation devices, scissors to cut away clothing, dressings and bandages, immobilization equipment, and ECG monitor/defibrillator.

As we near the scene, I pull on gloves. Anticipating blood spatter, I have mask and eye protection ready, too. I look around carefully to determine scene safety. All the nearby telephone poles appear undamaged (*So no electrical injuries, I'm*

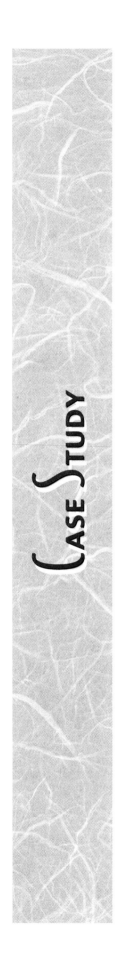

thinking), and the police already have traffic under control. I spot the vehicle and surmise from the damage that it has rolled several times. Out in the field, about 50 yards from where the vehicle finally landed, I observe a crowd of people surrounding someone lying on the ground. A police officer tells us this is the driver. There were no passengers and nobody else has been hurt, they say. However, the person who called in the accident seems to have left the scene, so there are no witnesses to interview.

I'm thinking: So there's only one patient, as far as we know. A roll-over and ejection—a significant mechanism of injury. It'll be a big surprise if this person hasn't suffered multiple major injuries. So it's really important for us to be systematic about our assessment. We don't want to get panicked and miss something.

As we approach the patient, I notice that he is in a supine position with his right leg flexed under him at an unnatural angle. He appears unresponsive to the crowd and the glare of flashlights. Any blood would be soaking into the ground, so it's hard to estimate how much he's lost. But the only blood I see on his clothing is a spreading stain on the pants legs where one leg is bent under the other.

I'm thinking: There must have been multiple impacts when he struck the inside of the car and then the ground. Maybe the car even rolled over on him at some point. From the angle of that right leg and the blood on his pants, I'm anticipating an open fracture of the right tibia, but that may be the least of his problems. I may find more external bleeding when I do the rapid trauma assessment. And with all that blunt trauma, there are likely to be internal injuries and internal bleeding, too. My general impression is that of a seriously injured male in his mid twenties.

When we reach the patient, my partner immediately stabilizes his head and neck. I call out to the patient but get no response. I squeeze his shoulder and he makes a slight pushing-away gesture. I open the airway, using a jaw thrust. The patient is breathing, but shallowly and only about 8 times a minute. My partner has already grabbed a BVM out of the jump kit and is ready to assist the patient's ventilations with supplemental oxygen.

Checking pulses, I find that the patient has no radial pulses but does have a carotid pulse, indicating that his systolic blood pressure is probably somewhere between 60 and 80 mmHg. His skin is pale, cool, and clammy. As I noted earlier, a considerable amount of blood is coming from an injury to his right leg where it is bent under him. Two EMT-basics have just arrived on the scene, and I assign one of them to quickly get the bleeding under control with direct pressure while I continue my assessment.

I'm thinking: Inadequate breathing . . . copious external bleeding . . . pale, cool, clammy skin, no peripheral pulses and a low, possibly falling, blood pressure, all indicating shock. . . . This is definitely a high priority patient. However, we mustn't get sidetracked by the apparent fracture and external bleeding. I'll complete the rapid trauma exam to be sure I've found all immediate life threats and so we can prioritize care, then prepare him for immediate transport.

I perform a head-to-toe rapid trauma assessment in less than 60 seconds, finding a reddened area over the right upper abdominal quadrant. When I palpate the area, the patient flinches. (*Reddening of the skin—the area hasn't had time to look bruised yet—tenderness on palpation. . . . These indicate internal injury and internal bleeding, making expedited transport an even more urgent priority.*)

As I expose and assess the extremities, I confirm an open right tibial fracture. I direct one of the EMTs to assess vital signs while the other EMT and I apply gentle traction to straighten the right leg. I quickly place a pressure dressing over the open wound. Then, the EMTs, my partner, and I log roll the patient and immobilize him to a long backboard.

I have found no medical ID medallion. The pulse is weak and rapid but steady. The patient has responded to painful stimulus with no indication of weakness or paralysis. There is a strong odor of alcohol on the patient's breath, and one of the policemen says they found an open container of bourbon in the car.

I'm thinking: No medical ID that would tell me he's diabetic, for instance. No indication of a heart attack or stroke. Other than alcohol intoxication, there's no evidence of a medical condition as the cause of the accident. So far, this seems to be a straightforward case of alcohol leading to trauma, external and internal bleeding, and shock.

Further assessment and emergency care will have to be done en route to the emergency department. We have been on the scene for approximately 8 minutes.

One of the EMTs offers to drive the ambulance to the hospital so my partner and I can both attend the patient. En route, I complete an ongoing assessment. The patient is stable, and I have time to perform a detailed physical exam but make no further findings. Meanwhile, my partner has started two IVs of lactated Ringer's. I complete another ongoing assessment. By the time we arrive at the emergency department, the patient has begun to respond when we call to him.

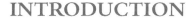

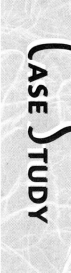

INTRODUCTION

The Case Study that opens this chapter demonstrates that a paramedic does more than just follow a standard sequence of assessment steps—scene size-up, initial assessment, focused history and physical exam, ongoing assessment, and detailed physical exam. While carrying out the assessment in a systematic way, a paramedic is constantly thinking and reasoning.

The kind of reasoning a paramedic needs to do has been described as an "inverted pyramid"—with the broad end at the top and the narrow point at the bottom (Figure 7-1). As soon as you receive the dispatch and the patient's chief

FIGURE 7-1 Follow an inverted pyramid format to avoid tunnel vision while working toward a field diagnosis.

DIFFERENTIAL DIAGNOSIS Form a mental list of possible causes of the patient's complaint. Consider as many causes as possible. Think broadly. Avoid tunnel vision.

NARROWING PROCESS Use information gathered during the assessment to eliminate some possible causes, support others based on patterns of signs, symptoms, and history. Begin narrowing toward a field diagnosis.

FIELD DIAGNOSIS Form a field diagnosis of the most probable cause or causes of the patient's complaint, based on information gathered during the assessment.

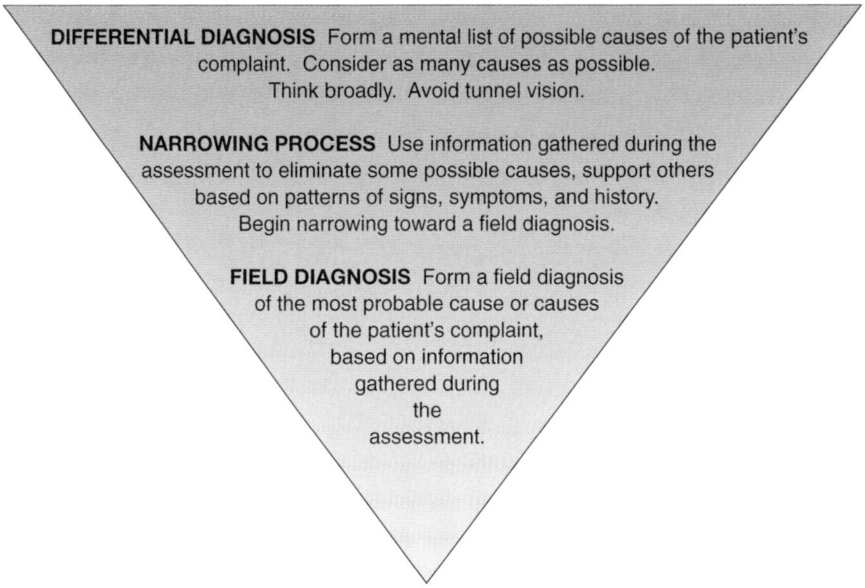

complaint, you try to form a mental list of all the possible causes of the patient's problem. (Such a list is often called a "differential diagnosis.") You want to keep your mind wide open, avoiding tunnel vision.

The patient in the Case Study was the victim of an auto crash and had an obvious open extremity fracture with associated external blood loss. Serious as it was, the paramedic resisted being distracted by this injury. Suppose the patient had suffered a heart attack or cardiac arrest prior to or following the crash. (The paramedic determined that he didn't.) Suppose the patient had other, more serious injuries. (The paramedic determined that he probably did—blunt abdominal trauma and internal bleeding.) What if the paramedic had not considered these other possibilities, had focused on the obvious leg injury, and had spent on-scene time splinting the fracture instead of completing the assessment and initiating rapid transport?

In this case, the paramedic used inverted-pyramid reasoning skills (which may also be called critical thinking, problem-solving, or clinical decision-making) to assess the patient and prioritize emergency care. The paramedic began by considering a wide variety of possible medical conditions and injuries. Then, while working through the standard sequence of assessment steps, the paramedic used the information gathered at each step of the assessment to eliminate some possibilities and support other possibilities. The paramedic considered pertinent negatives (signs that were *not* present, such as paralysis or an erratic pulse) as well as findings that were present (such as reddening and tenderness in one abdominal quadrant) to narrow in on a field diagnosis.

EFFECTIVE ASSESSMENT

Assessment forms the foundation for patient care.

Assessment forms the foundation for patient care. You can't treat or report a problem that is not found or identified. To find a problem, you must gather, evaluate, and synthesize information. Based on this process, you can then make decisions and take appropriate actions—formulate a management plan and determine the priorities for patient care.

A paramedic is entrusted with a great deal of independent judgment and responsibility for performing the correct actions for each individual patient, including such advanced skills as ECG interpretation, rapid sequence intubation,

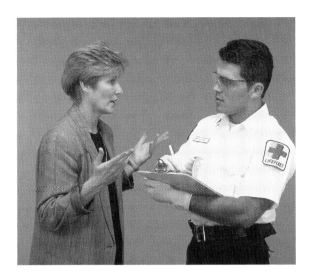

FIGURE 7-2   If the patient is unable to provide a history, gather information for the patient history from family members or bystanders.

and medication administration. Additionally, the medical director and hospital staff must rely on your experience and expertise as you describe the patient's condition and your conclusions about it. Consequently, the ability to reason and to reach a field diagnosis is critical to paramedic practice.

IMPORTANCE OF ACCURATE INFORMATION

The decisions that you make as a paramedic will only be as good as the information that you collect. To make accurate decisions, you need to gather accurate information.

The decisions you make as a paramedic will only be as good as the information you collect.

The History

A patient's history is a crucial part of the medical record, especially in medical conditions (as contrasted to trauma, where the physical exam takes precedence over the history). Very often, doctors will base 80 percent of their diagnosis upon the history. As a result, it is important for you to question the patient, family members, and bystanders (Figure 7-2). However, you must not allow your knowledge of the disease—or your suspicion of the underlying problem—to affect the quality of the history you gather. Just because a patient has had a heart attack in the past does not mean that the person is having one now. Focus your questioning on the present complaint and associated problems.

The Physical Exam

Never forget, or minimize, the importance of a thorough physical exam, especially when there is the possibility of trauma. Although the physical exam may be compromised by field conditions, it should never be done in a cursory manner. Even when you are dealing with angry family members or are in a bad physical environment, you must perform an effective examination. If field conditions make the exam difficult or nearly impossible, you may have to move the patient into the ambulance or some other controlled environment in order to perform the exam. If the patient is unresponsive or if there is a significant mechanism of injury, perform a complete head-to-toe assessment. If a patient is a responsive medical patient or has suffered minor trauma, focus your exam on the systems associated with the patient's chief complaint.

Pattern Recognition

In assessing a patient, remain alert to patterns. Compare the information that you gather with your knowledge base—what you have learned about the pathophysiology and presentation of various diseases and injuries. For example, a trauma patient with decreased mental status, unequal pupils, swelling or discoloration around the eyes, and bleeding from the ear is presenting a pattern typical of basilar skull fracture. A patient who complains of a cough, gradual onset of breathing difficulty, sharp chest pain, and shaking chills with an elevated temperature is displaying a pattern typical of pneumonia. There may be times when you don't recognize a pattern. Obviously, the greater your knowledge base, the greater the likelihood you will recognize patterns. The ability to recognize patterns also increases with experience, which is why new paramedics are generally assigned to work with experienced paramedics for a time.

Assessment/Field Diagnosis

Sometimes your field diagnosis will be based on a combination of pattern recognition and intuition, which is also based on experience. Once you have determined the problem, your next step is to formulate a plan of action, based upon the patient's condition and the environment.

BLS/ALS Protocols

All EMS systems have protocols devised by the medical director that guide both BLS and ALS patient care. However, protocols and standing orders do not replace the paramedic's judgment. For example, you must exercise judgment, based on your assessment and field diagnosis, to know which protocol to use. You must exercise judgment to know when and how to follow a protocol—and you must also exercise judgment about when to deviate from a protocol. If a patient is allergic to a medication, for example, you do not administer it, even though a protocol calls for its use.

FACTORS AFFECTING ASSESSMENT AND DECISION MAKING

A number of factors—both internal (for example, your personal attitudes) and external (for example, the patient's attitude, distracting injuries, or environmental factors at the scene)—can affect your assessment of the patient and ultimately your decisions on how to manage treatment. By keeping these factors in mind, you can avoid the limitations that they impose on your collection and evaluation of patient information.

Personal Attitudes

You must be as non-judgmental as possible to avoid "short circuiting" accurate data collection and the recognition of patterns.

Your attitude is one of the most critical factors in performing an effective assessment. You must be as nonjudgmental as possible to avoid "short circuiting" accurate data collection and pattern recognition by leaping to conclusions before completing a thorough assessment. Remember the popular computer mnemonic GIGO—garbage in/garbage out. You can't reach valid conclusions about your patient based on a hasty or incomplete assessment. You will be unable to provide good medical management if, for example, you base decisions on the patient's social standing or "likability."

Seek to identify any preconceived notions that you may have about a group and then work to eliminate them. As mentioned in Chapter 3, for example, a number of signs and symptoms have been mistakenly ascribed to aging when in

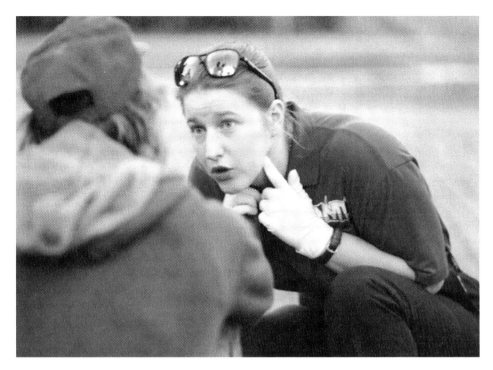

FIGURE 7-3   In treating substance abuse patients, maintain a nonjudgmental attitude.

fact they may point to serious medical conditions. A preconception that decreased mental acuity in an elderly patient is "normal" may lead you to miss what is really wrong with this patient and cause you to provide inadequate care.

Uncooperative Patients

Admittedly, uncooperative patients make it difficult to perform good assessments. All too often these patients are perceived as being "high," either on alcohol or drugs. However, you must remember that there are many other possible causes for patient belligerence.

Whenever assessing an uncooperative or restless patient, consider medical causes—hypoxia, hypovolemia, hypoglycemia, or a head injury, such as a concussion or a subdural hematoma. Be careful not to jump to the conclusion that this patient is "just another drunk" or a "frequent flyer." The frequent flyer that you have transported for alcoholic behavior in the past may, this time, be suffering from trauma or a medical emergency.

If the person is in fact a substance abuser, keep in mind that abuse or addiction is an illness. No matter how difficult these patients are to manage, they still deserve the best care that you can provide (Figure 7-3). If you treat every patient in the manner in which you would want your loved ones treated, you will seldom go wrong.

If you treat every patient in the manner in which you would want your loved ones treated, you will never go wrong.

Patient Compliance

Not all patients welcome the sight of an ALS team. Cultural and ethnic barriers—as well as prior negative experiences—may cause a patient to lack confidence in the rescuers. Such situations make it difficult for you to be effective at the scene, and the patients in fact may refuse to provide expressed consent for treatment or transport. It is your job to treat the patients in a way that will increase their confidence. If language is a barrier, try to speak through a friend, relative, or bystander who understands the patient's language, or in the case of deafness, signs. If you live in a community with a large ethnic population, try to become familiar with body language and customs of that culture. For example, some groups consider it rude to make eye contact. (For more on culturally diverse patients, see Chapter 5.) Again, don't permit yourself to make snap judgments about the patient.

Distracting Injuries

Yet another factor that can affect your assessment and decisions involves obvious, but distracting injuries. In the Case Study at the opening of this chapter, a nasty-looking tibial fracture might have caused the paramedic to overlook the less obvious signs of internal bleeding. Scalp lacerations usually look worse than they really are and could divert your attention from more serious injuries, such as an open chest wound. You must resist the temptation to form a field diagnosis too early. While paramedics often have to rely on their "gut instinct," it may also lead them to make snap judgments. An open, bleeding fracture of the femur may be so distracting that a paramedic rushes to treat it, missing the fact that the patient is also having difficulty breathing. Always take a systematic approach to patient assessment to avoid distractions and to find and prioritize care for all of the patient's injuries and conditions.

Environmental and Personnel Considerations

You've probably already experienced some of the environmental factors that can affect patient assessment and care. Among others, they include scene chaos, violent or dangerous situations, high noise levels, or crowds of bystanders. Even crowds of responders can be a problem, in some instances.

A large number of rescuers moving around can be just as distracting as a large number of bystanders.

While having enough help is crucial, it is also important to use personnel wisely (Figure 7-4). A large number of rescuers moving around can be just as distracting as a large number of bystanders. In such situations, some of the rescuers might be staged nearby and brought to the scene when and if necessary. Some may also be assigned to control bystanders.

As a rule, assessment is best achieved by one rescuer. A single paramedic can gather information and provide treatment sequentially. In the case of two paramedics, one paramedic can assess the patient, while the other provides simultaneous treatment. With multiple responders, however, assessment and history may take place by "committee," which often leads to disorganized management.

FIGURE 7-4   When multiple responders are on the scene, everyone should have a designated task.

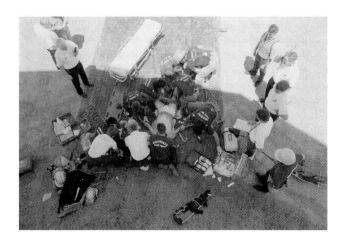

ASSESSMENT/MANAGEMENT CHOREOGRAPHY

While too many people, or multiple-tier responders, may make it hard to acquire a patient history and conduct a physical exam, it becomes even more difficult if the responders are all at the same professional level and have no clear direction. It is important to plan for these events so that personnel have predesignated roles. (See Chapter 9 on incident command.) These roles may be rotated among team members so no one is left out, but there must be a plan to avoid "freelancing." If there is only one paramedic, then that person must assume all ALS roles.

In the case of a two-paramedic team, an effective preplan involves the roles of team leader and patient care provider, assigned on an alternating basis. Paramedics who work together regularly may develop their own plan, but a universally understood plan allows for other rescuers to participate in a rescue without interrupting the flow. While the dynamics of field situations may necessitate changes in plans, a general "game plan" can go a long way toward preventing chaos. If field dynamics dictate a change in the preplanned roles, you are still working from a solid base. In setting up a two-person team, keep in mind the following descriptions of team leader and patient care provider roles.

Team Leader

The team leader is usually the person who will accompany the patient through to definitive care. The paramedic charged with this role should establish contact and maintain dialogue with the patient. He or she obtains the history, performs the physical examination, and presents the patient, in both verbal and written reports. During multiple casualty situations, the team leader acts as the initial EMS commander.

The team leader must maintain overall patient perspective and provide leadership to the team by designating tasks and coordinating transportation. While the team leader must actively participate in critical interventions, it is important that this person not fall into the trap of trying to do everything alone. During ACLS calls, for example, the team leader's tasks might include the following: reading the ECG, talking on the radio and giving drug orders, controlling the drug box, and keeping notes on drug administrations and effects. Actual treatment, however, would be left to the designated patient care provider.

Content Review

ROLES OF TEAM LEADER
- Obtains history
- Performs physical exam
- Presents patient
- Handles documentation
- Acts as EMS commander

Patient Care Provider

The patient care provider should ensure "scene cover"—i.e., watching the team leader's back. This person should gather scene information, talk to relatives and bystanders, and obtain vital signs. The patient care provider performs any skills or interventions requested by the team leader, such as attaching monitoring leads, administering oxygen, obtaining venous access, administering medications, and securing transportation equipment. In multiple casualty situations, the patient care provider acts as the triage group leader. During ACLS calls, he or she administers drugs, monitors tube placement, and oversees BCLS.

Content Review

ROLES OF PATIENT CARE PROVIDER
- Provides scene cover
- Gathers scene information
- Talks to relatives/bystanders
- Obtains vital signs
- Performs interventions
- Acts as triage group leader

THE RIGHT EQUIPMENT

Having the right equipment at the patient's side is essential. As a paramedic, you must be prepared to manage many conditions and injuries or changes in the patient's condition. As already mentioned, assessment and management must usually be done simultaneously. If you do not have the right equipment readily available, then you have compromised patient care and, in fact, the patient may die.

If you do not have the right equipment readily available, you have compromised patient care.

Think of your equipment as items in a backpack. Just like backpacking, you must downsize your equipment to minimum weight and bulk to facilitate rapid movement. At the same time, you need certain essential equipment to ensure survival—in this case, patient survival. The following is a list of the essential equipment for paramedic management of life-threatening conditions. You must bring these items to the side of every patient, regardless of what you initially think you may need:

- Infection Control
  - Infection control supplies—e.g., gloves, eye shields
- Airway Control
  - Oral airways
  - Nasal airways
  - Suction (electric or manual)
  - Rigid tonsil-tip and flexible suction catheters
  - Laryngoscope and blades
  - Endotracheal tubes, stylettes, syringes, tape
- Breathing
  - Pocket mask
  - Manual ventilation bag-valve-mask
  - Spare masks in various sizes
  - Oxygen tank and regulator
  - Oxygen masks, cannulas, and extension tubing
  - Occlusive dressings
  - Large bore IV catheter for thoracic decompression
- Circulation
  - Dressings
  - Bandages and tape
  - Sphygmomanometer, stethoscope
  - Note pad and pen or pencil
- Disability
  - Rigid collars
  - Flashlight
- Dysrhythmia
  - Cardiac monitor/defibrillator
- Exposure and Protection
  - Scissors
  - Space blankets or something to cover the patient

You may also pack some optional "take in" equipment, such as drug therapy and venous access supplies. The method by which these supplies are carried may depend upon how your system is designed—e.g., paramedic ambulances versus paramedics in non-transporting vehicles. It may also depend upon local protocols, flexibility of standing orders, the number of paramedic responders in your area, and the difficulty of accessing patients because of terrain or some other problem.

In most cases, venous access supplies should be carried with the drug box since venous access is required to administer most medications. The drug box should also contain any medications allowed in the formulary.

GENERAL APPROACH TO THE PATIENT

In addition to having the essential equipment, you need to have the essential demeanor to calm or reassure the patient. You must look and act the part of a professional, while exhibiting the compassion and understanding associated with an effective "bedside manner." While patients may not have the ability to rate your medical performance, they can certainly rate your people skills and service. Be aware of your body language and the messages it sends, either intentionally or unintentionally. Think carefully about what you say and how you say it—this includes your conversations with other members of the ALS team and anyone else at the scene.

Be aware of your body language and the messages it sends, either intentionally or unintentionally.

Once again, it helps to preplan your general approach to the patient. This will prevent confusion and improve the accuracy of your assessment. One team member should engage in an active, concerned dialogue with the patient. This same person should also demonstrate the listening skills needed to collect information and to convey a caring attitude. Taking notes may prevent asking the same question repeatedly, as well as ensure that you acquire and pass on accurate data.

By approaching the patient with the right equipment and the right attitude, you minimize confusion and stand ready to provide effective emergency care.

The following sections briefly review the steps of the assessment that you will perform systematically on all patients. To review the assessment steps in detail, see Volume 2 Chapter 3.

SCENE SIZE-UP

The scene size up has the following components:

- Body substance isolation—Be sure you are wearing disposable gloves and are wearing or have available other protective equipment that may be needed such as gown, mask, and eye protection.
- Scene safety—Observe the scene for any hazards to yourself, other rescuers, bystanders, and the patient. This is as important at a medical scene as at a trauma scene.
- Locate all patients, such as those who may have wandered away from a vehicle collision or additional patients in a household where the patient appears to be suffering from carbon monoxide or other toxic exposure.
- Mechanism of injury or nature of the illness—Determine this as well as possible at this stage of the call and remain observant for additional information as the call progresses.

If you determine that you may need additional equipment or support, now is the time to call for help.

INITIAL ASSESSMENT

After you size up the scene, you quickly begin the initial assessment for the purpose of detecting and treating immediate life threats. The components of the initial assessment are:

- Forming a general impression
- Mental status assessment (AVPU)
- Airway assessment
- Breathing assessment
- Circulation assessment
- Determining the patient's priority for further on-scene care or immediate transport

Depending on your findings during the initial assessment, you might determine that one of the following approaches is appropriate for the patient's priority status.

Resuscitative Approach

Take the resuscitation approach whenever you suspect a life-threatening problem, including:

- Cardiac or respiratory arrest
- Respiratory distress or failure
- Unstable dysrhythmias
- Status epilepticus (series of generalized motor seizures without an intervening return of consciousness)
- Coma or altered mental status
- Shock or hypotension
- Major trauma
- Possible C-spine injury

In these cases, you must take immediate resuscitative action (such as CPR and defibrillation and ventilation) or other critical action (such as supplemental oxygen, control of major bleeding, or C-spine immobilization). Additional assessment and care can be performed after resuscitation and the rapid trauma assessment and/or en route to the hospital.

Contemplative Approach

Use the contemplative approach when immediate intervention is not necessary, such as with stable chest pain or a mild allergic reaction. In such situations, the focused history and physical exam, followed by any required interventions, will be performed at the scene, before transport to the hospital.

Immediate Evacuation

In some situations, you will need to immediately evacuate the patient to the ambulance (Figure 7-5). For example, a patient with severe internal bleeding requires life-saving interventions beyond a paramedic's skills. You might also resort to immediate evacuation if the scene is too chaotic for rational assessment or if it is too unsafe or unstable.

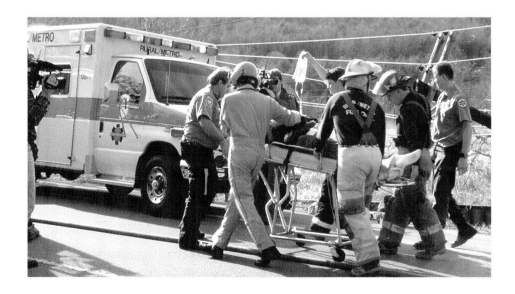

FIGURE 7-5   High-priority patients require immediate evacuation, with continued assessment and care done en route.

FOCUSED HISTORY AND PHYSICAL EXAM

Following the initial assessment, you will perform the focused history and physical exam. Based on the patient's chief complaint and the information you have gathered during the initial assessment, you should consider your patient to belong to one of the following four categories:

- Trauma patient with a significant mechanism of injury or altered mental status
- Trauma patient with an isolated injury
- Medical patient who is responsive
- Medical patient who is unresponsive

For a trauma patient with a significant mechanism of injury or altered mental status or for an unresponsive medical patient, perform a complete head-to-toe physical examination (rapid trauma assessment for the trauma patient, rapid medical assessment for the medical patient). For the trauma patient with an isolated injury or for the responsive medical patient, perform a physical exam focused on body systems related to the chief complaint.

For a medical patient, gather the history before performing the physical exam, unless the patient is unable to provide a history and there are no family members or bystanders who can provide information. For a trauma patient, gather the history after you have performed the physical exam. (Of course, elements of the history and the physical exam are often obtained simultaneously if partners are working together or as you talk to the responsive patient while examining him.)

THE ONGOING ASSESSMENT AND THE DETAILED PHYSICAL EXAM

The ongoing assessment must be performed on all patients to monitor and to observe trends in the patient's condition—every 5 minutes if the patient is unstable, every 15 minutes if the patient is stable. Ongoing assessments must be performed until the patient is transferred to the care of hospital personnel. The ongoing assessment includes evaluation of the following:

- Mental status
- Airway, breathing, and circulation (ABCs)
- Transport priorities
- Vital signs
- Focused assessment of any problem areas or conditions
- Effectiveness of interventions
- Management plans

The detailed physical exam is similar to but more thorough than the rapid trauma assessment. It is generally performed only on trauma patients and only if time and the patient's condition permit. The purpose is to find any injuries or conditions that may have been missed during earlier assessments. In a critical patient, continuing ongoing assessments are more important than a detailed physical exam.

IDENTIFICATION OF LIFE-THREATENING PROBLEMS

At all stages of the assessment, you must actively and continuously look for and manage any life-threatening problems.

At all stages of the assessment, from initial assessment through ongoing assessments, from the scene to the ambulance to arrival at the hospital, you must actively and continuously look for and manage any life-threatening problems.

You need to rapidly determine the chief complaint and to assess the distress in a systematic manner. Obtain baseline vital signs along with the focused physical exam, but if partners are working together, one may obtain the baseline vital signs earlier in the assessment. Focus on the relevant portions of the history and the physical findings. For example, a history of appendicitis would be relevant for a patient complaining of right lower quadrant pain, less relevant for a trauma patient with possible spinal injury.

If you have an educated suspicion of what you are looking for, then you will be able to ask more productive questions. However, you are less likely to find something if you don't suspect it. For this reason, throughout your assessment, keep in mind the mechanism of injury and the nature of the illness (as determined, starting with the initial assessment and the patient's chief complaint). Listen carefully to everything the patient says. With experience, you will develop skill at "multi-tasking"—asking questions, listening to answers, and caring for the patient almost simultaneously. However, until you gain that experience, and unless you are actively managing a life-threatening condition, ask questions and just listen. Allow your partner to perform necessary tasks so that you do not miss any important clues.

The underlying principle of assessment-based management is to rapidly and accurately assess the patient and then to treat for the worst case scenario.

The ability of a patient to describe symptoms and a paramedic's ability to listen greatly affect the quality and outcome of an assessment. The severity of pain does not always correlate well with the life-threatening potential of a condition. For example, a long splinter jammed under a fingernail will certainly cause pain, but few lives have been lost to such an injury. Conversely, some patients, especially the elderly, suffer myocardial infarctions with only vague symptoms that do not include chest pain. In addition, the location of pain and its source do not always correlate well, especially if it is visceral pain. For example, gall bladder attacks are often characterized by pain that is referred to the shoulder. As a paramedic, you must listen with your ears and then use your knowledge base about various illnesses and diseases to interpret what the patient says.

Basically your role as paramedic is to rapidly and accurately assess the patient and then to treat for the worst case scenario. This is the underlying principle of assessment-based management—your guide for providing effective emergency care.

PRESENTING THE PATIENT

The ability to communicate effectively is the key to transferring patient information, whether in an out-of-hospital setting or within the hospital itself. Although neither basic nor advanced life-support interventions may be required for every patient, a skill that will be used on every single patient is that of effective presentation, whether it is over the radio or telephone, in writing, or in face-to-face transfers at the receiving facility. Despite the frequency with which paramedics present patients, this is often the weakest link in patient care.

ESTABLISHING TRUST AND CREDIBILITY

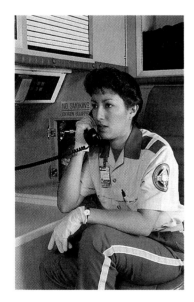

FIGURE 7-6   A clear, concise patient report will enable the hospital staff to prepare for the needs of the patient.

Effective presentation and communication skills help establish a paramedic's credibility (Figure 7-6). They also inspire the trust and confidence of patients and other medical personnel. If you present your assessment, your findings, and your treatment in a clear, concise manner, you give the impression of a job well done. A poor presentation, on the other hand, implies poor assessment and poor patient care.

Other health care providers have little time or interest in listening to rambling, disjointed presentations that cover unimportant details while omitting vital information. Use the SOAP format or some variation of it. Not only does SOAP help you organize your presentation, most health care providers have become accustomed to listening to it and know what to expect. (SOAP stands for subjective, *objective*, *assessment*, and *plan*. For a detailed description, see Volume 2, Chapter 6.)

The way in which you present the patient has direct implications for the person's care and recovery. Poor presentations compromise patient care. They lead to incomplete or even incorrect medical orders. If you do not communicate a patient's needs or status completely or accurately, a person may be denied some form of treatment based on the information that you have conveyed.

As a paramedic, you will be an extension of the supervisory physician, working under his or her license. No doctor is going to issue orders for medications or other patient care based on guesswork. You are the doctor's eyes and ears at the emergency scene, and it is essential that you provide accurate information about both the patient and the emergency situation.

Poor presentations compromise patient care.

DEVELOPING EFFECTIVE PRESENTATION SKILLS

The most effective oral presentations usually meet these guidelines:

• Last less than one minute
• Are very concise and clear
• Avoid extensive use of medical jargon
• Follow a basic format, usually the SOAP format or some variation
• Include both pertinent findings and pertinent negatives (findings that might be expected, given the patient's complaint or condition, but are absent or denied by the patient)
• Conclude with specific actions, requests, or questions related to the plan

The best way to become proficient at presenting patients is to plan ahead and to practice. Start with an end in mind—know what particular areas of information will be asked for or expected so that you can be ready with that information. As you become more experienced, the flow of information will become second nature to you. Until that time, use a pre-printed form to help you organize your thoughts and information and to take notes during the patient work-up. Practice presenting both simulated and real patients, perhaps at company or unit drills. Listen to other paramedics as they present patients and learn from them. Adopt their good habits and avoid their bad ones.

An ideal presentation should include the following:

Plan ahead. Know what particular areas of information will be asked for or expected so that you can be ready with that information.

• Patient identification, age, sex, and degree of distress
• Chief complaint (why a patient called)
• Present illness/injury
  – Pertinent details about the present problem
  – Pertinent negatives
• Past medical history
  – Allergies
  – Medications
  – Pertinent medical history
• Physical signs
  – Vital signs
  – Pertinent positive findings
  – Pertinent negative findings

- Assessment
  - Paramedic impression
- Plan
  - What has been done
  - Orders requested

Remember, the key to developing presentation skills is repetition and an understanding of the format being used. Once you have mastered this, you can transfer the patient with the satisfaction and confidence of a job well done. (For more detail on this topic, review Volume 2, Chapters 5 and 6 on communications and documentation.)

REVIEW OF COMMON COMPLAINTS

In order to develop as an entry-level practitioner at the paramedic level, it is important to participate in scenario-based reviews of commonly encountered complaints. As mentioned, you might take part in company or unit drills in which you will observe and work with experienced paramedics. You might also participate in laboratory-based simulations.

PRACTICE SESSIONS

The goal of practice sessions is to choreograph the roles and actions of the EMS response team. These sessions will give you the chance to practice assessment and decision making on cases that you are likely to encounter in out-of-hospital situations. They also give you the opportunity to provide intervention based upon your assessment and to reinforce the modalities in local and/or regional treatment protocols. Finally, you can practice patient presentation, both verbally and in written form. At all phases, you get the benefit of feedback from the team members and crew with whom you will be working.

LABORATORY-BASED SIMULATIONS

Laboratory-based simulations require you to assess a pre-programmed patient or mannequin. You will make decisions relative to interventions and transportation. You will also provide interventions, package the patient (or mannequin), and transport. Ideally, you will work as part of a team and practice the various roles assigned to team members, including that of patient.

SELF-MOTIVATION

The chance to practice does not stop at the classroom or at your unit. While a paramedic student or the new member of a team, take advantage of every opportunity to practice your new skills. Recruit family members or friends—or even a teddy bear—as volunteer patients. What is important is to practice, practice, practice until you feel comfortable with as many different situations as possible.

ʃUMMARY

Assessment forms the basis of patient care. In order to make correct decisions, you must gather information and then evaluate and synthesize it. A variety of factors may affect assessment and the decision-making process itself. Some of these factors include paramedic attitude; uncooperative patients; obvious, but distracting injuries; narrow, or tunnel, vision; the environment; patient compliance; and personnel considerations.

It is important to have the right equipment readily available to treat immediately life-threatening conditions. Effective communication and transfer of patient information—whether done face to face, over the telephone or radio, or in writing—is crucial to presenting the patient and assuring continuation of effective care.

Remember, the best way to develop good assessment skills is to practice until you become comfortable with a wide range of patient complaints.

YOU MAKE THE CALL

Begin your assessment practice with the following three scenarios. Each scenario follows a patient call in the sequence of assessment steps from the dispatch through the on-scene assessment and care to the patient presentation at the hospital. In each scenario, the actions of the paramedic are described in the column at left, the paramedic's reasoning in the column at right. In each case, the paramedic is exercising "inverted-pyramid" reasoning, starting by considering a variety of possible causes for the patient's complaint and gradually narrowing the possibilities to reach a field diagnosis.

As you read through each scenario, try to put yourself one step ahead of the printed information. Consider the information about the patient that is being disclosed at each step of the assessment and decide what your own reasoning would be about this patient before you read the paramedic's thoughts as we have provided them. Do you agree with what the paramedic in the scenario was doing and thinking? Would you have done something differently? Would you have reached different conclusions? Discuss each scenario with your instructor and your classmates.

Scenario 1

<u>Actions</u>	<u>Reasoning</u>
Dispatch	
It is 02:30 A.M. and the tones wake me up out of sleep for a "shortness of breath" call. Dispatch notifies us of a 68-year-old male who woke up with difficulty breathing.	68-year-old male having difficulty breathing. This could be any number of things . . . pneumonia . . . CHF . . . asthma . . . an allergic reaction. I'll have to be sure to grab the airway kit and suction along with the oxygen on my way in.
Scene Size-Up	
We arrive on scene at 02:37. There is already a squad car on location and the house and front porch are well lit. I see a short flight of steps leading up to the front door. They are in good condition. The two officers inside direct us down a brightly lit hallway to a rear bedroom.	I'm happy to see that the police have arrived ahead of me to make sure the scene is safe for my partner and me. The steps could have been a potential for injury, but they look OK. It looks like we can safely lift the stretcher up and down the stairs without having to call for help. The house has been lit up for us so I can see that there are no hazards between the doorway and the bedroom. I look around the bedroom but don't see any evidence of a chronic problem such as oxygen equipment or cigarettes. In other words, no indication so far of COPD, though I can't rule it out yet.

Initial Assessment

The patient is sitting up at the side of the bed in the "tripod" position. He is ashen and diaphoretic. He shifts his position frequently and looks like he is scared. He is coughing frequently and has nasal flaring. My partner grabs a quick O_2 sat and then places the patient on oxygen at 15 LPM via nonrebreather mask. I approach the patient to introduce myself and at the same time check a radial pulse, which I find is rapid. He tells me his name is Ronald Smith.

The patient has a patent airway, although the quality of his breathing is of concern. A patient in the tripod position is acutely short of breath. He is hypoxic as evidenced by his restlessness and a room air O_2 sat of 86%. I am concerned about his color. The fact that he is so sweaty leads me to think that this is not an asthma attack. A rapid pulse could be an indication that the problem is cardiac-related with respiratory complications, or he could have a fever due to some infectious process.

History

The patient tries to tell me why he called, but he cannot speak in complete sentences due to his shortness of breath, so his wife tells me the following history: "Over the past several weeks, my husband has become more and more short of breath. In the beginning, he would get short of breath after climbing the stairs but lately he has been resting after every little activity. The last couple of nights he has been having trouble sleeping because of the shortness of breath and a cough. Tonight he was trying to sleep propped up on some pillows because he was having trouble lying flat." She adds that lately he has also been having difficulty getting his shoes on and has taken to wearing his slippers all the time. He has also started to put on some weight in a short amount of time. He is scheduled for a doctor's appointment in the morning.

The progressive shortness of breath and pedal edema lead me to rule out pneumonia as a cause for the shortness of breath. All of these symptoms indicate congestive heart failure leading to pulmonary edema.

This new information confirms that I need to perform a respiratory assessment, which includes listening to breath sounds.

My partner starts taking vital signs, including a pulse ox with the patient on 100% oxygen as I start asking the patient's wife for some additional information using the SAMPLE method. I have learned that Mr. Smith has occasional chest pain that is relieved with rest, so he has never been to see a doctor for it. Aside from an appendectomy as a teenager, he has no significant medical history. He is allergic to penicillin and takes an occasional aspirin for chronic knee pain. He didn't have much of an appetite today, since he hasn't been feeling well, so he hasn't eaten much. Although he wasn't sleeping well all night, Mrs. Smith says that Mr. Smith was awakened from his sleep having difficulty breathing.

The fact that the patient has had chest pain that has gone untreated helps me to confirm that he is in CHF. Other than that, he has no significant medical history that will help me treat this episode of shortness of breath tonight.

My partner reports the patient's vital signs as follows: Pulse rate 120 and irregular, blood pressure 180/110, respiratory rate 44. His O_2 sat is now 95% on oxygen.

I can assume based on his new pulse ox reading that the oxygen is starting to help the hypoxia. His blood pressure and pulse rate indicate that his heart is still working very hard to compensate for the need to maintain oxygenation. His respiratory rate indicates that his breathing is still labored.

Physical Exam

I plan to perform a head to toe assessment while focusing on the patient's chief complaint of shortness of breath. Mr. Smith is still maintaining an airway and I note his color is starting to get a little better. His cough is producing pink, frothy sputum but he does not appear to be in danger of aspiration. I inspect his chest and find nothing abnormal about the anterior-posterior dimensions, nor can I palpate any crepitus. On percussion, I find his chest to sound dull. I begin to auscultate his breath sounds and find fine crackles all the way up all lung fields. He has jugular vein distention and I note that he has 3+ pitting edema to both extremities.

Interventions

Mr. Smith needs quick management of his pulmonary edema in order to prevent him from getting worse and possibly needing to be intubated. I am grateful that I work in a system that has extensive standing orders, so I am able to treat him quickly, without having to call medical direction. I explain to the patient exactly what I am going to do as I get ready to start a normal saline IV with microdrip tubing. My partner is placing the patient on a 3 lead ECG monitor at the same time and we note a sinus tachycardia with a rate in the 120's. The patient is still diaphoretic, so my partner uses benzoin to keep the leads in place. I proceed to place a nitroglycerin tablet under the patient's tongue and instruct him not to swallow it, just to let it dissolve. I warn him that this medicine may cause him to develop a headache. I then ask my partner to take another blood pressure as I prepare to give Mr. Smith Lasix at 40mg. I warn him that this medicine will make him need to urinate in a few minutes and we can assist with him that if necessary.

After this round of medicine, my partner and I agree that we should move Mr. Smith to the ambulance and finish treating him en route to the ED. Since it is the middle of the night, my partner and I agree that using the lights and sirens are not necessary and will only increase Mr. Smith's anxiety, so we choose to drive to the hospital non-emergent.

Ongoing Assessment

As my partner drives us to the hospital, I am constantly reassessing Mr. Smith's vital signs and respiratory status. His heart rate and his blood pressure are coming down slowly and his respiratory rate is slowing as well. His cough is becoming less frequent. In addition, I give him two more nitroglycerin tablets, 5 minutes apart. He has become less restless and is able to ask questions in complete sentences as we head to the ED.

The pink, frothy sputum indicates acute pulmonary edema. He has remained awake and alert so he is able to clear his own airway. The fact that his chest is symmetrical and I do not detect crepitus helps rule out COPD as the cause for his shortness of breath. The crackles in his lungs indicate fluid in the airways. I know that the fluid in his lungs and the pink, frothy sputum are evidence of left sided heart failure. This has led to his right sided heart failure, as evidenced by my patient's JVD and pedal edema.

I know that normal saline is the IV fluid of choice for congestive heart failure. I am concerned about his receiving an accidental fluid bolus so I place the IV on microdrip tubing.

Nitrates are used in CHF as a venodilator to decrease preload, and the diuretics decrease preload and afterload by decreasing circulating volume. I want to get him medicated as quickly as possible to decrease the workload on his heart. I may also consider giving morphine to Mr. Smith as an added vasodilator and to decrease the anxiety that he is feeling from being so critically ill, but I am concerned that morphine may act as a respiratory depressant.

I am concerned about dropping Mr. Smith's blood pressure too low or too fast with the nitroglycerin and Lasix. Therefore I know I need to recheck his vital signs before giving him any additional medication.

Mr. Smith remains awake, alert, and oriented. The fact that he isn't as restless indicates that he has begun oxygenating better. His respirations aren't as labored so he is having an easier time speaking to me.

Communications and Written Report

Mr. Smith's house is just a short ride from the hospital. I call ahead and let the nursing staff know that we are en route and will need a critical care bed upon our arrival. I have been keeping notes on my pad throughout my treatment of this patient so I can go back later and accurately document my treatment of Mr. Smith. I give the report to the receiving nurse and then head to the coffee pot so I can sit down and start writing out the trip sheet.

Follow-up

I call the ED in the morning as my shift is ending to see how Mr. Smith is doing. The nurse tells me that after a little more medication he did great and that he was admitted to a telemetry bed. He passed on a word of thanks to the paramedics, which is always nice to hear at the end of a long shift.

It is important to let the receiving hospital know when they will be receiving a critical patient so they can be prepared to continue his treatment upon his arrival.

Proper documentation is vital for the patient record and also for keeping me out of court. It is late and I am tired, but I know how important it is for me to get this trip sheet correct.

Scenario 2

Actions	Reasoning

Dispatch

At 3:30 P.M. my partner and I are sitting down to our first meal of the day and are having a heated discussion about which team was really the team of the Twentieth Century, the Yankees or the Braves, when the tones alert us to a call. We're being dispatched to an unconscious female on the floor of the local tool factory.

An unconscious female in a factory that is notorious for employees standing on their feet for hours at a time in a hot, unventilated environment. So much for my cheeseburger. As I get into the ambulance I'm trying to think of what this could be . . . heat exhaustion, diabetes, MI, seizure, stroke, head injury. It could be any one of a number of things. I really wish we had gotten more information on this dispatch.

Scene Size-Up

We arrive on the scene 6 minutes later, after dispatch has given us a little more information. Our patient is a female in her mid-to-late 30s who passed out while working on the assembly line floor. Security will be meeting us at the entrance to the work area with hard hats for both my partner and me. We look inside the door and see that the factory is still active, so we put on our safety goggles as well.

They tell us that this patient's problem doesn't appear to be job-related. We follow the security people carefully through the factory until we find our patient, who is lying still on the floor. A First Responder on the factory staff has been holding manual stabilization of the patient's head and neck in case she suffered a spine injury when she fell.

I am still concerned about the safety of treating a patient in an active factory, but security has assured us that as long as we stay behind them we aren't in any danger of being injured. They have stopped the machine that she was working on, but I decide to leave my goggles on just to be on the safe side.

On a quick scene size-up, I note that there isn't any blood on the floor and I don't see anything around me that could have caused a head injury. Still, if the initial fall wasn't caused by trauma, perhaps she struck her head when she hit the floor and that is why she is unconscious now. And, as the First Responder realized, she could also have suffered a spine injury. I ask the First Responder to maintain C-spine stabilization while my partner and I conduct the assessment.

Initial Assessment

The patient is lying on the ground, unconscious, profusely diaphoretic.

Due to the fact that I don't see any mechanism of injury and the fact that she is so sweaty, I think I can start to narrow in on a medical problem that could have caused her to become unconscious. I don't think this is heat stroke, because then she would most likely be hot and dry and this woman is soaked in sweat, but it could be heat exhaustion. It's even possible that she came to work drunk and passed out.

I get down on the floor beside the patient as my partner takes out the oxygen equipment. I see the woman has a patent airway and she is breathing adequately. I quickly assess the radial pulse and find it to be strong and regular.

Well, so far the ABCs are OK. I still can't rule out a cardiac event, although she looks kind of young for that, and the adequate breathing and strong, regular pulse makes a cardiac problem unlikely.

I try to arouse the patient with verbal and tactile stimuli, but I'm not having much luck. My partner places her on 100% oxygen via nonrebreather mask, but she remains unresponsive.

If this event is related to hypoxia, the oxygen should be helping with her level of consciousness, but it's not.

History

I get out my IV equipment as my partner starts asking if anyone saw what happened. One of her co-workers says that our patient, Jane, had been looking weak and that after she fell to the ground her body started to shake.

OK, this is a good clue. Maybe she has a seizure disorder. I'm also thinking that if her sugar is low she may have had a hypoglycemic seizure. I also can't rule out a stroke at this point. I look for a medical alert bracelet or necklace, but I don't find one.

As I'm setting up the IV equipment, one of Jane's supervisors comes over with her medical history form. It states that she is 38 years old and that she is an insulin-dependant diabetic.

I get an 18g IV started in the patient's right antecube, in case she needs a fluid bolus or $D_{50}W$. I get a drop of blood for the glucometer, and as I wait for the result I'm drawing blood off the IV and start a 500 mL bag of normal saline at a keep-open rate. I need to use a lot of tape to secure the IV because her arm is so sweaty.

The glucometer reads 29.

So there it is. My patient is hypoglycemic.

Interventions and Physical Exam

I get out some thiamine and draw up 100 mg while my partner opens up a box of $D_{50}W$. After the thiamine is on board, I begin to push the $D_{50}W$.

I've never seen it, but the thiamine is given to prevent Wernicke's syndrome, which can happen if the patient is thiamine deficient. This patient's glucose level is pretty low, but I'm hoping it won't take more than one 25 g dose of $D_{50}W$ to wake her up.

As I wait to see any results from my medication administration, I take Jane's blood pressure, which is 108/56.

Even though I know my patient's glucose level is low, I'm still worried that I may miss something else, like hypotension, which could have caused her syncope. This blood pressure is within normal limits, so I am not going to give a fluid bolus at this time.

Two minutes later, Jane starts to open her eyes and moves her arms and legs. I ask her not to move or try to get up yet.

After a few minutes, Jane becomes more alert and can answer my questions. She starts to complain of a headache and that she had been feeling really nauseated prior to falling on the floor. She tells me that she takes insulin twice a day. Lately she has been feeling tired and weak and when she checks her sugar it has been lower than usual, so she has been drinking juice to feel better. She has recently been dieting and exercising on a regular basis. She knows she needs to get to the doctor, but she doesn't have any time off from work.

I start a head-to-toe assessment and Jane complains of pain when I palpate her head. On the completion of the assessment, I don't find any other problems or complaints.

With the First Responder's assistance, my partner and I log-roll Jane on her side to place a long board underneath her. My partner holds her up on her side as I check the back of her head and palpate her back. I find a hematoma on the back of her head. We finish immobilizing her and transport her to the ambulance.

Ongoing Assessment

En route to the hospital, Jane becomes completely awake and her skin is starting to dry. I perform an ongoing assessment, including another set of vital signs, as we proceed non-emergent mode to the hospital.

Communications and Written Report

I call ahead to notify the receiving hospital that we are en route and to provide information about the patient. I then ask Jane some additional questions about her medical history that I will use to complete my patient report.

I am happy to see that the $D_{50}W$ is starting to work, but I am still concerned that Jane may have suffered a cervical spine injury from her fall, so I don't want her to move. I ask the First Responder to keep reminding her to stay still.

Jane's new diet and exercise program has caused her to need less insulin; she just hasn't gotten to the doctor so her dosages can be changed.

I am worried about her headache, since I don't know if it started before her fall, or if she hit her head when she fell.

Because of the danger of spine injury, and since Jane is still complaining of a headache, I know we need to immobilize her for transport.

I'm glad we decided to use C-spine precautions since Jane did suffer a head injury from the fall.

Since Jane has responded well to our treatment and her condition is not life threatening, we drive to the hospital without our lights and siren. I plan to tell Jane that this all would have been a lot easier if she had been wearing a medical alert ID or if any of her coworkers had been able to tell us that she was diabetic.

Even though Jane is a non-emergency transport, it is still a good idea to the let the hospital know we are coming. They have been pretty busy lately, and I want to make sure they have a bed waiting for us. As soon as I have transferred the patient to the hospital staff, I find a corner where I can complete my written documentation. I know how important documentation is, so I take the time to be sure my notes are complete and legible—even though I still haven't gotten to finish my lunch!

Follow-up

The hospital staff did a CT scan of Jane's head, which was negative. They alerted the factory personnel office that they were scheduling her for an outpatient appointment at the Diabetes Center, so Jane can learn how to manage her diabetes better and avoid incidents like this in the future. The factory management was supportive about her need to take time for this appointment.

Scenario 3

Actions	Reasoning
### Dispatch	
At 2300 my partner, Joe, and I are dispatched to a local residence for a behavioral emergency. Dispatch tells us that the caller was incoherent on the telephone, talking about seeing people with guns and how he needs to kill them all.	"What's this all about?" I'm thinking as I get into the passenger seat. It's my turn to treat the patient and Joe's turn to drive. We decide that we'll head over to the scene lights and siren, but then turn them off a couple of blocks away so we don't alarm the patient any further.
### Scene Size-Up	
We are the first to arrive on scene and have been instructed to wait for the police to clear the scene before entering.	Joe and I have been through this before. We know to park down the street so, in case the caller has a gun, he won't see us out there and decide to shoot at us.
Two police cars arrive one minute after we do and approach the dark house carefully. We watch the police as they enter the house. We will wait in the ambulance until we're radioed that the scene is safe.	Based on the dispatch, I'm concerned that this patient may really be violent. It's important for the police to clear the scene before we take any chances of getting hurt. If this guy really does have a gun, the police are the ones who need to handle the situation.
Ten minutes later, dispatch notifies us that it's safe to enter. The porch lights of the house get turned on and one of the police officers steps outside. The police officers tell us that they have searched the house and didn't find a gun. We go in, Joe bringing a Reeves stretcher and soft restraints in case they will be needed, which we hope they won't. (Our departmental policy states not to use handcuffs as restraints unless a patient is under arrest since they can cause further injury.) Joe leaves the stretcher and restraints in the hallway so the patient won't be upset by seeing them.	Although I trust the officers, I'll take a careful look around anyway. I need to see for myself that there is nothing that can be used as a weapon readily available. I also want to see if there are any medications around that could indicate what is going on with this patient.

Initial Assessment

We are directed to the living room where the patient, Mr. Allen, is sitting in the chair, speaking fast with his hands moving wildly. I approach Mr. Allen slowly and introduce myself. Since he is sitting up, in no acute distress, and talking to me, I know he has a patent airway and no difficulty breathing. I can also assume he has a good pulse rate for the same reason.

Although I normally like to place a hand on my patient's wrist when I introduce myself, to get a quick pulse assessment, I hesitate to do this with Mr. Allen. He might take my touch as an invasion of his space. I want to approach him slowly, so I don't startle him or cause him to become more agitated. From the way he is speaking, he appears to be very anxious. I'm still not sure what is going on here. Has he taken any drugs or medications that could have caused a reaction like this? Is he an alcoholic who is going through withdrawal and having hallucinations? Maybe he has a psychiatric history and this has happened before.

History and Physical Exam

I kneel down at the patient's level and speak slowly and quietly as I ask some questions. Mr. Allen tells me that he has seen the people out there who want to get him and if he had a gun he would get them first. The entire time he is talking to me he is wringing his hands together and looking around the room. He seems to want to get up at times, but then sits back in his chair.

Suddenly Mr. Allen looks at me and tells me that he isn't going back to that hospital with me. He starts to raise his voice and states repeatedly that he isn't going back to the hospital.

Joe has been looking around the kitchen and comes back with two empty pill bottles. One is for Clozaril and the other is for Xanax. They are both several months old.

After talking with him for several minutes and trying to get him to focus on what is wrong, Mr. Allen appears to be becoming even more agitated. He gets up and starts pacing the room, continuing to wring his hands. He is raising his voice, yelling at me that he won't let me take him back to that hospital. I continue to talk to him in a calm, soothing voice, reassuring him that I'm not going to hurt him. The police officers move in a little closer, ready to intervene if there is any violent outburst from the patient. By now, two more officers have arrived on the scene.

Mr. Allen doesn't have some of the hallmark signs of withdrawal, such as hand tremors, nausea, or sweating. So I'm inclined to think his behavior is not caused by withdrawal. I'm still wondering if this is a medication reaction or if he has a history of psychiatric problems. I am having trouble getting information from him because I can't get him to focus. I try to start over by introducing myself again and telling him why I am here.

I'm getting concerned because his agitation seems to be increasing. Since he mentions a history of previous hospitalization, I'm thinking that he may be suffering from a psychiatric problem. He seems to be exhibiting some of the signs of schizophrenia. He appears to be having hallucinations and is acting paranoid.

Well, that seems to answer that question. Mr. Allen is on an antipsychotic medication and an antianxiety medication. It seems that he hasn't been taking his meds for awhile. There is no family to tell us what is going on, and Mr. Allen isn't answering my questions.

I am getting concerned about our safety now. I have seen patients like this become violent. I hope Mr. Allen won't have to be restrained. We work closely with the local police, however, and I know they are ready to help us carry out a four-person restraint procedure if it's necessary.

Interventions

I make one last effort to speak quietly with the patient and assure him that I'm not going to hurt him. I tell him that I want to take him to the best place for him to get medical attention. In response, Mr. Allen runs toward the back door, but it's locked and he turns to face us. "I'm not coming with you," he yells. "I'm getting out of here."

I offer one final opportunity for him to cooperate with us and go to the hospital quietly. With that, Mr. Allen turns and tries to kick open the door. Then he turns to glare at us again.

Two of the officers, Joe, and I approach the patient to restrain him for transport. We move swiftly toward him, but I stay in front of him, speaking with him the entire time, since I have made initial contact with him.

Each of the four of us takes control of an extremity. We lay Mr. Allen on his side on the Reeves stretcher and use the soft restraints to tie his wrists and his legs. We check his distal pulses to be sure that the restraints are not too tight. We make sure that his airway is clear and he is breathing adequately.

Ongoing Assessment

Although Mr. Allen has stopped fighting the restraints, he continues to yell that he doesn't want to go to the hospital and that he knew that the people out there were going to get him. Even restrained, Mr. Allen is difficult to approach. Nevertheless, I conduct ongoing assessments en route.

Communications and Written Report

I call ahead to the hospital and notify the nursing staff that security should be waiting for us when we get there and that we will need a behavioral emergency room.

After we transfer Mr. Allen to hospital personnel, Joe and I thank the police officer and the security guards for their assistance and head to the EMS room so I can start writing my report. This is going to be a long one.

I was hoping it wouldn't come to this. The police hold him while Joe steps into the hallway to get the Reeves stretcher and the soft wrist and ankle restraints.

Although I am concerned about our safety, I am also concerned about Mr. Allen's safety. I know restraining him for transport is the safest thing to do for him and for us. We lower the Reeves stretcher onto our cot and the officers help us load him into the ambulance. One of the officers hands another officer his weapon, then hops in the back with me while Joe heads to the hospital. Our policy is not to use lights and sirens in a situation like this, as this may agitate the patient even more.

When transporting a patient in restraints, there is always a risk that the restraints will cause asphyxiation. Since Mr. Allen continues to yell, I know he is maintaining a patent airway. I frequently check his distal pulses for adequate circulation, but I decide not to check his blood pressure in order to avoid upsetting him even more.

Although we have a police officer with us, additional security will be needed when we transfer the patient from our stretcher to the hospital stretcher. An isolated room is needed for the patient to prevent him from harming himself or disturbing other people in the ED.

I know that my education officer will scrutinize this written report. My department is very concerned about proper use of restraints and patient safety. I take a lot of time documenting exactly what happened prior to restraining the patient and then reassessing what I did after the patient was restrained. Joe knows we are going to be here awhile, so he goes to take a break outside.

Follow-up

The hospital social worker is familiar with Mr. Allen and has had to commit him in the past. She tells me that he is often noncompliant with his medications and has been in out and out of psychiatric hospitals since his teens. She reassures us that we took proper action with him, since he has become violent in the past. She will make another attempt to place him in a situation where he can have more assistance and supervision but, given the shortage of available services, is not very optimistic about the outcome for Mr. Allen.

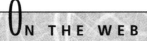

FURTHER READING

Dalton, A.L., D. Limmer, J.J. Mistovich, and H.A. Werman: *Advanced Medical Life Support*. Upper Saddle River, NJ: Brady/Prentice Hall, 1999.

Dalton, A.L.: "Enhanced Critical Thinking in Paramedic Continuing Education," *Prehospital and Disaster Medicine*, October–December 1996, Vol. 11, No. 4, pp. 246-253.

Farrell, M.: "Planning for Critical Outcomes," *Journal of Nursing Education*, September 1996, Vol. 35, No. 6, pp. 278-281.

Janing, J.: "Critical Thinking: Incorporation into the Paramedic Curriculum," *Prehospital and Disaster Management*, October–November 1994, Vol. 9, No. 4, pp. 238-242.

ON THE WEB

Visit Brady's Paramedic Website at www.bradybooks.com/paramedic.

CHAPTER 8

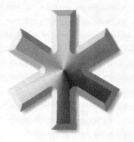

Ambulance Operations

Objectives

After reading this chapter, you should be able to:

1. Identify current local and state standards that influence ambulance design, equipment requirements, and staffing of ambulances. (pp. 318–320)
2. Identify the elements of a vehicle, equipment, and supply checklist. (pp. 320–321)
3. Describe the process for reporting vehicle or equipment problems/failure to the director of operations. (p. 321)
4. Identify the EMS equipment that needs routine service to assure proper field operation. (p. 321)
5. Discuss OSHA standards and other federal requirements for vehicle and equipment cleaning. (pp. 320–321)
6. Discuss the importance of completing an ambulance equipment/supply checklist. (pp. 320–321)
7. Discuss factors used to determine ambulance stationing and staffing within a community. (pp. 322–323)
8. Describe the advantages and disadvantages of air medical transport. (p. 332)
9. Identify conditions/situations that merit air medical transport. (pp. 331, 332–333)
10. Discuss strategies to help assure safe operation of ambulances when responding to or at an emergency. (pp. 323–330)

CASE STUDY

It's 6:00 A.M., the start of another shift. You and your partner have just arrived to relieve the overnight crew. As you check and sign out the narcotics with the outgoing paramedic, the tones go off for a priority one call on the other side of town. You quickly finish the paperwork and rush out the door. As you load your personal protection equipment, you shout to the outgoing crew: "How's the rig?" The paramedic responds, "Fine. We just restocked."

You feel confident that the ambulance has everything you will need. Your service is dedicated to ensuring that each shift fills in ambulance checklists and that replacement supplies are easily obtained. In this case, you arrive at the scene to find that the patient is complaining of breathing difficulty, most likely from an acute exacerbation of asthma. The call runs smoothly, and the patient actually improves en route to the hospital.

You quickly wrap up the paperwork and return to the station. En route, you and your partner recall the haphazard ambulance operations of a few years ago. The former management team looked the other way when some medics failed to restock the supplies and equipment that they used. Imagine not having enough oxygen or a bronchodilator for an asthma patient. You and your partner both agree, things have gotten a lot better since the new management has insisted that crews take the tour checklists seriously.

INTRODUCTION

Good ambulance operations involves some of the knowledge and skills that you've already established in your EMT-Basic training and through field experience. However, because the safety of so many people—the EMS team, the patient, and bystanders—depends upon effective ambulance maintenance and operation, it is important for you to review this information regularly so that it becomes second nature. In addition to the communication and dispatch skills learned in Volume 2, Chapter 5, you should keep in mind these five topics: ambulance standards, maintenance of ambulance equipment and supplies, ambulance stationing, safe ambulance operations, and the utilization of air medical transport.

AMBULANCE STANDARDS

✳ **deployment** strategy used by an EMS agency to maneuver its ambulances and crews in an effort to reduce response times.

Various standards, as well as administrative rules and regulations, influence the design of ambulances and the medical equipment carried on each unit. Similar guidelines determine staffing levels and **deployment** of EMS agencies (see information later in the chapter).

Because the oversight for EMS usually falls to state governments, many of the requirements for ambulance service are written in state statutes or regulations. However, national standards and trends do have an influence on the development of these laws. Typically, state laws are broad, while corresponding regulations provide more specific guidelines or rules. For example, a public health law may authorize the state department of health to issue regulations though its EMS Bureau. These regulations, known as the "state EMS code," might then handle such matters as the **essential equipment** to be carried on every ambulance.

✳ **essential equipment** equipment/supplies required on every ambulance.

In most cases, government standards tend to be generic enough so that they are "palatable," affordable, and politically feasible to all EMS agencies in the state. State standards usually set **minimum standards,** rather than a **gold standard,** for operation. In other words, they establish the lowest level at which units will be allowed to operate. When local and/or regional EMS systems get involved in regulation, their lists tend to be much more detailed and often approach a gold standard, which is the goal when ample resources are provided.

✳ **minimum standards** lowest or least allowable standards.

✳ **gold standard** ultimate standard of excellence.

AMBULANCE DESIGN

The U.S. General Services Administration–Automotive Commodity Center issues the federal regulations that specify ambulance design and manufacturing requirements. These specs—known as the **DOT KKK 1822D specs**—attempt to influence safety standards as well as standardize the look of ambulances.

✳ **DOT KKK 1822D specs** the manufacturing and design specifications produced by the Federal General Services Administrative Automotive Commodity Center.

Over the years, the "KKK specifications" have had a significant influence on ambulance manufacturing. The specs describe the following three basic ambulance designs.

- *Type I*—conventional truck cab-chassis with a modular ambulance body.
- *Type II*—standard van, forward control integral cab-body ambulance.
- *Type III*—specialty van, forward control integral cab-body ambulance.

In addition to these three designs, there is also a medium duty ambulance rescue vehicle (Figure 8-1). It is designed to handle heavier loads and has a gross weight of approximately 24,000 pounds.

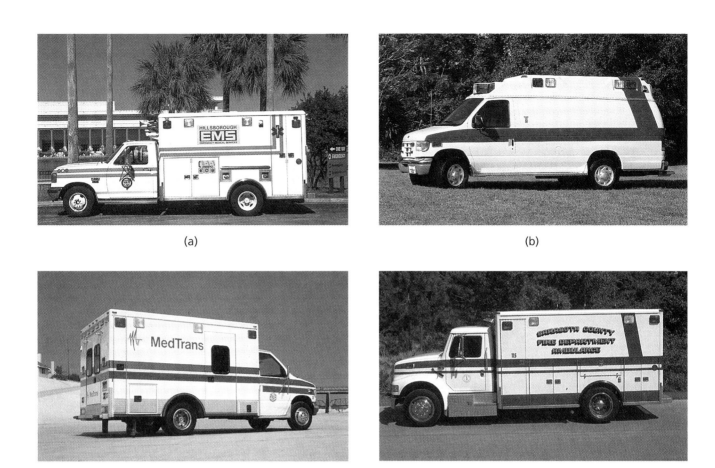

(a)

(b)

(c)

(d)

FIGURE 8-1   Four types of ambulances. (a) Type I. (b) Type II. (c) Type III. (d) Medium duty.

The federal specifications not only provide standards for the purchase of ambulances used by the federal government, they also provide guidelines for the states to follow. Massachusetts, for example, refers to the federal specifications in its own state regulations. In such cases, the federal specifications become the state standard for ambulance services to follow when purchasing vehicles.

Some states, including Connecticut, Vermont, and New Jersey, have chosen to develop their own standards. Often these states use the federal specifications as the basis or starting point for their own regulations. A few states, such as New York, use neither federal nor state specifications. Instead, the decisions for ambulance purchases are determined on a local or regional basis.

In addition to the DOT, other federal agencies and national organizations influence standards. Air ambulance standards, for example, are usually designed with input from representatives of the National Flight Nurses Association (NFNA) and the National Flight Paramedics Association (NFPA). The Federal Communications Commission (FCC), which is discussed in Volume 2, Chapter 5, specifies the radio bands and types of equipment that may be used in ambulances.

MEDICAL EQUIPMENT STANDARDS

With the advent of hazmat and increased awareness of infectious diseases, the Occupational Safety and Health Administration (OSHA) has gotten increasingly involved in ambulance standards. As the agency charged with protecting worker safety, OSHA has helped ensure equipment lists calling for disinfecting agents, sharps containers, red bag, HEPA masks, and personal protective equipment. The National Institute for Occupational Safety and Health (NIOSH) has established similar standards.

Other voluntary standards have been set by peer organizations, such as the National Fire Protection Association (NFPA). In many cases, these standards are referred to in local ordinances and thus have become the standard for a given municipality.

In addition to city, county, and/or district ambulance ordinances, local medical control boards sometimes list the medications that paramedics can carry. These boards, which issue indirect medical control, may also list the specific ALS equipment and supplies that should be on every ambulance. For example, in areas where the paramedics are trained to obtain a 12–lead ECG, the medical control board may have specified the actual brand of equipment in an effort to standardize care on a system-wide or regional basis.

ADDITIONAL GUIDELINES

At the national level, the Commission on Accreditation of Ambulance Services (CAAS) provides a voluntary "gold standard" for the EMS community to follow. CAAS requires that on-board medical equipment and supplies comply with state and local guidelines. In the absence of these guidelines, CAAS requires services to develop guidelines that meet or exceed those established by the American College of Surgeons (ACS). The ACS Committee of Trauma issued its first list of "essential equipment" to be carried on ambulances in 1970 and revised the list in 1994. Even the first version of the list included ALS equipment, emergency drugs, and fluids commonly used on ALS calls today.

CHECKING AMBULANCES

On each shift, an essential part of a paramedic's duties includes completion of the ambulance equipment and supply checklist. Aside from reminding the personnel exactly where all equipment and supplies are stored on the ambulance, the shift checklist helps assure that all equipment and supplies will be available and in working order when needed for patient care. The checklist also makes the work environment safer by assuring mechanical maintenance and the availability of personal protection equipment.

The components of a typical vehicle/equipment checklist include the following:

- Patient infection control, comfort, and protection supplies
- Initial and focused assessment equipment
- Equipment for the transfer of the patient
- Equipment for airway maintenance, ventilation, and resuscitation
- Oxygen therapy and suction equipment
- Equipment for assisting with cardiac resuscitation
- Supplies and equipment for immobilization of suspected bone injuries
- Supplies for wound care and treatment of shock
- Supplies for childbirth
- Supplies, equipment, and medications for the treatment of acute poisoning, snakebite, chemical burns, and diabetic emergencies
- Advanced Life Support equipment, medications, and supplies
- Safety and miscellaneous equipment
- Information on the operation and inspection of the ambulance itself

The shift checklist makes the work environment safer by assuring mechanical maintenance and the availability of personal protection equipment.

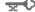

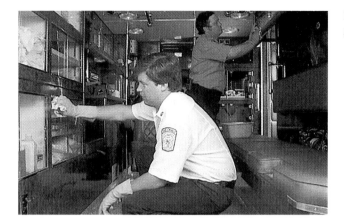

FIGURE 8-2 Disinfecting the ambulance.

Routine, detailed shift checks of the ambulance can minimize the issues associated with risk management. Many services, for example, hold a "stretcher day" once a week. By performing and documenting preventative maintenance on stretchers, it is less likely that a faulty stretcher will cause a patient to be dropped or EMS personnel to injure their backs. Medications carried on the paramedic unit expire. Therefore, expiration dates should be checked each shift, and the older, un-expired drugs marked appropriately so that they will be used first. In services that utilize scheduled medications such as narcotics, the paramedics should sign for these medications at the beginning and at the end of each shift.

As mentioned, the vehicle itself should be regularly checked so that it is always in safe working order. If the ambulance or any equipment needs repair, it is your responsibility to report the failure to your supervisor in a manner prescribed by the SOPs for your service.

To meet OSHA requirements, you must also make sure that the ambulance has been properly disinfected after the transport of any patients with potentially communicable diseases (Figure 8-2). Most services routinely clean the ambulance after every call, and some agencies document the procedure. All services are required, either by OSHA or the state equivalent of OSHA, to have an exposure control plan that specifies cleaning requirements and the methods of cleaning up blood spills in the ambulance. If there is no specific SOP in your agency, you should document cleaning and disinfecting on the shift checklist.

Finally, you should do all scheduled tests, maintenance, and calibrations on specific medical equipment. Items that should be regularly checked include:

- Automated external defibrillator (AED)
- Glucometer
- Cardiac monitor
- Oxygen systems
- Automated transport ventilator (ATV)
- Pulse oximeter
- Suction units
- Laryngoscope blades
- Lighted stylets
- Penlights
- Any other battery operated equipment

Expiration dates on medications should be checked each shift, and the older, un-expired drugs marked appropriately so that they will be used first.

It is your responsibility to report ambulance/equipment problems or failures to your supervisor in a manner prescribed by the SOPs for your service.

AMBULANCE DEPLOYMENT AND STAFFING

DEPLOYMENT FACTORS
* Location of facilities to house ambulances
* Location of hospitals
* Anticipated volume of calls
* Local geographic and traffic considerations

The strategy used by an EMS agency to maneuver its ambulances and crews in order to reduce response times is known as deployment. Deployment is based upon a number of factors: location of the facilities to house ambulances, location of hospitals, anticipated volume of calls, and the specific geographic and traffic considerations of your area.

Most services must develop deployment strategies based on current station locations. Few agencies are in a position where they can move their stations to better locations. Such moves require years of budgeting, land acquisition, community education, building design, and finance of a capital construction project.

The ideal deployment decisions must take into account two sets of data: past community responses and projected **demographic** changes. The highest volume of calls, or **peak load,** should be described both in terms of the day of the week and the time of day.

✱ **demographic** pertaining to population makeup or changes.

✱ **peak load** the highest volume of calls at a given time.

In communities that do not have multiple strategically located stations, services often deploy ambulances to wait for calls at specific high-volume locations. Such stationing locations are known as **primary areas of responsibility (PAR).** These same ambulances may be relocated throughout the day as the population moves—to work or to school—and as other ambulances in the community respond to calls. The size of a PAR may differ from a few city blocks to a larger location, such as "northeast sector of town." Size depends upon the number of ambulances available and the expected call volume.

✱ **primary area of responsibility (PAR)** stationing of ambulances at specific high-volume locations.

Some technologically sophisticated systems use computers to assist the dispatch center in relocating the ambulances. Vehicle tracking systems tell the computer exactly where each ambulance is located at a given time.

TRAFFIC CONGESTION

In determining deployment strategies, traffic congestion must be taken into account as well as special situations such as a ground-level railroad. Some communities, for example, must station an ambulance on the other side of the tracks before a freight train splits the town in half for perhaps 15 minutes or more. Other special considerations include daily activities within the community, especially commuter traffic and school bus schedules. Additional vehicles and crews may be required for these time periods. Other traffic (and potential patient) considerations include sporting events, VIP appearances, mass gatherings, community days, and so on.

One deployment strategy that has become popular in recent years is known as **system status management (SSM).** SSM is a computerized personnel and ambulance deployment system designed to meet service demands with fewer resources and to ensure appropriate response time and vehicle location.

✱ **system status management (SSM)** a computerized personnel and ambulance deployment system.

Appropriate response time must be determined by each community and its available resources. However, national guidelines set the standards for certain situations. For example, a cardiac arrest victim should receive defibrillation within the first four minutes and ALS within eight minutes. A system's standards for reliability must take into account the time frames for such high-priority calls. The medical director should have direct input into setting these standards. Response time can literally make the difference between life and death for the citizens of a community. An example of such a reliability standard might be response within four minutes to 90% of the priority one calls (cardiac arrests, respiratory complaints, and motor vehicle collisions).

To meet reliability standards, many communities use a **tiered response system** in which public safety agencies trained as first responders carry an AED to a patient's side. The first tier of response, which helps ensure arrival within four minutes, is then backed up by a second tier that brings an ALS unit to the patient within eight minutes. Some communities add a third tier of response by separat-

✱ **tiered response system** system that allows multiple vehicles to arrive at an EMS call at different times, often providing different levels of care or transport.

ing their paramedics from their ambulances. No one system works best for all communities. The system that is ideal for your specific area will depend upon such considerations as available personnel, available training, and many other factors.

OPERATIONAL STAFFING

For as long as paramedics have been trained, controversy has existed over the number of paramedics that should be assigned to a unit. This is a complex decision. Clearly, an ambulance with two paramedics onboard is limited in the amount of care these two highly trained personnel can provide if they are the only available responders to cardiac arrests (meaning no backup for simultaneous additional emergencies). As a result, some communities prefer to combine an EMT-Intermediate with a paramedic to make an ALS unit. Other communities, such as New York City, specify that an ALS unit must have two paramedics so that they can back each other up in making on-scene decisions. Because communities and available resources vary so widely, the controversy will in all likelihood be settled locally based upon the particular needs and available resources.

In general, ambulance staffing should take into account the peak load of the system. Some services vary shift times to assure ample coverage for the busiest days of the week and the busiest times of the day. Services should also take into account the need for **reserve capacity**—the ability to muster additional crews when all ambulances are on call or when a system's resources are taxed by a multiple casualty incident. Some services fulfill this need by asking off-duty personnel to carry pagers or to volunteer for backup. Whatever plan is adopted, each system must consider how they will deal with establishing a reserve of paramedics.

Finally, each service needs to determine standards for ambulance operators (drivers) and for driving the vehicle itself. As a rule, these standards are usually spelled out at the local service level.

✻ **reserve capacity** the ability of an EMS agency to respond to calls beyond those handled by the on-duty crews.

SAFE AMBULANCE OPERATIONS

Patients, family members, motorists, and other EMS providers are injured—sometimes fatally—in ambulance collisions. In addition to personal injuries, ambulance collisions exact a high toll: vehicle repair or replacement, lawsuits, down time from work, increased insurance premiums, and damage to your agency's reputation in the community.

There is no national database providing statistics on ambulance collisions in all 50 states. As a result, it is difficult to establish any form of "acceptable" ambulance collision rates per number of calls or miles driven. Furthermore, there are few published scientific studies that attempt to prove what, if any, strategies effectively reduce ambulance collisions. However, you can be certain of one thing. If your agency does experience a serious ambulance accident, it will undoubtedly be questioned on its training of drivers and on its accident prevention program.

EDUCATING PROVIDERS

The first part of any proactive education program is the recognition and definition of the problem. In the absence of a national database, this is easier said than done. However, some states do keep data, and their example can provide a starting point. The following statistics come from an analysis of 22 years of **reportable collisions**—accidents involving over $1,000 in vehicle damage or a personal injury—in New York State. The data is not intended to be scientific evidence that can be generalized to the other 49 states. It also does not include many of the crashes that have resulted from backing up the ambulances—crashes

✻ **reportable collisions** collisions that involve over $1,000 in damage or a personal injury.

that could be avoided by use of a **spotter.** Rather the data, which comes from a large number of cases, serves for purposes of illustration.

During the years 1974–1996, New York recorded 7,756 reportable ambulance collisions. They involved 64 fatalities and 10,636 injuries. Remember that the first rule in medical practice is "do no harm," and yet these collisions by emergency vehicles harmed a considerable number of people.

An analysis of the data collected by New York provides a profile of the typical ambulance collision. Inclement weather accounted for a relatively small number of the accidents. About 18% occurred on rainy days, 16% on cloudy days, and 6% on days with snow, sleet, hail, or freezing rain. The majority of collisions (55%) took place on clear days. Of all the collisions, some 67% took place during daylight hours.

Although head-on collisions can be very serious, they accounted for only 1% of the accidents. The largest number of collisions (41%) occurred when the ambulance struck another vehicle laterally or at a right angle or was struck itself. Approximately 21% of the collisions resulted from side swiping or overtaking another vehicle. Another 12% occurred while making a right or left turn.

Probably the most important observation from the data is that nearly three-quarters (72%) of all collisions took place at intersections. Most safety minded ambulance operators agree that the days of "blowing through" an intersection at high speeds with lights blaring and siren blasting have come and gone. Yet nearly half of all accidents took place at locations with a traffic control device. Another third took place at locations with no traffic device or sign at all.

Based on the statistics from New York, the profile of a typical ambulance collision might read as follows: *A lateral collision that takes place on a dry road during daylight hours on a clear day in an intersection with a traffic light.* Typically, when ambulance operators respond in poor weather conditions, they try to drive with a bubble of safety around the vehicle. Maybe the bubble should be there all the time, instead of reserving it for poor road conditions when ambulance collisions rarely occur!

REDUCING AMBULANCE COLLISIONS

So what is your EMS agency doing to reduce ambulance collisions? Do you have an aggressive proactive driver training program? Or does the agency follow a "we'll deal with it when it becomes a problem" kind of approach? All too often the latter approach can result in news bulletins such this one from the Associated Press: "Ambulance collides with car, killing three small children and seriously injuring their mother and sister; ambulance driver arrested on three counts of manslaughter."

As mentioned, such situations can be prevented by determining when and where they are most likely to occur. That is why the New York profile—or better yet, a profile from your own state—can be helpful in directing your own personal attitudes and training. Instead of confining your practice to skidding around wet or snowy parking lots, consciously practice safe driving under normal conditions.

If you have the opportunity to develop programs to reduce ambulance collisions in your community, consider implementing the following actions or standards:

- Routine use of driver qualification checklists and driver's license checks, either through the local police or the Department of Motor Vehicles
- Demonstrated driver understanding of preventive mechanical maintenance, including a vehicle operator checklist and a procedure for reporting any problems found during the check or while driving the vehicle
- Provision of plenty of hands-on driver training, using experienced and qualified field officers. (A 10,000–24,000 pound ambulance has a much longer stopping distance than the 2,500 pound pickup truck

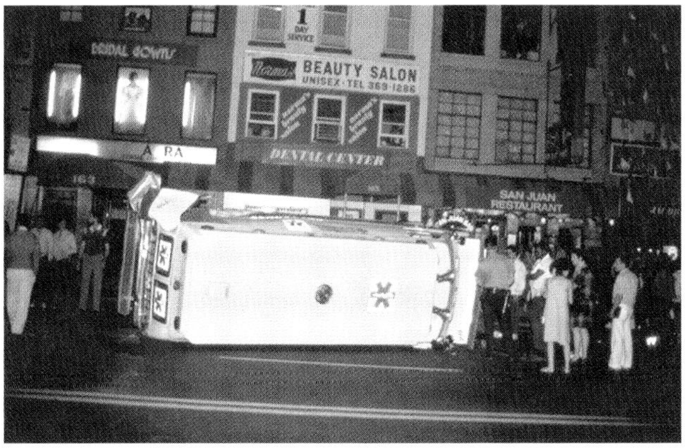

FIGURE 8-3 Ambulance collision.

that an operator drove to work. The goal is to prevent an inexperienced driver from being stopped by a light pole—or another car—after sliding through an intersection [Figure 8-3].)

- Implementation of a slow-speed course to assure that operators know how to use mirrors, back up, park, and handle ambulance-sized vehicles—including accurate estimation of braking distance and turn radius

- Training that ensures that operators know how to react to emergency situations such as the loss of brakes, loss of power steering, a stuck accelerator, a blown-out tire, or vehicle breakdown

- Demonstrated driver knowledge of both the primary and back-up routes to all hospitals in your service response area

- Demonstrated driver understanding of the rules, regulations, and laws that your Department of Motor Vehicles has established, for drivers in general and for ambulance operators in particular

STANDARD OPERATING PROCEDURES

Each EMS agency should have standard operating procedures (SOPs) pertaining to the operation of its vehicles. At a minimum, there should be SOPs that spell out the following:

- Procedure for qualifying as an ambulance operator
- Procedure for handling and reporting an ambulance collision
- Process for investigating and reviewing each collision
- Process for implementing quality assurance in the aftermath of a collision
- Method for using a spotter when backing up a vehicle (Figure 8-4)
- Use of seat belts in the ambulance, and the procedure for transporting a child passenger under 40 pounds
- Guidelines on what constitutes an emergency response and the exemptions that may be taken under state laws
- Guidelines on prudent speed; proper travel in, and the circumstances for using, oncoming lanes; and safe negotiation of intersections
- Circumstances and procedures for use of escorts
- A policy on zero tolerance for driving the vehicle under the influence of alcohol or any drugs

FIGURE 8-4 Use of a spotter.

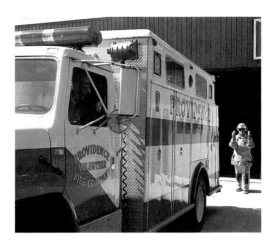

THE DUE REGARD STANDARD

The motor vehicle laws enacted by most states are based upon a model law. As might be expected, state laws pertaining to ambulance operation tend to be similar. One similarity centers on the legal concept of **due regard**. Essentially, due regard exempts ambulance drivers from certain laws but at the same time holds them to a higher standard.

State laws typically exempt ambulance drivers who are operating in an emergency from posted speed limits, posted directions of travel, parking regulations, and requirements to wait at red lights. There are, however, certain situations from which ambulances are rarely or never exempt. They include passing over a railroad crossing with the gates down and passing a school bus with flashing red lights. In the latter case, you should wait until the bus driver secures the safety of the children and turns off the red lights. Only then should you proceed past the bus.

While the laws are often liberal in their exemptions, they place the responsibility for deciding when and where these exemptions should be applied squarely on the shoulders of drivers. The laws often say, for example, "the foregoing provisions and exemptions do not relieve the operator of an emergency vehicle from acting with due regard for the safety of all persons." Such language sets a higher standard for ambulance operators than for almost any other driver on the road. Nowhere in the motor vehicle laws are other drivers held accountable for the safety of all other motorists!

To see how this higher standard might affect you, consider a situation that could occur in any community. It's 7:00 P.M. in a suburban neighborhood. After a dry, clear, warm day, the sun has started to set. A five-year-old child takes one last ride on a Big Wheel™ (a low-profile, plastic tricycle). The child peddles down a slightly inclined driveway past a pine tree obstructing the view of oncoming motorists and rolls into the street. A mid-sized car with four adults on their way to dinner and a movie is headed toward the driveway. The driver is sober, traveling the speed limit, and having a normal conversation. Suddenly the child darts into view from behind the pine tree. The driver immediately steps on the brakes, but it is too late. The car strikes the child, who later dies from multi-trauma in the emergency department.

When the police arrive, they take statements from all involved, assure the driver's sobriety, check the vehicle's inspection, and measure skid marks. In all likelihood, they issue no tickets. The family of the child may decide to sue the driver for the loss of their child, but the police usually take no action unless a specific motor vehicle law has been violated.

Now imagine the same situation, except it is your ambulance headed toward the child's driveway. An emergency call has brought you into the neighborhood. You

✱ due regard legal terminology found in the motor vehicle laws of most states that sets up a higher standard for the operators of emergency vehicles.

Ambulances are rarely or never exempt from passing over a railroad crossing with the gates down or passing a school bus with flashing lights.

have lights on, siren off, and are not exceeding the posted speed limit. As you and your partner search for house numbers, a child suddenly darts into view. You strike the brakes immediately, but unfortunately the child instantly dies from multi-trauma.

When the police arrive, they take statements from all involved, assure your sobriety, check the vehicle's inspection, and measure the skid marks. They then turn the case over to the county grand jury for further investigation. You will appear before the jury, which will scrutinize your personal and professional driving record, service SOPs, rules of the road, and perhaps even your personal habits. In the meantime, the local newspaper has run a front-page story, complete with your name and that of your service. The headline implies that you killed the child as you raced through town in your ambulance.

By now, some of your neighbors have begun to sneer while you empty your mailbox. The reputation of your service has been indelibly tarnished in the public's mind. Members of other crews say their patients have questioned the safety of riding in your service's ambulances. But you can't really respond. Your service has suspended you from driving pending the results of the hearing.

After more than a week of deliberations, the grand jury clears you of all responsibility. It has found that you were sober, attentive, and doing your job. There was nothing you could have done, says the jury, to have prevented the child's death. If the newspaper even carries the final chapter of the story, it appears inside the paper in a small follow-up piece.

The moral is this: As an ambulance driver, you will always be held to a higher standard than other drivers. You must be attentive and prepared to shoulder the responsibilities that come with the profession that you have chosen.

LIGHTS AND SIREN: A FALSE SENSE OF SECURITY

As a general rule, do not rely solely on lights and siren to alert other motorists of your approach. Studies have shown that most motorists do not see or hear your ambulance until it is within 50 to 100 feet of their vehicles. Even so, the siren is the most commonly used—and abused—audible warning device. Before you decide to turn on the siren, consider the following points:

- Motorists are less inclined to yield to an ambulance when the siren is continually sounded.
- Many motorists feel that the right-of-way privileges given to ambulances are abused when sirens are sounded.
- Inexperienced motorists tend to increase their driving speeds by 10 to 15 miles per hour when a siren is sounded.
- The continuous sound of a siren can possibly worsen sick or injured patients by increasing their anxiety.
- Ambulance operators may also develop anxiety from sirens used on long runs, not to mention the possibility of hearing problems.

Some states and services have specific laws and/or SOPs that address the use of sirens. Some useful guidelines include:

- Use the siren sparingly and only when you must.
- Never assume all motorists will hear your siren.
- Assume that some motorists will hear your siren, but choose to ignore it.
- Be prepared for panic and erratic maneuvers when drivers do hear your siren.
- Never use the siren to scare someone.

As a general rule, do not rely solely on lights and siren to alert other motorists of your approach.

The role of lights and siren in the modern emergency response situation has diminished. Recent data has shown that lights and siren only shave a few seconds off of response times, but significantly increase the possibility of injury to the responding crew.

Whenever the ambulance is on the road, day or night, turn on the headlights to increase its visibility. Alternating headlamps should only be used at night if they are installed in a secondary lamp. Probably the most useful light is the one in the center of the cowling on the front hood. This light can usually be easily seen in the rear view mirror of the car in front of you.

Each corner of the ambulance should have large flashers that blink in tandem or unison to help oncoming vehicles identify the location and size of the ambulance. Although the controversy over the use of strobes continues, consider the latest research on the subject when designing or picking the lighting on your ambulance. At present, recommendations lean toward the use of single beam bulbs and strobes instead of relying on one type of lighting system. The most important point is visibility. The vehicle must be clearly visible from 360 degrees to all other motorists and pedestrians.

ESCORTS/MULTI-VEHICLE RESPONSES

Most EMS agencies no longer suggest the use of a police escort for ambulances—except in those circumstances where the ambulance is providing service to an unfamiliar district and needs to be taken to the patient and/or the hospital. There are several reasons for this. First, ambulances and police cars have different braking distances. If an ambulance follows a police car too closely, it can easily rear end the car if they both stop quickly. Second, the two vehicles have different acceleration speeds. As a result, an ambulance operator may have trouble keeping up with a police car. A gap often develops, allowing other vehicles to pull in between. Finally, other motorists may not realize that the two emergency vehicles are traveling together. After the police car speeds by, a vehicle may pull in front of an ambulance, assuming the coast is clear.

In multi-vehicle responses, the dangers are the same as for an escort. In addition, another danger occurs when two emergency vehicles approach an intersection at the same time. Beside totally confusing motorists and pedestrians, the potential for an intersection collision increases dramatically. Often motorists fail to yield the right of way to the first emergency vehicle, the second emergency vehicle, or, in some instances, both vehicles.

It is a good idea to pay attention to other calls taken in your district. However, do not assume that you know all the responses that are taking place. To avoid warning the perpetrators of crimes, for example, the police often respond to incidents without announcing their approach. As a general rule, always negotiate an intersection assuming that you may meet another emergency vehicle.

PARKING AND LOADING THE AMBULANCE

Whenever you arrive first at the site of a motor vehicle collision, take steps to size up the scene for potential hazards to you, your crew, and the patients. Consider establishing a danger zone, parking at least 100 feet from the wreckage upwind and uphill (if possible) to avoid fire or any escaping hazardous liquids or fumes. If there is no fire or escaping liquids or fumes, park at least 50 feet from the wreckage. If possible, assign a member of the crew to handle traffic until the police arrive to take control of the task.

If your ambulance is the first emergency vehicle on the scene, make sure you park in front of the wreckage so your warning lights can alert approaching motorists.

If your ambulance is the first emergency vehicle on the scene, make sure you park in front of the wreckage so your warning lights can alert approaching motorists. Then set up flares, or non-incendiary warning devices, as quickly as possible.

If the scene has already been secured, park beyond the wreckage to prevent your ambulance from being exposed to traffic (Figure 8-5). If command has already been established by an on-scene EMS unit, you may receive pre-arrival

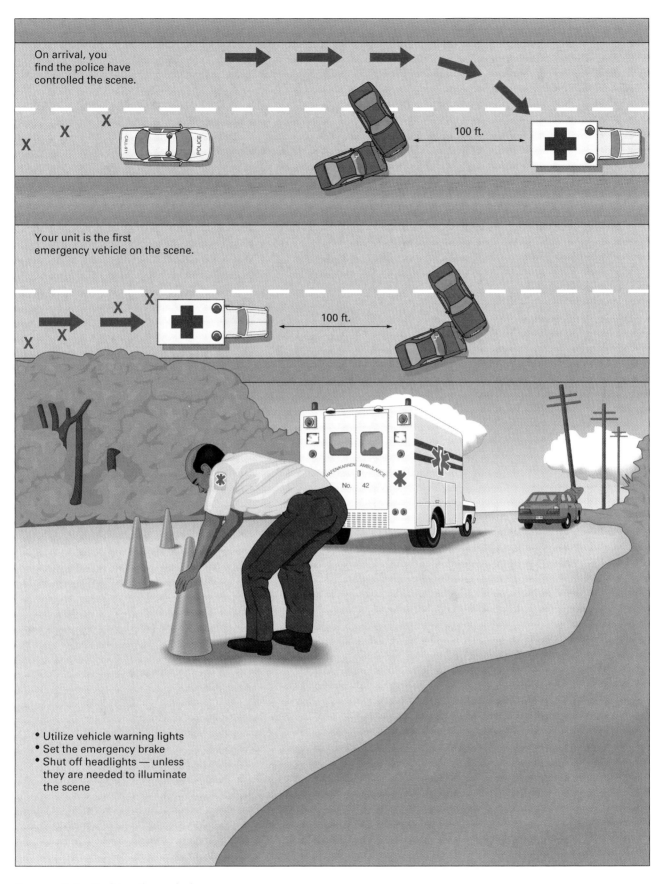

On arrival, you find the police have controlled the scene.

100 ft.

Your unit is the first emergency vehicle on the scene.

100 ft.

• Utilize vehicle warning lights
• Set the emergency brake
• Shut off headlights — unless they are needed to illuminate the scene

FIGURE 8-5   Parking the ambulance.

instructions. In the case of multiple casualty incidents, for example, the commander may tell you where to park and who you should report to.

Always be aware of potential traffic hazards at the scene of a call. Many EMS providers have been seriously injured—and some even killed—after being struck by passing motorists. As much as possible, try not to expose either your crew or your patient to traffic. Keep in mind that the rear ambulance doors often obstruct the warning lights when they are opened to load the patient. Also remember that studies have shown that red revolving lights attract drunk or tired drivers. Consider pulling off the road, turning off your headlights, and using just the amber rear sealed blinkers that flash in tandem or in unison. These lights, as noted, will help oncoming motorists to identify both the size and the location of your vehicle.

THE DEADLY INTERSECTION

Exercise extreme caution whenever you approach an intersection.

Recall that New York statistics reveal 72% of all ambulance collisions occur in intersections. Clearly the intersection is a very unsafe, if not deadly, place to be. Exercise extreme caution whenever you approach one of these hazards. Keep in mind the braking distance of your ambulance, the effectiveness of lights and siren, the rules of the road, the SOPs of your service, the acceleration needed to get through the intersection safely, and more. Helpful tips for negotiating an intersection include:

- Stop at all red lights and stop signs and then proceed with caution.
- Always proceed through an intersection slowly.
- Make eye contact with other motorists to assure they understand your intentions.
- If you are using any of the exemptions offered to you as an emergency vehicle, such as passing through a red light or a stop sign, make sure you warn motorists by appropriately flashing your lights and sounding the siren.
- Remember that lights and siren only "ask" the public to yield the right of way. If the public does not yield, it may be because they misunderstand your intentions, cannot hear the siren due to noise in their own vehicles, or cannot see your lights. Never assume that other motorists have a clue to what you plan on doing at the intersection.
- Always go around cars stopped at the intersection on their left (driver's) side. In some instances, this may involve passing into the oncoming lane, which should be done slowly and very cautiously. You invite trouble when you use a clear right lane to sneak past a group of cars at an intersection. If motorists are doing what they should do under motor vehicle laws, they may pull into the right lane just as you attempt to pass.
- Know how long it takes for your ambulance to cross an intersection. This will help you judge whether you have enough time to pass through safely.
- Watch pedestrians at an intersection carefully. If they all seem to be staring in another direction, rather than at your ambulance, they may well be looking at the fire truck headed your way.
- Remember that there is no such thing as a rolling stop in an ambulance weighing over 10,000 pounds or a medium-duty vehicle weighing some 24,000 pounds. Even at speeds as slow as 30 miles per hour, these vehicles will not stop on a dime. When negotiating an intersection, consider "covering the brake" to shorten the stopping distance.

UTILIZING AIR MEDICAL TRANSPORT

Air medical transport involves two types of air rescue units: fixed-wing aircraft and rotorcraft. Missions that use air rescue units are commonly referred to as **aeromedical evacuations,** or medevac.

FIXED-WING AIRCRAFT

As a rule, fixed-wing aircraft are primarily used for emergency medical transport in remote regions, such as parts of Alaska and Canada. These aircraft may also be used to bring patients injured while traveling away from their homes to hospitals nearer to where they live. Fixed-wing aircraft generally are employed when patients require transport over distances of more than 100 miles.

EMS units that have an airport in their primary operating territory may also respond to medical emergencies aboard commercial aircraft that have been forced to land. Most major airlines now carry AEDs as part of their first aid equipment so you can expect to find almost anything when called to a landing strip.

ROTORCRAFT

The type of air transport that you will most likely encounter as a paramedic will involve rotorcraft, or helicopters. The use of helicopters for medical rescue grew out of their proven benefit during the Korean war and the conflict in Vietnam. In Korea, Sikorsky YH-5 helicopters rescued downed soldiers at the front and evacuated them to aid stations. In Vietnam, helicopters, particularly the larger and more popular "Huey" (the UH-IH Iroquois) evacuated more than 349,000 patients. (Some of the Hueys can still be seen today, complete with bullet-hole patches!)

In 1969, Dr. R. Adams Cowley convinced the Maryland state legislature to fund the first statewide public safety medevac program operated by the state police. In the 1970s, St. Anthony's Hospital in Denver, Colorado, started the first hospital-based program. Today there are over 200 hospital-based air medical transport programs in the United States (Figure 8-6).

The growth of air medical transport provides an essential service to the EMS field provider agencies and the hospital community. Many agencies in the United States now have the ability to order medically equipped helicopters to traumatic incidents requiring rapid response. They also use helicopters to transport patients from the field, especially in rural areas, to specialized hospitals. Finally, helicopters can provide quick inter-hospital transport of critically ill or injured patients.

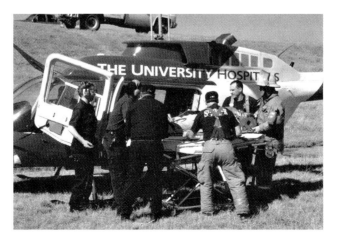

FIGURE 8-6   A hospital-based helicopter.

ADVANTAGES AND DISADVANTAGES OF AIR TRANSPORT

When compared with ambulances, aeromedical transport offers a number of advantages and disadvantages. Advantages include:

- Rapid transport in situations where the time required for ground transport poses a threat to the patient's survival or recovery
- Access to rural or remote areas
- Access to specialty units—e.g., neonatal intensive care units, replantation units, transplant centers, burn centers, and so on
- Access to personnel with specialized skills—e.g., surgical airway, thoracotomy, rapid sequence intubation, critical care, and more
- Access to specialty supplies—e.g., aortic balloon pumps

Disadvantages of aeromedical evacuation include weather and environmental restrictions to flying, altitude limitations, and airspeed limitations. Depending on the specific aircraft, cabin size can also restrict the number of crew members, the amount of equipment carried onboard, and the configuration of the stretcher. In smaller aircraft, such as the commonly used Bell LongRanger®, size limits the crew to the pilot and one flight-medic and/or flight nurse. It also restricts the procedures that can be done on the patient during flight.

In the case of helicopter transport, in-flight climate control systems may not meet with your normal expectations. The thin walls of the fuselage do not allow much space for thermal insulation. Expect the "ship" to be hot in summer and cool in winter. Inside lighting is limited, otherwise the glare might enter the pilot's compartment, severely affecting his or her vision. Even though there is a curtain between the patient's compartment and the pilot, the lights still must be kept low, making ongoing patient assessment a challenge for the flight crew.

Finally, helicopter transport costs a lot of money. Some communities simply cannot afford to have a program. Costs are pushed even higher when preventative maintenance and down time are taken into account.

ACTIVATION

Local and/or state guidelines may exist for the use of air medical transport in your area. Just as the public should access EMS by a single point (i.e., 911), ideally there should be a single access point for air medical transport in your region. In order for a helicopter program to be effective, the front-line First Responders, EMT-Basics, and Paramedics must be willing to consider the need for medevac as early as possible. The final decision should take into consideration the pilot's input, particularly on such factors as the safety of weather conditions, potential landing sites, and hazardous terrain.

INDICATIONS FOR PATIENT USE

The indications for patient transport by helicopter include medical emergencies, trauma emergencies, and search and rescue missions. Anatomic and physiologic compromising factors that may warrant the need for air medical transport include:

Clinical Criteria

- Trauma score < 12
- Glasgow Coma Scale < 10
- Penetrating trauma to abdomen, pelvis, chest, neck, or head

In order for a helicopter program to be effective, the front-line First Responders, EMT-Basics, and Paramedics must be willing to consider the need for medevac as early as possible.

Stable patients who are accessible to ground vehicles are best transported by ground vehicles.

- Spinal cord or spinal column injury or any injury producing paralysis or lateralizing signs
- Partial or total amputation or an extremity (excluding digits)
- Two or more long bone fractures or pelvis fracture
- Crush injury to abdomen, chest, or head
- Major burns or burns to face, hands, feet, or perineum; burns with respiratory involvement; electrical or chemical burns
- Patients in serious traumatic event < 12 or > 55 years of age
- Patients with near-drowning injuries
- Adult patients with:
  —Systolic BP < 90 mmHg
  —Respiratory rate < 10 or > 35 per minute
  —Heart rate < 60 or > 120 per minute
  —Unresponsive to verbal stimuli

The mechanism of injury may also indicate the need for air transport. However, keep in mind that a number of local programs require physiological abnormalities in addition to MOI findings. Injuries or accidents that may warrant air transport include:

Mechanism of injury
- Vehicle roll-over with unbelted passengers
- Vehicle striking pedestrian > 20 mph
- Falls > 10 feet
- Motorcycle victim ejected at > 20 mph
- Multiple victims

Difficult Assess Situations
- Wilderness rescue
- Ambulance egress or access impeded by road conditions, weather, or traffic

Time/Distance Factors
- Transport to trauma center > 15 minutes by ground ambulance
- Transport time to local hospital by ground ambulance greater than transport time to trauma center by helicopter
- Patient extrication time > 20 minutes
- Utilization of local ground ambulance results in absence of ground ambulance coverage for local community

Technically, the Federal Aviation Agency (FAA) does not license commercial operators to do rescue missions involving special means of access, such as rappelling out of a helicopter. Such missions are usually undertaken by highly trained teams who respond with police agencies under a public safety provision in a state or local regulation.

It is important to weigh the risks versus benefits before using a helicopter for EMS patient transport.

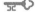

PATIENT PREPARATION AND TRANSFER

It is strongly suggested that EMS agencies set up in-service training so all employees become familiar with flight procedures prior to participating in any air missions. As with any training, review these procedures regularly so you know what to do whenever a patient is transported by air. Spend some time, for example, identifying any special considerations that must be taken into account prior to loading the patient. For example, you may need to immobilize the patient on a specific type of backboard. Smaller helicopters might accept only a certain size backboard, while larger helicopters might fit an entire stretcher. Also, some helicopter services limit the length of the patient when supine, which could alter your method of immobilizing a fractured femur. In this instance, a standard bipolar splint may extend the leg too long to fit inside the ship.

Methods of infection control and intubation will also be affected by air transport. Some agencies specify procedures to limit the spread of bloodborne pathogens in the helicopter. You might, for instance, be required to wrap the packaged patient in a disposable blanket or to place the patient in a body bag. It will also be necessary to convert IV bags to pressure infuser bags. Some flight crews may also need to intubate the patient prior to flight due to the limited area around the airway once the patient is onboard the aircraft. Depending on altitude, you may find it useful to put fluid in the air cuffs of tubes such as Foley catheters or endotracheal tubes, since the fluid will not expand or contract as gases do under certain flight conditions.

Remember that air pressure is changed by altitude, which affects IV bags, air cuffs of tubes, and the use of a PASG.

If you have employed a PASG, remember that it too may be affected by pressure changes. A problem may arise during descent, when the volume of gas in the chambers decreases. As a result, remember to maintain the pressure in the device as the plane or helicopter lands.

As already mentioned, it is difficult to assess a patient's lungs sounds in a helicopter. For this reason, ensure tube placement by visualization, observation of symmetrical chest expansion and condensation in the ET tube, positive color changes, or a reading with an end-tidal carbon dioxide detector. You might also use a pulse oximeter to assist in your ongoing patient assessment.

SCENE SAFETY AND THE LANDING ZONE

The medical helicopter industry has suffered a number of very serious crashes, especially in the mid 1980s. Over the past decade, great strides have been made in improving the safety of helicopter transport. An important factor in bringing about these changes has been the focus on safety among flight personnel. The Commission on Accreditation of Air Medical Services (CAAMS), for example, was developed as a voluntary agency dedicated to ensuring the safety of the air transport environment and to promoting the highest quality of patient care.

To fulfill the goals of CAAMS, flight crews should familiarize all EMS personnel in their region with their procedures and expectations. This will go a long way toward maintaining a safe scene and defining a safe landing zone (LZ) for the incoming helicopter.

All paramedics should be capable of selecting an appropriate LZ. As a rule, a helicopter requires a LZ of approximately 100-by-100 feet (about 30 large steps on each side) situated on ground with less than an eight-degree slope (Figure 8-7). Paramedics should also be able to describe the terrain, major landmarks, estimated distance to the nearest town, and other pertinent information to the helicopter pilot on a designated frequency. The LZ, as well as the approach and departure path, should be clear of wires, towers, vehicles, people, and loose objects.

FIGURE 8-7 Helicopter landing zone.

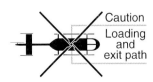

Caution
Loading and exit path

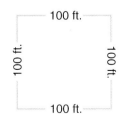

100 ft.
100 ft.
100 ft.
100 ft.

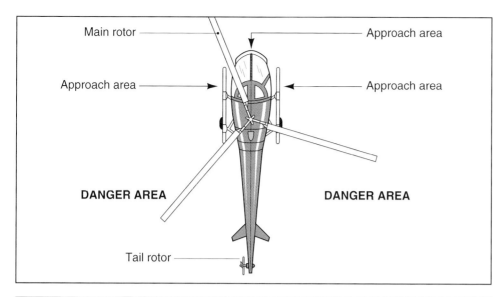

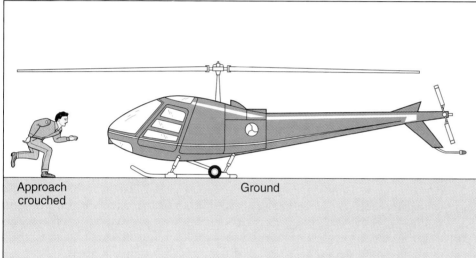

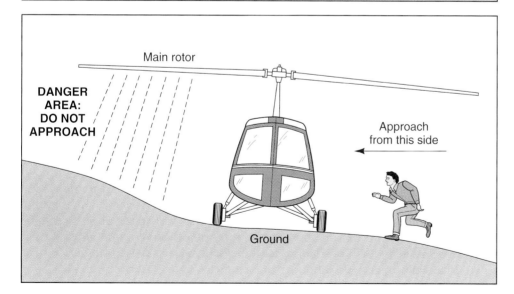

FIGURE 8-8 Danger areas around a helicopter.

A. The area around the tail rotor is extremely dangerous. A spinning rotor cannot be seen.

B. A sudden gust of wind can cause the main rotor of a helicopter to dip to a point as close as four feet from the ground. Always approach a helicopter in a crouch when the rotor is moving.

C. Approach the aircraft from the downhill side when a helicopter is parked on a hillside.

Most flight crews suggest that EMS crews mark the LZ with a single flare in an upwind position. During night operations, remember never to shine a light into the pilot's eyes. This could cause temporary blindness or interfere with depth perception.

Once the aircraft has landed, approach it with extreme caution and only upon approval of the flight crew. Make sure all loose objects, such as pillows and linens, are secured on the stretcher. Allow the flight crew to direct loading of the patient. Stay clear of the tail rotor at all times. Approach in a crouched-down position. (See Figure 8-8 on page 335.) A sudden gust of wind can cause the main rotor of a helicopter to dip to a point as close as four feet to the ground. If the helicopter has landed on a slight incline, approach it from the downhill side of the incline. Keep all traffic and vehicles away from the helicopter by a distance of at least 100 feet. Finally, do not allow anyone to smoke within 200 feet of the aircraft.

SUMMARY

Even though you have learned about ambulance operations and air medical transport in your EMT-Basic training and in your everyday experience, good safety habits grow stronger with review and practice. As a paramedic, you should be familiar with standards that influence ambulance design, equipment requirements, and staffing. You should also regularly complete all checklists, whether they apply to the vehicle, onboard equipment, or essential supplies. Be aware of items that require routine maintenance or calibration as well as the expiration dates on all drugs. Keep in mind OSHA requirements that promote the safety of personnel and patients and know how to report equipment problems or failures to your supervisor.

As you know, ambulance operators have a special responsibility whenever they take the wheel. It is your professional duty to recognize the profile of a typical ambulance collision and to develop strategies for preventing it from occurring. You should also be aware of the issues surrounding the staging and staffing of ambulances and determine your agency's policies on these matters.

Finally, after reading this chapter, you should appreciate the advantages and disadvantages of air medical transport. Know the conditions or situations that merit such transport and always remember the safety issues involved in packaging the patient, selecting a landing site, and approaching the aircraft.

YOU MAKE THE CALL

You and your partner are working on medic ambulance 622 covering the west portion of town. It's your turn to drive when a call comes in for an automobile collision. Responding priority one, lights and siren, you travel eastbound on Central Avenue, approaching the intersection of Wolf Road. You know that this is probably one of the busiest intersections in town. It has two through lanes and two turn lanes in each direction. As a result, there are almost always two moving lanes of traffic.

About 250 feet from the intersection, you notice that the light has turned red. There are stopped cars in both of the left turn lanes. There are a few cars in the center lane, and no cars at all in the right lane. As usual, there are a number of cars traveling northbound through the intersection. There are also southbound cars waiting to turn left and proceed eastbound.

1. Should you drive down the open eastbound right lane with your lights and siren on? Explain.
2. Should you enter the oncoming traffic by going around the left side of the vehicle that is currently stopped in the left hand, eastbound lane? Explain.
3. How can you best deal with this very dangerous intersection?

See Suggested Responses at the back of this book.

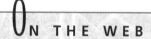

FURTHER READING

Browner, B.D.: (editor), *et. al. Emergency Care and Transport of the Sick and Injured*, 7th Edition. Sudbury, MA. Jones & Bartlett Publishers, Inc., 1999.

Elling, B., R. Guerin: *Ambulance Accident Prevention Seminar Student Workbook*. Albany, NY. Health Education Services, 1988.

Elling, B., R. Guerin: "Getting There," *Emergency,* October 1990.

Fitch, J., R. Keller, *et. al.: EMS Management: Beyond the Street,* 2nd ed. Carlsbad, CA. JEMS Publishing, 1993.

Holleran, R.S., *et. al.: Flight Nursing Principles and Practice,* 2nd ed. St. Louis, MO. Mosby, 1996.

Limmer, D., M. O'Keefe, *et. al.: Essentials of Emergency Care,* 2nd ed. Upper Saddle River, NJ. Prentice Hall, 1998.

MacDonald, M. (editor): *Guidelines for Air and Ground Transport of Neonatal and Pediatric Patients*. Washington, DC. American Academy of Pediatrics, 1999.

Peto, G.J., W.J. Medve: *EMS Driving: The Safe Way*. Upper Saddle River, NJ. Prentice Hall, 1996

ON THE WEB

Visit Brady's Paramedic Website at www.bradybooks.com/paramedic.

CHAPTER 9

Medical Incident Command

Objectives

After reading this chapter, you should be able to:

1. Explain the need for the incident management system (IMS)/incident command system (ICS) in managing emergency medical services incidents. (pp. 342, 343–344)

2. Define the terms multiple casualty incident (MCI), disaster management, open or uncontained incident, and closed or contained incident. (pp. 341, 346)

3. Describe essential elements of the scene size-up when arriving at a potential MCI. (pp. 345–346)

4. Describe the role of the paramedics and EMS system in planning for MCIs and disasters. (pp. 343, 362, 363–364)

5. Describe the functional components (command, finance, logistics, operations, and planning) of the incident management system. (pp. 343–351)

6. Differentiate between singular and unified command and identify when each is most applicable. (pp. 344–345)

7. Describe the role of command, the need for command transfer, and procedures for transferring it. (pp. 343–344, 345, 347–349)

Continued

Objectives Continued

8. Differentiate between incident command structures used at small, medium, and large-scale incidents. (pp. 343–349)
9. Explain the local/regional threshold for establishing command and implementation of the incident management system including MCI declaration. (pp. 343–345)
10. List and describe the functions of the following groups and leaders in ICS as it pertains to EMS incidents:
    a. Safety. (p. 350)
    b. Logistics. (p. 351)
    c. Rehabilitation (rehab). (p. 360)
    d. Staging. (pp. 346, 359)
    e. Treatment. (pp. 357–359)
    f. Triage. (pp. 354–357)
    g. Transportation. (pp. 359–360)
    h. Extrication/rescue. (p. 360)
    i. Disposition of deceased (morgue). (p. 357)
    j. Communications. (pp. 347, 361–362)
11. Describe the methods and rationale for identifying specific functions and leaders for the functions in ICS. (pp. 344–345, 347–348)
12. Describe the role of both command posts and emergency operations centers in MCI and disaster management. (pp. 345, 347, 361, 362)
13. Describe the role of the on-scene physician at multiple casualty incidents. (p. 359)
14. Define triage and describe the principles of triage. (pp. 354, 356)
15. Describe the START (simple triage and rapid transport) method of initial triage. (pp. 354–356)
16. Given color-coded tags and numerical priorities, assign the following terms to each:
    a. Immediate. (pp. 354, 356–357)
    b. Delayed. (pp. 354, 356–357)

c. Hold. (pp. 354, 356–357)
d. Deceased. (pp. 354, 356–357)
17. Define primary and secondary triage. (p. 354)
18. Describe when primary and secondary triage techniques should be implemented. (p. 354)
19. Describe the techniques used in tracking patients during multiple casualty incidents and the need for such techniques. (pp. 348–349, 356–357, 360)
20. Describe techniques used to allocate patients to hospitals and track them. (pp. 359–360)
21. Describe modifications of telecommunications procedures during multiple casualty incidents. (pp. 347, 361–362)
22. List and describe the essential equipment to provide logistical support to MCI operations to include:
    a. Airway, respiratory, and hemorrhage control. (p. 358)
    b. Burn management. (p. 358)
    c. Patient packaging/immobilization. (p. 358)
23. List the physical and psychological signs of critical incident stress. (pp. 360, 364)
24. Describe the role of critical incident stress management sessions in MCIs. (pp. 351, 364)
25. Describe the role of the following exercises in preparation for MCIs:
    a. Table top exercises. (pp. 363–364)
    b. Small and large MCI drills. (pp. 363–364)
26. Given several mass and multi-casualty incidents with preprogrammed patients, provide the appropriate triage, immediate care, and transport. (pp. 341–364)

Case Study

A chartered bus carrying 42 passengers is headed northbound on Interstate 85 when the driver loses control of the vehicle. The bus swerves off the roadway and strikes a tractor-trailer parked on the right shoulder. Several passing motorists use their cell phones to call the local 911 communications center. The dispatcher tones out the local EMS and fire departments and notifies the state police via landline.

The first ambulance arrives shortly after the first police unit. The paramedic in the passenger seat does a windshield survey. She then relays her observations to dispatch: "Central, 206 on the scene. We have a transit bus rear-end into a tractor-trailer, obvious rescue problem. 206 will be establishing Interstate 85 Command." The dispatcher acknowledges the message: "206, you're on the scene at 14:23, establishing Interstate 85 Command, moving communications to TAC-1."

The two paramedics now decide who will be the Incident Commander and who will be the Triage Officer. The Incident Commander walks the perimeter of the scene, surveying for rescue problems, hazards, and staging of resources. Meanwhile, the Triage Officer enters the bus through the damaged main door and does an approximate count of patients, relaying this information to the Incident Commander. Using the START system, the Triage officer moves quickly from patient to patient. She keeps a running count as she applies a triage tag to each person.

Outside the bus, the Incident Commander calls the dispatch center: "Central, Interstate 85 Command. We have a transit bus vs. tractor-trailer, estimating 40 patients, at least 15 category red. We are declaring an MCI, requesting 20 transport units. Staging instructions are for all EMS units to come southbound on I-85 and stage in the left lane. We also need fire and rescue units, who are to stage northbound just behind the accident scene."

The regional MCI plan immediately goes into effect. Local EMS agencies are mobilized, with remaining resources distributed around the area to ensure adequate coverage. Off-duty personnel are called in by pager system to staff additional units. Local hospitals are notified of the incident through this pager system, and immediately take a count of their available beds.

On the scene, the Triage Officer completes her first wave, resulting in 13 category red patients, 24 category yellow, 2 category green, and 4 category black. Five patients are entrapped, including the four category black patients.

Two more ambulances arrive and begin to treat the critical patients. Fire and rescue units arrive a short time later, initiating hazardous material control and rescue operations. The Field Supervisor arrives and meets with the Incident Commander, who provides a situation report and then transfers command. He alerts dispatch: "Central, Interstate 85 Command. Transferring command from 206 to Charlie-1." The paramedic remains with the Field Supervisor as an aide, answering the radio and recording information.

As additional EMS units arrive, the Field Supervisor assigns various functions, such as Treatment Manager, Transport Officer, and Safety Officer. Other personnel provide patient care, gather supplies, or transfer patients to waiting ambulances. Operations run smoothly, with IMS officers communicating with each other and personnel performing their assigned tasks.

Ambulances transport the first critical patients off the scene at 14:47, just 24 minutes after the first unit established command. The Transportation Officer distributes patients evenly among the five local hospitals, with the designated trauma center receiving the most critical ones. The last patients depart the scene 53 minutes after EMS Unit 206 established command. Although the incident is now terminated, coroner's units remain on the scene to transport the four fatalities.

During this incident, other EMS units in the region responded to 12 emergencies, including one multi-vehicle accident. Neither of the two multiple casualty incidents compromised response time or patient care within the system.

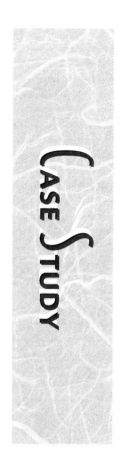

INTRODUCTION

Traditional paramedic training focuses on the relationship between one or two patient-care providers and a single patient. In this setting, a paramedic has the ability to concentrate on the assessment and treatment of the patient. Occasionally, however, paramedics are called upon to treat more than one patient at a time. The multi-patient incident may result from a motor vehicle collision (MVC), an apartment fire, a gang fight, or any number of other scenarios.

During your career as a paramedic, you can also expect to respond to a much larger **multiple casualty incident (MCI)**, also known as a mass casualty incident. The MCI can involve "everyday" incidents such as the bus vs. tractor-trailer collision described in the opening case study to disasters such as tornados, train wrecks, airline crashes, or even a terrorist event (Figures 9-1, 9-2a, and 9-2b). Definitions of an MCI vary with the district. Some districts define an MCI as any incident involving three or more patients. Other districts set the level for an MCI at five, seven, or more patients. In situations involving a disaster, the number of patients can reach into the hundreds or thousands.

In this chapter, you will learn about the EMS response to MCIs and disasters. The same techniques and tools used to respond to a multiple-patient MVC will be used to manage a major MCI. Command, organization, and communications procedures can be scaled up or down to fit the particular situation. The special considerations involved in **disaster management** will appear near the end of the chapter.

✱ **multiple casualty incident (MCI)** incident that generates large numbers of patients and that often make traditional EMS response ineffective because of special circumstances surrounding the event; also known as a mass casualty incident.

The same techniques and tools used to respond to a multiple-patient MVC will be used to manage a major MCI.

✱ **disaster management** management of incidents that generate large numbers of patients, often overwhelming resources and damaging parts of the infrastructure.

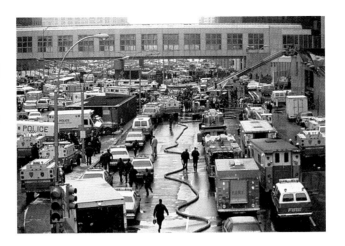

FIGURE 9-1 On February 26, 1993, use of the incident command system allowed crews from the police, fire, and medical services departments to respond to the bombing of the World Trade Center in New York City.

ORIGINS OF THE INCIDENT MANAGEMENT SYSTEM

✱ Incident Management System (IMS) national system used for the management of multiple-casualty incidents, involving assumption of responsibility for command and designation and coordination of such elements as triage, treatment, transport, and staging; sometimes called the Incident Command System.

Based on the confusion surrounding several major fires in the 1970s, the fire service took the lead in organizing responses to large-scale emergencies. The result was several versions of the Incident Command System (ICS)—a management program designed for controlling, directing, and coordinating emergency response resources. In recent years, the various ICS systems have been merged into the comprehensive, standardized **Incident Management System (IMS)**. It is a national system used for the management of multiple-casualty incidents, involving assumption of responsibility for command and designation and coordination of such elements as triage, treatment, transport, and staging. Although the Incident Command System was originally developed for use at major fires, the standardized IMS has been adopted by law enforcement, EMS, hospitals, and industry.

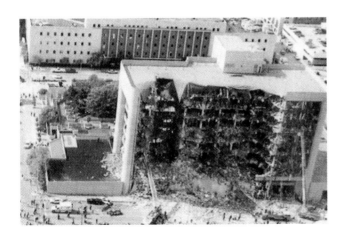

FIGURE 9-2a The scene of the April 19, 1995, bombing of the Alfred P. Murrah Federal Building in Oklahoma City. (Sygma)

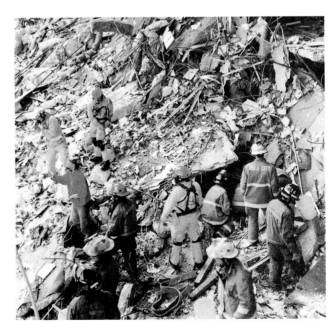

FIGURE 9-2b Crews with various kinds of protective gear attempting to locate—and extricate—victims from the debris. (Pool/Gamma Liaison)

REGULATIONS AND STANDARDS

The uniform practices followed at an MCI stem from a variety of sources. The only federal requirement for use of IMS falls under the OSHA regulations requiring "the use of a site-specific ICS" during an emergency response to the release of hazardous substances. Regulations by the Environmental Protection Agency (EPA), however, have picked up this wording so that even non-OSHA states must comply with this requirement.

National consensus standards, or widely agreed upon guidelines, have been developed by the National Fire Protection Association. Although these standards are not laws or regulations, they recommend practices for use at MCIs. Some of the standards with which you should be familiar include the ones that relate to hazardous materials incidents (Chapter 11), health and safety IMS, and disaster management.

In addition, various states have passed laws requiring the use of the Incident Management System. As a paramedic, you should research whether such laws exist in your state. Pay particular attention to the presence of a **scene-authority law**— a legal statute specifying who has ultimate authority at an MCI.

> ✱ **scene-authority law** legal state or local statute specifying who has ultimate authority at an MCI.

The national standard curriculum for implementing the Incident Management System is taught by the National Fire Academy in Emmitsburg, Maryland. However, California Firescope and several major urban fire departments have also developed programs. As already mentioned, IMS programs have become increasingly standardized in recent years. Nonetheless, you should become familiar with the specific type of IMS used within your jurisdiction.

A UNIFORM, FLEXIBLE SYSTEM

With its uniform terminology and approach, the Incident Management System has a number of advantages. First, an IMS can supersede jurisdictional and geographic boundaries to provide a well-organized response to routine and large-scale emergencies. Second, an IMS has the flexibility to respond to emergencies in both the public and the private sectors.

To familiarize you with the structure and practices of the Incident Management System, the following sections focus on its major functional areas. Use the mnemonic **C-FLOP** to keep these areas in mind as you read. The letters stand for:

> ✱ **C-FLOP** mnemonic for the main functional areas within the IMS—command, finance/administration, logistics, operations, and planning.

C—command

F—finance/administration

L—logistics

O—operations

P—planning

COMMAND AT MASS-CASUALTY INCIDENTS

The most important functional area in the Incident Management System is **command**. The Incident Commander (IC)—also known as the Officer in Command (OIC) or the Incident Manager (IM)—is the individual who runs the incident. Most agencies have a single person who is the highest-ranking official. However, establishing command at a multi-agency, multi-jurisdictional incident can be complicated. As already mentioned, state or local legislation may

> ✱ **command** the individual or group responsible for coordinating all activities and who makes final decisions on the emergency scene; often referred to as the Incident Commander (IC) or Officer in Charge (OIC).

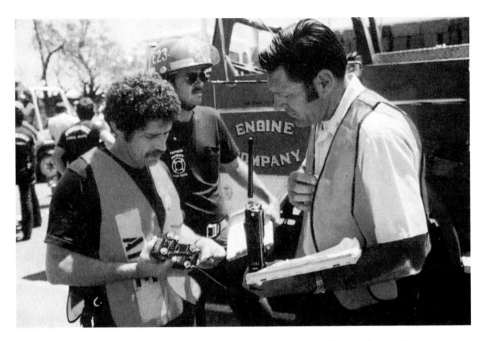

FIGURE 9-3   The first on-scene unit must assume command and direct all rescue efforts at a mass casualty incident (MCI).

decide the issue in such situations (Figure 9-3). Otherwise, the decision should be reached by a preexisting MCI or disaster plan. (The importance of planning will be discussed later in the chapter.)

The most critical concept to grasp in terms of IMS command is this: The ultimate authority for decision making rests with the Incident Commander. The IC is responsible for coordinating the many activities that occur on the emergency scene. Because it would be too confusing or impossible for all on-scene personnel to report directly to the IC, the person charged with command delegates certain functions and responsibilities to others. In this way, the IC maintains a reasonable **span of control,** or number of people or tasks that a single individual can monitor. Depending upon the scope of the incident, the span of control may range from three people to seven people. However, the average is around five.

SINGULAR VS. UNIFIED COMMAND

At small incidents with limited jurisdictions, **singular command** usually works best. Such incidents have a smaller scope and usually do not involve outside agencies. For example, a traffic accident may involve the local fire department, EMS, and police department. The three agencies might agree that the fire department should assume overall command, thus creating a singular command situation.

In many incidents, however, a singular command will not be feasible because of overlapping responsibilities or jurisdictions. Instead, a **unified command** will be established. Examples of such incidents include terrorist attacks, explosions, sniper or hostage situations, and large-scale disasters. In each of these examples, the managers from several jurisdictions—law enforcement, fire, and EMS—will coordinate their activities.

In establishing a unified command, the co-managers try to achieve balanced decision making. Together, they identify and access the appropriate agencies or specialized organizations that might be needed at the scene, such as the American Red Cross, health department, public works, and so on. They also select sec-

---

The ultimate authority for decision making rests with the Incident Commander.

✱ **span of control** number of people or tasks that a single individual can monitor.

✱ **singular command** process where a single individual is responsible for coordinating an incident; most useful in single-jurisdictional incidents.

✱ **unified command** process in which managers from different jurisdictions—law enforcement, fire, EMS—coordinate their activities and share responsibility for command.

tor leaders and seek to establish reasonable and unified spans of control. Finally, the commanders determine the need for public information officers and liaison with the media.

When the Incident Management System is expanded or the scene is large, co-managers set up a **command post (CP)**. The command post provides a place where command officers from various agencies can meet with each other and select a management staff. Because a command post may operate for weeks, the site should be selected carefully. Access to telephones, restrooms, and shelters should be taken into account. Also, the command post should be close enough to the scene so that officers can monitor operations, but far enough away so that they are outside the direct operational area. Persons operating on the scene, members of the media, and bystanders should not have routine access to the CP.

* command post (CP) place where command officers from various agencies can meet with each other and select a management staff.

ESTABLISHING COMMAND

As already mentioned, the determination of when to establish command and when to declare an MCI will vary from department to department. An MCI may be declared when an incident produces multiple patients, has circumstances that make scene management challenging, or significantly taxes the available resources of a system. Generally, when two or more units respond to an emergency or when casualties include two or more patients, you should implement the Incident Management System.

As a rule, the first arriving unit usually establishes command. EMS personnel survey the scene through the windshield of their vehicle as they arrive on-scene. As you already know, EMS providers should never exit the vehicle until they have identified all the elements of an incident and noted any potential hazards. At an MVC, for example, do not miss the vehicle partially hidden in the woods or the pool of gasoline near your vehicle. Once you have determined the visible scope of an incident and any obvious hazards, relay this information to dispatch.

Depending upon the scope of the incident and local protocols, you and your partner will most likely fill the roles of Incident Commander and Triage Officer—at least until other units arrive. Never forget the importance of assigning command early in an incident. Most MCIs are won or lost in the first ten minutes. Without use of incident command, emergency personnel may freelance. They may fail to prioritize patients, underestimate the severity of the incident, or delay requesting additional resources. Successful handing of any MCI involves coordination of all key personnel—whether two people, twenty, or more.

Generally, when two or more units respond to an emergency or when casualties include two or more patients, you should implement the Incident Management System.

Never forget the importance of assigning command early in an incident.

Successful handling of any MCI involves coordination of all key personnel—whether two people, twenty, or more.

INCIDENT SIZE-UP

The term "size-up," as you already know, applies to the formal evaluation of the situation surrounding an incident. As such, size-up is an integral part of establishing command. In managing an MCI, you must keep in mind three main priorities: life safety, incident stabilization, and property conservation.

Life Safety

Life safety is always your top priority. If you arrive first on the scene of a high-impact incident, you must observe and protect all rescuers, including yourself, from hazards. Then, and only then, will you attend to patients who are in immediate life-threatening situations. Keep in mind, however, that the needs of the many usually outweigh the needs of the few. If you commit to caring for the first patient that you encounter, you may neglect ten other critical patients lying nearby.

Content Review

INCIDENT PRIORITIES
- Life safety
- Incident stabilization
- Property conservation

If you are the Incident Commander, remember that responsibility for triage belongs to the Triage Officer. At a small-scale incident, the IC may end up triaging some patients. Even so, the Triage Officer assumes the main responsibility for sorting patients into categories based upon the severity of their injuries.

Incident Stabilization

While attending to life safety, you should also keep in mind your second priority—incident stabilization. To achieve this goal, quickly identify whether the situation is an **open incident** or a **closed incident**. An open incident, also known as an uncontained incident, has the potential to generate more patients at any time. A fire that traps people inside an office building is an example. You may find only several patients when you arrive on-scene. However, other patients—including fire fighters—may soon appear. As a result, the Incident Commander must anticipate the need for additional resources. Whenever you command an open incident, remember this point: It's better to call too many resources than too few.

In the case of a closed or contained incident, the injuries have usually already occurred by the time you arrive on-scene. An example might be a multi-vehicle collision. Yet even a so-called closed incident carries the potential for additional hazards—an undetected gas leak, a distraught family member who rushes into traffic, or further injury to patients wandering about the scene. As a result, it only makes sense for an IC to expend effort stabilizing an incident. Preventing further injuries—either of patients or rescue personnel—helps ensure a smoother and more successful management of an MCI.

Whenever you command an open incident, remember this point: It's better to call too many resources than too few.

Property Conservation

As with any other call, the third priority of an Incident Commander is conservation of property. At no time during an operation should rescue personnel damage property unless it is absolutely necessary for achieving the first two priorities—life safety and incident stabilization. Property conservation includes protection of the environment where operations are staged.

IDENTIFYING A STAGING AREA

Identification of a staging area goes hand-in-hand with the scene assessment. At MCIs involving hazardous materials or structural fires, for example, you must note wind speed and direction. Any Incident Commander must ensure that the staging area and command post lie well beyond the reach of any fumes, smoke, water, chemicals, or other hazardous materials.

Once you establish command of an MCI, you should also note both a primary and a secondary staging area. In picking a primary site, keep in mind the main purpose of a staging area—organization of resources in one place for quick and easy deployment. Position the primary staging area as close to the scene as possible without compromising safety. Make sure the site has good access and exit points to ensure the flow of emergency vehicles.

The secondary staging area should ideally lie in a different direction. This will provide you with a contingency plan in case the primary staging area becomes unusable. Conditions that may force a change in staging areas include altered traffic patterns, shifts in wind direction, or restricted access due to the deployment of fire hoses or other special equipment.

INCIDENT COMMUNICATIONS

Communications forms the cornerstone of the Incident Management System. Once command is established, the Incident Commander has a responsibility to relay this information to dispatch. Then, as soon as possible, the IC should transmit a preliminary report that includes the following data: type of incident, approximate number of patients by priority, request for additional resources, staging instructions, and a plan of action. If a fixed command post is required, the IC should communicate the location of this site as well.

Once an MCI has been declared, further communications should be moved to a secondary, or tactical, channel. The Incident Commander must be able to supply the information necessary to coordinate resources. That is the whole purpose of the Incident Management System. Use of a secondary channel will also prevent an Incident Commander from interfering with the communications by other jurisdictions or from overwhelming the primary EMS channel.

When acting as an Incident Commander, remember that communications will involve units from different jurisdictions and perhaps different districts. One of the foundations of incident management is the use of a common terminology. When communicating, you should eliminate all radio codes and use only plain English. A radio code may have different meanings in different places. As an Incident Commander, you must eliminate any unnecessary confusion in an already complicated situation. In fact, it may be preferable to avoid radio codes even in routine operations. Then there will be no need to even think about switching to plain English when you assume command of an MCI.

Communications are the cornerstone of the Incident Management System.

RESOURCE UTILIZATION

Few EMS departments have the resources to handle an MCI without outside help. Regardless of the nature of an incident, most units will need additional ambulances, personnel, equipment, and medical supplies. In many cases, they will also require specialized equipment and perhaps the help of public or private agencies.

The primary role of an Incident Commander is the strategic deployment of all necessary resources at an incident. Development of a strategy means setting goals and determining the tactics needed to accomplish these goals. Because of the complicated nature of an MCI, the Incident Commander must continually assess the effectiveness of a given strategy or plan.

To ensure flexibility, an Incident Commander should radio a brief progress report approximately every ten minutes until the incident has been stabilized. The report should state established goals, tactics and resources being used to meet these goals, and any progress or lack of progress. This forces an Incident Commander to monitor an operation, adapt tactics or resources to changing circumstances, and/or to eliminate ineffective tactics entirely. Subordinates should deliver similar reports to the Incident Commander so that he or she can properly evaluate the overall operation.

The primary role of an Incident Commander is the strategic deployment of all necessary resources at an incident.

COMMAND PROCEDURES

Several procedures help an Incident Commander to manage an MCI. First and foremost, all personnel must be able to recognize the IC. At smaller, single-agency events, everyone may know the IC simply by his or her voice over the radio. However, at medium or large-scale incidents, such recognition is often impossible. As a result, the Incident Management System calls for the IC and other officers to

FIGURE 9-4 Using command vests at a mass casualty incident (MCI) makes it easier to identify personnel. The Incident Commander directs the response and coordinates resources.

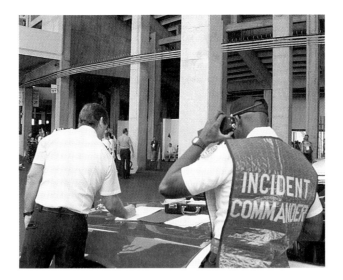

wear special reflective vests (Figure 9-4). The vests can be color-coded to functional areas and may have the officer's title on the front and back. Such vests should be worn whenever IMS is utilized, even at smaller incidents. By making a basic set of vests, especially for command and triage, available on every response unit, personnel will get in the habit of wearing and/or recognizing the vests prior to a major incident.

An Incident Commander can also benefit from the use of a worksheet or clipboard—two useful tools for tracking decisions (Figure 9-5). An IMS worksheet should include basic information on the incident, a small area to sketch the scene, and a checklist of important items to remember. It might also include a section

COLONIE EMS *Incident Tactical Worksheet*

Location_____
Med. Command_____

___ Establish unified command with fire & police
___ Place 2 cones on command vehicle
___ Put bib on
___ Designate triage office
___ Advise inbound units where to stage
___ Advise crews to stay with units until given instructions
___ Advise units to switch to EMS Admin., 265 or 715

LEVEL 1 (3-10 Patients)	LEVEL 2 (11-25 Patients)	LEVEL 3 (over 25 Patients)	FIRE	RESCUE
___ Declare MCI	___ Declare MCI	___ Declare MCI	___ Assess # of Units Needed	___ Establish Perimeter
___ EMS All Call	___ EMS All Call	___ EMS All Call	___ EMS All Call Req. 619	___ Request Speciality Units
___ Request # of Units Needed	___ Request # of Units Needed	___ Request # of Units Needed	___ Designate Triage	___ Triage Officer Handles Inner
___ Cover Town/Sr. Medic Act 615	___ Cover Town/Sr. Medic Act 615	___ Cover Town/Sr. Medic Act 615	___ Set up Rehab at Air Bank	Circle
___ Roll Call Hospitals	___ Roll Call Hospitals	___ Roll Call Hospitals	___ Use 619 as ALS Unit	
___ Transport Officer?	___ Get Mutual Aid Units	___ Get Mutual Aid Units		

			HAZ-MAT	
	___ Designate Treatment Officer	___ Designate Treatment Officer	___ Req. # of Units Needed	
	___ Designate Transport Officer	___ Designate Transport Officer	___ EMS All Call	___ Medical Baseline Assess-
	___ Designate Staging Officer	___ Designate Staging Officer	___ Est. Command in Cold Zone	ment of Team
	___ REMO MD to Scene	___ REMO MD to Scene	___ Designate Triage	___ Don Protective Barriers
	___ Consider Rehab & CISD	___ Request Bus to Scene	___ Identify Agent	___ Assist With Decontamination
(2-5 Amb. Needed)	(6-13 Amb. Needed)	(over 13 Amb. Needed)	___ Research Decontamination	___ Rehabilitate
			___ Research Med.	

HOSPITAL ROLL CALL	AMCH	St. PETERS	MEMORIAL	VA	ELLIS	St. CLARE'S	LEONARD	St. MARY'S	SAMARITAN
CAN TAKE									
# PATIENTS SENT									

# OF PATIENTS BY PRIORITY				
1 (Red)	2 (Yellow)	3 (Green)	0 (Black)	TOTALS

UNITS RESPONDING

620 621 622 ____ ____
630 631 632 ____ ____
640 641 642 ____ ____
650 651 652 ____ ____
610 611 605 ____ ____
TSU-1 TSU-2 ____ ____
619 ___ ___ ____ ____
Guild. ___ ___ ____ ____
CPHM ___ ___ ____ ____
Albany ___ ___ ____ ____
Mohawk ___ ___ ____ ____
Empire ___ ___ ____ ____

UNITS IN STAGING

620 621 622 ____ ____
630 631 632 ____ ____
640 641 642 ____ ____
650 651 652 ____ ____
610 611 605 ____ ____
TSU-1 TSU-2 ____ ____
619 ___ ___ ____ ____
Guild. ___ ___ ____ ____
CPHM ___ ___ ____ ____
Albany ___ ___ ____ ____
Mohawk ___ ___ ____ ____
Empire ___ ___ ____ ____

FIGURE 9-5 An incident tactical worksheet from the Town of Colonie, New York, EMS.

to record the on-scene units and personnel, their assignments, and relevant patient information, particularly transport data. Many commercial products are currently available for this purpose, including programs for generating worksheets by computer.

You will find a worksheet especially useful when transferring command, as often happens when higher-ranking officers arrive on scene. Command is only transferred face-to-face, with the current Incident Commander conducting a short but complete briefing on the incident status. A higher-ranking officer does not become IC simply by his or her arrival—a briefing must take place. The worksheet serves as an outline for the briefing.

TERMINATION OF COMMAND

As the incident progresses, resources will be reassigned or released. For example, an Incident Commander who transfers command to a higher-ranking officer may become an aide to the new IC or be assigned to a totally new IMS role. Eventually resources will be **demobilized,** or released for use elsewhere in the EMS system. Once the incident has progressed to the point where the IMS is no longer needed, command should be terminated. A final progress report should be delivered to the communications center. All units will then return to routine rules of operation.

The point at which command terminates depends upon the incident. Some high-impact incidents, such as natural disasters or terrorist events, may last for weeks. However, not all agencies may have a significant presence for the long-term. EMS may have a strong initial response, for example, but may simply have a single ambulance stand by for the long term. Other agencies may be released entirely from the incident if their services are no longer needed.

✱ **demobilized** release of resources—personnel, vehicles, and equipment—for use outside the incident when they are no longer needed at the scene.

SUPPORT OF INCIDENT COMMAND

Incident command is supported by four sections or functional areas: finance/administration, logistics, operations, and planning. Each section has a place within the Incident Management System and is headed by a **Section Chief.** However, all four areas may not be established at every incident. At small- or medium-sized incidents, for example, operations may be the only section implemented.

At large-scale or long-term incidents, the Incident Management System may activate the areas of finance/administration, logistics, and planning. Depending upon the type of incident and the structure of command, these sections may not be filled with EMS personnel. However, they may help coordinate some EMS activities.

In addition, several important officers may report directly to the Incident Commander. These officers handle public information, safety, outside liaisons, and critical stress debriefing. Together they are known as the **Management Staff,** or Command Staff. The combination of Management Staff and Section Chiefs comprise and carry out what are called **Staff Functions.**

As a paramedic, it is more important for you to know how the Incident Management System works than to be an expert in specific job functions. Figure 9-6 and the following sections give you a quick overview of the basic elements of the Incident Command System.

✱ **Section Chief** officer who supervises major functional areas or sections; reports to the Incident Commander.

✱ **Management Staff** officers that handle public information, safety, outside liaisons, and critical stress debriefing; also known as the Command Staff.

✱ **Staff Functions** officers who perform supervisory roles in the IMS rather than those who actually perform a task.

MANAGEMENT STAFF

The establishment and role of command has already been described. However, the Management Staff can play an important role in supporting the Incident Commander, particularly at major incidents or disasters. Therefore, you should be familiar with the role of the following officers or teams.

IMS LINE POSITIONS AND COMMAND STAFF

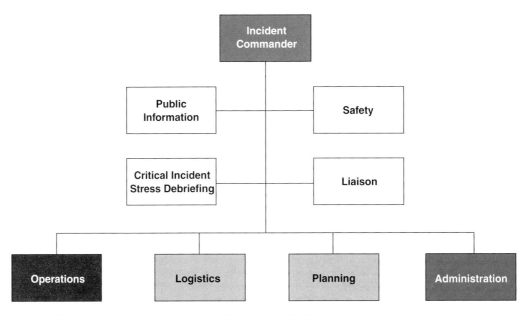

FIGURE 9-6   Basic elements of the Incident Management System.

Safety Officer

The **Safety Officer** may hold the most important role at an MCI. This person—or, in some cases, team of people—monitors all on-scene actions and ensures that they do not create any potentially harmful conditions. Because almost anything that happens at an incident is potentially harmful, the Safety Officer assumes an enormous responsibility. Some of the areas that must be monitored for safety compliance include infection control, use of personal protective equipment, crowd control, lifting of patients and equipment, and quality of scene lighting. Under the Incident Management System, the Safety Officer has the authority to stop any action that is deemed an immediate life threat.

Liaison Officer

The **Liaison Officer** coordinates all incident operations that involve outside agencies. These agencies may include other emergency services, disaster support networks, private industry representatives, government agencies, and more. As the title implies, the Liaison Officer makes sure these outside agencies are connected with the appropriate functional areas within the Incident Management System. This ensures, based on requests and reports from the Incident Commander, that specialized resources are deployed effectively.

Public Information Officer (PIO)

The **Public Information Officer** collects data about the incident and releases it to the press. Although you may not have a preexisting relation with the media in your community, a major incident will put your unit in the public spotlight. Your department's image depends upon favorable exposure in the media. As a result, it is important for an IMS to have an effective PIO.

Critical Incident Stress Management (CISM) Team

The **CISM Team** monitors the emotional status of all on-scene personnel. High-impact events may negatively affect the emotional health of public safety workers. The CISM Team will support these workers and attempt to reduce the stress. They may also conduct on-scene debriefings, if necessary. (The management of critical incident stress will be discussed in more detail later in the chapter.)

✳ Critical Incident Stress Management (CISM) Team monitors the emotional status of all on-scene personnel and provides the necessary support.

FINANCE/ADMINISTRATION

This section rarely operates on small-scale incidents. However, on large-scale or long-term incidents the staff supports command by assuming responsibility for all accounting and administrative activities. The section keeps personnel and time records. It also estimates costs, pays claims, and handles procurement of items required at the incident. These functions are usually performed by the jurisdictional government where the incident has occurred.

✳ Finance/Administration responsible for maintaining records for personnel, time, and costs of resources/procurement; reports directly to the IC.

LOGISTICS

The **logistics** section supports incident operations. One of its most critical functions is fulfilling the **Medical Supply Unit.** This unit coordinates procurement and distribution of equipment and supplies at an MCI.

Depending upon the structure of the IMS used, other units may be established as well. The **Facilities Unit,** for example, selects and maintains areas used for rehabilitation and command. It makes sure there is adequate food, water, restrooms, lighting, power, and so on. Other units might be set up to manage field communications, on-scene medical care for workers, and so on.

✳ Logistics supports incident operations, coordinating procurement and distribution of all medical resources.

✳ Medical Supply Unit coordinates procurement and distribution of equipment and supplies at an MCI.

✳ Facilities Unit selects and maintains areas used for rehabilitation and command.

OPERATIONS

Whatever work needs to be performed at an incident takes place under **Operations.** This section carries out tactical objectives, directs front-end activities, participates in planning, modifies the action plan, maintains discipline, and accounts for personnel. In short, Operations gets the job done.

As will be explained later in the chapter, Operations may have many **branches**—functional levels based upon primary roles or geographic locations. Branches organized by role might include sections within the various jurisdictions at an incident—EMS, rescue, fire, law enforcement, and so on. Branches based on geography might include the Operations at various locations. The IMS structure used at the bombing of the World Trade Center, for example, assigned a branch of Operations to each building in the complex.

✳ Operations fulfills directions from command and does the actual work at an incident.

✳ branches functional levels within the IMS based upon primary roles and geographic locations.

PLANNING

Planning provides past, present, and future information about an incident. The section helps formulate the overall action plan and oversees changes in that plan. It collects information such as weather reports, documents incident actions, and develops contingency plans. It ensures that written SOPs for **mutual aid**—agreements for sharing departmental resources—are activated or fulfilled.

The Planning section operates according to the principle of "anything that can go wrong will go wrong." The staff uses past incidents to anticipate troubles that might arise at the current incident. The section then acts accordingly. When Command and Operations must switch tactics, Planning stands ready to provide the necessary strategic support.

✳ Planning provides past, present, and future information about an incident.

✳ mutual aid agreements or plans for sharing departmental resources.

DIVISION OF FUNCTIONS

As already noted, getting organized quickly and early is essential to the success of any IMS operation. There are several ways to divide functions at an incident. The choice of organization depends upon the scope of an MCI, the structure of your department, the implementation of singular or unified command, and so on.

If you are an Incident Commander, one of your jobs will be to organize line functions—i.e., Operations—in the most effective manner. To do this, you should become familiar with the basic functional levels within the Incident Management System. Figure 9-7, for example, shows the functional levels within a typical EMS branch.

BRANCHES

You, or the co-managers in a unified command, may chose to establish any number of branches. As mentioned, these branches may be organized by primary role or by geography. Branches are supervised by Branch Directors, who report to the

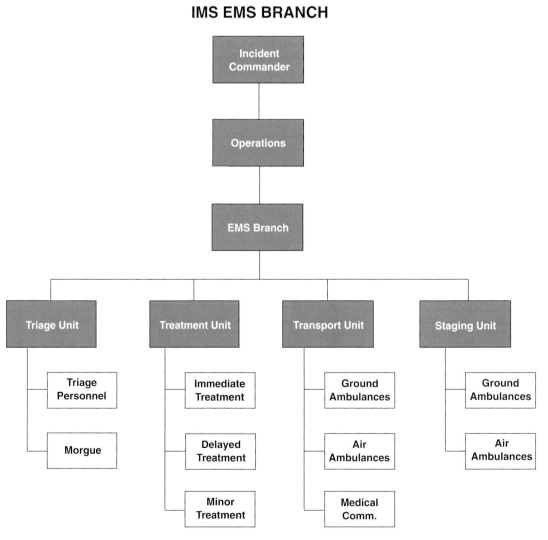

FIGURE 9-7 Example of branches that may operate in a major incident.

Section Chief for that particular functional area. The EMS Branch Director supervises all operations involved with patient care and transportation. Depending upon the system, rescue may be an independent branch or it may report to the director of EMS or fire.

GROUPS AND DIVISIONS

Branches may be further organized into groups or divisions—working areas of an incident where specific job tasks are accomplished. Groups are based upon function, while divisions are based upon geography. As an example, think of Triage as a group and the responders working on the third floor of a multi-floor incident as a division. Groups and divisions are managed by supervisors who in turn report to the Branch Director.

UNITS

Groups and divisions can be broken into even more task-specific groups known as units. They are supervised by Unit Leaders, who report to the supervisor of a group or division.

SECTORS

Depending on the type of Incident Management System in your area, you may hear the term **Sectors** used. A Sector is an interchangeable name for a branch, group, or division. However, it does not designate a functional or geographic area. Although there is no formal name for individuals who supervise a Sector, they are often called Sector Officers.

✱ **Sector** interchangeable name for a branch, group, or division; does not, however, designate a functional or geographic area.

FUNCTIONAL GROUPS WITHIN AN EMS BRANCH

The Incident Management System operates under the so-called "tool box" theory. Do not remove a tool from the toolbox unless you actually need to use it. The flexibility of IMS is founded on the ability to only implement the areas of IMS that are needed at an incident. This theory holds for all areas of IMS, including branches, groups, sectors, divisions, and specific areas where EMS operates. At many EMS incidents, the basic IMS organization in Figure 9-8 will be all the "tools" that you need.

The flexibility of the Incident Management System is founded on the ability to only implement the areas that are needed at an incident.

BASIC IMS ORGANIZATION
EMS OPERATIONS

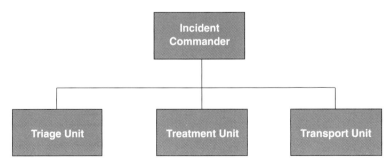

FIGURE 9-8   Organization for a small to medium-sized incident.

TRIAGE

As you have read, **triage** is the act of sorting patients based upon the severity of their injuries. The object of emergency medical services at an MCI is to do the most good for the most people. For this reason, you need to determine which patients need immediate care to live, which patients will live despite delays in care, and which patients will die despite receiving medical care.

Because triage will direct subsequent operations, it is one of the first functions performed at an MCI. As a result, all personnel should be trained in triage techniques and all response units should carry triage equipment. The Triage Group Supervisor may act independently or may supervise the Triage Group/Sector.

Primary and Secondary Triage

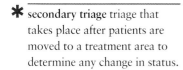
Triage occurs in phases. **Primary triage** takes place early in the incident, when you first contact patients. The action provides a basic categorization of sustained injuries. It must be done quickly and efficiently so that command can determine on-site treatment needs and resources. Universally recognized triage categories include the following:

Category	Color	Priority
Immediate	Red	Priority-1 (P-1)
Delayed	Yellow	Priority-2 (P-2)
Hold	Green	Priority-3 (P-3)
Deceased	Black	Priority-0 (P-0)

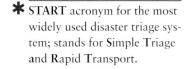
Secondary triage takes place throughout the incident as patients are collected, moved to treatment areas, and receive appropriate medical care. A patient's condition may change over time, requiring you to upgrade or downgrade his or her triage category.

The START System

The most widely used triage system is **START**, an acronym standing for **S**imple **T**riage **a**nd **R**apid **T**ransport. The system was developed at Hoag Memorial Hospital in Newport Beach, California. START's easy-to-use procedures allow for rapid sorting of patients into the preceding categories. START does not require a specific diagnosis on the part of the responder. Instead it focuses on these signs or symptoms (Figure 9-9):

- Ability to walk
- Respiratory effort
- Pulses/perfusions
- Neurological status

Ability to Walk You initiate the START system by asking patients who can walk to get up and come to you. Any patients who can complete these acts, despite their injuries, will be categorized "green." Either you or another member of triage group should place the appropriate tag on the patients. Because patients who can walk will walk, you should make every effort to confine them to one site. There is already enough confusion at an MCI without having the "walking wounded" wandering around the scene.

Respiratory Effort Next, you begin to triage the non-walking patients. Remember to keep the focus on tagging patients. Your only treatment effort should be directed toward correction of airway problems and severe bleeding.

START TRIAGE SYSTEM

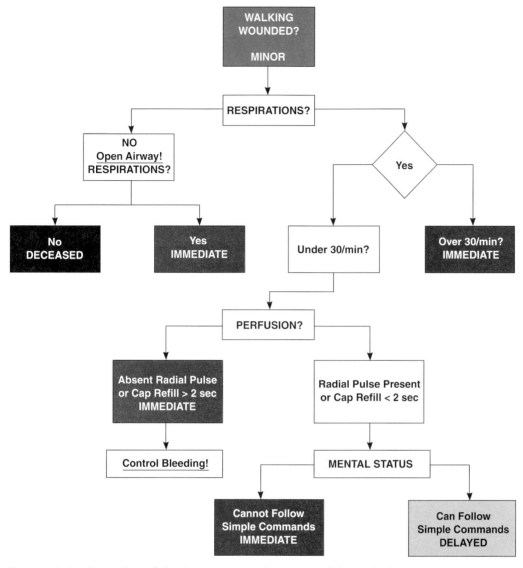

FIGURE 9-9 Operation of the START system, the most widely used triage system.

Begin by assessing breathing effort. If patients are not breathing, open their airway manually. Categorize those patients who start to breath spontaneously as "red." Tag those who fail to respond as "black." For those patients who are breathing, quickly assess their respiratory rate. Patients with respirations above 30/minute should be tagged "red." If respirations are less than 30/minute, go to the next assessment step.

Pulse/Perfusion Assessment of circulatory status can be accomplished in two ways: radial pulses and capillary refill. The presence of a radial pulse indicates a systolic blood pressure of at least 90 mmHg. However, delayed capillary refill (over 2 seconds) is a poor indicator of perfusion in adults. It can be compromised by cold weather or be normally delayed in certain people. Therefore, the preferred method of assessing perfusion is the radial pulse. Patients with absent radial pulses will be triaged "red." If patients have respirations less than 30/minute *and* a present radial pulse, go to the next assessment step.

- Can get up and walk
- Open airway
- Respirations over 30/minute
- Radial pulse
- Follows commands

Neurological Status You now quickly assess mental status. Use this quick test. Ask patients to grip both of your hands. If they can perform this simple task, categorize them Priority-2 or "yellow." If they cannot follow such simple commands, categorize them Priority-1 or "red."

Triage Tagging/Labeling

As already mentioned, you should attach a color-coded tag to each patient that you have triaged. Tagging offers these advantages:

- Alerts care providers to patient priorities—i.e., provides organization of treatment
- Prevents re-triage of the same patient
- Serves as a tracking system during transport and/or treatment

Commercial tags are available, such as the METTAG (Figure 9-10). However, you can also use colored surveyor's tape. Each has its advantages and dis-

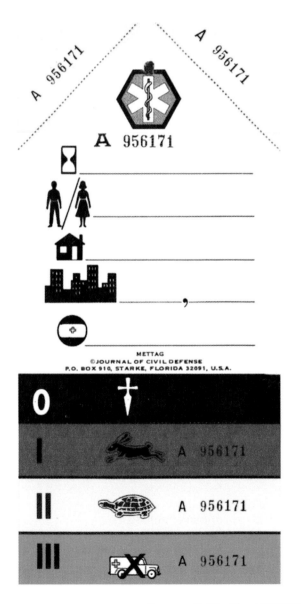
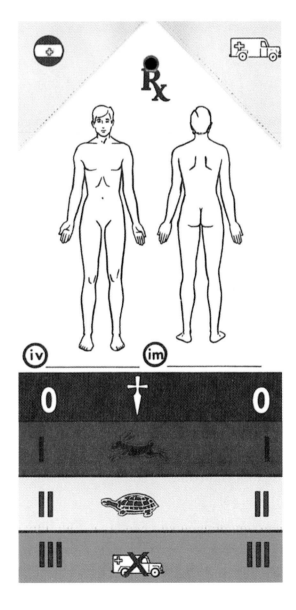

FIGURE 9-10 The METTAG.

advantages. Tags provide tear-off strips that help you count patients in each triage category. Tags also make it easier to track patients, record treatment information, and indicate a patient's location in a transportation accident. But tags can be damaged in wet weather, and tear-off strips can make it difficult to change patient categories. Surveyor's tape costs less money, but does not allow you to count patients during triage. Also, black tape cannot be easily seen at night.

Some systems combine the use of both tags and tape. Others use tags only when immediate transport is unavailable and/or when patients need to be sorted into separate treatment areas. Whatever method of tagging that you use, it must meet these two criteria:

- Be easy to use
- Provide rapid visual identification of priorities

The Need for Speed

As stated on several occasions, you must not become committed to one-on-one patient care during triage. However, that does not mean that you do nothing. Simple care—opening airways and direct pressure on profuse bleeding—can save lives early in an incident. As a result, the Triage Officer should carry certain medical equipment—infection control supplies, oral airways, and trauma dressings. Other essential items for the Triage Officer include tags or tape, a portable radio to communicate with the Incident Commander, a command vest, and a flashlight (at night).

Ideally, it will take you less than 30 seconds to triage each patient. However, that means it will take you five minutes to triage ten patients, more than 20 minutes to triage 40 patients, and so on. As a result, other personnel will often assist the Triage Officer in MCIs with a large number of patients. The simple decision to add personnel can dramatically reduce triage time and speed treatment and transport. Triage personnel can act individually or be assigned to units. Either way, they report to the Triage Officer, who in turn relays necessary information to the IC. After completing the task of triage, personnel can be reassigned to other units, such as treatment.

The simple decision to add personnel can dramatically reduce triage time and speed treatment and transport.

Morgue

You should collect patients who are triaged "black," or deceased (Priority-0), in an area away from treatment. This area, known as the **morgue,** should be access-controlled so that bystanders or the media cannot enter it. In determining the disposition of the deceased, you will need to work closely with the medical examiner, coroner, law enforcement, and other appropriate agencies. (If possible, attempt to leave the deceased victims until a decision and plan for the disposition of their bodies can be determined.)

Once a morgue is established, it will be supervised by a **Morgue Officer.** This person may report to the Triage Officer or the Treatment Officer. In many cases, these supervisors will in fact assist in selecting and securing an area for the morgue.

Keep in mind the importance of having a preexisting plan for managing situations with large numbers of fatalities. Special facilities may be required to care for the victims. In addition, responders may require the support of a CISM Team or members of the clergy.

✱ morgue area where deceased victims of an incident are collected.

✱ Morgue Officer person who supervises the morgue; may report to the Triage Officer or the Treatment Officer.

Treatment

When the number of patients exceeds the number of ambulances available for transportation, you will need to collect patients into treatment areas (Figure 9-11). The **Treatment Group Supervisor** controls all actions in the Treatment Group/Sector.

✱ Treatment Group Supervisor controls all actions in the Treatment Group/Sector.

FIGURE 9-11 Treatment sector at a multiple casualty incident (MCI).

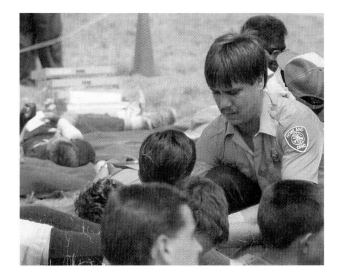

The responders who carry patients to the treatment area should be organized into teams of four to prevent lifting injuries. As patients arrive in the treatment area, you should conduct or oversee secondary triage to determine if their status has changed. Patients should then be separated into functional treatment areas based on their category: red (immediate, P-1), yellow (delayed, P-2)), or green (hold, P-3).

You will also need medical equipment to operate a treatment area properly. Essential equipment includes airway maintenance supplies, oxygen and delivery devices, bleeding control supplies, and burn management supplies. In addition, you will need patient immobilization and transportation devices such as stretchers, long spine boards, or other equipment to move patients.

Red Treatment Unit

This area provides care for all critical patients. As a result, Command and/or Logistics will assign the bulk of medical resources to this unit. Providers with ALS skills usually report to the red treatment area so they can stabilize patients and prepare them for transport. Because medical resources can be quickly used, a supply system is necessary to support this operation. Finally, this is the place where any on-scene physicians or nurses should be utilized.

Yellow Treatment Unit

Teams of responders carry all non-critical patients to this unit for stabilization. Although these patients are not as critical as those in the red area, ALS procedures may still be necessary. A patient with an isolated femur facture, for example, will probably be categorized yellow. Although this patient does not require immediate intervention or transport, he or she may still require an intravenous line and eventual surgical intervention.

Green Treatment Unit

Ambulatory patients report to the green area, where they are prepared for transport. Very little care is necessary in this area, but these patients still require monitoring in case their condition deteriorates. In such instances, they will be triaged and moved to the appropriate treatment area.

Supervision of Treatment Units

Each of the preceding units is supervised by a **Treatment Unit Leader,** who reports to the Treatment Group Supervisor. The leader's job requires extreme flexibility to ensure that patients receive adequate care. Patient conditions can change and responders, equipment, or supplies may not be available in the sub-area. As a result, communications must be carefully coordinated. The Treatment Group Supervisor must be apprised of activities in each sub-area. He or she must also help coordinate operations with other functional areas, particularly command, triage, and transport.

✳ **Treatment Unit Leaders** EMS personnel who manage the various treatment units and who report to the Treatment Group supervisor.

ON-SCENE PHYSICIANS

At some high-impact or long-term incidents, physicians may be utilized outside the hospital to support EMS. Physicians may use their advanced medical knowledge and skills in several ways at an MCI. For example, they may be better able to make difficult triage decisions, perform advanced triage and treatment in the treatment area, or perform emergency surgery to extricate a patient as a last resort. Physicians also provide direct supervision and medical direction over paramedics in the treatment area, removing the need to operate under standing orders or radio contact. You should establish a contingency plan outlining when and how physicians respond to and operate at an MCI.

STAGING

Ambulances may be the most precious resource at a mass casualty incident. As a result, ambulances must be staged as they arrive to allow proper access to the scene and, more important, egress with the patients. If ambulances arrive before they are needed to treat patients, they should be kept in a staging area under a **Staging Officer.** This area may be a roadway, a parking lot, or some other site where the units can wait until they are deployed by command.

Depending upon local protocols, drivers or crew members will be required to wait with the vehicles until they are needed for transport. A staging pool keeps personnel from "freelancing" and ensures their availability for quick deployment. It also prevents premature commitment of resources. If ambulances are required for immediate transport, the staging area can serve as a loading area for patients.

✳ **Staging** location where ambulances, personnel, and equipment are kept in reserve for use at an incident.

✳ **Staging Officer** supervises the staging area and guards against premature commitment of resources and freelancing by personnel; reports to the branch director.

TRANSPORT

The **Transportation Supervisor** coordinates operations with the Staging Officer and the Treatment Supervisor. His or her job is to get patients into the ambulances and routed to hospitals. If you are assigned to this role, you will need to be flexible in determining the order in which patients are packaged and loaded. You may, for example, elect to place two critical patients in one ambulance for transport to a trauma center. If you decide that the ambulance provider cannot adequately care for two critical patients, you may instead decide to transport one critical and one non-critical patient. You may also take into account the facilities at a given hospital and avoid overwhelming its resources with critical patients.

The routing of patients to hospitals is as important as getting them into the ambulances. Early in the incident, your communications center should contact local hospitals and determine how many patients in each triage category they can handle. You must take this information into account. You must also consider any specialties that a hospital may have—trauma centers, burn units, neurological teams, and so on. Keep in mind, too, that many patients may have left the scene before the arrival of EMS and transported themselves to the closest hospital.

✳ **Transportation Supervisor** coordinates operations with Staging Officer and the Transportation Supervisor; gets patients into the ambulance and routed to hospitals.

The routing of patients to hospitals is as important as getting them into an ambulance.

Depending upon the scope and nature of the incident, you may have to factor in such self-transport as well.

As you might suspect from this discussion, a Transportation Supervisor needs to implement some type of tracking system or destination log. Ideally, the tracking sheet or log should include the following data:

- Triage tag number
- Triage priority
- Patient's age, gender, and major injuries
- Transporting unit
- Hospital destination
- Departure time
- Patient's name, if possible

The tracking sheet not only helps to organize activities at an MCI, it also proves invaluable in reconstructing the incident at a later time. In addition, this record will help document on-scene patient care.

EXTRICATION/RESCUE

✽ Extrication group or branch responsible for removing patients from entanglements and transferring them to the treatment area; also known as Rescue.

Depending upon your system, **Extrication** or Rescue may be a branch or a group. If this operation is considered an EMS function, it will be a group (sector) under the EMS branch. If it is a fire department function, it may be under the fire branch. If the rescue is extensive or long-term, the operation may be separated into its own branch within the IMS.

In general, the Extrication/Rescue group removes patients from entanglements at the incident and arranges for them to be carried to treatment areas. The operation has many facets and may require specialized personnel and equipment. During extended operations, treatment personnel will need to work in this area and begin patient care prior to removal.

Depending on the circumstances, personnel operating in this area will need personal protective equipment, including helmets, eye protection, gloves, breathing apparatus, and/or protective clothing (Figure 9-12). Some of the rescue tools may also require specific support materials, such as gasoline, electricity, or compressed air. Extrication/rescue is a very dangerous area, and all efforts should be taken to ensure that operations are well supervised and safe.

REHABILITATION

At extended operations, a special rehabilitation area should be established to support on-scene responders. Arrangements should be made with Logistics to ensure the necessary food, water, and medical monitoring supplies.

A predetermined threshold should be established so that rescuers with abnormal vitals are removed from the operation.

Ideally, rescuers should regularly rotate through a dedicated rehabilitation area away from the incident. The site should provide thermal control and shelter from fumes, crowds, or the media. In this environment, rescuers can rest and hydrate themselves. Medical personnel operating in this area will take the vital signs of rescuers and watch for signs of fatigue or incident stress. A predetermined threshold should be established so that rescuers with abnormal vitals are removed from the operation. This is especially important during extremely hot or cold conditions.

✽ Rapid Intervention Team ambulance and crew dedicated to stand by in case a rescuer becomes ill or injured.

Provision should also be made for a **Rapid Intervention Team.** If possible, an ambulance and crew should be dedicated to stand by outside the staging area. The Incident Commander can then contact the unit if a rescuer becomes ill or injured. Unfortunately, the demands of a large-scale MCI sometimes prevent implementation of this aspect of the IMS.

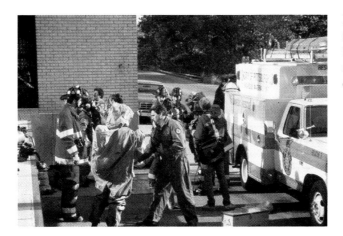

COMMUNICATIONS

The chapter has already covered size-ups, progress reports, frequency use, and more. However, it cannot be said too often: Communications forms the cornerstone of the Incident Management System. Therefore, it helps to review some basic rules of communications within the system's EMS branch.

First, think about what you are going to say before you say it. Does the message really need to be transmitted over the radio? Remember that the frequencies at an MCI will already be congested with messages. As a result, you should try to prevent as much unnecessary radio traffic as possible.

Second, key up your radio before transmitting. Wait one second after pressing the button to speak. This allows your radio to begin transmitting effectively—and all other radios to begin listening—before you begin your message. Keep in mind that missed messages mean missed chances at increased coordination and efficiency.

Third, acknowledge each message with feedback to ensure that you understood it. For example, the message "Staging from Transport, please send two ambulances to pick up patients" should not be acknowledged with "Staging received." It should be answered with "Staging received, two ambulances to pick up patients."

Other rules include points already covered in the chapter: the use of plain English instead of radio codes; the need for a common radio channel between command, groups (sectors), divisions, and units; face-to-face communications when appropriate; and respect for the lines of communication established by the IMS. In other words, report to the person you are supposed to report to.

EMS Communications Officer

At large-scale incidents, the Incident Management System provides for an **EMS Communications Officer,** also known as the EMS COM or the MED COM. This person works closely with the Transportation Supervisor to notify hospitals of incoming patients. A dedicated radio channel works best for this purpose. The EMS COM will not deliver complete patient reports, which would increase the communications traffic. Instead, he or she will transmit the basic information collected by the Transportation Supervision, such as the number of Priority 1 patients en route to a hospital, the expected arrival time, and so on.

Alternative Means of Communication

Remember that your primary radio system may not always work at an MCI. Disasters can knock out radio towers and power. Frequencies can be overwhelmed. Telephone lines can be down. Radio batteries can fail. As a result,

✱ **EMS Communications Officer** notifies hospitals of incoming patients from an MCI; reports to the Transportation Officer and may also be called the EMS COM or MED COM.

alternative means of communication should be included in every MCI preplan and should be practiced regularly. You might use cellular phones, mobile data terminals, alphanumeric pagers, fax machines, or other technology to overcome the failure of your primary radio system. When all else fails, runners can be used to hand deliver messages around the incident scene. Although there are obvious limitations to this method, it may be your last resort. So know how to use it.

DISASTER MANAGEMENT

Disasters can alter the routine operating procedures used at high-impact events. For example, disasters can damage a region's infrastructure, preventing the operation of railroads, hospitals, radio systems, and so on. If a disaster occurs in your jurisdiction, you will be a victim as much as a responder, which is why outside assistance is often required. As a rule, disaster management occurs in the following four stages: mitigation, planning, response, and recovery.

MITIGATION

Mitigation involves the prevention or limiting of disasters in the first place. For example, the public safety community tries to prevent people from building houses on flood plains or from putting up structures unable to withstand the impact of natural phenomena or terrorist attacks. In addition, most communities today have early warning systems to alert people to weather emergencies such as hurricanes and tornadoes or to geological emergencies such as volcanic eruptions or earthquakes.

PLANNING

As already indicated, planning is integral to the successful management of all high-impact emergencies. Every community, including your own, should take part in a hazard analysis and then rate these hazards according to their likelihood. For more on this analysis, see the last section of this chapter.

Depending upon your hazard analysis, devise relocation plans and/or evacuation procedures as needed. When possible, every effort should be made to keep people in their natural social groupings. That is, provide home-based relocation instead of removing people to hospitals and clinics when they are not injured. If you must evacuate people, use whatever means you have to spread the message frequently and with urgency. Alert people to the nature of the disaster, its estimated time of impact, and description of its expected severity. Advise people of safe routes out of the area and the appropriate destinations for those people who must leave an area.

Critical to any successful disaster plan will be provision for an efficient communication system in case the primary system fails. Decide, for example, where a central communications center might be established for people needing help. Set up guidelines on the use of radios by all EMS personnel. Make arrangements for portable radios and recorders as necessary.

RESPONSE

In a disaster, there is a great disparity between the casualties and resources. The event overwhelms the natural order and causes a great loss of property and/or life. As a result, a disaster almost always requires outside assistance and alternative operating plans. In general, you will follow the guidelines set up by the Incident Management System.

RECOVERY

Recovery involves the return of your department, your jurisdiction, and your community to normal as soon as possible. Actions taken will vary with the nature of the disaster and/or the disaster plan under which you operate. You may be involved with the reunion of families, follow-up care, and support of the personnel charged with handling potential hazards such as collapsed buildings, highways, and so on.

MEETING THE CHALLENGE OF MASS CASUALTY INCIDENTS

As implied by the preceding sections, you will never be more challenged in your EMS career than when you respond to an MCI. The routine actions that you do every day will suddenly become more difficult or, in some cases, impossible because of the stress of the incident. For this reason, you should anticipate various problems and work to overcome them.

COMMON PROBLEMS

Things can—and do—go wrong at MCIs and disasters. One way to avert or minimize complications is to anticipate them. As the saying goes, "To be forewarned is to be forearmed." Studies of past incidents have revealed the following common problems. Any one of these can hinder the success of a rescue operation.

- Lack of recognizable EMS command in the field
- Failure to provide adequate widespread notification of an event
- Failure to provide proper triage
- Lack of rapid "initial" stabilization of patients
- Failure to move, collect, and organize patients rapidly into a treatment area
- Overly time-consuming patient care
- Premature transportation of patients
- Improper or inefficient use of in-field personnel
- Improper distribution of patients to medical facilities
- Failure to establish an accurate patient-tracking system
- Inability to communicate with on-scene units, regional EMS agencies, or other personnel
- Lack of command vests for all IMS officers or supervisors
- Lack of adequate training and/or practice of rescuers at an MCI
- Lack of drills among regional agencies involved in the IMS
- Lack of proper community assessment, preplanning, and contingency plans

PREPLANNING, DRILLS, AND CRITIQUES

As mentioned several times, planning for an MCI or disaster makes response much smoother. Anticipate any problems that may occur and work towards removing them. Anything that can be planned in advance should be planned in advance.

The first step involves a complete assessment of the potential hazards—both natural and human—that could occur in your area. If you live in Kansas, for example, you might not worry about hurricanes, but tornados are a very real possibility. Sites of potential incidents in almost any community include chemical or nuclear plants, factories or mines, schools, jails, sporting arenas, entertainment centers, railroads, airports, and so on.

Once you have completed the assessment, your agency should develop a plan that outlines the SOPs and protocols for potential incidents. You will not, of course, be able to plan for every possible scenario. If you develop 100 preplans, for example, you can expect to be summoned to scenario 101 or 102—i.e., the unscripted event. For this reason, you must develop contingency plans for worse-case scenarios. For example, how would you communicate with ambulances if something or someone knocked out the dispatch center? What would you do if the local hospital suddenly became unusable because of chemical contamination?

After you have completed a preplan, test it. Start small. Tabletop drills, for example, are a good place to begin. Once you have worked out the wrinkles, distribute the plan to everyone in your department, the surrounding departments, local police, fire departments, hospitals—in short, to anyone who could be involved in the IMS in your area. Use the plan to ensure that the necessary mutual aid agreements are in place and that the appropriate personnel within the IMS know about these agreements.

Then make sure that all personnel who could show up at an MCI have received proper training in use of the IMS. As you have learned, the first responders on the scene will often determine the course of an event. Run or take part in drills so that you can gain practice in MCI operations and large-scale use of the Incident Management System. Again, start out small. Use local drills within your department to help familiarize personnel with the system. Then, aim for large-scale drills that involve outside agencies.

<table>
<tr><td>Never say "It will never happen here."
〰⊙</td></tr>
</table>

Finally, never say "It will never happen here." Experience has proven time and again that mass casualty incidents and disasters can occur almost anywhere and at any time. Make it part of your professional training to be ready to act as an Incident Commander—the person charged with establishing and organizing the IMS.

CRITICAL INCIDENT STRESS MANAGEMENT

As you already know, every EMS professional faces the possibility of critical incident stress (CIS)—the powerful emotional response to a catastrophic event. The response can begin during the event or immediately after. There can also be a delayed response, such as a flashback during a later call. Reactions can be physical, emotional, behavioral, or a combination of all three.

✱ Trauma Intervention Programs (TIP) a national non-profit organization that establishes and operates local chapters of citizen volunteers specially trained to provide assistance to anyone emotionally traumatized by a crisis event.

For this reason, you or your agency should make provisions for use of specially trained Critical Incident Stress Management (CISM) Teams of a local chapter of **Trauma Intervention Programs (TIP)**. Such resources will provide access to mental health workers or other specially trained personnel who are familiar with emergency operations. As noted earlier, CISM team members should circulate around the scene of a high-impact incident to spot anyone exhibiting a stress reaction. Other CISM members should be available for debriefing after an event.

At smaller incidents, a CISM team will probably not be activated. For this reason, you and other members of your crew should be aware of the signs or symptoms of a stress reaction. Be ready to help each other. For more on the management of stress within an EMS agency or unit, see Volume 1, Chapter 2.

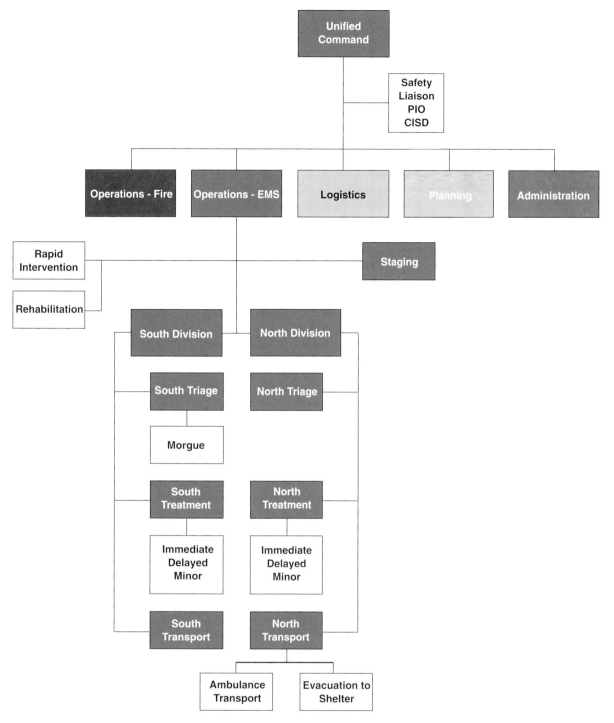

FIGURE 9-13   Sample command structure for a mass casualty incident (MCI) at a rest home.

SUMMARY

The principles covered in this chapter are just an overview of the Incident Management System. Every paramedic should be thoroughly familiar with the procedures used at a typical IMS. As a paramedic, you should follow these procedures at every multi-patient, multi-unit response—from the smallest incident to the largest incident. Keep in mind the saying, "We play as we practice." If you do, you will be prepared for the MCI or disaster that puts the Emergency Medical System to one of its biggest tests. Sometimes, departments or personnel fail to learn from the lessons of the past, saying "It can't happen here." Just the opposite is true: Expect to respond to several MCIs during your EMS career. A good preplan, regular use of the IMS, and MCI training will allow you to handle this event calmly and professionally.

YOU MAKE THE CALL

At 17:15 hours on a hot and humid Thursday afternoon, the Smith County dispatch center receives several calls from businesses surrounding the Shady Acres Rest Home. The calls all report hearing a loud explosion at or near the facility. The dispatcher immediately tones out the police department, fire department, and Smithville EMS. Smithville responds with two ambulances and the Field Supervisor (Figure 9-13, p. 365).

You arrive in the first ambulance. You do a windshield survey and observe heavy fire and smoke coming from the south wing of the rest home. Part of the roof is missing, and debris clutters the nearby parking lot. You notice several staff members jumping and waving at you from the facility's main entrance.

After you make your approach, you ask one of the aides for a census count. You learn at the time of the explosion, the facility housed 68 patients and 7 staff members. There were 30 patients in the south wing at the time of the explosion and 38 in the north wing. The south wing is heavily involved with fire and partially collapsed. Smoke is beginning to fill the north wing.

1. What two roles in the Incident Management System will you and your partner fill?
2. How would you size-up the incident?
3. What additional resources would you anticipate, and what instructions would you provide for them?
4. How would you use the Incident Management System to organize this incident?
5. What problems would you anticipate, and how would you protect against them?

See Suggested Responses at the back of this book.

FURTHER READING

Anderson, C.: "Countdown to Disaster: How to Plan an Effective Disaster Drill," *Emergency Medical Services*, April 1998, p. 59.
ASTM F 1288-90: *Standard Guide for Planning and Responding to a Multiple Casualty Incident*.

Auf der Heide, E.: *Disaster Response: Principles of Preparation and Coordination.* St. Louis: C.V. Mosby Company, 1989.

Christen, H. and P. Maniscalco: *The EMS Incident Management System: EMS Operations for Mass Casualty and High-Impact Incidents.* Upper Saddle River, NJ: Brady Publishing, 1998.

Emergency Program Manager, Federal Emergency Management Agency, Emergency Management Institute IS-1.

Final Report: Alfred P. Murrah Federal Building Bombing, April 19, 1995. The City of Oklahoma. Stillwater, OK: Fire Protection Publications, 1996.

Goldfarb, Z. and S. Kuhr: "EMS Response to the Explosion," in W. Manning, *The World Trade Center Bombing: Report and Analysis,* Federal Emergency Management Agency, United States Fire Administration, National Fire Data Center.

Heightman, A.J.: "The MCI Tool Bag," *Rescue,* January–February 1996, p. 34.

Incident Command System for Emergency Medical Services, Student Manual. Federal Emergency Management Agency, United States Fire Administration, National Fire Academy.

Larson, R.D.: "Incident Dispatcher Teams," *APCO Bulletin,* September 1997, p. 40.

Lilja, G. P., M.A. Madsen, and J. Overton: "Multiple Casualty Incidents," in A.E. Kuehl, *Prehospital Systems & Medical Oversight,* Second Edition. St. Louis, MO: Mosby Lifeline, 1994.

Ludwig, G.: "Multi-Casualty Incident: The Ultimate Test," *9-1-1 Magazine,* January-February, 1993, p. 42.

Maniscalco, P. and H. Christen: "EMS Incident Management: Creating Organization Out of Chaos," *Emergency Medical Services,* May 1998, p. 55.

Maniscalco, P.: "Terrorism Hits Home," *Emergency Medical Services,* May 1993, p. 31.

Morris, G.: "Common Errors in Mass Casualty Management," *JEMS,* February 1986, p. 34.

NFPA 1500: *Standard on Fire Department Occupational Safety and Health,* 1995 Edition.

NFPA 1561: *Standard on Fire Department Incident Management System,* 1995 Edition.

NFPA 1600: *Recommended Practices for Disaster Management,* 1995 Edition.

Page, J.: "Silly Vests and Dunce Caps: Which Would You Rather Wear as an Incident Commander?" *Rescue,* January-February 1996, p. 6.

Sachs, G.: "Multiple Casualty Incident Management, Part 1," *Fire Engineering,* December 1997, p. 73.

Story, C.: "Preplanning for an MCI," *JEMS,* November 1993, p. 52.

Streger, M.: "Prehospital Triage," *Emergency Medical Services,* June 1998, p. 25.

ON THE WEB

Visit Brady's Paramedic Website at www.bradybooks.com/paramedic.

CHAPTER 10

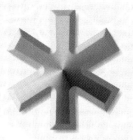

Rescue Awareness and Operations

Objectives

After reading this chapter, you should be able to:

1. Define the term rescue, and explain the medical and mechanical aspects of rescue operations. (pp. 371–372)
2. Describe the phases of a rescue operation, and the role of the paramedic at each phase. (pp. 378–383)
3. List and describe the personal protective equipment needed to safely operate in the rescue environment to include:
   a. Head, eye, and hand protection. (pp. 373, 374)

b. Personal flotation devices. (p. 375)
c. Thermal protection/layering systems. (pp. 374–375)
d. High visibility clothing. (p. 373)

4. Explain the risks and complications associated with rescues involving moving water, low head dams, flat water, trenches, motor vehicles, and confined spaces. (pp. 386, 388–389, 393–396, 396–399)
5. Explain the effects of immersion hypothermia on the ability to survive

Continued

sudden immersion and self rescue. (pp. 384–385)

6. Explain the benefits and disadvantages of water-entry or "go techniques" versus the reach-throw-row-go approach to water rescue. (p. 386)

7. Explain the self rescue position if unexpectedly immersed in moving water. (p. 385)

8. Describe the use of apparatus placement, headlights and emergency vehicle lighting, cones and flare placement, and reflective and high visibility clothing to reduce scene risk at highway incidents. (p. 397)

9. List and describe the design element hazards and associated protective actions associated with autos and trucks, including energy-absorbing bumpers, air bag/supplemental restraint systems, catalytic converters, and conventional and non-conventional fuel systems. (pp. 397–399)

10. Given a diagram of a passenger auto, identify the A, B, C, and D posts, fire wall, and unibody versus frame construction. (pp. 399–400)

11. Explain the difference between tempered and safety glass, identify its locations on a vehicle, and describe how to break it. (p. 400)

12. Explain typical door anatomy and methods to access through stuck doors. (pp. 400–401)

13. Describe methods for emergency stabilization using rope, cribbing, jacks, spare tires, and come-a-longs for vehicles found in various positions. (p. 402)

14. Describe electrical and other hazards commonly found at highway incidents (above and below the ground). (pp. 397–399)

15. Define low-angle rescue, high-angle rescue, belay, rappel, scrambling, and hasty rope slide. (pp. 403–404)

16. Describe the procedure for Stokes litter packaging for low-angle evacuations. (pp. 404–406)

17. Explain anchoring, litter/rope attachment, and lowering and raising procedures as they apply to low-angle litter evacuation. (pp. 404, 406)

18. Explain techniques used in non-technical litter carries over rough terrain. (p. 406)

19. Explain non-technical high-angle rescue procedures using aerial apparatus. (p. 406)

20. Explain assessment and care modifications (including pain medication, temperature control, and hydration) necessary for attending entrapped patients. (pp. 407–409)

21. List the equipment necessary for an "off road" medical pack. (pp. 375, 409)

22. Explain the different types of "Stokes" or basket stretchers and the advantages and disadvantages associated with each. (pp. 404–406)

23. Given a list of rescue scenarios, provide the victim survivability profile and identify which are rescue versus body recovery situations. (pp. 371–410)

24. Given a series of pictures, identify those considered "confined spaces" and potentially oxygen deficient. (pp. 392–396)

CASE STUDY

A call comes into Fire Unit 1204, a volunteer-operated paramedic ambulance, to assist an injured person in a rural state park approximately 15 miles from the station. You hear the call over your radio and respond promptly, along with another volunteer.

Because of distance and the winding roadways leading to the park, it takes nearly 30 minutes to arrive on scene. At the park entrance, one of the rangers informs you that a rock climber fell while trying to rappel down a popular cliff to meet his climbing partner on a rock ledge. Using a four-wheel-drive vehicle, the ranger takes you to the trail leading to the patient. Since the portable radio will not reach dispatch from the park, your partner stays with the ambulance.

From a vantage point along the trail, you spot the patient through binoculars. You see a young man lying on a rock ledge, about 55 feet below the trail. The climber's partner waves frantically to catch your attention, but seems unharmed. The cliff above the ledge is nearly vertical with a smooth rock face. You quickly determine the need for a high-angle rescue team and possibly a helicopter for rescue and medical evacuation.

You relay the size-up information to the ambulance. Your partner, in turn, calls dispatch and requests the necessary resources. Dispatch arranges for two members of a regional high-angle rescue team to fly with the helicopter, which has been placed on standby.

Upon arrival, rangers lead the team to the emergency site. The two specially trained paramedics quickly confer with you, size up the situation, and assure scene and personal safety. They then prepare their equipment for descent and access to the patient.

When the first rescuer rappels to the ledge, the uninjured climber blurts out: "I don't know what happened. He's such a good climber. Did you see all those leaves and pebbles near the anchor? I think he must have slipped while setting up his rappel. He's breathing but hasn't really moved since landing. A hiker saw the fall and called the ranger station with her cell phone—but that was so long ago. Please help—he's my best friend!"

To avoid having two patients, the rescuer directs the uninjured climber to "tie in" at a safe spot on the ledge. Due to the significant mechanism of injury, she performs an initial assessment on the patient and a rapid trauma exam. Her assessment reveals an unresponsive patient with multiple fractures. Nonetheless, blood pressure and pulse appear stable at this time.

Due to the heavy forest canopy, rescuers decide not to do a short haul with the helicopter. While the other high-angle rescuer rigs the ropes and rescue system, the paramedic immobilizes the patient and establishes an IV of lactated Ringer's solution. Because she anticipates a prolonged removal time, the paramedic collects some of the patient history from the uninjured climber and begins the detailed physical exam. She starts a second IV, cleans and dresses all wounds, and splints all fractures.

It takes approximately 25 minutes for the team to rig the rescue and haul the patient off the ledge in a Stokes basket stretcher. Although badly shaken, the uninjured climber is hoisted to the top and turned over to your care. Meanwhile, the high-angle team carries the patient to the helicopter, which is waiting in a clearing about 200 yards down the trail. He is then flown to the nearest trauma unit for treatment. About one hour later, a violent thunder storm hits the area. Without use of the high-angle team, the patient might still be lying unprotected on the ledge.

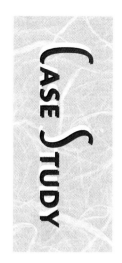

INTRODUCTION

EMS personnel usually have no trouble reaching their patients—that is, unless they're pinned beneath a vehicle, trapped in a collapsed building, or injured climbing a rock face or crawling into a cave. When people get injured or stranded in such situations, often somebody must first rescue the patients before emergency medical care can even begin.

So what does rescue mean? According to the dictionary, it is "the act of delivering from danger or imprisonment." In the case of EMS, rescue means extricating and/or disentangling the victims who will become your patients. Without rescue, there are no patients and vice versa.

ROLE OF THE PARAMEDIC

Rescue is a patient-driven event, and EMS is a patient-driven profession. However, not all EMS crews have the training to perform rescue. In most cases, it is simply not practical to train every paramedic in the detailed knowledge or operational skills necessary for each rescue specialty (Figure 10-1). It is possible, though, to instruct paramedics in the concept of rescue and to train them to what is known as an "awareness level." Awareness training imparts enough knowledge to recognize hazards and to realize the need for additional expertise at the scene. Failing to train paramedics in rescue awareness will eventually end in the injury or death of EMS personnel, patients, or both.

Rescue involves a combination of medical and mechanical skills with the correct amount of each applied at the appropriate time. Think of the medics who serve in the military. There is no army in the world that does not train and deploy medical people into combat. Even if the medics do not fire a weapon, they have enough military and medical training to treat patients in a combat situation. It's the same with the paramedics who serve on high-angle teams, SCUBA teams, and other specialized rescue units. If a rescue unit does not have medical training, your unit provides the balance.

In any rescue situation, treatment begins at the site of the incident. If the patient can be accessed in any way, treatment may in fact start before the patient is actually released from entrapment. Once medical care begins, it continues throughout the incident. The trick is to balance the medical and mechanical rescue skills to ensure that the patients obtain effective and timely extraction. Teams

Failing to train paramedics in rescue awareness will eventually end in the injury or death of EMS personnel, patients, or both.

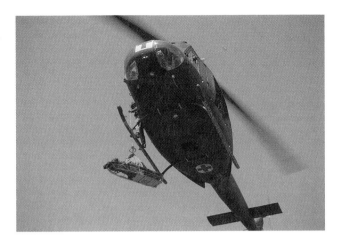

FIGURE 10-1 Rescue is a dangerous activity and safety is the number one priority. It is impossible for an individual paramedic to be highly trained in all types of rescue. Instead, specialized rescue teams should be utilized.

must work together to provide a well-coordinated effort to meet the patient's medical and physical needs.

The role of EMS in a rescue operation varies from area to area. Some localities, for example, may require additional training beyond the awareness level. In general, however, all paramedics should have the proper training and personal protective equipment (PPE) to allow them to access the patient, provide assessment, and establish incident command.

As first responders, paramedics should understand the hazards associated with various environments—e.g., extreme heat or cold, potentially toxic atmospheres, unstable structures, and so on. They should also be able to recognize when it is safe and unsafe to access the patient or attempt a rescue. If you deem an environment safe and if you have the training to effect a rescue, you should at least participate in the rescue under the guidance of individuals with additional expertise. You should also understand the rescue process so that you can decide when various treatments are indicated or contraindicated. In the climbing accident in the case study, for example, you would direct all parties not to move the patient until he was immobilized.

Because the field of rescue entails so many specialties, a single chapter cannot provide a step-by-step list of procedures and equipment for all the various scenarios you may encounter. Although practice scenarios can be found in related course materials, this chapter focuses on considerations that apply to most rescue situations. It discusses rescuer PPE and safety, presents the seven general phases of a rescue operation, and provides an "awareness level" of rescue operations in the following environments:

- Surface water—e.g., "low head" dams, flat water, moving water
- Hazardous atmospheres—e.g., confined spaces, trenches, hazmat incidents
- Highway operations—e.g., unstable vehicles, hazardous cargoes, volatile fuels
- Hazardous terrains—e.g., high-angle cliffs, off-road wilderness areas

The application of safety equipment—both to the rescuers and the patient—is paramount in any rescue situation.

PROTECTIVE EQUIPMENT

Personal and patient safety equipment must be paramount in any rescue situation. To prepare for a rescue response, you must develop a PPE cache. Without the appropriate protective gear, you will jeopardize both your own safety and the safety of the patient. Some of the equipment listed in the following sections has

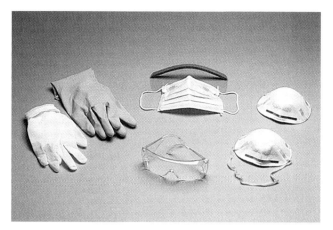

FIGURE 10-2 Your personal protection equipment (PPE) helps to minimize the risk of exposure to infectious diseases. For more specialized operations, such as water rescues, you need more specialized equipment.

application in many rescue situations. Other pieces of gear are appropriate to specific environments or conditions.

RESCUER PROTECTION

In all rescue environments, EMS personnel should wear highly visible clothing so they can be spotted easily. Ideally, PPE should fit the situation, but gear can be adapted, if necessary. For example, your PPE may not completely prevent exposure to infectious disease. Nonetheless, it minimizes the risk of infection (Figure 10-2). In fact, most PPE has not been specifically designed for EMS use. Instead, it has been borrowed from other fields, such as firefighting, mountaineering, caving, occupational safety, and more.

The use of adapted gear has resulted from the lack of a national uniform reporting system to identify risk-related exposures for EMS personnel. Future risk management and PPE design should be driven by such data. As a minimum, you should have at least the following equipment available:

- **Helmets:** The best helmets have a four-point, non-elastic suspension system (Figure 10-3). Most of the four-point suspension helmets are designed to withstand a greater impact than the two-point system found in construction hard hats. Avoid helmets with non-removable "duck bills" in the back—this will compromise your ability to wear the helmet in tight spaces. A compact firefighting helmet that meets NFPA standards is adequate for most vehicle and structural applications. Climbing helmets work better for confined space and technical rescues, while padded rafting or kayaking helmets are more appropriate for water rescues.

- **Eye Protection:** Two essential pieces of eye gear include goggles, vented to prevent fogging, and industrial safety glasses. These should be ANSI approved. Do not rely on the face shields found in fire helmets. They usually provide inadequate eye protection.

- **Hearing Protection:** From a purely technical standpoint, high-quality earmuff styles provide the best hearing protection. However, you must take into account other factors such as practicality, convenience, availability, and environmental considerations. In high-noise areas, for example, you might use the multi-baffled rubber earplugs used by the military or the sponge-like disposable earplugs.

- **Respiratory Protection:** Surgical masks or commercial dust masks prove adequate for most occasions. These should be routinely carried on all EMS units.

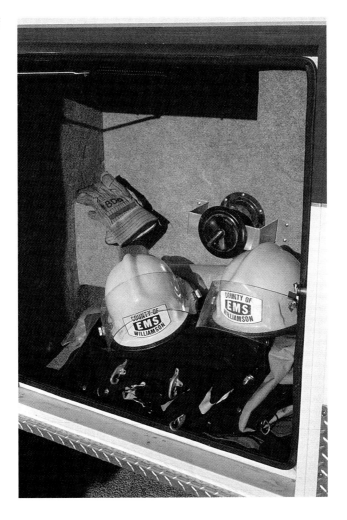

FIGURE 10-3 The quantity of safety and rescue equipment that can be carried on a standard ambulance is limited. However, helmets should be among the minimum types of rescue gear aboard each unit.

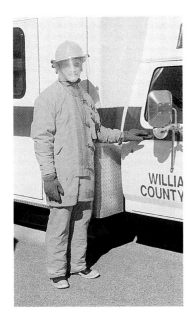

FIGURE 10-4 Full protective gear, including turnout gear, eye protection, helmet, and gloves.

- **Gloves:** Leather gloves usually protect against cuts and punctures. They allow free movement of the fingers and ample dexterity. As a rule, heavy, gauntlet-style gloves are too awkward for most rescue work.
- **Foot Protection:** As a rule, the best general boots for EMS work are high-top, steel-toed and/or shank boots with a coarse lug sole to provide traction and prevent slipping. For rescue operations, lace-up boots offer greater stability and better ankle support by limiting the range of motion. They also don't come off as easily as pull-on boots when walking through deep mud. Insulation may be useful in some colder working environments.
- **Flame/Flash Protection:** Every service should have an SOP calling for the use of flame/flash protection whenever the potential for fire exists. Turnout gear, coveralls, or jump suits all offer some arm and leg protection and help prevent damage to your uniform (Figure 10-4). They also have the added advantage of quick and easy application. For protection against the sharp, jagged metal or glass found at many motor vehicle accidents or structural collapses turnout gear generally works best. For limited flash protection, select gear made from Nomex®, PBI®, or flame-retardant cotton. For high visibility, pick bright colors such as orange or lime and reflective trim or symbols. Some services, for example, have an SOP calling for highly visible gear

and/or orange safety vests at all highway operations—both day and night. Insulated gear or jumpsuits are helpful in cold environments, but they can also increase heat stress during heavy work or in high ambient temperatures.

- **Personal Flotation Devices (PFDs):** If your service includes areas where water emergencies can result, your unit should carry PFDs that meet the U.S. Coast Guard standards for flotation. They should be worn whenever operating on or around water. The Type III PFD is preferred for rescue work. You should also attach a knife, strobe light, and whistle to the PFD so that they are easily accessible.

- **Lighting:** Depending upon the type and location of the rescue, you might also consider portable lighting. Many rescuers carry at least a flashlight or, better yet, a headlamp that can be attached to a helmet for hands-free operation. Consider the long-burning headlamps commonly worn by mountaineers and found through catalogs, the Internet, or climbing/camping stores.

- **Hazmat Suits or SCBA (self-contained breathing apparatus):** These items should only be made available to the personnel trained to use them. Most services or regions have special hazmat units to provide the highly specialized support required at rescue situations involving toxic substances. (For a discussion of hazmat training and equipment, see Chapter 11.)

- **Extended, Remote, or Wilderness Protection:** If your unit provides service to a remote or wilderness area, you might need to hike into—or even be air transported into—a rugged environment. In such cases, you would be advised to have a backcountry survival pack as part of your gear. This backpack should be pre-loaded with PPE for inclement weather (cold, rain, snow, wind), provisions for personal drinking water (iodine tables/water filter), snacks for a few hours (energy gels or bars), temporary shelter (tent/tarp/bivouac ["bivy"] sack), butane lighter, and some redundancy in lighting in case of light source failure.

Personal flotation devices should be worn whenever operating on or around water.

Content Review

CHECKLIST FOR BACKCOUNTRY SURVIVAL PACK
- PPE for inclement weather
- Provisions for drinking water
- Snacks for a few hours
- Temporary shelter
- Butane lighter
- Redundant light sources

PATIENT PROTECTION

Many of the considerations for rescuer safety also apply to patients, with several significant differences. A patient protective equipment cache should include at least the following items:

- **Helmets:** Patients usually do not require the same heavy-duty helmets as rescuers. As a result, the less expensive, construction-style hard hats often provide adequate protection against minor hazards. However, if you anticipate greater danger, as in climbing or caving rescues, outfit patients with the same high-grade helmets as rescuers would use in the same or similar environments.

- **Eye Protection:** Vented goggles, held in place by elastic bands, are ideal. They are not as easily dislodged as safety glasses. You might also use workshop face shields.

- **Hearing and Respiratory Protection:** Apply the same considerations for hearing protection as you would for yourself. Earplugs are usually adequate.

- **Protective Blankets:** You should have a variety of protective blankets to shield patients from debris, fire, or weather. Inexpensive vinyl

Always be sure to avoid covering the victim's mouth and nose during rescue operations.

tarps do a good job of protecting patients from water, weather, and most debris. Aluminized rescue blankets protect from fire, heat, or glass dust. Commercially available wool blankets provide excellent insulation from the cold. Plastic shielding (the kind used by landscapers) and plastic trash bags of many sizes and weights are also very useful. One 55-gallon-drum liner is large enough to cover a single patient. It can serve as a disposable blanket, poncho, vapor barrier, or, in a wilderness situation, bivy sack.

- **Protective Shielding:** Circumstances may call for protective equipment more substantial than blankets or plastic sheets. All rescue teams should be trained to use backboards and other commonly found equipment as shields to protect patients from fire, weather, falling rock or debris, glass, or other sharp-edged objects. Shields specifically designed for a Stokes basket should be available. Keep in mind that a device that shields a patient from debris or the elements may also limit rescuers' access to the patient. The more securely that you package a patient, the more difficult it will be for you to monitor him or her. As patient care becomes more complicated, changing patient conditions may be overlooked.

SAFETY PROCEDURES

As you already know, safety—your own and that of your crew—is your first priority. Yet, in rescue situations a number of factors prod you to take action—your own desire to access the patient for treatment, the urging of people to "do something," the patient's cries for help, the presence of media, frustration at rescuers' lack of medical experience, and more. However, one mistake can spell disaster for you, your crew, and/or the entrapped victim. One way to curb "heroics" is by establishing rescue SOPs, determining crew assignments, and, above all else, preplanning scenarios well in advance of actual rescues.

RESCUE SOPS

Standard operating procedures (SOPs) are the nuts and bolts of effective EMS practice. At rescue situations, all teams should have written safety procedures familiar to everyone. Contents should include sections on all types of anticipated rescues. Each section should specify required safety equipment, required or prohibited actions, and any rescue-specific modifications in assignments. SOPs should include a statement requiring a Safety Officer and an explanation of that person's relationship to Incident Command. Ideally, the Safety Officer should be someone with the knowledge and authority to intervene in unsafe situations. This person makes the "go/no go" decision in the operation. (For more on the role of Safety Officers, see Chapter 9.)

CREW ASSIGNMENTS

EMS units must anticipate crew assignments and special needs before the rescue operation takes place.

In addition to SOPs, an EMS unit must anticipate crew assignments and special needs *before* the rescue operation. This task can be done through personnel screening, careful preplanning, and regular practice of any dangerous rescue techniques that members of your unit may be trained to perform (Figure 10-5).

Search-and-rescue planners often use personnel screening to determine the participants in the rescue process. Programs exist to identify the physical capabilities of crew members. Findings of these programs could have a significant impact

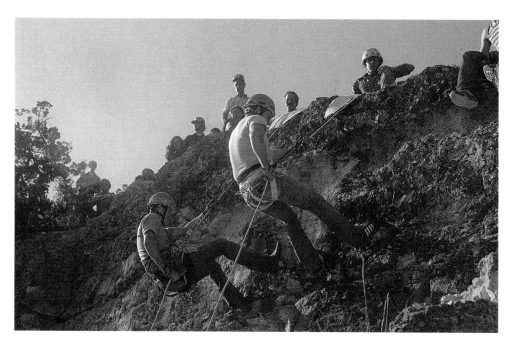

FIGURE 10-5   Dangerous rescue techniques, such as vertical rescue, should be frequently practiced to ensure utmost safety.

on personnel assignments. In addition, psychological testing is recommended. It may even be desirable to screen for specific traits, such as phobias. For example, a rescuer's inordinate fear of heights or small spaces should be taken into account when assigning duties.

PREPLANNING

As stressed in Chapter 9, one of the most critical factors in promoting safety and operational success is preplanning. Preplanning starts with the identification of potential rescue locations, structures, or activities within your area. Effective preplanning then evaluates the specific training and equipment needed to manage each of these events. The preplan also generates ideas on efficient use of existing resources and anticipates the need for additional equipment, rescuers, and/or expertise.

Due to the intensity and length of many rescue operations, provisions must be made for the maintenance and rotation of rescue personnel. Plans should be made for "stand-by" or staging sites that offer protection from the weather. Sites should be away from the immediate operations area and secure from bystanders and the media. Personnel should be rotated at controlled intervals. Predetermined policies should be set regarding food and hydration of crews. On-scene diets should be high in complex carbohydrates and low in sugars and fats. Fluid replacement should consist of diluted (at least 50%) electrolyte solutions such as those found in sports drinks. The classic coffee-and-donuts regimen should be avoided altogether.

The preplanning should be the basis of a broader regional emergency rescue plan, to be tested and modified in practice exercises. When possible, other specialized rescue agencies, such as high-angle teams, should take part in the exercises. These "test-run" scenarios will give you and other members of your unit ample opportunity to utilize the IMS as it applies to rescue situations.

Practice exercises with specialized rescue teams will give you and your unit ample opportunity to utilize the IMS as it applies to rescue situations.

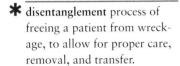

✱ **disentanglement** process of freeing a patient from wreckage, to allow for proper care, removal, and transfer.

As already mentioned, there are several types of rescue operations, each of which includes technically difficult procedures, very specialized equipment, or both. *They should be attempted only by personnel with special training and experience in these areas.* Some of these special rescue operations will be examined later in the chapter. But first you need to be aware of the general approach to most rescue situations.

Like any other EMS incident, rescue operations go through phases. Although specific procedures vary from area to area and from rescue to rescue, most calls will go through seven general phases: arrival and size-up, hazard control, patient access, medical treatment, **disentanglement**, patient packaging, and removal/transport.

PHASE 1: ARRIVAL AND SIZE-UP

Size-up begins with the dispatcher's call and subsequent arrival at the scene (Figure 10-6). Although the dispatcher's message may indicate a rescue situation, you must still understand the environment and potential risks. Upon arrival, you or another paramedic must quickly establish Medical Command and appoint a Triage Officer. You must also conduct a rapid scene-size up, determine the number of patients, and notify dispatch of the magnitude of the event. Now is the time to implement the IMS, any mutual-aid agreements, and the procedures for contacting off-duty personnel or backup ALS units.

Prompt recognition of a rescue situation and identification of the specific type of rescue are essential. You may be summoned to a structural collapse, vehicle rollover, or climbing accident. Each of these situations holds out the potential for entrapment and the need for specialized crews and equipment. Often, you must make a quick "risk-versus-benefit" analysis based upon the conditions found upon arrival. Be careful not to overestimate your capability to handle a rescue situation. As indicated, individual acts of courage may be called for, but safety comes first. If in doubt, err on the side of safety.

In calling for backup, follow this precaution: "Don't undersell overkill." Remember that it is always easier to send back a rescue crew than to rectify a personal tragedy caused by too few rescuers or hasty heroics. Also keep in mind the realistic time needed to access and evacuate an entrapped patient. Make use of the IMS to shave off valuable response minutes in what may be a life-threatening situation.

PHASE 2: HAZARD CONTROL

On-scene hazards must be identified with speed and clarity. You must often deal with these hazards before even attempting to reach the patient. To do otherwise would place you and other personnel at risk. Control as many of the hazards as possible, but don't attempt to manage any condition beyond your training or skills. Some situations, for example, involve chemical spills, radiation, gas leaks, explosives, or other dangerous substances. You will need to employ a hazmat team and confine your actions to a safe area. (For more on setting up zones at a hazmat scene, see Chapter 11.) Electric wires hold a "double threat" for fire and shock.

The very environment in which you stand can be risk-filled. Look around to determine the possibility of lightning, avalanches, rock slides, cave-ins, and so on. Manage and minimize the risks from uncontrollable hazards as soon as possible to avoid other injuries. Ensure that all personnel, for example, wear appropriate PPE. Never forget the dangers of traffic. EMS providers have been killed at highway accidents by drunks attracted to the bright lights striking crew members in non-reflective gear. The following are some other potential hazards that

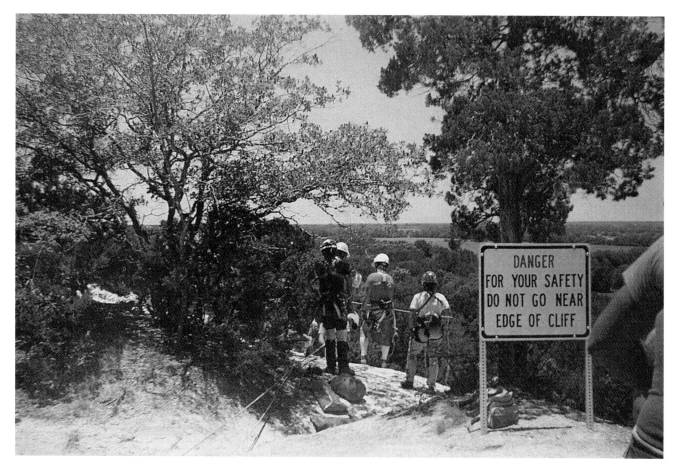

FIGURE 10-6 The first step of a rescue operation is arrival and scene size up. If the scene assessment reveals any hazards, efforts must be taken to control them, the second step of a rescue operation.

you may encounter. As you skim this list, keep in mind that these are only a sampling of the conditions you may encounter.

- Poisonous or caustic substances
- Biological agents or germ-infected materials
- Swift moving currents, floating debris, or water contaminated with toxic agents
- Confined spaces such as vessels, trenches, mines, or caves
- Extreme heights or icy rock faces, especially in mountainous situations
- Possible psychological instability, as often experienced in hostage crises, urban violence, mass hysteria, or individual emotional trauma on either the part of the patient or the crew (Recall the need for pre-assessment of crew members.)

PHASE 3: PATIENT ACCESS

After controlling hazards, you will then attempt to gain access to the patient or patients (Figure 10-7). Begin by formulating a plan. Determine the best method to gain access and deploy the necessary personnel. Make sure that you take steps to

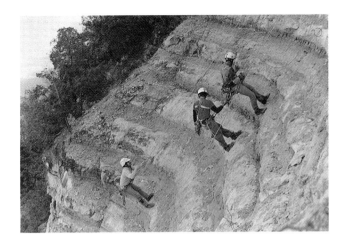

FIGURE 10-7 The third step of a rescue operation is gaining access to the patient. In specialized rescues, such as vertical rescue, this can be a long process.

Access triggers the technical beginning of the rescue.

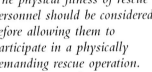

The physical fitness of rescue personnel should be considered before allowing them to participate in a physically demanding rescue operation.

stabilize the physical location of the patient. For example, look for threats of structural collapse, cave-ins, or vehicle rollover.

Access triggers the technical beginning of the rescue. While gaining access, you must use appropriate safety equipment and procedures. This is the point when you and/or the Command and Safety Officer must honestly evaluate the training and skills needed to access the patient. Untrained, poorly equipped, or inexperienced rescue personnel must not put their safety—and the safety of others—at risk by attempting foolhardy, heroic rescues.

During the access phase, key medical, technical, and command personnel must confer with the Safety Officer on the strategy they will use to accomplish the rescue. To assure that everyone understands and supports the rescue plan, a formal briefing should be held for rescue personnel before the operation begins. Even with well-trained personnel and adequate equipment, rescue efforts can be poorly executed because team members do not understand the "big picture" or they do not know what is expected of each member of the team.

PHASE 4: MEDICAL TREATMENT

After devising a rescue plan, medical personnel can begin to make patient contact. Remember: No personnel should enter an area to provide patient care unless they are physically fit, protected from hazards, and have the technical skills to reach, manage, and remove patients safely. The interests of both rescuer and patient may be served by a first responder with expertise in the type of rescue required. However, if a first responder does not have the required fitness or skills, he or she may need to be rescued because of some hasty, ill-advised effort to treat the patient.

In general, a paramedic has three responsibilities during this phase of operation. They include:

- Initiation or patient assessment and care as soon as possible
- Maintenance of patient care procedures during disentanglement
- Accompaniment of the patient during removal and transport

Again, whether or not you actually fulfill each of these responsibilities depends upon the medical expertise of the special rescue team. Recall, for example, the opening case study in which a trained high-angle paramedic accessed AND treated the patient.

If you are treating the patient, take these actions if the conditions allow. Quickly conduct an initial assessment (MS-ABC and C-spine status) on each patient (Figure 10-8). The next critical steps include rapid trauma assessment for the patient with a significant MOI, detailed physical exam, and medically oriented recommendations to the evacuation team.

Because a long time may elapse before transport, a patient's condition may change dramatically during disentanglement and removal. As a result, you should perform patient assessment with two goals in mind. First, identify and care for existing patient problems. Second, anticipate changing patient conditions, and determine the assistance and equipment needed to cope with those changes.

Continually evaluate risks to both rescuers and the patient. In many situations, the best overall patient care requires rapid stabilization and immediate removal. Final positive patient outcome may depend upon initial sacrifice of definitive patient care so that the patient and rescuers can be removed from imminent danger. Examples of such situations might include:

- Injured, stranded high-rise window cleaners; workers on water, radio, or TV towers; high-rise construction workers
- Workers or bystanders involved in a trench cave-in
- Persons stranded in swift-running, rising water
- Patients entrapped in vehicles with an associated fire
- Patients overcome by life-threatening atmospheres
- Victims entrapped with unstable and/or volatile hazardous materials

In such cases, rapid transport of a non-stabilized patient to a safer location may be justified by the risk of injury to the rescuers and exposure of the patient to even greater complications. Rapid movement might be required even though the transport will aggravate existing patient injuries. Generally, management for the entrapped patient has the same foundation as all emergency care. Steps include:

- Initial assessment of the MS-ABCs
- Management of life-threatening airway, breathing, and circulation problems
- Immobilization of the spine
- Splinting of major fractures
- Packaging with consideration to patient injuries, **extrication** requirements, and environment conditions
- Ongoing reassessment during the transport phase

Specifics of patient management during a rescue often follow the same or similar protocols to those used "on the street." However, some specifics may be, or should be, significantly different. Differences result mainly from the lengthy time periods often required to access, disentangle, and/or evacuate the patient. EMS personnel are trained in rapid stabilization and transport, particularly with trauma patients. However, during a rescue mission, the desire to achieve speedy transport, as well as obey the "Golden Hour" rule, may be impossible to fulfill. As a result, you must be able to "shift gears" mentally to an extended-care situation. (For some background on time-related changes in treatment, see the discussion of distance in Chapter 13, "Rural EMS.")

In addition to extended field time, you must be prepared to provide more in-depth psychological support for rescue patients than might otherwise be required. This is especially true in situations where a patient has already been entrapped for a considerable amount of time. Establish a solid rapport with the patient, striking up a constant and reassuring conversation. In quieting the fears of rescue patients, keep in mind the following tips:

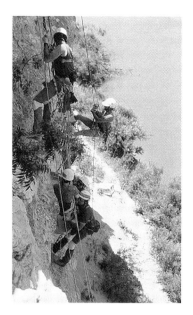

FIGURE 10-8 The fourth step in a rescue operation is patient treatment. Assessment and care may need to be modified, depending upon the on-scene environment and any special hazards.

Content Review

GOALS OF RESCUE ASSESSMENT

- Identify and care for existing patient problems
- Anticipate changing patient conditions and determine in advance the assistance and equipment needed

✱ extrication use of force to free a patient from entrapment.

In responding to rescues, you must be prepared to "shift gears" mentally to an extended-care situation.

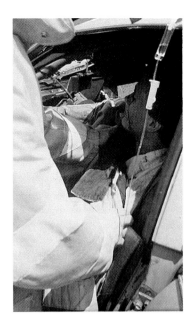

FIGURE 10-9 The fifth step in a rescue operation is disentanglement. It can be prolonged, as in the case of auto entrapment.

- Learn and use the patient's name.
- Be sure the patient knows your name and knows that you will not abandon him or her.
- Be sure that other team members know and use the patient's correct name. The term "it" should never be substituted for the patient's name in any prehospital setting.
- Avoid negative or fearful comments regarding the operation, the causes of the operation, or the patient's condition within earshot of the victim.
- Explain all delays to the patient and identify steps that will be taken to remedy the situation.
- Ask special rescue teams to explain any technical aspects of the operation that could frighten or impact upon the patient's condition. Translate these operations into clear, simple terms for the patient.
- Don't lie to the patient. If something may hurt during rapid movement, acknowledge it. If the patient suspects an unstable environment, acknowledge that too. However, be sure to explain what will be done to mitigate the situation—i.e., the pain or the unstable environment.
- Above all else, stay calm and act every bit the professional. If you don't know the answer to a question, find somebody who does. Remember: Rescues are driven by patient needs.

PHASE 5: DISENTANGLEMENT

Disentanglement may be the most technical and time-consuming portion of the rescue.

✱ **active rescue zone** area where special rescue teams operate; also known as the "hot zone" or "inner circle."

Disentanglement involves the actual release from the cause of entrapment, such as the dashboard of a wrecked automobile, a concrete slab from a structural collapse, or the blocked entry to a cave. This phase may be the most technical and time-consuming portion of the rescue (Figure 10-9). If assigned to patient care during this phase of the rescue, you have three responsibilities. They are:

- Personal and professional confidence in the technical expertise and gear needed to function effectively in the **active rescue zone**—sometimes referred to as the "hot zone" or "inner circle"
- Readiness to provide prolonged patient care—i.e., medical support of technical efforts
- Ability to call for and/or use special rescue resources

If you or another member of the rescue team cannot fulfill these requirements, reassess available rescue personnel and call for backup. Disentanglement is not a time for the claustrophobic—extrication may involve crawling into a tight space. Disentanglement is also not a time for the squeamish—in some cases, an amputation may be required.

Methods used to disentangle the patient must be constantly analyzed on a risk-to-benefit basis. You and/or other members of the rescue team must balance the patient's medical needs with such concerns as the time it will take to perform treatment, the safety of the environment, and so on. If a patient has a severely crushed extremity and it will take an inordinate amount of time to release the extremity, the patient may in fact bleed to death without an amputation. This is only one of the hard treatment decisions that may be faced during the disentanglement phase of the operation.

PHASE 6: PATIENT PACKAGING

After disentanglement, a patient must be appropriately packaged to ensure that all medical needs are addressed. You must consider such things as the means of egress—e.g., a litter carry through the woods versus walking a patient out. You must also factor time based upon the patient's medical conditions—e.g., rapid extrication techniques versus application of a Kendrick Extrication Device (KED). Some forms of patient packaging can be more complex than others, depending upon the specialized rescue techniques required to extricate the patient—e.g., being lifted out of a hole in a Stokes by a ladder truck, being vertically hauled through a manhole in a Sked® stretcher, and so on. In situations where the patient may be vertical or suspended in a Stokes basket, it is paramount that the rescuer know how to properly package the patient to prevent additional injury.

It is paramount that the rescuer know how to properly package the patient to prevent further injury.

PHASE 7: REMOVAL/TRANSPORT

Removal of the patient may be one of the most difficult tasks to accomplish or it may be as easy as placing the person on a stretcher and wheeling it to a nearby ambulance (Figure 10-10). Activities involved in the removal of a patient will require the coordinated effort of all personnel. Transportation to a medical facility should be planned well in advance, especially if you anticipate any delays. Decisions regarding patient transport—whether it be by ground vehicle, by aircraft, or by physical carry-out—should be coordinated based on advice from medical direction (Figure 10-11). En route to the hospital, perform the ongoing assessment, repeating vitals every 5 minutes for an unstable patient and every 15 minutes for a stable patient. Update the patient's condition and administer additional therapy per medical direction.

SURFACE WATER RESCUES

As previously mentioned, there are a number of different categories of rescue operations in which you may apply the principles and practices described thus far in the chapter. Water emergencies are among the most common. Because people are attracted to water in such great numbers and for such a wide variety of activities, accidents can take many different forms.

Most water rescues are resolved without the involvement of EMS personnel—e.g., bystanders jump into a pool to pull out a struggling swimmer, other boaters rescue someone whose canoe has overturned, and so on. However, some water

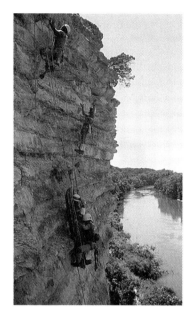

FIGURE 10-10 The sixth step in a rescue operation is packaging and removal of the patient. Again, this can be a time-consuming process, as in the case of a vertical rescue.

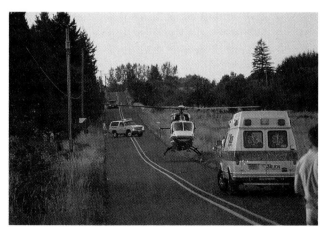

FIGURE 10-11 The seventh, and final step, in a rescue operation is transport of the patient. This can be either by helicopter or ground ambulance, depending upon the situation and the condition of the patient.

emergencies require that the rescuers have special training and equipment. In such cases, the temperature and dynamics of flat or moving water place both the victim and the rescuer at high risk of entrapment. Although all the possible scenarios for water-rescue training cannot be supplied in a single section of a chapter, the following are some general concepts and methods to raise your "water rescue awareness."

GENERAL BACKGROUND

Water rescues may involve many kinds of water bodies—pools, rivers, streams, lakes, canals, flooded gravel pits, or even the ocean. Some communities also have drainage systems that remain dry until flash floods turn them into raging rivers.

Most people who get injured or drown in these water bodies never intended to get into trouble. But one or more factors conspire to create an emergency—the weather changes, swimmers underestimate the water's power, non-swimmers neglect to wear a PFD and fall in, people develop a muscle stitch or cramp while in the water, submerged debris knocks waders off their feet, boats collide, and more.

Nearly all incidents in and around water are preventable. It is important for you to become familiar with safe aquatic practices. First and foremost, know how to swim and make swimming part of your physical exercise. Second, remember that even the strongest swimmer can get into trouble. Therefore, always carry PFDs aboard your unit and always wear a PFD whenever you are around water or ice (Figure 10-12). (Make sure your crew does the same.) Third, you might consider taking a basic water rescue course.

Water Temperature

Since the human body temperature is normally 98.6°F, almost any body of water is colder and will cause heat loss. Water temperature in smaller bodies of water varies widely with the seasons and the amount of runoff. Yet, even on warm days, water temperature can be quite cold in most places. As a result, water temperature and heat loss figure in the demise of most victims and ill-equipped rescuers.

FIGURE 10-12 A personal flotation device (PFD) is mandatory equipment for any water-related rescue.

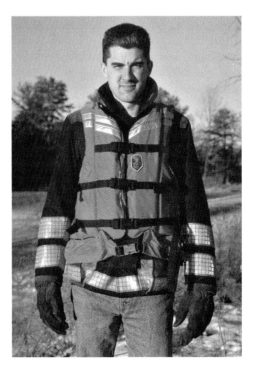

As implied, immersion can rapidly lead to hypothermia, a condition discussed in Volume 3, Chapter 10. As a rule, people cannot maintain body heat in water that is less than 92°F. The colder the water, the faster the loss of heat. In fact, water causes heat loss 25 times faster than the air. Immersion in 35°F water for 15 to 20 minutes is likely to kill a person. Factors contributing to the demise of a hypothermic patient include:

- Incapacitation and an inability to self rescue
- Inability to follow simple directions
- Inability to grasp a line or flotation device
- Laryngospasm (caused by sudden immersion) and greater likelihood of drowning

There are a number of actions that can delay the onset of hypothermia in water rescues. The use of PFDs slows heat loss and lessens the energy required for flotation. If people suddenly become submerged, they can also assume the **Heat Escape Lessening Position (HELP).** This position involves floating with the head out of water and the body in a fetal tuck. Researchers estimate that someone who has practiced with HELP can reduce heat loss by almost 60%, as compared to the heat expended when treading water. If a group of victims find themselves in the water, researchers also suggest huddling together. This technique not only prevents heat loss, but provides a better target for members of a rescue team.

Basic Rescue Techniques

Basic rescue techniques vary with the dynamics of the water—i.e., moving water versus non-moving (flat) water. If your unit responds to frozen bodies of water, you may also add techniques for ice rescue and include the proper cold water entry dry suits as part of your PPE cache (Figure 10-13).

✳ Heat Escape Lessening Position (HELP) developed by Dr. John Hayward. It is an in-water, head-up tuck or fetal position designed to reduce heat loss by as much as 60%.

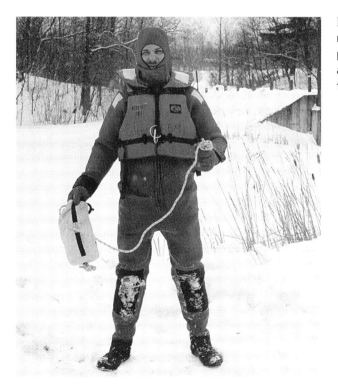

FIGURE 10-13   Safe ice rescue requires proper equipment and protective clothing, particularly a dry suit and water-sealed footwear.

The water rescue model is REACH-THROW-ROW-GO. All paramedics should be trained in reach-and-throw techniques. A PFD is useless if it is not worn. So all EMS personnel should put it on, even for shore-based rescues.

If at first, you are unable to talk the patient into a self-rescue, then reach with a pole or long rescue device. If this is not effective or if the victim is too far out, try throwing a flotation device. All paramedics should become proficient with a water-throw bag for shore-based operations. Remember: Boat-based techniques require specialized rescue training. Water-entry ("go") is only the last resort— and is an action best left to specialized water rescuers.

MOVING WATER

By far the most dangerous water rescues involve water that is moving. Competency at handling the power and dynamics of swift-water rescues comes only with extensive training and experience. The force of moving water can be very deceptive. The hydraulics of moving water change with a number of variables, including water depth, velocity, obstructions to flow, changing tides, and more. Only specially trained rescuers can readily recognize these factors.

To train for swift-water entry, rescuers must develop a proficiency in many specialized skills. In preparation for technical rope rescues, they must master the skills required for high-angle rope rescues. They must also become well-practiced in such skills as crossing moving water bodies, defensive swimming, use of throw bags and boogy boards, shore-based swimming, boat-based rescue techniques, management of water-specific emergencies, the capability to package the patient with water-related injuries, and more.

Four swift-water rescue scenarios present a special challenge and danger to rescuers. They include recirculating currents ("drowning machines"), strainers, foot/extremity pins, and dams or hydroelectric intakes.

Recirculating Currents

* **recirculating currents** movement of currents over a uniform obstruction; also known as a "drowning machine."

Recirculating currents result from water moving over a uniform obstruction to flow such as a large rock or low head dam. The movement of currents can literally create what is known as a "drowning machine" (Figure 10-14).

Upon first appearance, recirculating currents can look very tame. Anglers, for example, often fish on the downstream portion of a low head dam, casting their lines into the recirculating waters. This is a good place to catch fish because they can often be seen just below the dam. But think about it. If fish with their natural ability to swim get stuck in the recirculating currents, imagine what would happen to humans if they got too close to the dam. Once caught in the recirculating currents, people find it very difficult to escape. The resulting rescue can be extremely hazardous—even for specially trained rescuers.

Strainers

* **strainers** a partial obstruction that filters, or strains, the water such as downed trees or wire mesh; causes an unequal force on the two sides.

When moving water flows through obstructions such as downed trees, grating, or wire mesh, an unequal force is created on the two sides of the so-called "strainers" (Figure 10-15). Currents can literally force a patient up against a strainer, making it difficult to be removed due to the power of the current. In some cases, the current might be flowing into a drainage pipe under the surface, which is in turn covered by a rebar (metal) grate. Victims can get sucked into the grate and are then pinned against it.

This too can be a hazardous rescue. If you get stuck floating downstream and see the potential of getting pinned against a strainer, attempt to swim over the object. Whatever you do, don't put your feet on the bottom of the river—your

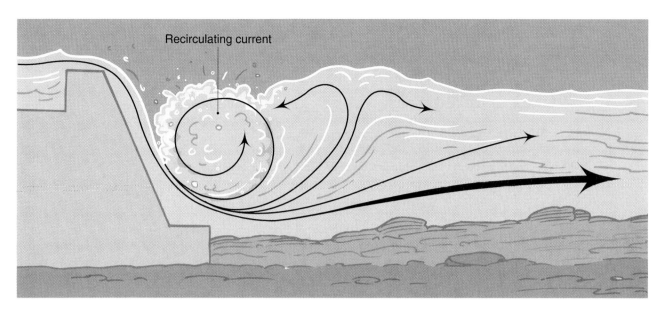

FIGURE 10-14   When water flows over a large uniform object, it can create a hydraulic or hole with a recirculating current that moves against the river's flow and can trap people.

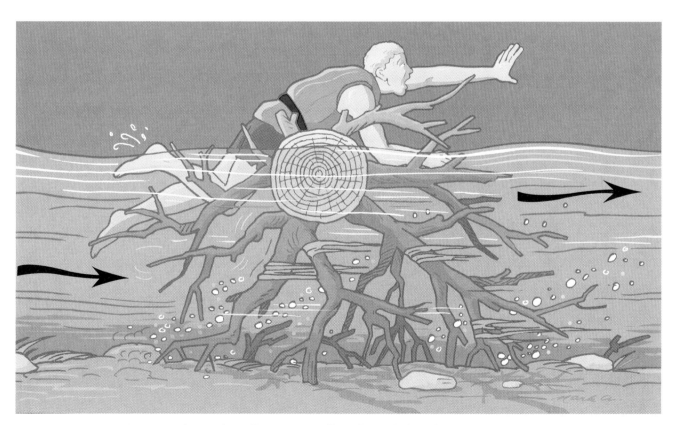

FIGURE 10-15   Strainers are objects that allow water to flow through them but that will trap other objects—and people.

feet could get stuck or, even worse, you could get swept off your feet and slammed into the obstruction.

Foot/Extremity Pins

It is always unsafe to walk in fast-moving water over knee depth because of the danger of entrapping a foot or extremity.

For the sake of safety, keep this point in mind: It is always unsafe to walk in fast-moving water over knee depth because of the danger of entrapping a foot or extremity. When this occurs, the weight and force of the water can knock you below the surface of the water. In order to remove the foot or extremity, it must be extracted the same way it went in. Water currents often make this extremely difficult. Again, this is a hazardous rescue because of the need to work below the surface of already dangerous water conditions.

Dams/Hydroelectric Intakes

Yet another dangerous situation involves dams and hydroelectric intakes, such as those often found along rivers. The height of the dam is no indication of the degree of hazard. As already indicated, low head dams can create powerful drowning machines. As a result, assume that all dams have the ability to form recirculating currents. Hydroelectric intakes, on the other hand, serve as dangerous strainers with all the accompanying hazards.

Self-Rescue Techniques

Some water survival techniques have already been mentioned—such as wearing PFDs, the use of HELP, and so on. However, if you suddenly fall in swift-running water (or flat for that matter), keep these suggestions in mind:

- Cover your mouth and nose during entry.
- Protect your head and, if possible, keep your face out of the water.
- Do not attempt to stand up in moving water.
- Float on your back, with your feet pointed downstream.
- Steer with your feet, and point your head towards the nearest shore at a 45-degree angle or continue to float downstream until you come to an area where the water slows enough for you to swim to the edge.
- If the water turns a bend, remember that the outside of the curve moves faster that the inside of the curve.
- Look for large objects, such as rocks, that can block the water and cause recirculating currents or strainers.
- Learn to identify **eddies**—water that flows around especially large objects and, for a time, flows upstream around the downside of the obstruction. These back currents move more slowly and can actually sweep you toward the edge—and safety.
- Above all else, take precautions not to fall into the water in the first place. Remember: reach-throw-row-go, with "go" being the absolutely last resort.

✱ **eddies** water that flows around especially large objects and, for a time, flows upstream around the downside of an obstruction; provides an opportunity to escape dangerous currents.

FLAT WATER

The greatest problem with flat water is that it looks so calm. Yet, a large proportion of drowning or near-drowning incidents take place in flat or slow-moving water (Figure 10-16). Some of the factors in these deaths were mentioned earlier. In a significant number of cases, alcohol plays a role in the accident.

Three caveats apply to the vast majority of drowning and near-drowning incidents (see table).

- *Children should be under constant supervision if a lake, pool, or pail of water of any size is nearby.*
- *Water sports and alcoholic beverages never mix.*
- *Life preservers or life jackets should always be worn when boating.*

Where people drown	
Type of water or site	Drownings (%)
Salt water	1%–2%
Fresh water	98%–99%
Swimming pools	
Private	50%
Public	3%
Lakes, rivers, streams, storm drains	20%
Bathtubs	15%
Buckets of water	4%
Fish ponds or tanks	4%
Toilets	4%
Washing machines	1%

Adapted with permission from Orlowski JP: Drowning, near-drowning, and ice-water submersions. *Pediatr Clin North Am* 1987;34(1):77.

These and other standard water safety precautions for swimming, diving, and boating should be made clear and repeated frequently.

Effective prevention in children requires constant supervision and common sense. A young child can find and fall into water in just a minute or two — less time than anyone would realize he or she is gone unless attention is continuous — and fences are not always effective in keeping children out of places where they should not go. A fence may appear to enclose a pool completely, but the gate may not be self-closing or the lock may be broken. The vast majority of children who drown in swimming pools do so in the backyards of their own homes, usually in the later afternoon on summer weekends. And isn't it sensible to require that baby sitters know CPR?

Programs that claim to "drown–proof" or teach young children to swim are controversial, and many experts feel they provide a false sense of security. The American Academy of Pediatrics does not recommend teaching children younger than 3 years of age to swim, although some regional programs take children as young as 6 months. Drown-proofing programs fail — studies indicate that a significant number of children have submersion accidents despite their training — because the sequential patterning approach used to teach the very young child in a structured environment engenders, in effect, learned helplessness. The cues a child learns in the class or pool setting are missing in the real-life crisis.

A large number of adult drowning victims have detectable levels of blood alcohol. Swimmers should be warned about diving into shallow or unexplored water. Boating precautions should be heeded by all boaters. Seizure disorders are an important but easily overlooked risk factor in persons of all ages.

FIGURE 10-16   Preventing water accidents.

Nearly 50% of boating fatalities, for example, result from alcohol intoxication or impairment. As a result, many states have enacted tough laws to restrict the operation of boats while under the influence of alcohol—a drug that impairs the ability to think, reason, and survive in an alcohol-related water accident.

Factors Affecting Survival

A number of factors help determine the demise or survival of a patient. A person's "survivability profile" is affected by age, posture, lung volume, water temperature, and more. Two especially important factors are include the presence of PFDs and what is known as the "cold-protective response."

Personal Flotation Devices

Many recreational water users associate "life preservers" with rough water or people who can't swim. But PFDs should be essential items for all water-related activities. One study, for example, linked nearly 89% of all boating fatalities to the lack of a PFD. This fact is a reminder of why you should don a PFD whenever you approach water.

Content Review

FACTORS AFFECTING SURVIVAL
- Age
- Posture
- Lung volume
- Water temperature
- Use of PFDs
- Mammalian diving reflex

Every system should have a strict SOP mandating the use of PFDs for all EMS personnel. Even services in arid regions can be involved in water rescues. They can be called to swimming pool accidents or river-rafting accidents. In some places, especially in the southwest, they can respond to flash-flooding in canyons that can trap or kill hikers or "canyoneers." The same flash flooding can overload drainage systems, creating hazardous conditions for the public and rescuers alike.

Cold Protective Response

The same cold water that can kill people also triggers a protective response known as the "mammalian diving reflex." This is how it works: When the face of a human, or any mammal, is plunged into cold water less than 68°F, the parasympathetic nervous system is stimulated. The heart rate rapidly decreases to a bradycardic rhythm. Meanwhile, blood pressure drops and vacoconstriction occurs throughout the body. Blood is shunted from less vital organs to the heart and brain, temporarily delivering life-sustaining oxygen. As a general rule, the colder the water, the more oxygen is diverted.

The mammalian reflex, along with the length of time the head was above water during the cooling process, can significantly delay death. Some patients have been resuscitated after 45 minutes under water. The record is 66 minutes for a patient rescued in Salt Lake, Utah, on June 10, 1989. As a rule, the reflex is more pronounced in children than in adults.

Location of Submerged Victims

Because of protective physiologic responses, rescuers must make every effort to locate submerged victims. Interview witnesses to establish a relative location. Ask each witness, for example, to locate an object across the water to form a line. Repeat this process with each witness. Use the point of convergence among lines to target the most accurate "last seen" location. Start searching from this point and fan out in larger and larger circles, forming a radius equal to the depth of the water.

Rescue Versus Body Recovery

A number of conditions determine when a rescue turns into a body recovery. Some factors are length of time submerged, any known or suspected trauma, age and physical condition of the victim, water temperature and environmental conditions, and estimated time for rescue or removal.

Once a patient is recovered, you should attempt resuscitation on any hypothermic and/or pulseless, nonbreathing patient who has been submerged in cold water. (Some experts advise providing resuscitation to every drowning patient, regardless of water temperature, even those who have been in the water for some time.) A patient must be rewarmed before an accurate assessment can be made. Remember: water-rescue patients are never dead until they are warm and dead. (For more on drowning and near-drowning, see Volume 3, Chapter 10.)

Remember: water-rescue patients are never dead until they are warm and dead.

In-Water Patient Immobilization

In flat water where you are able to safely stand, it is important that you know how to perform in-water immobilization (Figure 10-17). In general, the procedure mirrors the application of a long board, with the following modifications:

- **Phase One: In-Water Spinal Immobilization**
    1. Apply the head-splint technique. (There are other techniques, but they do not work as well because of the use of PFDs by the rescuers.)

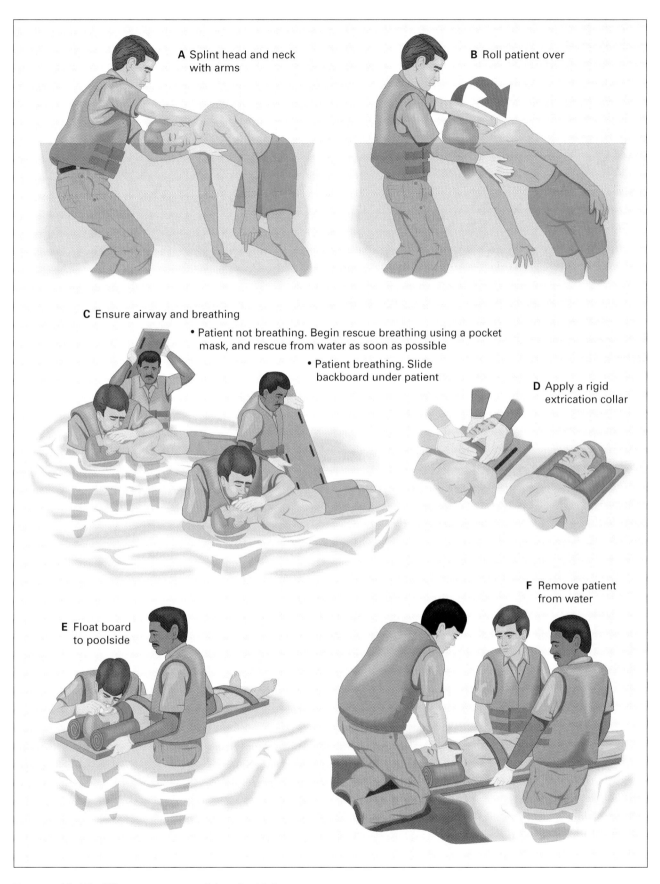

A Splint head and neck with arms

B Roll patient over

C Ensure airway and breathing

• Patient not breathing. Begin rescue breathing using a pocket mask, and rescue from water as soon as possible

• Patient breathing. Slide backboard under patient

D Apply a rigid extrication collar

E Float board to poolside

F Remove patient from water

FIGURE 10-17   Water rescue, possible spinal injury.

2. Approach the patient from the side.
3. Move the patient's arms over the head.
4. Hold the patient's head in place by using the patient's arms as a "splint."
5. If the patient was found in a face-down position, perform steps 1-4, then rotate the patient toward the rescuer in a face-up position.
6. Assure an open airway.
7. Maintain this position until a cervical collar is applied.

- Phase Two: Rigid Cervical Collar Application
  1. A second rescuer determines the proper collar size.
  2. This second rescuer then holds the open collar under the victim's neck.
  3. The primary rescuer maintains immobilization and a patent airway.
  4. The second rescuer brings the collar up to the back of the patient's neck and the primary rescuer allows the second rescuer to bring the collar around the patient's neck while the primary rescuer maintains the airway.
  5. The second rescuer secures the fastener on the collar while the primary rescuer maintains the airway.
  6. The second rescuer secures the patient's hands at the waist of the patient.

- Phase Three: Back Boarding and Extrication from the Water
  1. Secure the necessary personnel—two rescuers in the water and additional rescuers at the water's edge—and the correct equipment. It is strongly urged that rescuers use a floating backboard for water rescue.
  2. Submerge the board under the patient's waist.
  3. Never lift the patient to the board. Instead, allow the board to float up to the victim. (If the board does not float, lift it gently to the victim.)
  4. Secure the patient with straps, cravats, or other devices.
  5. Move the patient to an extrication point along the shore or boat.
  6. Always extricate the patient head first, so the body weight does not compress possible spinal trauma.
  7. If possible, avoid extrication of the patient through surf, as the board could capsize and dump the patient back into the water. Consider using bystanders who can swim as a breakwall behind the patient.
  8. Maintain airway management during extrication.

HAZARDOUS ATMOSPHERE RESCUES

Confined-space rescues present any number of potentially fatal threats, but one of the most serious is an oxygen-deficient environment. At first glance, most confined spaces appear relatively safe. As a result, you might mistakenly think rescue procedures will be easier and/or less time-consuming and dangerous than they really are. Here's where rescue awareness comes in. According to NIOSH, nearly 60% of all fatalities associated with confined spaces are people attempting to rescue a victim.

While "confined space" can have a variety of interpretations, OSHA regulation CFR 1910.146 interprets the term to mean any space with limited access/egress that is not designed for human occupancy or habitation. In other words, confined spaces are not safe for people to enter for any sustained period of time. Examples of con-

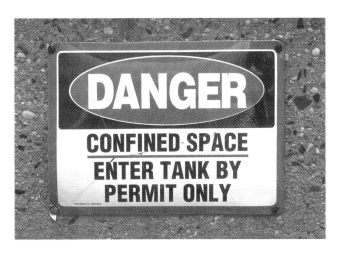

FIGURE 10-18a Look for clues to potentially hazardous atmospheres and confined spaces, such as warning signs.

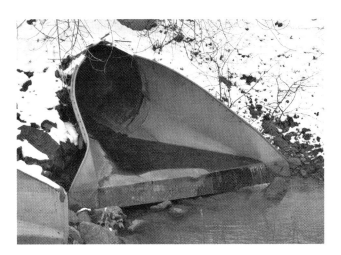

FIGURE 10-18b Treat a culvert for what it is—a dangerous confined space.

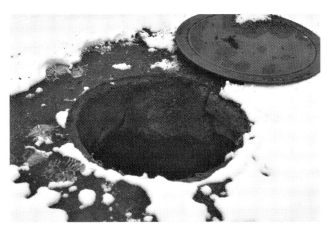

FIGURE 10-18c Manholes provide access to underground utility vaults. The vault may have a limited or hazardous atmosphere and may offer the potential for entrapment.

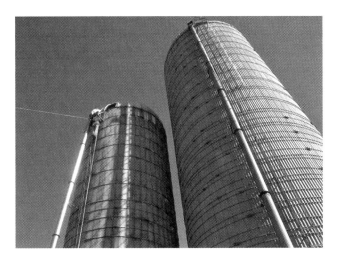

FIGURE 10-18d Rescuers should never be permitted to enter confined spaces, such as silos, unless they have training, equipment, and experience in this environment.

fined spaces are: transport or storage tanks, grain bins and silos, wells and cisterns, manholes and pumping stations, drainage culverts, pits, hoppers, underground vaults, and mine or cave shafts (Figures 10-18a–d).

CONFINED-SPACE HAZARDS

As already mentioned, confined spaces present a wide range of hazards. You may confront one or more these hazards in any given confined-space rescue. As a first responder, it is your responsibility to identify these hazards as soon as possible, both for purposes of scene safety and for summoning the necessary support. Some of the most common risks include:

- **Oxygen-Deficient Atmospheres:** Untrained rescuers may not readily think of oxygen deficiency. It simply is not a "visible" threat. Special entry teams know otherwise. Before going into a confined space,

Confined-space rescues carry a high risk of oxygen deficiency.

FIGURE 10-19 Rescuers exposed to toxic or hazardous materials will need to go through decontamination.

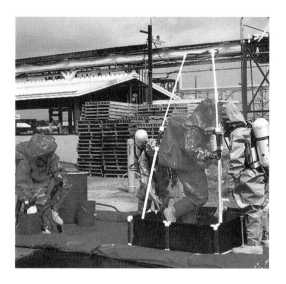

they monitor the atmosphere to determine the following: oxygen concentration, levels of hydrogen sulfide, explosive limits, flammable atmosphere, or toxic contaminants. They are also aware that increases in oxygen content for any reasons—e.g., a gust of wind—can give atmospheric monitoring meters a false reading. The bottom line is this: Confined spaces often mean hazardous atmospheres.

- **Toxic or Explosive Chemicals:** Many chemicals found in confined spaces can be toxic, especially if inhaled (Figure 10-19). Some of the poisonous fumes contain gases that displace oxygen in the red blood cells. Other chemicals are highly explosive. Dangerous chemical gasses commonly found in confined spaces include: hydrogen sulfide (H_2S), carbon dioxide (CO_2), carbon monoxide (CO), exceptionally low or high oxygen concentrations, Chlorine (Cl_2), ammonia (NH_3), and nitrogen dioxide (NO_2).

- **Engulfment:** Some confined spaces contain physical substances—grain, coal, sand, and so on—that can literally bury a patient or a rescuer who falls into the space. Dust from these materials can also create a highly explosive atmosphere.

- **Machinery Entrapment:** Confined spaces come with all sorts of machinery or equipment that can entrap a person. Augers or screws can also entrap a victim.

- **Electricity:** Confined spaces often contain motors or material—management equipment powered by electricity. In addition to the risk of shock or electrocution, these machines contain the potential for stored energy. To ensure safe entry, rescue crews will have to take a number of steps. First, it may be necessary to blank out the flow of all power into the site. Second, stored energy should be dissipated, following lock out/tag out procedures. Third, the space may need to be ventilated to ensure against oxygen deficiency or explosive dust particles. Remember: It only takes one spark to trigger an explosion.

- **Structural Concerns:** Structure supports and shapes further complicate confined-space rescues. Some confined spaces have "I" beams that can cause injury due to limited light and height. Other

It only takes one spark to trigger an explosion. Be careful of all potential sources of electricity.

confined spaces have non-cylindrical shapes that present difficult extrication problems. Confined spaces can be shaped in the form Ls, Ts, Xs, and any combination thereof. Because of limited access, rescuers may find it difficult or even impossible to use standard SCBA. They may have to resort to supplied air breathing apparatus—i.e., oxygen lines. They may also need to be lowered into the space with a full-body harness or other system to make retrieval easier in case something goes wrong.

CONFINED-SPACE PROTECTIONS IN THE WORKPLACE

Fortunately, state and federal laws require most industries to develop a confined-space rescue program. This means that employers must provide a training program for all employees who work in or around confined spaces. These employees may be called upon to perform on-site rescues and may indeed be an important part of the emergency response.

OSHA also requires a permit process before workers may enter a confined space such as a trench. In addition, most industries must fulfill strict requirements such as ongoing atmospheric monitoring, posted warnings, and work-site permits with detailed data on hazard management. The area must be made safe or workers must don PPE. Retrieval devices must also be in place whenever workers enter the spaces. Non-permitted sites are the most likely locations for emergencies because of the oxygen deficiencies that result from inadequate atmospheric monitoring.

The types of confined-space emergencies most commonly encountered in the workplace include falls, medical emergencies (often hazmat-related), oxygen deficiencies or asphyxia, explosions, and entrapment. You should never allow rescuers into a confined space unless they have the training, equipment, and experience specific to this environment. You will almost always summon outside specialized agencies for support.

CAVE-INS AND STRUCTURAL COLLAPSES

As earthquakes in California have proven, it can be very dramatic to watch rescues from cave-ins or structural collapses. But it doesn't take an earthquake to produce this type of confined-space emergency. Collapsed trenches or cave-ins can occur in almost any community. In fact, most trench collapses occur in trenches less than 12 feet deep and 6 feet wide, particularly in trenches that do not comply with OSHA regulations (Figure 10-20).

To understand the medical magnitude of a collapsed trench, consider these facts. A typical cubic foot of soil weights 100 pounds. As a result, just two feet of soil on the chest or back can weigh between 700 to 1,000 pounds. People are literally buried alive. Unless uncovered quickly, they suffer death by asphyxiation.

Reasons for Collapses/Cave-Ins

Trenches collapse or cave in for a number of reasons. The most common reasons include:

- Contractors disregard safety regulations, either out of negligence or out of efforts to save money. (Federal law requires either shoring or a trench box for excavations deeper than 5 feet. Anything less is an invitation for trouble.)

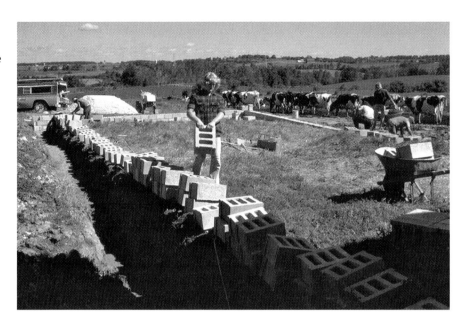

- The lip of one or both sides of the trench caves in.
- The wall shears away or falls in entirely.
- The "spoil pile," or dirt removed from the hole, is placed too close to the edge of the trench.
- Water seepage, ground vibrations, intersecting trenches, or previously disturbed soil weaken the structural integrity.

Rescue From Trenches/Cave-Ins

If a collapsed trench or cave-in has caused a burial, a secondary collapse is likely.

If a collapse has caused burial, a secondary collapse is likely. Therefore, your initial actions should be geared toward safety. Secure the scene, establish command, secure a perimeter, and immediately summon a team specializing in trench rescue. While waiting for the team to arrive, do not allow entry in the area surrounding the trench or cave-in. Safe access can take place only when proper shoring is in place.

HIGHWAY OPERATIONS AND VEHICLE RESCUES

As you already know, the most common rescue situations encountered by EMS personnel involve motor vehicle accidents. These incidents generally go through the phases covered at the start of this chapter. However, certain modifications must be made to meet the special hazards associated with traffic control and the extrication of patients from wrecked vehicles.

HAZARDS IN HIGHWAY OPERATIONS

To prepare for highway rescues, you must size up the scene, identify all hazards, and assure scene safety—i.e., control any potentially dangerous situations. In the case of highway operations, this means reducing traffic-related hazards and identifying hazards related to the vehicle crash itself.

Traffic Hazards

Traffic flow is the largest single hazard associated with EMS highway operations. You may have to respond to incidents on roads with limited access and to incidents on highways with unlimited access. In either situation, you will need to work closely with police to avoid unnecessary congestion and yet other accidents. Remember: back-ups impede the flow both to and from the scene.

Traffic flow is the largest single hazard associated with EMS highway operations.

An even bigger personal danger results from the risk of vehicles hitting EMS apparatus or personnel. Studies have shown that drivers who are tired, drunk, or drugged actually drive right into the emergency lights. Spectators can worsen the situation by getting out of their cars to watch or even "help."

At this point in your career, you probably already know some of the things you can do to reduce traffic hazards. Here are a few tried-and-tested techniques:

- **Staging:** Staging is always critical at any MCI, but it takes on added importance on limited-access roads or highways. Always consider staging emergency vehicles away from the scene. Then have Command bring the vehicles in whenever there is an appropriate place and/or assignment for the crews. The staging area should be within a minute or two of the scene, ideally in a large parking lot or less congested area. Some situations simply cannot accommodate the entire response at once.

- **Positioning of Apparatus:** When apparatus does arrive, ensure that it causes the minimum reduction of traffic flow. As much as possible, apparatus should be positioned to protect the scene. The ambulance loading area should NOT be directly exposed to traffic. Also, DO NOT rely solely on ambulance lights to warn traffic away. These lights are often obstructed when medics open the doors for loading.

DO NOT rely solely on ambulance lights to warn traffic away.

- **Emergency Lighting:** Use only a minimum of warning lights to alert traffic of a hazard and to define the actual size of your vehicle. Too many lights can confuse or blind drivers, causing yet other accidents. Experts strongly advise that you turn off all headlights when parked at the scene and rely instead on amber scene lighting.

- **Redirection of Traffic:** Be sure traffic cones and flares are placed early in the incident. If the police are not already on scene, this is your responsibility. As a first responder, you must redirect traffic away from the collision and away from all emergency workers. In other words, you need to create a safety zone. Make sure that you do not place lighted flares too near any sources of fuel or brush, otherwise you risk an explosion or fire. Once you light the flares, allow them to burn out. DO NOT try to extinguish them. Attempting to pick up a flare can cause a very severe thermal burn.

- **High Visibility:** As already mentioned, all rescuers should be dressed in highly visible clothing. Since many EMS, police, and fire agencies wear dark-colored uniforms, you should don a brightly colored turnout coat or vest with reflective tape. You can directly apply the tape at the scene.

Other Hazards

Other hazards besides traffic control exist at highway operations. In some communities, paramedics receive training to manage these hazards. In other communities, they receive "awareness training" and learn to summon specialized

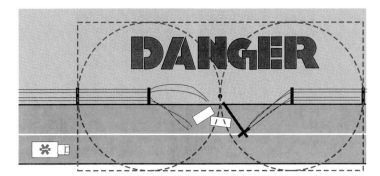

Downed Lines
In accidents involving downed electrical wires and damaged utility poles, the danger zone should extend beyond each intact pole for a full span and to the sides for the distance that the severed wires can reach. Stay out of the danger zone until the utility company has deactivated the wires, or until trained rescuers have moved and anchored them.

FIGURE 10-21 Establish a danger zone in motor vehicle collisions involving electrical hazards.

rescue personnel. Regardless of the procedure in your service area, you must be able to recognize all non-traffic hazards (Figure 10-21). Otherwise, you risk injuring yourself, your crew, the patient, or even passing motorists. Some of these non-traffic hazards include:

Bystanders who are smoking can cause a bigger problem than the original crash if they flick ashes into a fuel leak.

- **Fire and Fuel:** Fuel spilled at the scene increases the chances of fire. Be very careful whenever you smell or see pools of liquid at a collision. Keep in mind that bystanders who are smoking can cause a bigger problem than the original crash if they flick lighted ashes into a fuel leak. DO NOT drive your emergency vehicle over a fuel spill—or worse yet, park on one! Remember that all automobiles manufactured since the 1970s have catalytic converters. They run at a temperature of around 1,200°F—hot enough to heat fuel to the point of ignition. Be especially careful when a vehicle has gone off the road into dry grass or brush. The debris can be just as dangerous as spilled fuel, especially when brought into contact with a blazing hot catalytic converter.
- **Alternative Fuel Systems:** Be equally cautious of vehicles powered by alternative fuel systems. High-pressure tanks, especially if filled with natural gas, are extremely volatile. Even vehicles powered by electricity can be dangerous. The storage cells possess the energy to spark, flash, and more.
- **Sharp Objects:** Automobile collisions mean lots of sharp objects—whether they be glass, metal, plastic, or fiberglass. Be sure to wear appropriate protective gear, such as heavy leather gloves and eyewear.
- **Electric Power:** Contact with downed power lines or underground electrical feeds can be lethal. If a vehicle is in contact with electrical lines, consider it to be "charged" and call the power company immediately. In most newer communities, electric lines run underground. However, a vehicle can still run onto a transformer or an electric feed box. As a result, make sure you look under the car and all around it during your scene size up. DO NOT touch a vehicle until you have ruled out all electrical hazards.
- **Energy-Absorbing Bumpers:** The bumpers on many vehicles come with pistons and are designed to withstand a slow-speed collision.

DO NOT touch a vehicle until you have ruled out all electrical hazards.

The intent is to limit front- or rear-end damage. Sometimes, however, these bumpers become "loaded" in the crushed position and do not immediately bounce back out. When exposed to fire or even just tapped by rescue workers, the pistons can suddenly unload their stored energy. Some bumpers have been thrown a hundred feet from the vehicle when they unload. As a result, you must examine bumpers for loading. If you discover a loaded bumper, stay away from it unless you are specially trained to deal with this hazard.

- **Supplemental Restraint Systems (SRS)/Air Bags:** Air bags also have the potential to release stored energy. If they have not deployed during the collision, they may do so during the middle of an extrication. As a result, these devices must be deactivated prior to disentanglement. Auto manufacturers can provide information about power removal or power dissipation for their particular brand of SRS. Also, keep in mind that many new model vehicles come equipped with side impact bags.

- **Hazardous Cargoes:** An incredible amount of hazardous materials travel across the highways of North America. You will learn much more about the role of EMS in highway accidents involving hazmat in Chapter 11. For your personal safety, suspect hazmat at any scene involving commercial vehicles.

- **Rolling Vehicles:** As you already know, you must size up the position of a vehicle whenever you arrive at the scene of a collision. Don't overlook the subtle situations that can occur at any accident. You might arrive on the scene and see the vehicle on all four wheels and consider it stable. Then someone from your crew jumps into the rear seat to stabilize the patient's neck manually. Suddenly the vehicle starts rolling down the street. This situation is not only embarrassing, it is dangerous! As a result, always check that the transmission is in park. Make sure the parking brake is on, the ignition is off, and any key rings with remote ignition starters are removed.

- **Unstable Vehicles:** Motor vehicles can land in all kinds of unstable positions. They can roll onto their side or roof. They can stop on an incline or unstable terrain. They can be suspended over a cliff or river. They can come to rest on a patch of ice or an on-site spill or leak. In such situations, you need to request the necessary stabilization crews or equipment. You should also know how to apply proper techniques for temporary stabilization, using ropes, chocks, or a come-a-long. Under no circumstances should you allow rescuers to access the patient until the vehicle is stabilized.

For your personal safety, suspect hazmat at any scene involving commercial vehicles.

AUTO ANATOMY

Motor vehicle collisions present EMS personnel with the most common access and/or extrication problems. As a result, you must know some basic information about automobile construction or "anatomy." Obviously, vehicles can differ greatly, both in terms of manufacture and design. However, most recent automobiles have certain features in common that can guide you in simple access situations.

Basic Constructions

Vehicles can have either a unibody or a frame construction. Most automobiles today have a unibody design, while older vehicles and light-weight trucks have a frame construction. For unibody vehicles to maintain their integrity all the following features must remain intact: roof posts, floor, firewall, truck support, and windshield.

Both types of constructions have roofs and roof supports. The support posts are lettered from front to back. The first post, which supports the roof at the windshield, is called the "A" post. The next post is the "B" post. The third post, found in sedans or station wagons, is the "C" post. Station wagons have an additional rear post, known as the "D" post.

If you remove the plastic molding on the posts, the remaining steel can be easily cut with a hacksaw. Application of power steering fluid helps reduce the heat produced by cutting. In the case of unibody design, remember that cutting a post will interrupt the vehicle's construction.

Firewall and Engine Compartment

The firewall separates the engine compartment and the occupant compartment. Frequently, the firewall can collapse on a patient's legs during a high-speed, head-on collision. Sometimes, a patient's feet may go through the firewall. Movement on other parts of the vehicle, such as cutting a rocker panel or roof support post, can place additional pressure on the feet.

The engine compartment usually contains the battery. This can cause a fire hazard so many rescue teams cut the battery cables to eliminate this risk. Before disconnecting the power, it's a good idea to move back electric seats and lower power windows. Otherwise, you might needlessly complicate the extrication.

Glass

Vehicles have two types of glass: safety glass and tempered glass. Safety glass is made from three layers of fused materials: glass–plastic laminate–glass. It is found in windshields and designed to stay intact when shattered or broken. However, safety glass can still produce glass dust or fracture into long shards. These materials can easily get into a patient's eyes, nose, or mouth and/or create cuts. As a result, be sure to cover a patient whenever you remove this type of glass.

Tempered glass has high tensile strength. However, it does not stay intact when shattered or broken. It fractures into many small beads of glass, all of which can cause injuries and cuts.

Doors

The doors of most newer vehicles contain a reinforcing bar to protect the occupant in side-impact collisions. They also have a case-hardened steel "Nader" pin. Named after consumer advocate Ralph Nader, these pins help keep the doors from blowing open and ejecting the occupants. If the Nader pin has been engaged, it will be difficult to pry open the door. You must first disengage the latch or use hydraulic jaws.

Before attempting to assist a patient through a door, you should be trained in proper extrication techniques. In general you should follow these steps:

- Try all four doors first—a door is the easiest means of access.
- Otherwise, gain access through the window farthest away from the patient(s).
- Alternatively, use simple hand tools to peel back the outer sheet of metal on the door, exposing the lock mechanism. Unlock the lock and pry the cams from around the Nader pin. Then pry out the door.

These steps can be highly useful in situations in which the patient must be promptly removed from the vehicle or the vehicle rescue team is delayed for some reason. Before removing a patient, keep in mind the earlier points about deactivating or dissipating front and/or side air bags.

RESCUE STRATEGIES

In managing highway operations or vehicle rescues, you should use the following general strategies:

- **Initial Scene Size-Up:** Establish command, call for appropriate backup, locate and triage the patients. Triage may be delayed until hazards are controlled.
- **Control Hazards:** This topic has already been covered. But always remember this point: Traffic can be your worst enemy at a collision.
- **Assess the Degree of Entrapment and Fastest Means of Extrication:** Try all doors. If they can't be opened, decide whether it is advisable and/or necessary to break glass. Although you may not have the training or responsibility to use extrication equipment, you should observe their use so you know what technical skills are available should you need them (Figure 10-22). Be aware of the considerations and techniques for door removal, roof removal, dashboard or firewall rollup, and construction of a new door.
- **Establish Circles of Operation:** Set up two circles of operation early in the incident. The inner circle is the area where the actual rescue takes place. Limit the number of workers in this area to team members operating rescue tools and/or charged with actual patient care. If two different units must work in the inner circle—e.g., a fire department extrication crew and an EMS crew—you will need to maintain a good working balance between the crews to avoid "over rescuing." The outer circle is where staging takes place. Hold all additional equipment and personnel in this area until they are assigned a duty.
- **Treatment, Packaging, Removal:** As a rule, the role of EMS personnel in vehicle stabilization and removal is that of patient care provider.

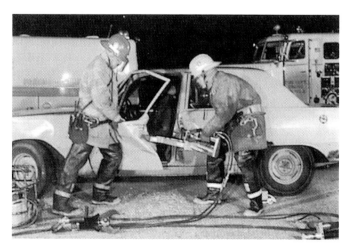

FIGURE 10-22 Modern extrication equipment is essential for a fast, efficient rescue. Paramedic skill in using these devices will depend upon local protocols and the location of extrication units.

Table 10-1	VEHICLE STABILIZATION EQUIPMENT
Type	**Description and Use**
Airbag	Synthetic bag, available in various shapes and sizes, which, when inflated, has great lifting capability
Come-along	Ratcheting cable device used to pull in a straight direction
Cribbing	4×4 or 2×4 blocks of hardwood cut to approximately 18-inch long sections
Hydraulic cutter	Hydraulic power tool used to cut metal
Hydraulic ram	Hydraulic power tool used to push or pull in a straight direction
Hydraulic spreader	Hydraulic power tool used to open, spread, or separate items such as vehicle doors
Jack	Manual device used much as ram would be used
Step chock	Set of several 2×6 blocks of hardwood cut to varying lengths and secured together to form "steps"
Wedge	4×4 piece of cribbing tapered to an edge on one end
Winch	Powered cable reel usually electrically or hydraulically driven and mounted to a truck, which is used to pull

Patient care always precedes removal from the vehicle unless delay would endanger the life of the patient, EMS personnel, or other rescuers.

Once specialized rescue personnel assure you that the vehicle is stable and the scene is safe to enter, you may approach the patient, initiate assessment, and administer emergency care. Patient care always precedes removal from the vehicle unless delay would endanger the life of the patient, EMS personnel, or other rescuers. Again, work with rescuers in any way possible to minimize risk, both to the patient and to on-scene personnel. You should be well-practiced in the application of long spineboards for rapid removal of the patient through the doors or vertical extrication through removed roofs.

RESCUE SKILLS PRACTICE

Depending upon local protocols, you should practice or observe the use of the rescue skills and equipment needed for initial vehicle stabilization. Some of the common tools used for vehicle stabilization can be found in Table 10-1.

You should also make a point of practicing and/or observing the various disentanglement or extrication skills commonly used with vehicle rescues, many of which have already been mentioned. Know how to gain access using hand tools through non-deformed doors, deformed doors, safety and tempered glass, trunks, and floors. Become familiar with the use of heavy hydraulic equipment employed by special rescue teams in your area and take part in practice scenarios to build agency cooperation. Again, preplan and prepare so that you are ready when this all-too-common type of rescue occurs.

HAZARDOUS TERRAIN RESCUES

In recent years, outdoor activities—mountain climbing, rock climbing, ice climbing, mountain biking, cross-country skiing, snowboarding, and hiking—have drawn more and more people into rugged areas. Inevitably accidents happen, and they happen in places that can be difficult to reach. You don't have to live in the wilderness to take part in a hazardous terrain rescue. For example, a mountain biker can get injured along the trails that run along many power lines or a rock climber can get injured on an outcropping in a relatively populated area. Some climbers even scale the sides of buildings!

As a paramedic, you must know how to take part in rugged terrain rescues. At a minimum, you should know how to perform litter evacuations without causing additional injury to patients. Even more important, you should develop a "rescue awareness" so that you know when to call specialized teams and how to work with those teams once they arrive on scene.

TYPES OF HAZARDOUS TERRAIN

In general, there are three types of hazardous terrain: steep slope or "low-angle" terrain, vertical or "high-angle" terrain, and flat terrain with obstructions. Low-angle terrains typically can be accessed by walking or **scrambling**—climbing over boulders or rocks using both hands and feet. Footing can be difficult, and it may be hazardous to carry a litter even with multiple people. As a result, low-angle teams use ropes to counteract gravity and/or may set a rope to act as a hand line. Any error can result in a fall or tumble. Depending upon the presence of boulders, brush, downed trees, and so on, injuries can be quite serious.

High-angle terrain usually involves a cliff, gorge, side of a building, or terrain so steep that hands must be used when scaling it. Crews depend on rope and/or aerial apparatus for access and litter movement. Errors are likely to cause serious, life-threatening injuries. In many cases, falls can be fatal upon impact.

Flat terrain with obstructions includes trails, paths, or creek beds. Obstructions can take many forms such as downed trees, rocks, slippery leaves or pine needles, and **scree**—the loose pebbles or rock debris that can form on the slopes or bases of mountains.

Although this is the least hazardous type of rugged terrain, it is still possible to slip while carrying a patient, causing injury.

PATIENT ACCESS IN HAZARDOUS TERRAIN

Unless you have been trained in high-angle or low-angle rescue, patient access and removal should be left to specialized teams. Even if you have the skills to perform the rescue, you will in all likelihood need additional resources to provide the necessary balance of technical and medical support for the patient.

High-Angle Rescues

High-angle, or vertical, rescuers must constantly contend with the effects of gravity. Any organization that could be assigned a vertical technical rescue must have extensive initial training, additional advanced training, frequently supervised practice sessions, and top-of-the-line equipment (Figure 10-23a). Each member of a high-angle team must have complete competency in knot tying, use of ladders and/or ropes to ascend and descend a steep face, ability to rig a hauling system, and the skills for packaging a patient for evacuation by litter and rope. Some of the specialized terms that you will hear high-angle rescuers use include:

- **aid**—using means other than hands, feet, and body to get up a vertical face, such as in "aided ascent."
- **anchor**—technique for securing rescuers to a vertical face; an anchor may be rope or a combination of rope and other special hardware or "gear."

Develop the "rescue awareness" to know when to call specialized rescue teams and how to work with those teams when they arrive on scene.

Content Review

THREE TYPES OF HAZARDOUS TERRAIN
- Steep slope or "low-angle" terrain
- Vertical or "high-angle" terrain
- Flat terrain with obstructions

* **scrambling** climbing over rocks and/or downed trees on a steep trail without the aid of ropes. This can be especially dangerous when the surface is wet or icy.

* **scree** loose pebbles or rock debris that can form on the slopes or bases of mountains; sometimes used to describe debris in sloping dry stream beds.

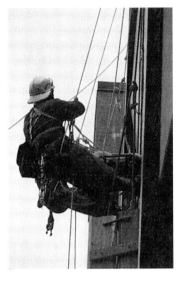

FIGURE 10-23a   High-angle rescue is dangerous and difficult. It should be deferred to persons trained and experienced in high-angle rescue techniques.

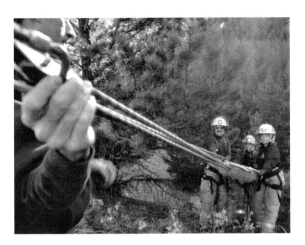

FIGURE 10-23b   Low-angle situations are not the same as high-angle situations. Therefore, many EMS agencies have trained their paramedics in the skills of low-angle rescue.

- **belay:** procedure for safeguarding a climber's progress by controlling a rope attached to an anchor. The person controlling the rope is sometimes also called the belay.
- **rappel:** to descend by sliding down a fixed double rope, using the correct anchor, harness, and gear.

Low-Angle Rescues

Many EMS systems have trained their paramedics in the skills of low-angle rescue or "off-the-road" rescue. Like high-angle rescues, crews require rope, harnesses, hardware, and the necessary safety systems (Figure 10-23b). Low-angle rescues may be up to 40°, except if the face is overly smooth. Then a high-angle team will be better able to handle the more technical access and evacuation.

Each member of a low-angle crew must know how to assemble a hasty harness tied from two-inch tubular webbing (or don a climbing harness), rappel and ascend by rope, package a patient in a litter, and rig a simple hauling system to assist the litter team up the embankment. Teams must also know how to set up a hasty rope slide to assist with balance and footing on rough terrain. Although low-angle rescues involve less technical skill than high-angle rescues, they still require ongoing practice and proper equipment.

PATIENT PACKAGING FOR ROUGH TERRAIN

Packaging a patient is a critical aspect of any hazardous terrain rescue. The Stokes basket stretcher is the standard litter for rough terrain evacuation (Figures 10-24a and 10-24b). It provides a rigid frame for patient protection and is easy to carry with an adequate number of personnel. Alternative spinal immobilizers

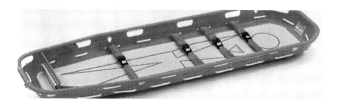

FIGURE 10-24a A basket stretcher.

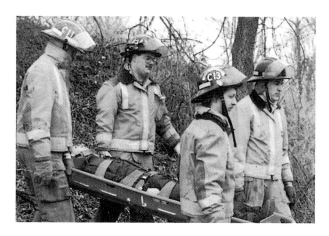

FIGURE 10-24b A basket stretcher is often used to carry patients over rough terrain.

can be used in a Stokes basket such as the KED, "halfback" backboard (extrication/rescue vest), or the Sked®. As a last resort, the Stokes can be used as spinal immobilizer itself.

Stokes baskets came in wire and tubular as well as plastic styles. The older "military style" wire mesh Stokes basket will not accept a backboard. Newer models, however, offer several advantages. They included:

- Generally greater strength
- Less expense per unit
- Better air/water flow through the basket
- Better flotation, an important concern in water rescues

Plastic basket stretchers are usually weaker than their wire mesh counterparts. They are often rated for only 300 to 600 pounds. However, they tend to offer better patient protection. In general, Stokes baskets with plastic bottoms and steel frames are best. These versatile units can also be slid in snow, when necessary.

Most Stokes baskets, regardless of their style, are not equipped with adequate restraints. As a result, they will require additional strapping or lacing for rough terrain evacuation and/or extrication. A plastic litter shield can be used to protect the patient from dust and objects that may fall on the person's face. When moving across flat terrain, lace the patient into the Stokes basket to limit movement. When using a Stokes basket for high-angle or low-angle evacuation, take the following additional steps:

- Apply a harness to the patient.
- Apply leg stirrups to the patient.
- Secure the patient to a litter to prevent movement.
- Tie the tail of one litter line to the patient's harness.
- Use a helmet or litter shield to protect the patient.
- Administer fluids (IV or orally).
- Allow accessibility for taking BP, performing suction, and assessing distal perfusion.

- Ensure adequate padding—a crucial consideration.
- Consider use of a patient heating/cooling system, especially for prolonged evacuations.
- Provide for an airway clearing system via a gravity "tip line," if necessary.

PATIENT REMOVAL FROM HAZARDOUS TERRAIN

When removing the patient from a hazardous terrain, a non-technical/non-rope evacuation is usually faster. In other words, when possible, walk the patient out. Remember: carrying a patient on a litter over flat ground can be a strenuous task even under ideal conditions. As the terrain becomes rougher, the litter carry becomes more demanding.

Flat Rough Terrain

When removing a patient in a litter from a flat rough terrain, make sure you have enough litter carriers to "leapfrog" ahead of each other to save time and to rotate rescuers. An adequate number of litter bearers would be two or, better yet, three teams of six. Litter bearers on each carry should be approximately the same height.

Several devices exist to ease the difficulty of a litter carry. For example, litter bearers can run webbing straps over the litter rails, across their shoulders, and into their free hands. This will help distribute the weight across the bearers' backs. Another helpful device is the litter wheel. It attaches to the bottom of a Stokes basket frame and takes most of the weight of the litter. Bearers must keep the litter balanced and control its motion. As you might suspect, the litter wheel works best over flatter terrain.

Low-Angle/High-Angle Evacuation

As already mentioned, low-angle and high-angle evacuations require specialized knowledge and skills. Before beginning patient removal, rescuers must ensure that all anchors are secure. They must check their own safety equipment and recheck patient packaging. They must also have the necessary lowering and hauling systems in place, again doing the recommended safety checks.

Materials, especially ropes, should never be used if there is any question of their safety. If you see a frayed rope or any stressed or damaged equipment, do not hesitate to point it out to the rescuers in a polite, but professional manner. Also, because hauling sometimes requires many "helpers," you may be asked to assist. Make sure you understand all directions given by the rescuers. Evacuation is a team effort.

Some high-angle units, especially fire departments, make use of aerial apparatus such as tower-ladders or bucket trucks to assist in the removal of a patient in a Stokes basket. These units are usually employed in structural environments but can be adapted to hazardous terrain if there is room for a truck.

When using aerial apparatus, it is necessary to provide a litter belay during movement to a bucket. Litters, of course, must then be correctly attached to the bucket. Use of aerial ladders can be difficult because upper sections are usually not wide enough to slot the litter. The litter must always be properly belayed if being slid down the ladder. Finally, ladders or other aerial apparatus should NOT be used as a crane to move a litter. They are neither designed nor rated for this work. Serious stress can cause accidents resulting in patient death.

Use of Helicopters

Helicopters can be useful in hazardous terrain rescues, especially when hospitals lie at a distant location (see Chapter 13). You must understand the capabilities of local helicopter systems and know who provides helicopter rescue in your region. Be aware of the difference in mission, crew training, and capabilities of helicopters that do air medical care versus helicopters that do rescue. You should be familiar with the advantages, disadvantages, and local restrictions for each of the following practices or techniques BEFORE you summon a helicopter from the field:

- Boarding and deboarding practices
- Restrictions on carrying non-crew members
- Use of cable winches for rescues
- Weight restrictions
- Restrictions on hovering rescues
- Use and practice of one-skids and toe-ins
- Use of **short hauls** or sling loads of equipment and/or personnel, as opposed to the more dangerous rappel-based rescues

Be aware of the difference in mission, crew training, and capabilities of helicopters that do air medical care versus helicopters that do rescue.

✳ short haul a helicopter extrication technique where a person is attached to a rope that is, in turn, attached to a helicopter. The aircraft lifts off with the person attached to it. Obviously this means of evacuation requires highly specialized skills.

Packaging/Evacuation Practice

Depending upon local protocols, you should practice the packaging and evacuation techniques expected of EMS personnel in your region. You should familiarize yourself with the specific types of basket stretchers and litters available to your unit and the proper packaging, immobilization, and restraint techniques for use with each type. You should also practice with other equipment used for rough-terrain rescues, including the Sked® and appropriate half-spine devices.

Practice or observe the skills required for low-angle and high-angle rescues. When possible, take part in exercises with the rescue units that you would summon to perform these evacuations. By fully understanding the capabilities of the rescue response teams in your area, you will circumvent any "turf" issues. You will also know how to work together whenever a multi-jurisdictional event occurs.

EXTENDED CARE ASSESSMENT AND ENVIRONMENTAL ISSUES

As you learned in Volume 3, Chapter 10, environmental emergencies can present their own special challenges. For rescue operations, at least some personnel should have formal training in managing patients whose injuries have been aggravated by prolonged lack of treatment, often under extreme conditions. If SOPs do not already exist, procedures adopted from wilderness medical research will prove useful. Position papers written by the Wilderness Medical Society or the National Association for Search and Rescue can serve as guidelines for protocols.

Regardless of the source, you will discover that many protocols for extended care vary substantially from standard EMS procedures. If your agency anticipates involvement in some of the rescue situations described in this chapter, you should consider protocols that at least address the following areas:

- Long-term hydration management
- Repositioning of dislocations

- Cleansing and care of wounds
- Removal of impaled objects
- Non-pharmacological pain management—utilizing proper splinting, distracting the patient by talking or asking questions, scratching or creating sensory stimuli when doing painful procedures
- Pharmacological pain management—utilizing pharmacological agents with isolated trauma such as amputation or fracture or with multiple trauma such as crushing or pinning of more than an extremity
- Assessment and care of head and spinal injuries
- Management of hypothermia or hyperthermia
- Termination of CPR
- Treatment of crush injuries and compartment syndromes. (For a review of these trauma injuries, see Volume 4.)

A number of environmental issues can affect your assessment during a rescue situation. Some of the most important issues include the following:

- **Weather/Temperature Extremes:** Extreme weather or temperature conditions increase the risk of patient hypo/hyperthermia. These conditions also make it difficult or impossible to expose the patient completely for full assessment and treatment. As a result, your physical examination may be compromised. Use of tarps, blankets, plastic sheeting may help in some cases, but your assessment will usually be limited at best.

- **Limited Patient Access:** Parts of the patient may not be accessible for examination because they are pinned beneath debris or stuck in a confined space. Cramped space and low-lighting conditions also make assessment difficult. For this reason, it is important that you carry a headlamp with extended battery packs.

- **Difficulty Transporting Street Equipment:** Hazardous terrain often makes it difficult to transport typical street equipment to the patient. Tackle boxes and heavy equipment may be inappropriate to take into a confined space, the back woods, or down a hasty rappel. As a result, equipment usually must be downsized. Often you will utilize a backpack to keep your hands free for carrying. Essential equipment for the MS-ABCs of initial assessment and management include:
  - *Airway*—oral and nasal airways, manual suction, intubation equipment
  - *Breathing*—thoracic decompression equipment, small oxygen tank/regulator, masks/cannulas, pocket mask/BVM
  - *Circulation*—bandages/dressings, triangular bandages, occlusive dressings, IV administration equipment, BP cuff and stethoscope
  - *Disability*—extrication collars
  - *Expose*—scissors
  - *Miscellaneous*—headlamp/flashlight, space blanket, padded aluminum splint (SAM® splint), PPE (leather gloves, latex gloves, eye shields)

- **Cumbersome PPE:** Necessary, but cumbersome, PPE can restrict rescuer mobility. In certain instances, some of the PPE might be removed to perform care steps. For example, the heavy outer gloves worn in extremely cold conditions might be taken off during administration of an IV. However, all PPE should be reapplied as soon as possible.

- **Patient Exposure:** Patients should be quickly covered to assure thermal protection. During the extrication, place hard protection, such as a spine board, and take steps to prevent patient contact with sharp objects or debris. For example, use an aluminized blanket to prevent glass shards from contacting the patient.

- **Use of ALS Skills:** Good BLS skills are mandatory in hazardous terrains, but limit ALS skills to those that are really essential. More wires and tubing complicate the extrication process. Continuous oxygenation and definitive airway control and volume may be essential. However, rescuers can't carry lots of oxygen tanks into rugged terrains. As a result, you may have to use your tank at a slower flow rate so that it will last a longer period of time.

- **Patient Monitoring:** Hazardous terrain can alter your use of monitoring equipment. In high noise areas, for example, you may have to take BP by palpation or use a compact pulse oximetry unit. An ECG monitor can be cumbersome during extrication and will be more difficult to use than in a street situation.

- **Improvisation:** Improvisation is common in rescue situations. To minimize the amount of equipment carried over hazardous terrain, you may want to consider such techniques as tying upper extremity fractures to the torso or tying lower extremity fractures to the uninjured leg. Lightweight SAM® splints can be very useful in the backwoods and should be part of your downsized medical gear. Whatever you do, continue talking to the patient and explain exactly what is happening. Answer any questions, particularly if you are improvising. The patient is already frightened by the entrapment. Don't worsen the situation by making the patient feel even more out of control.

Good BLS skills are mandatory in hazardous terrains, but limit ALS skills to those that are really needed. Do not complicate any already complicated operation.

SUMMARY

All rescue operations can be divided into at least seven functional stages: arrival and size-up, hazard control, patient access, medical treatment, disentanglement, patient packaging, and removal/transport. Whenever you function in any of one of these phases, you must be properly outfitted with protective equipment. You must also have training specific to the assigned rescue.

In any rescue, you must access the scene quickly so assessment and management may begin. Situational threats to the rescuer and/or patient should be identified and remedied as thoroughly as conditions permit. Patients should be reassessed throughout the rescue and repackaged as extrication and removal progresses.

During the operational phases of the rescue, you must provide direct patient care and work with technical teams to assure optimal patient management. Any paramedic assigned to rescue duties should have training in the care of patients who may require prolonged management. Such training results from the increased time to locate, access, remove, and/or transport a rescue patient.

Either you or a paramedic on your crew must accompany the patient throughout the transportation phase. This person should constantly monitor any changes in condition, while coordinating patient transport to an appropriate medical facility. If a specialized rescue team includes a trained paramedic, this person may fulfill these functions.

YOU MAKE THE CALL

You and your partner are working on the medic ambulance 642 covering the north portion of town. You receive a call for a motor vehicle collision on Interstate I-94. Upon arrival, you quickly determine that the collision involves more than the average complications. Apparently, the vehicle swerved off the road and rolled down an embankment. Traffic is already backed up for about a half mile. Several motorists have gotten out of their cars.

When you look over the embankment, you discover that two bystanders have climbed down the hill and are standing near the overturned automobile. They yell up: "There's just one guy inside. He's breathing, so we know he's alive. But we can't get any response out of him. Do you want us to do something?" While you're directing the bystanders to stand clear of the car, "rubbernecking" in the other lane causes a low-speed collision directly in the highway.

1. What are your immediate considerations as you size up the scene?
2. Why would you consider this a rescue operation?
3. What additional resources would you request?

See Suggested Responses at the back of this book.

FURTHER READING

Kidd, J.S. and J.D. Czajkowsi: *Vehicle Extrication—a Training Manual*. Saddlebrook, NJ: Fire Engineering, 1991.

Merrick, C., Editor: *Rescue Technician: Operational Readiness for Rescue Provides*. St. Louis, MO: Mosby-Year Book, 1998.

Moore, R.E.: *Vehicle Rescue and Extrication*. St. Louis, MO: Mosby Lifeline, 1991.

NFPA 1983 Standard on Fire Service Life Safety Rope and System Components, 1500 Standard on Fire Department Occupational Safety and Health Program, 1521 Standard on Fire Department Safety Officer, 1582 Standard on Medical Requirements for Firefighters.

OHSA 29—Labor, Code of Federal Regulations—Excavation Requirements 1926.650, Specific Excavation Requirements 1926.651, Requirements for Protective Systems 1926.652, Working on or Near Water 1926.106, Permit Required Confined Spaces 1910.146, The Control of Hazardous Energy (Lock-out/Tag-out) 1910.147, Personal Protective Equipment 1910.132, Bloodborne Pathogens 1910.1030, Hazardous Communications 1910.1200, Hazardous Materials Response 1910.120, Respiratory Protection 1910.134, Fire Brigade 1910.156.

Ray, S.: *Swiftwater Rescue: A Manual for the Rescue Professional*. Ashville, NC: CPS Press, 1997.

Smith, D.S. and S.J. Smith: *Water Rescue: Basic Skills for Emergency Responders*. St. Louis, MO: Mosby Lifeline, 1994.

Tilton, B. and F. Hubbell: *Medicine for the Backcountry*, 2nd Edition. Merrillville, IN: ICS Books, 1994.

Vines, T.: *High-Angle Rescue Techniques*, 2nd Edition. St. Louis, MO: Mosby, 1999.

Wilkerson, J.A.: *Medicine for Mountaineering & Other Wilderness Activities*, Fourth Edition. Merced, CA: The Mountaineers, 1992.

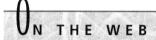

ON THE WEB

Visit Brady's Paramedic Website at www.bradybooks.com/paramedic.

CHAPTER 11

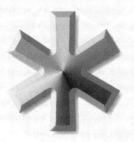

Hazardous Materials Incidents

Objectives

After reading this chapter, you should be able to:

1. Explain the role of the paramedic/EMS responder at the hazardous material incident in terms of the following:
   a. Incident size-up. (pp. 417–426)
   b. Assessment of toxicologic risk. (pp. 420–426, 429–433)
   c. Appropriate decontamination methods. (pp. 433–437)
   d. Treatment of semi-decontaminated patients. (pp. 431–433, 435)
   e. Transportation of semi-decontaminated patients. (p. 437)
2. Identify resources for substance identification, decontamination, and treatment information. (pp. 423–426)

3. Identify primary and secondary decontamination risk. (pp. 429–430)
4. Describe topical, respiratory, gastrointestinal, and parenteral routes of exposure. (p. 430)
5. Explain acute and delayed toxicity, local versus systemic effects, dose response, and synergistic effects. (pp. 430–431)
6. Explain how the substance and route of contamination alters triage and decontamination methods. (p. 434)
7. Explain the employment and limitations of field decontamination procedures. (pp. 436–437)

Continued

Objectives Continued

8. Explain the use and limitations of personal protective equipment (PPE) in hazardous material situations. (pp. 437–439)
9. List and explain the common signs, symptoms, and treatment of the following substances:
    a. Corrosives (acids/alkalis). (p. 431)
    b. Pulmonary irritants (ammonia/chlorine). (pp. 431–432)
    c. Pesticides (carbamates/organophosphates). (p. 432)
    d. Chemical asphyxiants (cyanides/carbon monoxide). (pp. 432–433)
    e. Hydrocarbon solvents (xylene, methlyene chloride). (p. 433)
10. Describe the characteristics of hazardous materials and explain their importance to the risk assessment process. (pp. 415, 416, 435–436)
11. Describe the hazards and protection strategies for alpha, beta, and gamma radiation. (pp. 428–429)
12. Define the toxicologic terms and their use in the risk assessment process. (pp. 428–429)
13. Given a specific hazardous material, research the appropriate information about its physical and chemical properties and hazards, suggest the appropriate medical response, and determine the risk of secondary contamination. (pp. 420–426)
14. Identify the factors that determine where and when to treat a hazardous material incident patient. (pp. 426, 434–436)
15. Determine the appropriate level of PPE for various hazardous material incidents including:
    a. Types, application, use, and limitations. (pp. 437, 438)
    b. Use of a chemical compatibility chart. (p. 439)
16. Explain decontamination procedures including:
    a. Critical patient rapid two-step contamination process. (p. 436)

b. Non-critical patient eight-step decontamination process. (pp. 436–437)
17. Identify the four most common solutions used for decontamination. (p. 436)
18. Identify the body areas that are difficult to decontaminate. (p. 436)
19. Explain the medical monitoring procedures for hazardous material team members. (p. 439)
20. Explain the factors that influence the heat stress of hazardous material team personnel. (p. 439)
21. Explain the documentation necessary for hazmat medical monitoring and rehabilitation operations. (p. 439)
22. Given a simulated hazardous substance, use reference material to determine the appropriate actions. (pp. 423–424, 426)
23. Integrate the principles and practices of hazardous materials response in an effective manner to prevent and limit contamination, morbidity, and mortality. (pp. 415–440)
24. Size up a hazardous material (hazmat) incident and determine:
    a. Potential hazards to the rescuers, public, and environment. (pp. 417–420)
    b. Potential risk of primary contamination to patients. (p. 429)
    c. Potential risk of secondary contamination to rescuers. (pp. 429–439)
25. Given a contaminated patient, determine the level of decontamination necessary and:
    a. Level of rescuer PPE. (pp. 437–438)
    b. Decontamination methods. (pp. 433–437)
    c. Treatment. (pp. 431–433)
    d. Transportation and patient isolation techniques. (p. 437)
26. Determine the hazards present to the patient and paramedic given an incident involving a hazardous material. (pp. 415–440)

CASE STUDY

The radio dispatches your unit to a chemical burn incident at the Acme Chicken Processing Plant. You jump aboard the ambulance and travel to the address given by the dispatcher. Upon arrival, you observe about 50 workers standing in the parking lot. A security guard approaches the ambulance and points toward the loading dock. He tells you, "A couple of people were sprayed with refrigerant when the hose broke open. Some of them got burned."

You proceed to the loading dock and find six patients. All of them are experiencing shortness of breath. Several have burns, including one patient with obvious facial injuries. Bystanders have already begun flushing his eyes with water. The plant supervisor tells you the refrigerant was anhydrous ammonia. You relay the initial scene size-up to the dispatch center. Then you request additional ambulances, a supervisor, the fire department, and a local hazmat team.

As the first on-scene unit, you initiate the Incident Management System. You assume the role of Incident Commander, while your partner acts as Triage Officer. She quickly tags three patients red and three patient yellow. She reports one patient with some facial burns and possible eye injuries. Two other patients have chemical burns on their backs and extremities and are suffering respiratory distress. The remaining three patients have no burns, but are having difficulty breathing.

You instruct the patients to immediately remove all their clothing for decontamination. By this time, additional units have already begun to arrive. The fire chief requests a quick report and then initiates gross decontamination with large amounts of water. Meanwhile, you relocate all personnel to avoid contact with the run-off dilution.

You assign the patient with facial burns and eye injuries to a crew from one of the ALS ambulances. They complete decontamination and begin treatment. Other crews decontaminate and treat the remaining patients in the order established by triage. All patients receive oxygen. Paramedics establish intravenous lines and administer albuterol by small-volume nebulizer to the patients who are wheezing. Crews also apply dressings to the burn patients as necessary.

By now the supervisor has arrived, and you complete a face-to-face transfer of command. The supervisor oversees hazmat operations, and notifies hospitals of incoming patients. The hazmat team dons the necessary equipment and provides paper garments for the patients. Because decontamination is not very demanding, transport begins quickly. Your ambulance remains on-scene as a dedicated unit for the hazmat team.

You assess two hazmat crew members before they enter the plant. In analyzing the damage, the hazmat team determines that the anhydrous ammonia must be cleaned up by a contractor. However, if nobody enters the building, the chemical poses no immediate hazard to the workers, the public, or the environment.

You now perform a post-entry evaluation of the hazmat team. You find that they have not suffered significant heat loss during their entry. The supervisor then terminates the incident and orders the plant closed until the contractor completes the clean-up operation.

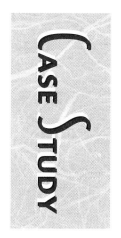

INTRODUCTION

Hazardous materials (hazmat) exist all around us. Companies in the United States manufacture more than 50 billion tons of hazardous materials a year. Some 4 billion tons of them are shipped throughout the United States by truck, pipeline, railroad, and tankers (Figure 11-1). They can exist as solids, liquids, or gases. They can irritate, burn, poison, corrode, or asphyxiate.

You learned about some hazardous materials in the chapters on toxicological and environmental emergencies in Volume 3 of *Paramedic Care: Principles and Practice*. This chapter deals with the hazardous materials spilled or released as a result of an accident, equipment failure, human error, or an intentional violation of the laws and regulations that govern their manufacture, use, and disposal.

For purposes of this chapter, keep in mind the definition of a hazardous material offered by the U.S. Department of Transportation (DOT). A hazardous material can be regarded as "any substance which may pose an unreasonable risk to health and safety of operating or emergency personnel, the public, and/or the environment if not properly controlled during handling, storage, manufacture, processing, packaging, use, disposal, or transportation."

✳ **hazardous material (hazmat)** any substance that causes adverse health effects upon human exposure.

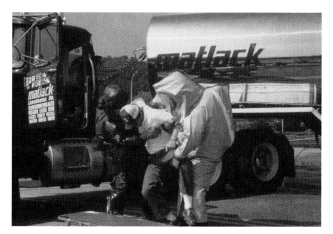

FIGURE 11-1   A hazardous materials emergency can involve countless substances and occur in many situations. Warning placards on a truck should immediately alert you to the possible need of a "hazmat" team.

ROLE OF THE PARAMEDIC

Hazardous materials, or hazmat, incidents present some of the most challenging situations that you will face as a paramedic. As mentioned, a hazmat event can involve all kinds of substances—corrosive chemicals, pulmonary irritants, pesticides, chemical asphyxiants, hydrocarbon solvents, and radioactive wastes. The exposure to hazardous materials may be limited to just a few victims, or it may cause widespread destruction and loss of many lives. However, as the opening case study shows, even a small-scale incident is almost always a multi-jurisdictional event. As such, EMS agencies should train all of their personnel how to respond to hazmat incidents and how to interact with other agencies that might be summoned to the scene.

Traditionally, paramedics do not perform defensive (containment) and offensive (control) functions at a hazardous material response. Even so, paramedics are still an integral part of a community's hazmat response system. As you will learn in this chapter, EMS personnel fulfill a variety of tasks at a hazmat incident. As first responders, they may size up the incident, assess the toxicological risk, and activate the Incident Management System needed to handle the event. They will also be called upon to evaluate decontamination methods, treatment and transport of exposed patients, and medical monitoring of hazmat teams who enter the area.

Even a small-scale hazmat incident almost always turns into a multi-jurisdictional event, thus triggering use of the IMS.

Content Review

EMS HAZMAT FIRST RESPONDERS

- Size up incident
- Assess toxicological risk
- Activate the IMS
- Establish command

Content Review

HAZMAT REQUIREMENTS/ STANDARDS

- OSHA publication CFR 1910.120
- EPA regulation 40 CFR 311
- NFPA standard 473

REQUIREMENTS AND STANDARDS

Two federal agencies—the Occupational Safety and Health Administration (OSHA) and the Environmental Protection Agency (EPA)—have set forth a number of regulations and standards for dealing with hazmat emergencies. The most important of these are found in OSHA publication CFR 1910.120, "Hazardous Waste Operations and Emergency Response Standard (1989)." This standard provides specific response procedures, including use of an Incident Management System (IMS), use of personal protective equipment (PPE), use of a Safety Officer, and special training requirements. The EPA has published a mirror regulation, called 40 CFR 311, that applies to those agencies that fall outside of OSHA.

In addition, the National Fire Protection Association (NFPA) has published NPFA 473, *Standard for Competencies for EMS Personnel Responding to Hazardous Materials Incidents*. This standard, along with two other NPFA standards for hazmat response, deals with the training standards for EMS personnel assigned to hazmat incidents.

LEVELS OF TRAINING

The above documents set forth three levels of training appropriate to EMS response at hazmat incidents—Awareness Level, EMS Level 1, and EMS Level 2. The Awareness Level applies to responders who may arrive first at a scene and discover a toxic substance. Training focuses on recognition of hazmat incidents, basic hazmat identification techniques, and individual protection from involvement in the incident. All EMS personnel, as well as police officers and firefighters, need to be trained to the Awareness Level.

EMS Level 1 training, or the "operations level," is required for those people who may perform patient care in the cold zone on patients who do NOT present a significant risk of secondary contamination. This training focuses on hazard assessment, patient assessment, and patient care for previously contaminated patients.

EMS Level 2 training, or the "technician level," is required for those people who may perform patient care in the warm zone on patients who still present a significant risk of secondary contamination. This training focuses on personal protection, decontamination procedures, and treatment for patients who are beginning or undergoing decontamination.

The level of training required for each individual depends on their role in the hazmat response system. All systems require some individuals trained in both the EMS Level 1 and Level 2 standard. In this way, patient care can begin during decontamination and continue after the patient has been cleaned of contaminants.

INCIDENT SIZE-UP

Sizing up a hazardous materials incident is a very difficult task. You often receive inaccurate or incomplete information. Plus events tend to develop very quickly during each phase of the incident. As already indicated, you can also expect a number of agencies to be involved in the response. As a result, you should be skilled in the use of the Incident Management System (IMS) discussed in Chapter 9 and practice it regularly with the other agencies that typically respond to a hazmat call.

IMS AND HAZMAT EMERGENCIES

Priorities for a hazmat incident are the same as for any other major incident: life safety, incident stabilization, and property conservation. However, you should be prepared for the special circumstances surrounding most hazmat emergencies. Some incidents, for example, will require immediate evacuation of patients from a contaminated area. Other incidents will have ambulatory contaminated patients who seek out EMS personnel as soon as you arrive on scene. In performing early hazmat interventions, you face the challenge of avoiding exposure to the hazardous material yourself. As a result, never compromise scene safety during the early phase of a hazmat operation. Otherwise, you risk becoming a contaminated patient. (The subject of "self-rescued" patients will be discussed later in the chapter.)

In setting priorities, you must also quickly determine whether the hazmat emergency is an open incident or a closed incident. That is, does the event have the potential for generating more patients? As you learned in Chapter 9, the answer to this question will determine the resources that you request, how you stage them, and the way in which you deploy personnel. In reaching your decision, remember that some chemicals have delayed effects. Triage must be ongoing, as patient conditions can change rapidly.

Finally, in employing the IMS at a hazmat incident, you must take into account certain special conditions when choreographing the scene. The most preferable site for deploying resources will be uphill and upwind. This will help prevent contamination from ground-based liquids, high vapor density gases, runoff water, and vapor clouds.

The basic IMS at a hazmat incident will require a command post, a staging area, and a decontamination corridor. Depending upon the event, the Incident Commander may also establish separate areas—such as treatment areas and personnel staging areas—to prevent unnecessary exposure to contamination. A backup plan for areas of operations must be determined early in the event. For example, what would you do if the wind direction suddenly shifted and a cloud of chlorine gas headed toward your staging area?

Priorities for a hazmat incident are the same as for any other major incident: life safety, incident stabilization, and property conservation.

Never compromise scene safety during the early phase of a hazmat operation. Otherwise, you risk becoming a patient yourself.

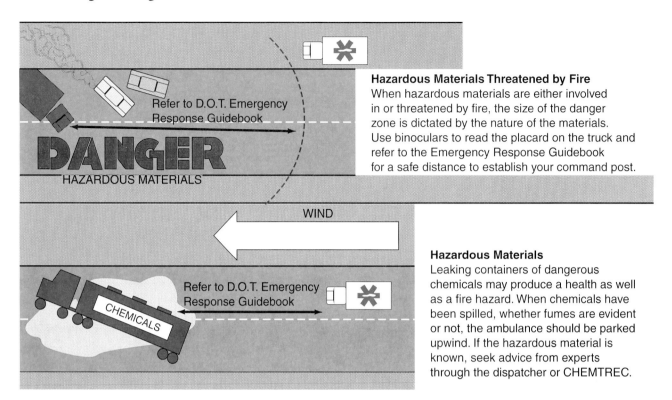

Figure 11-2   Transportation incidents involving hazardous materials.

INCIDENT AWARENESS

One of the most critical aspects of any hazmat response is the simple awareness that a dangerous substance is present.

One of the most critical aspects of any hazmat response is the simple awareness that a dangerous substance may be present. Virtually, every emergency site—residential, business, or highway—possesses the potential for hazardous materials. For example, most households keep ammonia and liquid bleach in the kitchen or laundry room. When combined, these substances can produce a toxic gas. Homes with kerosene heaters or blocked flues can be filled with carbon monoxide. Don't take any chances. Always keep the possibility of dangerous substances in mind whenever you approach the scene of an emergency. If you suspect the presence of hazardous materials, use binoculars to inspect the scene from a distance (Figure 11-3).

Transportation

Do not rule out the presence of hazmat at a MVC just because you do not see a warning placard.

* **warning placard** diamond-shaped graphic placed on vehicles to indicate hazard classification.

Any transportation accident—automobile, truck, or railroad—should raise a suspicion of hazardous materials (Figure 11-2). Maintain a high degree of hazmat awareness whenever you are summoned to MVCs involving commercial vehicles, pest control vehicles, tanker trucks, tractor-trailers, or cars powered by alternative fuels. Do not rule out the presence of hazardous materials just because you do not see a **warning placard.** Hospitals and laboratories, for example, routinely and legally transport medical radioactive isotopes in unmarked passenger cars. You might look in the back seat of a crashed automobile and see a container with a label indicating radioactive contents.

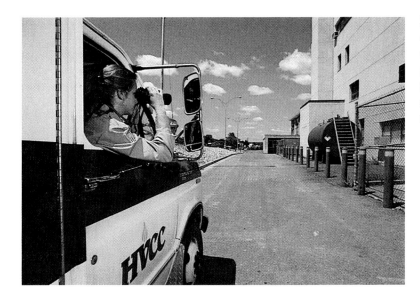

FIGURE 11-3 Don't take any chances. Use binoculars to make a visual inspection of potentially hazardous situation—such as a suspicious storage tank—from a safe distance.

Railroad accidents merit special attention for two reasons. First, railroad cars can carry large quantities of hazardous materials. The largest tanker truck, for example, has about a 14,000-gallon capacity, while a railroad tank car, can carry up to 34,000 gallons. Second, there may be several tank cars hitched together on a freight train. Obviously, there is a greater chance for a major incident if one or more of these tanks are ruptured in an accident. Fortunately, railroads run along fixed lines, which means you can preplan your response in case a railroad accident occurs within your jurisdiction.

Fixed Facilities

Hazmat incidents can also take place at fixed facilities where dangerous substances are produced or stored. Chemical plants and all manufacturing operations have tanks, storage vessels, and pipelines used to transport products and/or wastes. Additional fixed sites with possible hazardous materials include warehouses, hardware or agricultural stores, water treatment centers, and loading docks. If you work in a rural area, keep in mind the number of places where you can find hazardous materials on a farm or ranch—silos, barns, greenhouses, and more. (For information on rural hazmat emergencies, see Chapter 13.)

Finally, remember that many communities have some kind of fixed pipelines, especially in urban settings. These pipelines can be damaged by acts of nature (earthquakes), by construction crews, or, if above ground, by vehicle crashes. A rupture or leak in a gas or oil pipeline can spell disaster, especially if ignited.

Terrorism

Unfortunately, a new type of hazmat incident has emerged in recent years in the form of terrorism. The terrorists may use any variety of chemical, biological, or nuclear devices to strike at government or high-profile targets. These **weapons of mass destruction (WMD)** can be manufactured from materials as simple as those found on most farms, as was the case in the bombing of the Alfred P. Murrah Federal Building in Oklahoma City (see Chapter 9). The perpetrators can come from within the United States or from abroad.

✳ **weapons of mass destruction (WMD)** variety of chemical, biological, or nuclear devices used by terrorists to strike at government or high-profile targets; designed to create a maximum number of casualties.

POTENTIAL TERRORIST
TARGETS

• Public buildings
• Multinational
  headquarters
• Shopping centers
• Workplaces
• Sites of assembly

At terrorist incidents, remember that a secondary device may exist.

✱ **UN number** a four-digit identification number specific to a given chemical; some UN numbers are assigned to a group of related chemicals, but with different characteristics, such the UN 1203 designation for diesel fuel, gasohol, gasoline, motor fuels, motor spirits, and petrol. (The letters *UN* stand for "United Nations." Sometimes the letters *NH* for "North American" appear with or instead of the UN designation.)

The most frightening aspect of terrorism is the lack of predictability on when or where an attack might take place. Lacking a clear verbal or written threat, it can happen almost anyplace. However, terrorists usually select their targets by activity, particularly government or industrial, and by the number of people present. Potential targets include: public buildings, multinational headquarters, shopping centers, workplaces, and sites of assembly such as arenas, stadiums, and transportation centers, or places of worship. All of these locations should be identified in any mass casualty or disaster plan for your community.

In responding to a suspected terrorist incident, look for potential clues. Patients in a closed environment, such as a subway or an office building, will exhibit similar symptoms if they have been exposed to a chemical or biological WMD. In the case of an explosion, remember that a secondary device may exist. Take every precaution not to fall victim to a terrorist attack yourself. Make full use of the Incident Management System and all specialized agencies able to respond to the scene of suspected terrorism.

RECOGNITION OF HAZARDS

To aid in the visual recognition of hazardous materials, two simple systems have been developed. The Department of Transportation (DOT) has implemented placards to identify dangerous substances in transit, while the National Fire Protection Association (NFPA) has devised a system for fixed facilities.

Placard Classifications

While many vehicles are required by law to carry placards (Figure 11-4), the absence of a placard does not mean the absence of a hazmat threat. Regulations depend upon the type of substance and/or the amount of substance in transit.

When placards are used, you can spot them easily by their diamond shape (Figure 11-5). Each placard indicates hazmat classifications through use of a color code and hazard-class number. Some placards also carry a **UN number**—a

FIGURE 11-4 Vehicles carrying hazardous materials are required to display placards indicating the nature of their contents. Even if you have studied these placards earlier in your EMS career, you should regularly review the symbols, color-codes, and hazard class numbers so that you can identify dangerous materials.

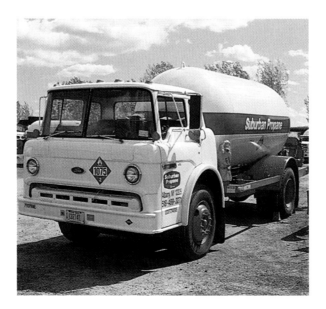

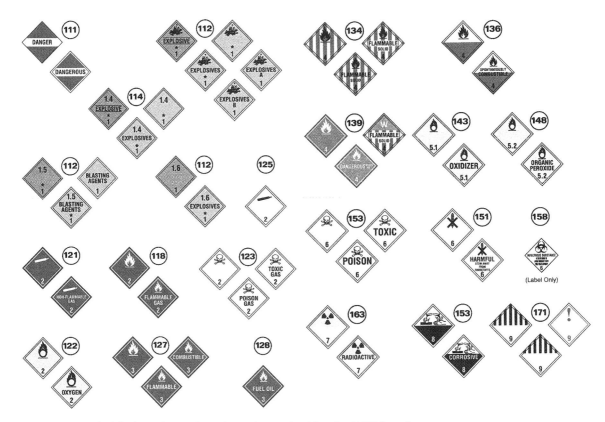

FIGURE 11-5 Sample labels and warning placards required by the DOT for all packages, storage containers, and vehicles containing hazardous materials.

four-digit number specific to the actual chemical. For quick reference, keep in mind the general classifications in Table 11-1.

In addition to numbers and colors, placards also use symbols to indicate hazard types. For example, a flame symbol indicates a flammable substance, a ball-on-fire symbol indicates an oxidizer, a propeller symbol indicates a radioactive substance, and a skull-and-crossbones symbol indicates a poisonous substance. When combined with numbers and colors, these symbols help you to recognize the specific nature of the hazardous material. For instance, a red placard with the

Table 11-1 HAZARD CLASSES AND PLACARD COLORS

Hazard Class	Hazard Type	Color Code
1	explosives	orange
2	gasses	red or green
3	liquids	red
4	solids	red and white
5	oxidizers and organic peroxides	yellow
6	poisonous and etiologic agents	white
7	radioactive materials	yellow and white
8	corrosives	black and white
9	miscellaneous	black and white

number 2 and a flame symbol means that the vehicle is carrying a flammable gas. Over time, you will become more familiar with these and other important symbols such as a "W" with a line through it, which means "reacts with water."

In using the placard system, keep in mind several shortcomings. Although some substances need to be placarded in all quantities, others need to be placarded only if they are transported in large quantities. This means that there may be hazardous materials onboard a truck, but they fall below the quantity required for placarding. Also, the "Dangerous" placard means that there are two or more substances onboard between 1,000 and 5,000 pounds total weight. However, the generic placard tells you nothing about the hazardous nature of the materials. Finally, people can remove placards or fail to apply them in the first place. In this case, you have no immediate indication at all of a dangerous hazmat situation.

Placards may only provide minimal information about a hazardous substance. Some materials, when shipped in smaller quantities, may not require a placard at all.

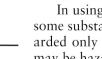

NFPA 704 System

The NFPA 704 System identifies hazardous materials at fixed facilities. Like the DOT placards, the system uses diamond-shaped figures, which are placed on tanks and storage vessels. The diamond is divided into four sections and color coded (Figures 11-6a and 11-6b). The top segment is red and indicates the flammability of the substance. The left segment is blue and indicates the health hazard. The right segment is yellow and indicates the reactivity. The bottom segment is white and indicates special information. The information may include water reactivity, oxidizer, or radioactivity.

Flammability, health hazard, and reactivity are measured on a scale of 0 to 4. A designation of 0 indicates no hazard, while a designation of 4 indicates extreme hazard.

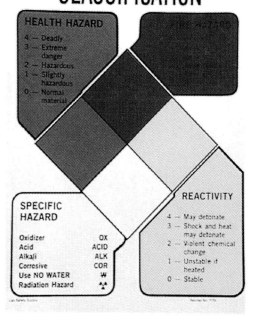

FIGURE 11-6a   NFPA 704 hazardous materials classification.

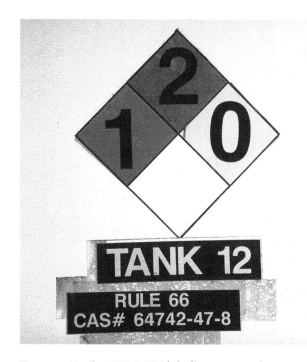

FIGURE 11-6b   NFPA 704 labeling on a tank.

IDENTIFICATION OF SUBSTANCES

Once you have determined that an incident involves hazardous materials, you must next try to identify the particular substance. This is the "crux," or most difficult aspect, of dealing with a hazmat incident. You will often lack adequate on-scene information to make a positive identification, or you will get conflicting preliminary information. For this reason, you must be familiar with the resources that can assist you in identification of a hazardous material and become skilled at using each of them.

To prevent dangerous interpretations, try to locate two or more concurring reference sources. Do not take action until you find this information—otherwise you risk making mistakes and providing incorrect patient treatment.

Emergency Response Guidebook (ERG)

You have already read about UN numbers—the four-digit numbers specific to actual chemicals. Some placards will include the UN number as well as the hazard class information. For example, you may see a tanker truck with a red (3) placard with the number 1203 in the middle. Based on what you already know, you can determine that the incident involves a flammable liquid. To identify the specific flammable liquid, you will need the *North American Emergency Response Guidebook* (Figure 11-7).

The ERG—published by the U.S. Department of Transportation, Transport Canada, and the Secretary of Communications and Transportation of Mexico—should be carried on every emergency vehicle. It lists more than a thousand hazardous materials, along with placards, UN numbers, and chemical names. It also cross-references each identification number to specific emergency procedures related to the chemical. The ERG includes, for example, a list of evacuation distances for the most hazardous substances. It is revised every three years, and the most up-to-date version should be readily available to all crew members.

When using the ERG, keep in mind two shortcomings. First, the reference only provides basic generic information on medical treatment. One recommendation, for instance, involves calling EMS. Obviously, this is not very helpful for EMS personnel. Second, more than one chemical often has the same UN number.

Identification of a specific hazardous substance forms the "crux," or most problematic part, of a hazmat incident.

Content Review

HAZMAT REFERENCES

- *Emergency Response Guidebook* (ERG)
- Shipping papers
- Material safety data sheets
- Monitors/chemical tests
- Databases (CAMEO®)
- Hazmat telephone hotlines (CHEMTREC; CHEMTEL, Inc.)
- Poison control centers
- Toxicologists
- Reference books

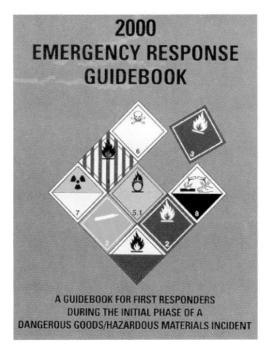

FIGURE 11-7 Have the *Emergency Response Guidebook* in your vehicle at all times.

For example, UN 1203 may be diesel fuel, gasohol, gasoline, motor fuels, motor spirits, or petrol. The difference between a gasoline leak and a diesel fuel leak is dramatic, highlighting the need to use other methods of positive identification.

Shipping Papers

* **shipping papers** documents routinely carried aboard vehicles transporting hazardous materials; ideally should identify specific substances and quantities carried; also known as bills of lading.

The most accurate information about a transported substance can be found in the **shipping papers,** or bill of lading. Trucks, boats, airplanes, and trains routinely carry these documents. Ideally, they should list the specific substances and quantities carried. However, drivers, pilots, or engineers may not take these papers when they exit the vehicle or craft, and you may find the scene too unstable to retrieve the documents yourself. In some cases, the papers may be incomplete or inadequate, requiring you to consult additional sources of identification.

Material Safety Data Sheets (MSDS)

* **material safety data sheets (MSDS)** easily accessible sheets of detailed information about chemicals found at fixed facilities.

In the case of fixed facilities, employers are required by law to post **material safety data sheets** (**MSDS**). These sheets contain detailed information about all potentially hazardous substances found on site. The sheets typically list the following data: the names and characteristics of the materials; what types of health, fire, and reactivity dangers the materials pose; any specific equipment or techniques required for safe handling of the materials; and suggested emergency first-aid treatment.

Even simple chemicals, such as window cleaners, should have material safety data sheets posted in an easily accessible location. Figure 11-8 shows the MSDS posted for a familiar chemical—chlorine bleach. Among other information, it indicates possible adverse reactions in cases of accidental exposure, spills, leaks, and so on. Note, too, the range of substances that can produce toxic fumes if mixed with the bleach.

Monitors and Testing

If you are unable to secure positive identification using the preceding sources, you may have to rely on monitors and other means of testing. If you do not have the training and equipment to do the reconnaissance, leave testing to the hazmat team. Monitoring devices or materials typically include:

- *Air and gas monitors*—typically determine the percentage of oxygen in the air and measure the presence of explosive gases, carbon monoxide, and toxic gases such as hydrogen sulfide
- *Litmus paper*—measures the approximate pH of a liquid, indicating whether it is an acid or a base
- *Colormetric tubes*—suction the air and search for specific chemicals

Other Sources of Information

* **CAMEO®** Computer-Aided Management of Emergency Operations; website developed by the EPA and NOAA as a source of information, skills, and links related to hazardous substances.

Once you have identified the hazardous substance, you will need to determine its specific chemical or physical properties. You can consult textbooks, handbooks, or technical specialists. You might also make use of a computerized database such as **CAMEO®**—Computer-Aided Management of Emergency Operations. Developed by the Environmental Protection Agency (EPA) and the National Oceanic and Atmospheric Administration (NOAA), this web site provides answers to technical questions, opportunities for skills practice, copies of software, links for networking, and more. Yet another source of information includes your local or regional poison control center. (For more on use of poison control centers, see Volume 3, Chapter 8.

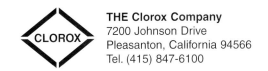

THE Clorox Company
7200 Johnson Drive
Pleasanton, California 94566
Tel. (415) 847-6100

Material Safety Data Sheets

Health	2+
Flammability	0
Reactivity	1
Personal Protection	B

I – CHEMICAL IDENTIFICATION

Name	regular Clorox Bleach	CAS No.	N/A
Description	clear, light yellow liquid with chlorine odor	RTECs No.	N/A

Other Designations	Manufacturer	Emergency Procedure
EPA Reg. No. 5813-1 Sodium hypochlorite solution Liquid chlorine bleach Clorox Liquid Bleach	The Clorox Company 1221 Broadway Oakland, CA 94612	• Notify your supervisor • Call your local poison control center OR • Rocky Mountain Poison Center (303)573-1014

II – HEALTH HAZARD DATA

• Causes severe but temporary eye injury. May irritate skin. May cause nausea and vomiting if ingested. Exposure to vapor or mist may irritate nose, throat and lungs. The following medical conditions may be aggravated by exposure to high concentrations of vapor or mist: heart conditions or chronic respiratory problems such as asthma, chronic bronchitis or obstructive lung disease. Under normal consumer use conditions the likelihood of any adverse health effects are low. FIRST AID: EYE CONTACT: Immediately flush eyes with plenty of water. If irritation persists, see a doctor. SKIN CONTACT: Remove contaminated clothing. Wash area with water. INGESTION: Drink a glassful of water and call a physician. INHALATION: If breathing problems develop remove to fresh air.

III – HAZARDOUS INGREDIENTS

Ingredients	Concentration	Worker Exposure Limit
Sodium hypochlorite CAS# 7681-52-9	5.25%	not established

None of the ingredients in this product are on the IARC, NTP or OSHA carcinogen list. Occasional clinical reports suggest a low potential for sensitization upon exaggerated exposure to sodium hypochlorite if skin damage (e.g., irritation) occurs during exposure. Routine clinical tests conducted on intact skin with Clorox Liquid Bleach found no sensitization in the test subjects.

IV – SPECIAL PROTECTION INFORMATION

Hygienic Practices: Wear safety glasses. With repeated or prolonged use, wear gloves.

Engineering Controls: Use general ventilation to minimize exposure to vapor or mist.

Work Practices: Avoid eye and skin contact and inhalation of vapor or mist.

V – SPECIAL PRECAUTIONS

Keep out of reach of children. Do not get in eyes or on skin. Wash thoroughly with soap and water after handling. Do not mix with other household chemicals such as toilet bowl cleaners, rust removers, vinegar, acid or ammonia containing products. Store in a cool, dry place. Do not reuse empty container; rinse container and put in trash container.

VI – SPILL OR LEAK PROCEDURES

Small quantities of less than 5 gallons may be flushed down drain. For larger quantities wipe up with an absorbent material or mop and dispose of in accordance with local, state and federal regulations. Dilute with water to minimize oxidizing effect on spilled surface.

VII – REACTIVITY DATA

Stable under normal use and storage conditions. Strong oxidizing agent. Reacts with other household chemicals such as toilet bowl cleaners, rust removers, vinegar, acids or ammonia containing products to produce hazardous gases, such as chlorine and other chlorinated species. Prolonged contact with metal may cause pitting or discoloration.

VIII – FIRE AND EXPLOSION DATA

Not flammable or explosive. In a fire, cool containers to prevent rupture and release of sodium chlorate.

IX – PHYSICAL DATA

Boiling point..................................212°F/100°C (decomposes)
Specific Gravity (H_2O = 1).............1.085
Solubility in Water.........................complete
pH..11.4

FIGURE 11-8   An example of a Material Safety Data Sheet (MSDS).

Two other sources of information are **CHEMTREC**—the Chemical Transportation Emergency Center—and **CHEMTEL, Inc.** Established by the Chemical Manufacturer's Association, CHEMTREC maintains a 24-hour, toll-free hotline. It provides information on the chemical properties of a substance and explains how the material should be handled. If necessary, CHEMTREC will even contact shippers and manufacturers to find out more detailed information about the incident and provide field assistance. In the United States and Canada, the toll-free number for CHEMTREC is 800-424-9300. For collect calls and calls from other points of origin, contact 703-527-3887. CHEMTREC can also refer you to the proper agencies for emergencies involving radioactive materials.

CHEMTEL, Inc., maintains another 24-hour, toll-free emergency response communications center for the United States and Canada. In addition to providing support for chemical emergencies, CHEMTEL also supplies the names of state and federal authorities for dealing with radioactive incidents. For toll-free calls, dial 800-255-3024. For collect calls and calls from other points of origin, contact 813-979-0626.

HAZARDOUS MATERIALS ZONES

As already mentioned, your main priority at a hazmat incident is safety. First, you protect your own safety and the safety of your crew. Then you attend to the safety of the patient(s) and the public. To ensure that expert help arrives, request it right away—just as you would under the IMS. Establish command and hold it until relieved by somebody higher in the chain of command.

While waiting for additional support, keep a bad situation from becoming worse by evacuating people from the area around the incident. Do not risk anyone's safety by allowing "heroic" rescues. The result can only be an increased number of contaminated patients. Prepare for the arrival of additional resources by setting up the control zones shown in Figure 11-9. They are:

While waiting for additional help, keep a bad situation from becoming worse by evacuating uncontaminated people from the area around the incident.

✱ **hot zone** location at a hazmat incident where the actual hazardous material and highest levels of contamination exist; also called the red zone or the exclusionary zone.

✱ **warm zone** location at a hazmat incident adjacent to the hot zone; area where a decontamination corridor is established; also called the yellow zone or contamination reduction zone.

✱ **cold zone** location at a hazmat incident outside the warm zone; area where incident operations take place; also called the green zone or the safe zone.

- *Hot (red) zone:* The hot zone, also known as the exclusionary zone, is the site of contamination. Prevent anyone from entering this area unless they have they have the appropriate high-level personal protection equipment (PPE). Hold any patients that escape from this zone in the next zone, where decontamination and/or treatment will be performed.

- *Warm (yellow) zone:* The warm zone, also called the contamination reduction zone, lies immediately adjacent to the hot zone. It forms a "buffer zone" in which a decontamination corridor is established for patients and EMS personnel leaving the hot zone. The corridor has both a "hot" and a "cold" end.

- *Cold (green) zone:* The cold zone, or "safe zone," is the area where the incident operation takes place. It includes the command post, medical monitoring and rehabilitation, treatment areas, and apparatus staging. The cold zone must be free of any contamination. No people or equipment from the hot zone should enter until undergoing the necessary decontamination. You and your crew should remain inside this zone unless you have the necessary training, equipment, and support to enter other areas.

SPECIALIZED TERMINOLOGY

To prevent conflicts between the personnel or departments working at a hazmat incident, everyone should use the same terminology. This helps to eliminate dangerous misunderstandings during operations and treatment.

Hot (Contamination) Zone

- Contamination is actually present.
- Personnel must wear appropriate protective gear.
- Number of rescuers limited to those absolutely necessary.
- Bystanders never allowed.

Warm (Control) Zone

- Area surrounding the contamination zone.
- Vital to preventing spread of contamination.
- Personnel must wear appropriate protective gear.
- Life-saving emergency care is performed.

Cold (Safe) Zone

- Normal triage, stabilization, and treatment are performed.
- Rescuers must shed contaminated gear before entering the cold zone.

TERMS FOR MEDICAL HAZMAT OPERATIONS

The following are the general terms that you can expect to encounter during a medical hazmat operation. They apply to situations involving chemical and/or radioactive materials.

- *Boiling point*—temperature at which a liquid becomes a gas.
- *Flammable/explosive limits*—range (upper and lower) of vapor concentration in the air at which an ignition will initiate combustion. The lower explosive limit (LEL) is the lowest concentration of chemical that will burn in the air. Below the LEL, there is not enough chemical to support combustion. The upper explosive limit (UEL) is the highest concentration of chemical that will burn in the air. Above the UEL, there is too much chemical and not enough oxygen to support combustion.
- *Flash point*—lowest temperature at which a liquid will give off enough vapors to ignite.
- *Ignition temperature*—lowest temperature at which a liquid will give off enough vapors to support combustion; slightly higher than the flash point.

- *Specific gravity*—the weight of a volume of liquid compared with an equal volume of water. Chemicals with a specific gravity greater than one will sink in water, while chemicals with a specific gravity less than one will float on water.
- *Vapor density*—the weight of a vapor or gas compared with the weight of an equal volume of air. Chemicals with a vapor density greater than one will fall to the lowest point possible, while chemicals with a vapor density less than one will rise.
- *Vapor pressure*—pressure of a vapor against the inside walls of a container. As temperatures increase, so do vapor pressures.
- *Water solubility*—ability of a chemical to dissolve into solution in water.
- *Alpha radiation*—neutrons and protons released by the nucleus of a radioactive substance (Figure 11-10). This is a very weak particle and will only travel a few inches in the air. Alpha particles are stopped by paper, clothing, or intact skin. They are hazardous if inhaled or ingested.
- *Beta radiation*—electrons released with great energy by a radioactive substance. Beta particles have more energy than alpha particles and will travel 6 to 10 feet in the air. Beta particles will penetrate a few millimeters of skin.
- *Gamma radiation*—high-energy photons, such as x-rays. Gamma rays have the ability to penetrate most substances and to damage any cells within the body. Heavy shielding is needed for protection against gamma rays. Because gamma rays are electromagnetic (instead of particles), no decontamination is required. (For more information on the hazards and protection strategies of the three types of radiation, see Volume 3, Chapter 10.)

TOXICOLOGICAL TERMS

It is equally important to learn the terminology related to the toxic effects of hazardous materials. Here are the most important toxicological terms used in the field:

- *Threshold limit value/time weighted average (TLV/TWA)*—maximum concentration of a substance in the air that a person can be exposed to for eight hours each day, forty hours per week, without suffering any adverse health effects. The lower the TLV/TWA, the more toxic the substance. The *Permissible Exposure Limit (PEL)* is a similar measure of toxicity.
- *Threshold limit value/short-term exposure limit (TLV/STEL)*—maximum concentration of a substance that a person can be exposed to for 15 minutes (time-weighted); not to be exceeded or repeated more than four times daily with 60-minute rests between each of the four exposures.
- *Threshold limit value/ceiling level (TLV-CL)*—maximum concentration of a substance that should never be exceeded, even for a moment.
- *Lethal concentration/lethal doses (LCt/LD)*—concentration (in air) or dose (if ingested, injected, or absorbed) that results in the death of 50% of the test subjects. Also referred to as the LCt50 or LD50.
- *Parts per million/parts per billion (ppm/ppb)*—representation of the concentration of a substance in the air or a solution, with parts of

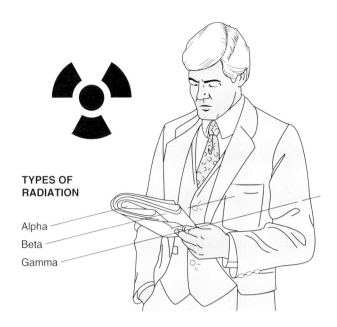

FIGURE 11-10 Alpha, beta, and gamma rays.

TYPES OF
RADIATION

Alpha
Beta
Gamma

the substance expressed per million or billion parts of the air or solution.

- *Immediately dangerous to life and health (IDLH)*—level of concentration of a substance that causes an immediate threat to life. It may also cause delayed or irreversible effects or interfere with a person's ability to remove himself or herself from the contaminated area.

CONTAMINATION AND TOXICOLOGY REVIEW

You have already covered some of the following material in Volume 3, Chapter 8. These points serve as a review, highlighting topics of particular relevance to haz-mat situations. Keep this material in mind whenever you come upon any scene in which you suspect the presence of dangerous substances.

TYPES OF CONTAMINATION

Whenever people or equipment come in contact with a potentially toxic sub-stance, they are considered to be contaminated. The contamination may be ei-ther primary or secondary.

Primary contamination occurs when someone or something is directly ex-posed to a hazardous substance. At this point, the contamination is limited—i.e., the exposure has not yet harmed others.

Secondary contamination takes place when a contaminated person or ob-ject comes in contact with an uncontaminated person or object—i.e., the con-tamination is transferred. Touching a contaminated patient, for example, can result in a contaminated care provider. Although gas exposure rarely results in secondary contamination, liquid and particulate matter are much more likely to be transferred.

To understand the difference between primary and secondary contamination, consider this example. A chemical pipeline ruptures and sprays several people

* **primary contamination** direct exposure of a person or item to a hazardous substance.

* **secondary contamination** transfer of a hazardous sub-stance to a non-contaminated person or item via contact with someone or something already contaminated by the substance.

Although gas exposure rarely results in secondary contamination, liquid and particulate matter can be easily transferred.

with a hazardous substance. This is primary contamination. One of these patients walks out of the area and calls an ambulance. Upon arrival, this same patient climbs into the back of the ambulance, exposing the paramedics and the ambulance to the contaminant. This is secondary contamination. As a member of the EMS crew, you must make every effort not to become part of the incident through such secondary contamination.

ROUTES OF EXPOSURE

As you know, there are four ways in which a person can be exposed to a hazardous substance. The most common method is respiratory inhalation. Gases, liquids, and particulate solids can all be inhaled through the nose or mouth. Once substances enter the bronchial tree, they can be quickly absorbed, especially in oxygen deficient atmospheres. The substance then enters the central circulation system and is distributed throughout the body. As a result, inhaled substances often trigger a rapid onset of symptoms.

Toxic substances may also be introduced into the body through the skin, either by topical absorption or parenteral injection. Any toxic substance placed topically on intact skin and transferred into the person's circulation is considered a medical threat. In the case of injections, poisons directly enter the body via a laceration, a burn, or a puncture.

In hazmat situations, the least common route of exposure is through gastrointestinal ingestion. In occupations involving hazardous materials, people can be exposed to poisons by eating, drinking, or smoking around deadly substances. Foodstuffs can be exposed to a chemical and then eaten. People can forget to wash their hands and introduce the substance in their mouths.

CYCLES AND ACTIONS OF POISONS

Absorption—the rate at which a substance is delivered into the blood stream—varies with the type and dosage of the poison. In general, the higher the dose, the greater the effect the substance will have on the body. Because of the wide variety of toxic substances, you will need to rely on the resources mentioned earlier to determine a given substance's actions, distribution to target organs, likely areas of deposit, and so on.

Basically, a poison's actions may be acute or delayed. **Acute effects** include those signs and symptoms that manifest themselves immediately or shortly after exposure. **Delayed effects** may not become apparent for hours, days, weeks, months, or even years. If a person is exposed to chlorine gas, for example, he or she immediately develops shortness of breath—an acute effect. If a person is exposed to a carcinogen, on the other hand, it may take many years before a malignancy develops—a delayed effect. Some substances, such as mustard gas (a military blister agent) cause immediate damage, but victims do not develop symptoms for many hours.

Once a substance is introduced into the body, it is distributed to target organs. Effects from a chemical may be local or systemic. **Local effects** involve areas around the immediate site and should be evaluated based upon the burn model. You can usually expect some skin irritation (topical) or perhaps acute bronchospasm (respiratory). An acid sprayed on the skin, for example, creates immediate skin damage at the point of contact.

Systemic effects occur throughout the body. They can affect the cardiovascular, neurologic, hepatic, and/or renal systems. Although hydrofluoric acid may cause local skin burns upon contact, for example, it can also trigger hypocal-

In hazmat situations, the least common route of exposure is through gastrointestinal ingestion. The most common routes are inhalation and topical absorption.

✱ **acute effects** signs and/or symptoms rapidly displayed upon exposure to a toxic substance.

✱ **delayed effects** signs, symptoms, and/or conditions developed hours, days, weeks, months, or even years after the exposure.

✱ **local effects** effects involving areas around the immediate site; should be evaluated based upon the burn model.

✱ **systemic effects** effects that occur throughout the body after exposure to a toxic substance.

cemia and dysrhythmias. As a result, exposure to this substance can be potentially fatal.

The organs mostly commonly associated with toxic substances are the liver and the kidneys. The liver metabolizes most substances, by chemically altering them through a process known as **biotransformation.** The kidneys can usually excrete the substances through the urine. However, both the liver and kidneys may be adversely affected by chemicals as are other organ systems. In such situations, the body may not be able to eliminate the toxic substances, creating a life-threatening situation.

When treating patients exposed to toxic substances, keep in mind that two substances or drugs may work together to produce an effect that neither of them can produce on its own. This effect, known as **synergism,** is part of the standard pharmacological approach to medicine. Before administering any medication, be sure to consult with medical direction or the poison control center on possible synergistic effects or treatments.

TREATMENT OF COMMON EXPOSURES

As noted several times, patients may be exposed to an incredibly large number of chemicals. Their treatment may range from supportive care to specific antidotes. After ensuring your own safety, all patients should receive the necessary supportive measures—airway support and suctioning, respiratory support, supplemental oxygen, circulatory support, and intravenous access. Before administering specific pharmacological treatment, at least two sources should agree on the medication. In addition, you should confer with medical direction, as previously mentioned.

The following are several of the most common classifications of chemicals to which patients may be exposed. A brief overview of effects and treatment procedures is provided for each circumstance. Keep in mind that this is a generic discussion and is not intended to replace the specific identification resources already described.

Corrosives

Corrosives—acids and alkalis (bases)—can be found in many everyday materials. Most drain cleaners, for example, contain the alkali sodium hydroxide. Depending upon the concentration, these substances can damage skin and other tissues. Corrosives can be inhaled, ingested, absorbed, or injected. Primary effects include severe skin burns and respiratory burns and/or edema. Some corrosives may also have systemic effects.

When decontaminating a patient exposed to solid corrosives, brush off dry particles. In the case of liquid corrosives, flush the exposed area with large quantities of water. Tincture of green soap may help in decontamination. Irrigate eye injuries with water, possibly using a topical ophthalmic anesthetic such as tetracaine to reduce eye discomfort. In patients with pulmonary edema, consider the administration of furosemide (Lasix) or albuterol. If the patient has ingested a corrosive, DO NOT induce vomiting. If the patient can swallow and is not drooling, you may direct the person to drink 5cc/kg water up to 200 cc. As with other injuries, maintain and support the ABCs.

Pulmonary Irritants

Many different substances can be pulmonary irritants, including the fumes from chlorine and ammonia. When inhaled, chlorine mixes with respiratory secretions

* **biotransformation** changing a substance in the body from chemical to another; in the case of hazardous materials, the body tries to create less toxic materials.

* **synergism** a standard pharmacological principle in which two substances or drugs work together to produce an effect that neither of them can produce on its own.

Before administering any medication to a hazmat patient, be sure to obtain at least two independent sources of agreement. Also consult with medical direction or the poison control center on possible synergistic effects or treatments.

If a patient has ingested a corrosive, DO NOT induce vomiting.

to produce hydrochloric acid. Ammonia mixes with respiratory secretions to produce ammonium hydroxide, an alkali. In addition to tissue damage, these chemicals can cause pulmonary edema. The substances can also injure intact skin. Liquid ammonia, for example, will cause cold burns.

Primary respiratory exposure cannot be decontaminated. However, you should remove the patient's clothing to prevent any trapped gas from being contained near the body. You should also flush any exposed skin with large quantities of water. Irrigate eye injuries with water, possibly using tetracaine to reduce eye discomfort. Treat pulmonary edema with furosemide, if indicated. Again, treatment includes maintaining and supporting the ABCs.

Pesticides

Toxic pesticides or insecticides primarily include carbamates and organophosphates. Patients may come in contact with these chemicals through all four routes of exposure—inhalation, absorption, ingestion, or injection. The substances can act to block **acetylcholinesterase (AChE)**—an enzyme that stops the action of acetylocholine, a neurotransmitter. The result is overstimulation of the muscarinic receptors and the SLUDGE syndrome: salivation, lacrimation, urination, diarrhea, gastrointestinal distress, and emesis. Stimulation of the nicotinic receptor may also trigger involuntary contraction of the muscles and pinpoint pupils.

These chemicals will continue to be absorbed as long as they remain on the skin. As a result, decontamination with large amounts of water and tincture of green soap is essential. Remove all clothing and jewelry to prevent the chemical from being trapped against the skin. Maintain and support airway, breathing, and circulation. Secretions in the airway may need to be suctioned.

The primary treatment for significant exposure to pesticides is atropinization. The dose should be increased until the SLUDGE symptoms start to resolve. For carbamates, Pralidoxime is NOT recommended. If an adult patient presents with seizures, administer 5 to 10 mg of diazepam. Do NOT induce vomiting if the patient has ingested the chemical. However, if the patient can swallow and has an intact gag reflex, you can administer 5 cc/kg up to 200 ml of water.

Chemical Asphyxiants

The most common chemical asphyxiants include carbon monoxide (CO) and cyanides such as bitter almond oil, hydrocyanic acid, potassium cyanide, wild cherry syrup, prussic acid, and nitroprusside. Keep in mind that both CO and cyanides are byproducts of combustion, so patients who present with smoke inhalation may need to be assessed for these substances as well. Most patients are exposed to CO and cyanides through inhalation. However, keep in mind that cyanides can also be ingested, absorbed, or injected.

These two chemicals have different actions once inhaled. Carbon monoxide has a very high affinity for hemoglobin—approximately 200 times greater than oxygen. As a result, it displaces oxygen in the red blood cells. Cyanides, on the other hand, inhibit the action of **cytochrome oxidase.** This enzyme complex, found in cellular mitochondria, enables oxygen to create the adenosine triphosphate (ATP) required for all muscle energy. Primary effects of CO exposure include changes in mental status and other signs of hypoxia such as chest pain, loss of consciousness, or seizures. Primary effects of cyanides include rapid onset of unconsciousness, seizures, and cardiopulmonary arrest.

Primary respiratory exposure cannot be decontaminated. However, you should remove the patient's clothing to release any trapped gases.

✳ acetylcholinesterase (AChE) enzyme that stops the action of acetylcholine, a neurotransmitter.

Most pesticides will continue to be absorbed as long as they are on the skin. Decontamination with large amounts of water and tincture of green soap is essential.

The primary pharmacological treatment of significant exposure to pesticides is atropinization. The dose should be increased until the SLUDGE symptoms start to resolve.

Assess patients who present with smoke inhalation for the presence of carbon monoxide and cyanides—two byproducts of combustion.

✳ cytochrome oxidase enzyme complex, found in cellular mitochondria, that enables oxygen to create the adenosine triphosphate (ATP) required for all muscle energy.

Decontamination of patients exposed to CO and cyanide asphyxiants is usually unnecessary. However, they must be removed from the toxic environment without exposing rescuers to inhalation. Take off the patient's clothing to prevent entrapment of any toxic gases, while maintaining airway, breathing, and circulatory support. Definitive treatment for CO inhalation is oxygenation. In some cases, it may be provided through hyperbaric therapy, which increases the displacement of carbon monoxide from hemoglobin molecules by oxygen.

Definitive treatment for cyanide exposure can be provided by several interventions carried in a cyanide kit. First, administer amyl nitrite. This short-acting vasodilator has the ability to convert hemoglobin to methemoglobin, which forms a nontoxic complex with cyanide ions. Wrap an ampule in gauze or cloth and crush it between your fingers. Then place it in front of a spontaneously breathing patient for 15 seconds. Repeat at one-minute intervals until an infusion of sodium nitrite is ready. Keep in mind that amyl nitrite is volatile and highly flammable when mixed with air or oxygen.

Next, administer the sodium nitrite, 300 mg IV push over 5 minutes. (Sodium nitrite also produces methemoglobin.) Quickly follow the sodium nitrite with an infusion of sodium thiosulfate, 12.5 g. IV push over 5 minutes. The sodium thiosulfate converts the cyanide/methemoglobin complexes into thiocyanate, which can be excreted by the kidneys. If the signs and symptoms reappear, the process should be repeated at half the original doses.

Hydrocarbon Solvents

Many different chemicals can act as solvents, including xylene and methylene chloride. Usually found in liquid form, they give off easily inhaled vapors. Primary effects include dysrhythmias, pulmonary edema, and respiratory failure. Delayed effects include damage to the central nervous system and the renal system. Exposure to these chemicals may be intentional, such as among drug abusers seeking the CNS effects (euphoria) produced by the fumes. If the patient ingests the chemical and vomits, aspiration may lead to pulmonary edema.

Treatment varies with the route of exposure. In cases of topical contact, decontaminate the exposed area with large quantities of warm water and tincture of green soap. If the patient has ingested the solvent, DO NOT induce vomiting. If the adult patient presents with seizures, administer 5–10 mg diazepam. In the case of inhalation, maintain and support the ABCs.

APPROACHES TO DECONTAMINATION

Decontamination, as you have read, attempts to reduce or remove hazardous substances from people and/or equipment to prevent adverse health effects. Decontamination can be accomplished by physical or chemical means. Physical decontamination involves the removal of chemicals by separating them from the person or equipment, while chemical decontamination focuses on changing the hazardous substance into something less harmful.

There are several purposes for performing decontamination (decon) procedures. First, decon reduces the dosage of the material to which patients are exposed. Second, it reduces the risk of secondary contamination of rescuers, on-scene personnel, bystanders, hospital personnel, the families of rescuers, and the general public.

Definitive treatment for CO inhalation is oxygenation.

Keep in mind that amyl nitrite is volatile and highly flammable. When mixed with air or oxygen, it can be easily ignited.

Content Review

USE OF CYANIDE KIT

- Administer ampule of amyl nitrite for 15 seconds.
- Repeat at one-minute intervals until sodium nitrite is ready.
- Administer infusion of sodium nitrite, 300 mg IV push over 5 minutes.
- Follow with infusion of sodium thiosulfate, 12.5 g. IV push over 5 minutes.
- Repeat at half original doses, if necessary.

Content Review

HAZMAT CHEMICAL CLASSIFICATIONS

- Corrosives—acids and bases
- Pulmonary irritants—fumes from chlorine and ammonia
- Pesticides—carbamates and organophosphates
- Chemical asphyxiants—carbon monoxide and cyanides
- Hydrocarbon solvents—xylene and methylene chloride

METHODS OF DECONTAMINATION

There are four methods of decontamination—dilution, absorption, neutralization, and isolation. The method used depends upon the type of hazardous substance and the route of exposure. In many instances, rescuers will use two or more of these methods during the decontamination process.

Dilution

Dilution involves the application of large quantities of water to the contaminated person or item. Water is considered the universal decon solution, especially for reducing topical absorption. It may be aided by use of a soap, such as tincture of green soap. Mixing hazardous substances with water significantly reduces their concentration, hopefully to a level where they are no longer dangerous. Be aware that a small number of chemicals should never be mixed with water.

Absorption

Absorption entails the use of pads or towels to "blot" up the hazardous material. The process is usually applied after washing with water—i.e., as a means of drying the patient. Absorption further reduces the contamination levels, but is not usually a primary method of decon. Absorption is more commonly used during environmental clean up.

Neutralization

Neutralization is almost never used by EMS personnel as a method of decontamination. Be aware of its risks—possible misidentification of the chemical or neutralizing agent and potential for exothermic reactions.

Neutralization occurs when one substance reduces or eliminates the toxicity of another substance, such as adding an acid to a base. Although this is a third method of patient decontamination, it is almost never used by EMS personnel. In a field setting, it is difficult to identify the exact hazardous substance and the proper neutralizing agent. In addition, neutralization often produces an exothermic reaction, or release of large quantities of heat. The heat can be just as damaging, or even more damaging, than the original chemical. Lavage usually dilutes and removes the chemical faster and is more practical given the typical on-scene equipment.

Isolation/Disposal

Isolation and/or disposal involves separating the patient or equipment from the hazardous substance. Isolation begins by establishing zones at the incident to prevent any further contamination or exposure. Next, hazmat teams remove patients from the hot zone to the warm zone. Lastly, any items that might contain or trap a hazardous substance should be removed, including a patient's clothing and jewelry. All contaminated items should be properly disposed of or stored.

DECONTAMINATION DECISION MAKING

If life threats exist, the patients come first, environmental considerations last.

In performing decontamination, always recall the priorities of incident management: life safety, incident stabilization, and property conservation. These priorities should guide your decision making throughout the incident. For example, you should try to prevent any run-off waters used for decontamination from damaging the environment. However, environmental considerations form a major concern only in cases where there are no life threats—i.e., patients are stable and not expected to deteriorate during the decon process. If life threats exist, the patients come first, environmental considerations come last.

Modes of Operation

In general, EMS personnel engage in one of two modes of operation at hazmat incidents that generate patients: "fast-break" or long-term decision making. Fast-break decision making occurs at incidents that call for immediate action to prevent rescuer contamination and/or to handle obvious life-threats. Long-term decision making takes place at extended events in which hazmat teams retrieve patients, identify substance, and determine methods of decontamination and treatment.

Fast-Break Decision Making At hazmat incidents where patients are conscious, contaminated victims will often self-rescue. They will walk themselves from the primary incident site to the EMS units. In such cases, you must make fast-break decisions to prevent rescuer contamination. Keep in mind that it may take time for a hazmat team to arrive and set up operations. In the interim, the conscious, contaminated patients may try to leave the scene entirely. As a result, all EMS units must be prepared for gross decontamination. Basic personal protective equipment should be on board and all personnel should be familiar with the two-step decontamination procedures covered later in this chapter.

All EMS units must be prepared for gross decontamination procedures.

Implement this mode of decision making at all incidents with critical patients and unknown or life-threatening materials. Fire apparatus often respond very quickly and carry large quantities of water that can be used for decon. Remove patient clothing, treat life-threatening problems, and wash with water. While it is preferable to use warm water to prevent hypothermia, this option is not always available. Please remember that the first rule of EMS is NOT TO BECOME A PATIENT! At no time should you or other crew members expose yourselves to contaminants—even to rescue a critically injured patient. Instead, contain and isolate the patient as best possible until the proper support arrives.

At no time should you or other crew members expose yourselves to contaminants—even to rescue a critically injured patient.

When treating critically injured hazmat patients, it is important to perform a rapid risk-to-benefit assessment. Ask yourself these questions: How much risk of exposure will I incur by intubating a patient during decon? Does the patient really need an intravenous line established right now? Few ALS procedures will truly make a difference if performed rapidly, but one mistake can make any rescuer into a patient. Take a few moments, and think before you act.

At incidents where patients are non-critical, rescuers can take a more contemplative approach, especially if they can identify the substance. Decontamination and treatment proceed simultaneously, following the general steps already mentioned. However, depending upon whether the substance has been identified and the type of substance involved, you may be able to give special attention to other matters. For example, you might contain run-off water. You might better protect patient privacy, grossly decontaminating ambulatory patients in a more controlled setting. You might also spend time on patient monitoring, reclothing patients, isolating or containing patients, and so on.

Long-Term Decision Making At more extended events, you will engage in long-term decision making. This mode of operation most often occurs when patients remain in the hot zone and have not self rescued. Traditionally, EMS personnel have not been trained or equipped to enter the hot zone to retrieve these patients. Instead, a hazmat team is summoned promptly, and the EMS crew awaits the team's arrival. The team will not make their entry until you or members of your crew perform the necessary medical monitoring and establish a decontamination corridor. It often takes 60 minutes or more for actual team deployment.

This mode of operation provides a number of advantages: a better opportunity for thorough decontamination, better PPE, less chance of secondary decontamination, greater consideration of the environment, and more detailed research

Content Review

ADVANTAGES OF LONG-
TERM DECISION MAKING

• More complete
  decontamination
• Better PPE
• Less secondary
  contamination
• Greater property
  conservation
• More thorough substance
  research
• Less room for error

Self-rescued patients often decide the mode of operation at a hazmat incident. Be prepared for fast-break operations whenever you suspect the presence of a toxic substance.

Content Review

TWO-STEP DECON

• Removal of clothing and
  personal effects
• Gross decontamination
  (two times)

Content Review

FOUR MOST COMMON
DECONTAMINATION
SOLVENTS

• Water
• Tincture of green soap
• Isopropyl alcohol
• Vegetable oil

of the actual hazardous substance. Obviously, long-term decision making presents less opportunity for error and is preferable to fast-break decision making. Unfortunately, self-rescued patients often decide the mode of operation the minute you arrive on the scene. Be prepared for fast-break operations whenever you suspect a potential hazmat incident.

FIELD DECONTAMINATION

As mentioned, the decontamination method and type of PPE depend upon the substance involved. If in doubt, assume the worst case scenario. When dealing with unknowns, do not attempt to neutralize. Brush dry particles off the patient before the application of water to prevent possible chemical reactions. Next, wash with great quantities of water—the universal decon agent—using tincture of green soap if possible. Isopropyl alcohol is an effective agent for some isocyanates, while vegetable oil can be used to decon water-reactive substances.

Two-Step Process

Use the two-step decon process for gross decontamination of patients who cannot wait for a more comprehensive decon process, usually patients at a fast-break incident. As noted, remove all clothing, including shoes, socks, and jewelry. (Remember to have some method of accounting for personal effects BEFORE hazmat incidents occur.) Wash and rinse the patients with soap and water, making sure that they do not stay in the run-off. Repeat the process, allowing the fluid to drain away each time. Pay special attention to difficult contamination areas such as the scalp and hair, ears, nostrils, axilla, fingernails, naval, genitals, groin, buttocks, behind the knees, between the toes, and toenails.

Eight-Step Process

The eight-step process takes place in a complete decontamination corridor and is much more thorough. To leave the hot zone, the hazmat rescuers follow these steps:

- **Step 1:** Rescuers enter the decon area at the hot end of the corridor and mechanically remove contaminants from the victims.
- **Step 2:** Rescuers drop equipment in a tool-drop area and remove outer gloves.
- **Step 3:** Decon personnel shower and scrub all victims and rescuers, using gross decontamination. As surface decontamination is removed, the dilution is conducted into a contained area. Victims may be moved ahead to Step 6 or Step 7.
- **Step 4:** Rescuers remove and isolate their SCBA. If re-entry is necessary, the team dons new SCBA from a non-contaminated side.
- **Step 5:** Rescuers remove all protective clothing. Articles are isolated, labeled for disposal, and placed on the contaminated side.
- **Step 6:** Rescuers remove all personal clothing. Victims who have not had their clothing removed have it taken off here. All items are isolated in plastic bags and labeled for later disposal or storage.
- **Step 7:** Rescuers and victims receive a full-body washing, using soft scrub brushes or sponges, water, and mild soap or detergent. Cleaning tools are bagged for later disposal.
- **Step 8:** Patients receive rapid assessment and stabilization before being transported to hospitals for further care. EMS crews medically monitor rescuers, complete exposure records, and transport rescuers to hospitals as needed.

These procedures are not set in stone. Small variations may exist from system to system. You should become familiar with the specific procedures in the jurisdiction where you practice.

Transportation Considerations

Remember that no patient who undergoes field decontamination is truly decontaminated. Field-decontaminated patients, sometimes called **semi-decontaminated patients,** may still need to undergo a more invasive decon process at a medical facility. Depending on the type of exposure, wounds may need debridement, hair or nails may need to be trimmed or removed, and so on. However, it is always better to deliver a grossly decontaminated living patient to the hospital than a perfectly decontaminated corpse. Just make sure that field-decontaminated patients are transported to facilities capable of performing more thorough decon procedures.

When transporting field-decontaminated patients, always recall that they may still have some contamination in or on them. For example, a patient may have ingested a chemical, which can be expelled if the patient coughs or vomits. As a result, use as much disposable equipment as possible. Keep in mind that any airborne hazard will not only incapacitate the crew in the back of the ambulance, but will affect the driver as well. Although it is not practical to line the ambulance in plastic, you can isolate the patient using a stretcher decon pool. The pool can help contain any potentially contaminated body fluids. Plastic can also be used to cover the pool, adding yet another protective barrier.

HAZMAT PROTECTION EQUIPMENT

As you know, the personal protective equipment used at a hazmat incident is specifically designed to prevent or limit rescuer injuries (Figures 11-11a to 11-11e). Hard hats, for example, protect rescuers against impacts to the head. There are basically four levels of hazmat protective equipment, ranging from Level A (the highest level) to Level D (the minimum level).

- *Level A*—provides the highest level of respiratory and splash protection. This hazmat suit offers a high degree of protection against chemical breakthrough time and fully encapsulates the rescuer, even covering the SCBA. The sealed, impermeable suits are typically used by hazmat teams entering hot zones with an unknown substance and a significant potential for both respiratory and dermal hazards.

- *Level B*—offers full respiratory protection when there is a lower probability of dermal hazard. The Level B suit is non-encapsulating, but chemically resistant. Seams for zippers, gloves, boots, and mask interface are usually sealed with duct tape. The SCBA is worn outside the suit, allowing increased maneuverability and greater ease in changing SCBA bottles. The decon team typically wear Level B protective equipment.

- *Level C*—includes a non-permeable suit, boots, and gear for protecting eyes and hands. Instead of SCBA, Level C protective equipment uses an **air-purifying respirator (APR)**. The APR relies on filters to protect against a known contaminant in a normal environment. As a result, the canisters in the APR must be specifically selected and are not usually implemented in a hazmat emergency response. Level C clothing is usually worn during transport of patients with the potential for secondary contamination.

- *Level D*—consists of structural firefighter, or turn-out, gear. Level D gear is usually not suitable for hazmat incidents.

No patient who undergoes field decontamination is ever truly decontaminated.

* semi-decontaminated patient
another name for field-decontaminated patient.

It is always better to deliver a grossly decontaminated living patient to the hospital than a perfectly decontaminated corpse.

When possible, protect the crew from secondary decontamination by placing a semi-decontaminated patient in a stretcher decon pool.

* air-purifying respirator (APR)
system of filtering a normal environment for a specific chemical substance using filter cartridges.

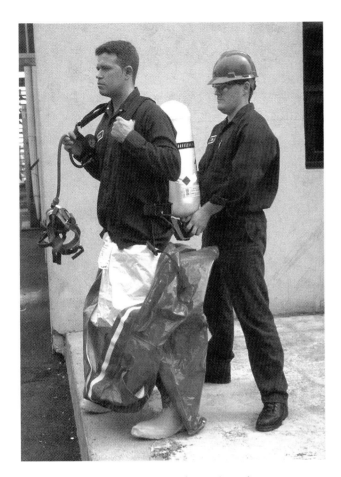

FIGURE 11-11a Assisting with an air tank.

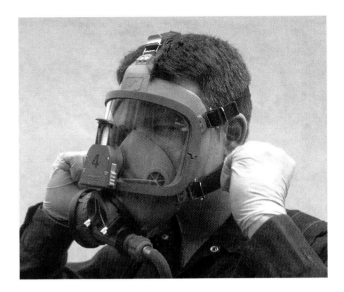

FIGURE 11-11b Putting on a mask.

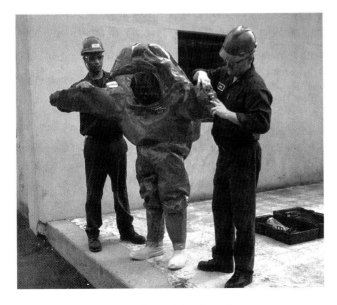

FIGURE 11-11c Assisting with a hood.

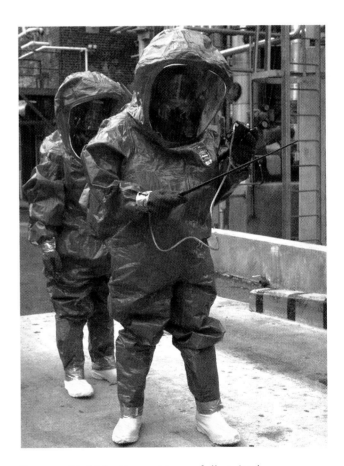

FIGURE 11-11d Hazmat team, fully suited.

The level of hazmat protective gear depends upon the chemical or substance involved. Ideally, the chemical should be identified so a permeability chart can be consulted to determine the breakthrough time. No single material is suitable to all hazmat situations. Some materials are resistant to certain chemicals and non-resistant to others.

EMS personnel should not become involved in any hazmat situation without the proper PPE. All ambulances carry some level of PPE, even if not ideal. If the situation is emergent and the chemical unknown, use as much barrier protection as possible. Full turnout gear (Level D) or a Tyvek suit is better than no gear at all. HEPA filter masks and double or triple gloves offer good protection against some hazards. Keep in mind that latex gloves are not chemically resistant. Instead, use nitrile gloves, which have a high resistance to most chemicals. Also remember that leather boots will absorb chemicals permanently, so be sure to don rubber boots.

When chemicals can be identified, consult a permeability chart to determine the breakthrough time on a hazmat suit.

If the situation is emergent and the chemical is unknown, use as much barrier protection as possible, even if less than ideal.

MEDICAL MONITORING AND REHABILITATION

As noted, one of the primary roles of EMS personnel at a hazmat incident is the medical monitoring of entry personnel. All hazmat team members should undergo regular annual physical examinations, with baseline vital signs placed on file.

ENTRY READINESS

Prior to entry, you or other EMS crew members will assess rescuers and document the following information on an incident flow sheet: blood pressure, pulse, respiratory rate, temperature, body weight, ECG, and mental/neurologic status. If you observe anything abnormal, do not allow the hazmat team member to attempt a rescue.

Hazmat team members will only enter the hot zone in groups of two, with two more members in PPE remaining outside the hot zone as a backup team. The PPE used at hazmat incidents can cause significant stress and dehydration. As a result, entry team personnel should prehydrate themselves with 8 to 16 ounces of water or sport drink. Because sport drinks are more effective at half strength, dilute them with 50% water when possible.

If you observe anything abnormal during pre-entry medical monitoring, do not allow the hazmat team member to attempt a rescue.

AFTER-EXIT "REHAB"

After the hazmat entry team exits the hot zone and completes decontamination, they should report back to EMS for post-entry monitoring (Figure 11-12). Measure and document the same parameters on the flow sheet. Rehydrate the team with more water or diluted sports drink. You can use weight changes to estimate any fluid losses. Check with medical direction or protocols to determine fluid replacement by means of PO or IV. Entry team members should not be allowed to re-enter the hot zone until they are alert, non-tachycardic, normotensive, and within a reasonable percentage of their normal body weight.

HEAT STRESS FACTORS

In evaluating heat stress, you will need to take into account many factors. Primary considerations include temperature and humidity. Prehydration, duration and degree of activity, and the team member's overall physical fitness will also have a bearing on your evaluation. Keep in mind that Level A suits protect a rescuer, but prevent cooling. A rescuer essentially works inside an encapsulated sauna. The same suit that seals out hazards also prevents heat loss by evaporation, conduction, convection, and radiation. Therefore, place heat stress at the top of your list of tasks for post-exit medical monitoring.

> **Content Review**
>
> ### PRE-ENTRY/POST-EXIT DOCUMENTATION
> - Blood pressure
> - Pulse
> - Respiratory rate
> - Temperature
> - Body weight
> - ECG
> - Mental/neurologic status

FIGURE 11-12 Rescuers involved in the decontamination process.

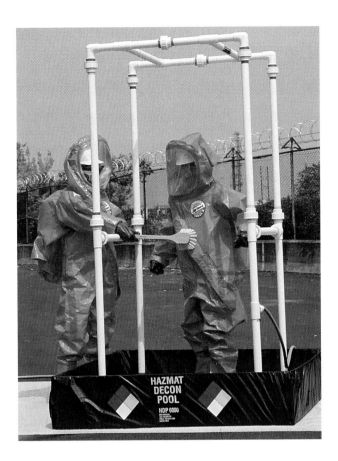

IMPORTANCE OF PRACTICE

As a paramedic, you will play an important role at any hazmat incident. You may establish command, make the first incident decisions, and help protect all on-scene personnel, including the hazmat team. As a result, you should practice skills that you can expect to use in most EMS systems.

Here are some things you should routinely do. Put on and take off Level B hazmat protective equipment. Set up a rapid two-step decontamination process and an eight-step decontamination process, preferably with the help of the local hazmat team. With a crew member, identify a simulated chemical, determine the correct PPE, and establish the proper decontamination methods. Practice pre-entry and post-exit medical monitoring and documentation. Prepare a patient and ambulance for transport. As these skills may be rarely used except in the busiest EMS systems, you should work closely with your local hazmat team to practice these skills on a regular basis.

SUMMARY

Every member of an EMS team should be prepared to face the challenges of the hazmat incident. At all times, keep in mind the high potential for rescuer involvement in a hazmat incident, especially during the early phases. As with any EMS operation, the primary consideration is your own safety. No patient's life is worth your own. This is especially true at a fast-break incident in which you must resist heroic efforts that will place you in contact with ambulatory, self-rescued patients. You become useless at a hazmat incident if you become contaminated yourself.

YOU MAKE THE CALL

You are dispatched to a motor vehicle collision on an interstate highway. You arrive on-scene and find that a car has rear ended a tractor-trailer. Two people exit the cab of the truck and begin to walk toward the ambulance. Both have obvious respiratory distress. You note that the driver of the car appears to be unresponsive behind the steering wheel.

You do a quick windshield size-up for hazards and see a black-and-white placard on the rear of the truck. The placard bears a skull and crossbones and two numbers—6 and 2783. You notice some liquid dripping from the rear door of the truck onto the hood of the car.

The occupants of the truck walk up to the side of the ambulance. You observe that they are drooling, tearing, and sweating profusely. One of them knocks on your window and says, "Please help us. We can't breathe."

1. What do you suspect has happened based on your quick scene size-up?
2. What are your initial priorities?
3. How will you identify the substance involved in the accident?
4. What additional resources would you request?
5. Is this a fast-break or a long-term incident? Explain.
6. What are your first actions?

See Suggested Responses at the back of this book.

FURTHER READING

29 CFR 1910.120, Hazardous Waste Operations and Emergency Response Standard (1989).

Christen, H. and P. Maniscalco: *The EMS Incident Management System: EMS Operations for Mass Casualty and High-Impact Incidents.* Upper Saddle River, NJ: Brady Publishing, 1998.

De Lorenzo, R.A. and R.S. Porter: *Weapons of Mass Destruction: Emergency Care.* Upper Saddle River, NJ: Prentice Hall, 2000.

EMS Safety: Techniques and Applications. Federal Emergency Management Agency, United States Fire Administration, 1994.

Hankins, D.G.: "Hazardous Materials," in Kuehl, A.E., *Prehospital Systems & Medical Oversight*, Second Edition. St. Louis, MO: Mosby Lifeline, 1994.

Lesak, D.M.: *Hazardous Materials: Strategies and Tactics.* Upper Saddle River, NJ: Brady Publishing, 1999.

NFPA 473: *Standard Competencies for EMS Personnel Responding to Hazardous Materials Incidents*, 1997 Edition.

NFPA 704: *Standard for Identification of the Fire Hazards of Materials*, 1996 Edition.

Noll, G.G., M.S. Hildebrand, and J.G. Yvorra: *Hazardous Materials: Managing the Incident.* Stillwater, OK: Fire Protection Publications, 1995.

Stutz, D.R. and S. Ulin: *Haztox: EMS Response to Hazardous Materials Incidents.* Miramar, FL: GDS Communications, 1994.

ON THE WEB

Visit Brady's Paramedic Website at www.bradybooks.com/paramedic.

CHAPTER 12

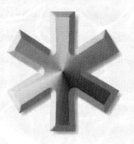

Crime Scene Awareness

Objectives

After reading this chapter, you should be able to:

1. Explain how EMS providers are often mistaken for the police. (pp. 445–446, 451)
2. Explain specific techniques for risk reduction when approaching the following types of routine EMS scenes:
   a. Highway encounters. (pp. 448–449)
   b. Violent street incidents. (pp. 449–450)
   c. Residences and "dark houses." (pp. 446, 447)
3. Describe the warning signs of potentially violent situations. (pp. 445, 446, 448–453)
4. Explain emergency evasive techniques for potentially violent situations, including:
   a. Threats of physical violence. (pp. 448–449, 453–454, 455)
   b. Firearms encounters. (pp. 446, 454–455)
   c. Edged weapon encounters. (pp. 453–454, 455)
5. Explain EMS considerations for the following types of violent or potentially violent situations:
   a. Gangs and gang violence. (pp. 450–451)
   b. Hostages/sniper situations. (pp. 456, 457–458)

Continued

CASE STUDY

At 10:30 PM, your paramedic unit receives a call for an unknown problem at 4926 Magnolia Boulevard. The residence lies in a well-kept part of the city. As you turn onto Magnolia, you shut off the vehicle's emergency lights. Before arriving on scene, you request further information from dispatch. The dispatcher tells you an older male requested an ambulance because "someone is sick and needs help, now!" He then quickly hung up without providing any further details. Computer aided dispatch (CAD) shows no prior calls at the residence and no history of violence at the location.

Your partner stops the ambulance two houses away from the scene. You both observe the quiet single-family residence. Since you see no signs of danger, your partner moves the rig closer. Both you and your partner exit the vehicle and approach the residence with only the necessary equipment. The two of you take separate, unpredictable paths to the residence, keeping each other in sight. This provides a better view of the dwelling.

Your partner looks in the front window and observes an older man standing over a woman about the same age. She seems to be very ill. There are no signs of fighting, intoxication, or other unusual behavior.

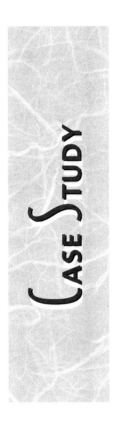

You and your partner decide that it is safe to approach the door. You knock, and the man urges you to enter quickly. "My wife is so sick," he exclaims. "I don't know what to do. Please follow me."

You introduce yourself and immediately notice that the man has difficulty hearing you. He is older than you had suspected and is obviously distraught. The combination of factors explains why he may have failed to provide adequate information to dispatch.

You learn that the patient is experiencing chest discomfort and has been vomiting. You treat her according to ALS protocols and then transport both the patient and her husband to the hospital.

Neither you nor your partner has any doubt about your cautious approach to the call. You have learned from experience that quiet calls can be just as worrisome as those made with loud voices. At least with loud voices, you have some reason to suspect trouble. Although you discovered a reasonable explanation for this suspicious call, you know all too well that your personal safety depends upon your ability to detect potentially violent situations before you even step outside your ambulance.

INTRODUCTION

Violence can occur anywhere. Regardless of where you work as a paramedic—the inner city, the suburbs, or rural America—you can be affected by violence. The violence can take all forms, from interpersonal abuse in the home to gang activities in the street. The violence can also involve any number of weapons ranging from fists to guns to explosives.

While people of all ages and backgrounds commit acts of violence, the last two decades have seen a dramatic increase in violence among youth. According to the Division of Violence Prevention at the National Center for Injury Prevention and Control, arrest rates for homicide, rape, robbery, and aggravated assault are consistently higher for people ages 15 to 34 than for all other age groups. Even more alarming, an average of 20 youth homicides occur in the United States every day.

Approximately one of six victims of violent crimes requires medical attention, often by the emergency medical services. Several studies suggest that a substantial number of these victims fail to report the violence to the police. As a result, the emergency medical services may be a victim's only contact with professionals who can intervene to prevent further harm.

Yet despite the increased presence of violence, EMS providers find it almost impossible to predict exactly when and where a violent incident will occur. Nearly all calls that you or any other paramedic handle on a given day will progress without any threat of danger. In fact, you have a higher risk of being injured by oncoming traffic than by a violent act. Even so, you cannot let down your "crime scene awareness." Otherwise, you risk becoming a victim or hostage of a violent situation.

As this chapter will show, your most important safety tactic is an ability to identify potentially violent situations as soon as possible. While you can't predict violence hours in advance, you can remain alert to signs of danger. You can also become aware of local issues that hold a potential for violence, such as the presence of street gangs or a known area of drug activity.

Equally as important, you should familiarize yourself with standard operating procedures (SOPs) for handling violent situations and/or the specialized resources that you can call upon for backup. Find out, for example, whether your unit has access to a **Tactical Emergency Medical Service (TEMS)**—a unit that provides on-site medical support to law enforcement. If so, know how and when to access it. Above all else, remain alert to the signs of danger from the start of a call to the time you return your ambulance to service.

 Tactical Emergency Medical Services (TEMS) a specially trained unit that provides on-site medical support to law enforcement.

APPROACH TO THE SCENE

Your safety strategy begins as soon as you are dispatched on a call. Even the most basic information can provide important tactical clues. Emergency medical dispatchers try to keep callers on the line to obtain as much information as possible. They remain alert to background noises such as fighting or intoxicated persons and in turn warn incoming units of these dangers. Modern computer aided dispatch (CAD) programs provide instant information on previous calls at a particular location and display "caution indicators" to notify dispatchers when a location has a history of violence.

Your safety strategy begins as soon as you are dispatched on a call.

Even in the age of computers, however, some of your best information can still come from your own experience and that of other crews. Your memory of previous calls can serve as an important indicator of trouble. For example, if a bar or club has a reputation for fights and you are summoned there, you will already have a high suspicion of danger before you arrive.

POSSIBLE SCENARIOS

There are three possible scenarios in which you might observe violence during an EMS call. The dispatcher may advise you of a potentially violent scene en route to the call. Obviously, you will be alert to danger from the start. In other cases, you may not spot danger until you arrive on the scene and begin your size-up and approach. In yet a third scenario, you may not face danger until the start of patient care or transport.

Advised of Danger En Route

When the dispatcher reports possible danger, do not approach the scene until it is secured by law enforcement personnel. Remember that lights and sirens can draw a crowd and/or alert the perpetrator of a crime. So use them cautiously or not at all.

Never follow police units to the scene. To do so might place you at the center of violence. If you arrive first, keep the ambulance out of sight so that the rig does not attract the attention of bystanders or any of the parties involved in the incident. While you wait for police to secure the scene, set up a staging area.

Never follow police units to the scene. To do so, might place you at the center of violence.

Management of the incident depends upon interagency cooperation. Communicate with the police—you are in this together. Be sure you understand any differences in dispatch terminology. For example, what is a code 1 emergency for police units is a code 3 emergency for EMS units. Work with police to determine if and when you should approach the scene.

Keep in mind that violence can occur or resume even with the police present. Furthermore, depending upon your uniform colors and the use of badges, people might mistake you for the police—especially if you exit from a vehicle with flashing lights and siren. They might expect you to intervene in a violent situation, or

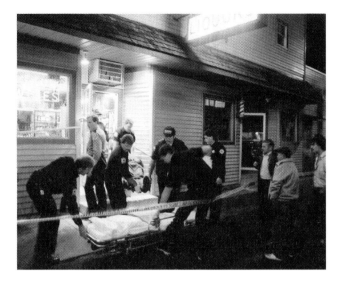

FIGURE 12-1   Never approach the scene until you are advised that the scene is secure. Remember, even if a scene has been declared secure, violence may still erupt.

they might direct aggression toward you as an authority figure. If the scene cannot be made safe, retreat immediately (Figure 12-1).

Observing Danger Upon Arrival

Even if dispatch has not alerted you to danger, you must still keep this possibility in mind once you arrive on scene. One of the main purposes of the scene size-up is to search for any possible hazards. This includes non-violent dangers such as downed power lines, dangerous pets, unstable vehicles, or hazmat. As you look for these dangers, observe for other signs of trouble such as crowds gathering on the street, an unusual silence, or a darkened residence. Obviously, you will adopt a different approach for a confirmed medical emergency than for an "unknown problem, caller hang-up." Even so, do not exit the vehicle until you have ruled out all immediate hazards.

   If you have any doubts about a call, park away from the scene. If you must park in view of the location, take an unconventional approach to the door (Figure 12-2). People will expect you to use the sidewalk. So approach from the side, on the lawn, or flush against the house. Avoid getting in between a residence and the lighted ambulance so you do not "backlight" yourself. Also, hold your flashlight to the side rather than in front of you (Figure 12-3). Armed assailants often fire at the light.

   Before announcing your presence, listen and observe for signs of danger. If you can, look in windows for evidence of fighting, the presence of weapons, or the use of alcohol or drugs. Gradually make your way to the doorknob side of the door, or the side of the door opposite the hinges (Figure 12-4). Listen for any signs of danger such as loud noises, items breaking, incoherent speech, or the lack of any sounds at all.

   If you spot danger at any time during your approach, immediately stop and reevaluate the situation. Decide whether it is in the interest of your own safety to continue or retreat until law enforcement officials can be summoned. Rather than risk becoming injured or killed, err on the side of safety.

Rather than risk becoming injured or killed, err on the side of safety.

Eruption of Danger During Care or Transport

Remain alert throughout a call, especially in areas with a history of violence. You may enter the scene and spot weapons or drugs. Additional combative people may arrive on scene. The patient or bystanders may become agitated or threatening.

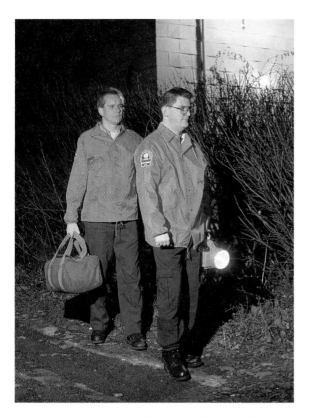

FIGURE 12-2 Approach potentially unstable scenes single file along an unconventional path.

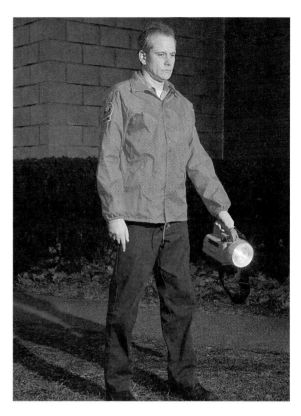

FIGURE 12-3 Hold a flashlight to the side of your body, not in front of it. Armed assailants usually aim at the light.

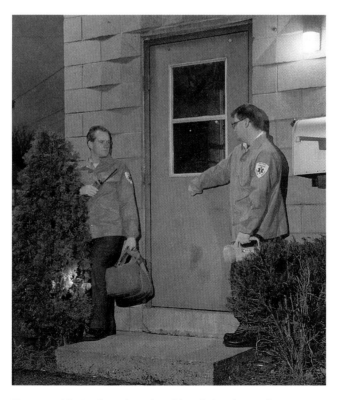

FIGURE 12-4 Stand to the side of the door when knocking. Do not stand directly in front of a door or window, making yourself an unwitting target.

Even if treatment has begun, you must place your own safety first. You now have two tactical options: (1) quickly package the patient and leave the scene with the patient or (2) retreat without the patient.

Your choice of action depends upon the level of danger. Abandonment is always a concern. However, in most cases, you can legally leave a patient behind when there is a *documented* danger. As discussed later in the chapter, keep accurate records of incidents involving violence. If you must defend yourself, use the minimum amount of force necessary. Immediately summon police and retreat as needed.

Regardless of the situation, always have a way out. Your failure to plan will undoubtedly lead to an emergency at some point in time. Make sure that SOPs include an "escape and strategic escape plan." Then adhere to this plan so you do not become a victim of violence yourself.

In most cases, you can legally leave a patient behind when there is a documented danger.

Content Review

POTENTIALLY DANGEROUS SCENES

- Highway encounters
- Violent street incidents
- Murders, assaults, robberies
- Dangerous crowds
- Street gangs
- Drug-related crimes
- Clandestine drug labs
- Domestic violence

SPECIFIC DANGEROUS SCENES

Most out-of-hospital services were developed to meet the needs of individual patients in controlled situations. However, in recent years, EMS personnel trained for this limited role have been pressed increasingly into service in potentially hazardous situations. The result has been the employment of specialized resources with the tactical judgment and skills not normally taught in EMS programs. Your ability to survive a violent street encounter depends upon recognition of threats and an understanding of some the things that can be done to provide for rescuer and patient safety. The following are some of the known dangers that you may face while "on the street." (A discussion of tactical safety strategies appears later in the chapter.)

HIGHWAY ENCOUNTERS

The preceding examples of known dangers have focused largely on residences. However, EMS units frequently report to roadside calls involving motor vehicle collisions, disabled vehicles, or sick and/or unresponsive people inside a car—e.g., "man slumped over wheel" calls. Chapters 8 and 10 have already indicated the dangers of highway operations and the steps that you should take to protect yourself. However, highway operations also hold the risk of violence from occupants who may be fleeing felons, intoxicated or drugged, or in possession of weapons. Some potential warning signs of danger include:

- Violent or abusive behavior
- An altered mental state
- Grabbing or hiding items inside the vehicle
- Arguing or fighting among passengers
- Lack of activity where activity is expected
- Physical signs of alcohol or drug abuse—e.g., liquor bottles, beer cans, or syringes
- Open or unlatched trunks—a potential hiding spot for people or weapons
- Differences among stories told by occupants

To make a safe approach to a vehicle at a roadside emergency, follow these steps:

- Park the ambulance in a position that provides safety from traffic.

- Notify dispatch of the situation, location, the vehicle make and model, and the state and number of the license plate.
- Use a one-person approach. The driver should remain in the ambulance, which is elevated and provides greater visibility.
- The driver should remain prepared to radio for immediate help and to back or drive away rapidly once the other medic returns.
- At nighttime, use the ambulance lights to illuminate the vehicle. However, do not walk between the ambulance and the other vehicle. You will be backlighted, forming an easy target.
- Since police approach vehicles from the driver's side, you should approach from the passenger's side—an unexpected route.
- Use the A, B, and C door posts for cover.
- Observe the rear seat. Do not move forward of the C post unless you are sure there are no threats in the rear seat or foot wells.
- Retreat to the ambulance (or another strategic position of cover) at the first sign of danger.
- Make sure you have mapped out your intended retreat and escape with the ambulance driver.

VIOLENT STREET INCIDENTS

You can encounter many different types of violence while working on the streets. You see examples on the news all the time. Incidents can range from random acts of violence against individual citizens to organized efforts at domestic or international terrorism. The following are some of the dangerous street situations that you may face at some point in your EMS career.

Murder, Assault, Robbery

Although the overall crime rate has dropped in recent years, millions of violent acts still occur annually. They take place at residences, at schools, and at commercial establishments. However, according to the U.S. Department of Justice, the most common location for violent crimes is on the streets—often within five miles of the victim's home. In order of occurrence, the most frequent crimes include simple assaults, aggravated assaults, rapes and sexual assaults, robberies, and homicides.

In one-quarter of the incidents of violent crime, offenders used or threatened the use of a weapon. Homicides are most commonly committed with handguns, but knives, blunt objects, and other types of guns or weapons may also be used. About one in five violent victimizations involve the use of alcohol.

While motives vary, the late 1990s and early 2000s saw a rise in **hate crimes**—crimes committed against a person solely on the basis of the individual's actual or perceived race, color, national origin, ethnicity, gender, disability, or sexual orientation. A number of states or communities have passed legislation on the management of hate crimes, including the steps to be taken on scene. Determine whether these laws exist in your area, and establish protocols that your agency should follow. Crew assignments, for example, should be well thought out in advance of the response to a hate crime. You should also know the specific type of information that must be documented for later use by the courts.

In responding to the scene of any violent crime, keep these precautions in mind:

- Dangerous weapons may have been used in the crime.
- Perpetrators may still be on-scene or could return to the scene.

✱ **hate crimes** crimes committed against a person solely on the basis of the individual's actual or perceived race, color, national origin, ethnicity, gender, disability, or sexual orientation.

Crew assignments should be well thought out in advance of the response to a hate crime.

- Patients may sometimes exhibit violence toward EMS, particularly if they risk criminal penalties as a result of the original incident.

Dangerous Crowds and Bystanders

As mentioned earlier, you must remain aware of crowd dynamics whenever you respond to a street incident. Crowds can quickly become large and volatile, especially in the case of a hate crime. Violence can be directed against anyone or anything in the path of an angry crowd. Your status as an EMS provider does not give you immunity against an out-of-control mob.

Whenever a crowd is present, look for these warning signs of impending danger:

- Shouts or increasingly loud voices
- Pushing or shoving
- Hostilities toward anyone on scene, including the perpetrator of a crime, the victim, police, and so on
- Rapid increase in the crowd size
- Inability of law enforcement officials to control bystanders

To protect yourself, constantly monitor the crowd and retreat if necessary. If possible, take the patient with you so that you do not have to return later. Rapid transport may require limited or tactical assessment at the scene with more in-depth assessment done inside the safety of the ambulance. Be sure to document reasons for the quick assessment and transport.

Street Gangs

Gangs include groups of people who band together for a variety of reasons—fraternization, self protection, creation of a surrogate family, and most frequently for the pursuit of criminal enterprises. Street gangs can be found in big cities, suburban towns, and lately in rural America. No EMS unit is totally immune from gang activity. In fact, some organized gangs have purposely branched out into smaller towns in an effort to escape surveillance and expand their illicit businesses.

Youth gangs account for a disproportionate amount of youth violence across the nation. Gang activity is associated with high levels of delinquency, illegal drug use, physical violence, and possession of weapons. Young people from all demographic backgrounds report some knowledge of gangs or gang activity.

Some of the largest and best-known gangs include the Crips, Bloods, Almighty Latin King Nation (Latin Kings), Hell's Angels, Outlaws, Pagans, and Banditos. Local variations of these and other gangs can be found throughout the country. In some places, gangs have used firebombs, Molotov cocktails, and, on a limited basis, military explosives (hand grenades) as weapons of revenge and intimidation. Links have been drawn between street gangs and the sale of drugs, which in turn finance gang activities.

Commonly observed gang characteristics include the following:

- **Appearance**—Gang members frequently wear unique clothing specific to the group. Because the clothing is often a particular color or hue, it is referred to as the gang's "colors." Wearing a color, even a bandana can signify gang membership. Within the gang itself, members sometimes wear different articles to signify rank.
- **Graffiti**—Gangs have definite territories, or "turfs." Members often mark their turf with graffiti broadcasting the gang's logo, warning away intruders, bragging about crimes, insulting rival gangs, or taunting police.

- **Tattoos**—Many gang members wear tattoos or other body markings to identify their gang affiliation. Some gangs even require these tattoos. The tattoos will be in the gang's colors and often contain the gang's motto or logo.
- **Hand signals/language**—Gangs commonly create their own methods of communication. They give gang-related meanings to everyday words or create codes. Hand signs provide quick identification among gang members, warn of approaching law enforcement, or show disrespect to other gangs. Gang members often perform signals so quickly that an uninformed outsider may not spot them, much less understand them.

EMS units venturing into gang territory must be extremely cautious because of the potential for violence. Danger is increased if your uniform looks similar to the uniform worn by police. Gangs with a history of arrest may in fact make every effort to prevent you from transporting one of their members to a hospital or any other place beyond the reach of the gang. Do not force the issue if your safety is at stake.

EMS uniforms should not resemble law enforcement uniforms.

DRUG-RELATED CRIMES

The sale of drugs goes hand-in-hand with violence (Figure 12-5). Hundreds of people die each year in drug deals gone bad. In addition, drug dealers protect their drug stashes and "shooting galleries" with booby traps, weapons, and abused dogs likely to attack. The combination of a high-cash flow, addiction, and automatic weapons threaten anyone who unwittingly walks onto the scene of a drug deal or threatens to uncover an illicit drug operation.

There are a number of signs that can alert you to the involvement of drugs at an EMS call. These include:

- Prior history of drugs in the neighborhood of the call
- Clinical evidence that the patient has used drugs of some kind
- Drug-related comments by bystanders

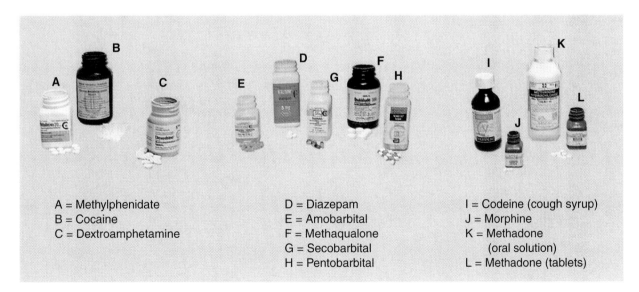

A = Methylphenidate
B = Cocaine
C = Dextroamphetamine

D = Diazepam
E = Amobarbital
F = Methaqualone
G = Secobarbital
H = Pentobarbital

I = Codeine (cough syrup)
J = Morphine
K = Methadone
    (oral solution)
L = Methadone (tablets)

FIGURE 12-5 Substances abused and sold come in all forms. Some of the most common prescribed substances sold or used on the streets are shown here. Persons that abuse or deal in drugs may exhibit violent behavior.

- Drug paraphernalia visible at the scene such as the following:
  - tiny zip-top bags or vials
  - sandwich bags with the corners torn off (indicating drug packaging) or untied corners of sandwich bags (indicating drug use)
  - syringes or needles
  - glass tubes, pipes, or homemade devices for smoking drugs
  - chemical odors or residues

Whenever you observe any of the preceding items, assume the use or presence of drugs at the scene. Even if the patient is not involved, others at the scene may still pose a danger. Keep in mind that not all patients who use drugs will be seeking to harm you. Some may, in fact, be looking for help. Evaluate each situation carefully. Above all else, remember to retreat and/or request police backup at the earliest sign of danger.

CLANDESTINE DRUG LABORATORIES

Drug dealers often set up "laboratories" to manufacture controlled substances or to otherwise refine or convert a controlled substance to another more profitable or useable form such as tablets. One of the most common types of substances manufactured in drug laboratories is methamphetamine, also known by street names such as "crank," "speed," or "crystal." Other drugs include LSD, "crack," and more.

Clandestine drug laboratories, or "clan labs," have three requirements: privacy, utilities, and equipment such as glassware, chemical containers, and heating mantles or burners. Most clan labs are uncovered by neighbors who report suspicious odors, deliveries, or activities.

Drug raids on clan labs have a way of turning into hazmat operations. All too often, the labs contain toxic fumes and volatile chemicals. The people on scene complicate matters by fighting or shooting at the rescuers who come to extricate them from the toxic environment. As they retreat, drug dealers may also trigger booby traps or wait for police or EMS personnel to trigger them. If you ever come upon a clan lab, take these actions:

- Leave the area immediately.
- Do not touch anything.
- Never stop any chemical reactions already in progress.
- Do not smoke or bring any source of flame near the lab.
- Notify the police.
- Initiate ICS and hazmat procedures.
- Consider evacuation of the area.

Remember that laboratories can be found anywhere—on farms, in trailers, in city apartments, and more. They may be mobile, roaming from place to place in a camper or truck. Or they may be disassembled and stored in almost any variety of locations. The job of raiding clan labs belongs to specialized personnel—not EMS crews.

DOMESTIC VIOLENCE

Domestic violence involves people who live together in an intimate relationship. The violence may be physical, emotional, sexual, verbal, or economic. It may be directed against a spouse or partner, or it may involve children and/or older relatives who live at the residence.

When called to the scene of domestic violence, the abuser may turn on you or other members of the crew. You have two main concerns: your own personal safety and protection of the patient from further harm. For more on the indications of domestic violence and the appropriate actions of EMS crews, see Chapter 4, "Abuse and Assault."

TACTICAL CONSIDERATIONS

As mentioned on several occasions, your best tactical response to violence is observation. Know the warning signs and stay out of danger in the first place. If the dispatcher alerts you to hazards, resort to staging until the appropriate authorities can resolve the situation.

That said, you still may find yourself in situations with a potential for danger—a suspicious call that you must check out, the eruption of violence during treatment, and so on. In such instances, you must have a "game plan" in place. This section presents some of the actions you can take to protect your own safety while attempting to provide tactical patient care.

SAFETY TACTICS

Dangerous situations mean extreme stress. As a result, your response to danger will be most effective if you practice tactical options frequently. Even on routine calls, think about safety, contact and cover, escape routes, and other strategies that can help you make a better decision when you are faced with actual danger. Borrowing a phrase from professional sports: "You will play the game the way you practice." If you have rehearsed the responses to danger before you actually need them, you will be more likely to use them successfully. The following sections describe some proven methods for EMS safety in dangerous situations.

Content Review

SAFETY TACTICS
- Retreat
- Cover and concealment
- Distraction and evasion
- Contact and cover
- Warning signals and communication

Retreat

The prudent strategy is to retreat whenever you spot indicators of violence or potential physical confrontations, particularly with fleeing criminals or emotionally disturbed people (Figure 12-6). Retreat in a calm, but decisive manner. Be aware that the danger is now at your back and integrate cover into your retreat.

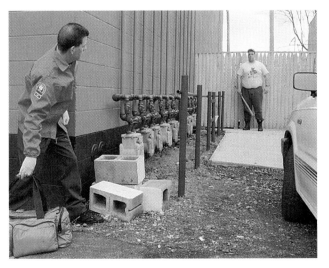

FIGURE 12-6 A patient's stance and position can indicate a potential for violence. If you suspect such a situation, put your own personal safety first. Retreat and request police backup.

Ideally you will retreat to the ambulance so that you can summon help. However, if a dangerous obstacle—such as a crowd—blocks access to your rig, retreat by foot or by whatever means possible. Nothing in the ambulance is worth your life.

In deciding how far to retreat, your primary goal is to protect yourself from any potential danger. You must be out of the immediate line of sight. You must also seek cover from gunfire. Finally, you must allow enough distance to react if a person or crowd attempts to move toward you again. You need time and space to respond to changing situations.

As soon as possible, notify other responding units and agencies of the danger. Activate appropriate codes, SOPs, and/or interagency agreements, particularly with law enforcement departments. Be sure to document your observations of danger and your specific responses. Include information such as the following:

- Actions taken while on scene
- Reasons you retreated
- Time at which you left and/or returned to the scene
- Personnel or agencies contacted

Also keep in mind that retreat does not mean the end of a call. As already mentioned, you should seek to stage at a safe area until police secure the scene and you can respond once again. Staging, along with thorough documentation, will reduce liability and provide evidence to refute charges of abandonment.

Cover and Concealment

concealment hiding the body behind objects that shield a person from view but that offer little or no protection against bullets or other ballistics.

cover hiding the body behind solid and impenetrable objects that protect a person from bullets.

When faced with danger, two of your most immediate and practical strategies are cover and concealment (Figures 12-7a & 12-7b). **Concealment** hides your body, such as when you crouch behind bushes, wallboards, or vehicle doors. However, most common objects do not stop bullets. During armed encounters, seek **cover** by hiding your body behind solid and impenetrable objects such as brick walls, rocks, large trees or telephone poles, and the engine block of vehicles.

For cover and concealment to work, they must be used properly. In applying these safety tactics, keep in mind the following general rules.

- As you approach any scene, remain aware of the surroundings and any potential sources of protection in case you must retreat or are "pinned down."

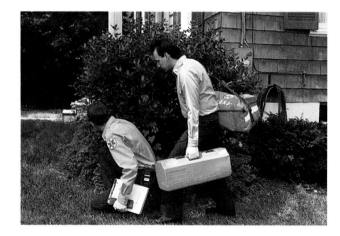

FIGURE 12-7a   Concealing yourself is placing your body behind an object that can hide you from view.

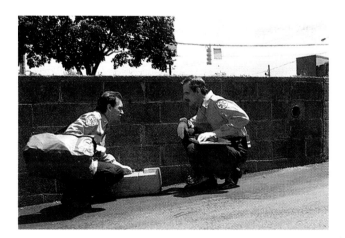

FIGURE 12-7b   Taking cover is finding a position that both hides you and protects your body from projectiles.

- Choose your cover carefully. You may have only one chance to pick your protection. Select the item that hides your body adequately, while shielding you against ballistics.
- Once you have made your choice of cover, conceal as much of your body as possible. Be conscious of any reflective clothing that you may be wearing. Armed assailants can use it as a target, especially at night.
- Constantly look to improve your protection and location.

Distraction and Evasion

Distraction and evasion can be integrated into any retreat. Some specific techniques to avoid physical violence include:

- Throwing equipment to trip, slow, or distract an aggressor
- Wedging a stretcher in a doorway to block an attacker
- Using an unconventional path while retreating
- Anticipating the moves of the aggressor and taking counter moves
- Overturning objects in the path of the attacker
- Using preplanned tactics with your partner to confuse or "throw off" an aggressor

Key to the success of these safety tactics is your own physical well-being. Regular exercise and good health ensure that you will have the strength to outrun or, if necessary, defend yourself against an attacker. Some units provide basic training in self-defense or have protocols on its use. Make sure you take advantage of this training and/or know the protocols related to the application of force.

Contact and Cover

The concept of contact and cover comes from a police procedure developed in San Diego, California, where several officers were injured or killed while interviewing suspects. Studies of the incidents revealed that the officers focused directly on the suspect, reducing their ability to observe the "big picture." This left them exposed to threats of physical violence and/or encounters with edged weapons or firearms.

To solve this problem, the San Diego police department adopted an interview approach in which one officer "contacts" the suspect while another officer stands 90 degrees to the side. By standing at a different angle, the second officer can provide "cover" to the officer dealing with the suspect.

When adapted to EMS practice, the procedure assigns the roles shown in Table 12-1. As with any tactic adopted from another discipline, contact and cover has obvious correlations and drawbacks. The tactic is ideal for street encounters

Table 12-1 CONTACT AND COVER

Contact Provider	Cover Provider
Initiates and provides direct patient care.	Observes the scene for danger while the "contact" provider cares for the patient.
Performs patient assessment.	Generally avoids patient care duties that would prevent observation of the scene.
Handles most interpersonal scene contact.	In small crews, may perform limited functions such as handling equipment.

with intoxicated persons or subjects acting in a suspicious manner. An obvious drawback is that two medics working on a cardiac arrest will not be able to designate one person to act solely as a "cover" medic.

Perhaps the best application of this police procedure to EMS is its emphasis on the importance of observation and teamwork. A crew that works well together will assign roles—formally or informally—to guarantee safety and patient care. In its most basic form, contact and cover means that you will watch your partner's back while he or she watches yours.

Warning Signals and Communication

Communication forms a vital part of EMS regardless of the situation. In the case of "street survival," it is an invaluable safety tool. Every team or crew should develop methods of alerting other providers to danger without alerting the aggressor. Devise prearranged verbal and nonverbal clues and then practice them.

Be sure to involve dispatch in the process. Choose signals that will indicate a variety of circumstances while sounding harmless to an attacker. This can be a life-saving technique in situations where you find yourself, the crew, and/or the patient held hostage. Your so-called "routine" radio reports can spell out the nature of the trouble and summon help from a **Special Weapons and Tactics (SWAT) Team**—a trained police unit equipped to handle hostage holders or other difficult law enforcement situations.

✱ Special Weapons and Tactics (SWAT) Team a trained police unit equipped to handle hostage holders and other difficult law enforcement situations.

TACTICAL PATIENT CARE

The increased involvement of care providers in violent situations has raised discussion and debate over the tactical training and protection offered to the EMS community. Interagency planning is essential, especially for clarifying the duties and roles of EMS and law enforcement agencies at crime scenes, riots, or terrorist events. Other aspects of tactical patient care include the use of body armor by EMS providers and the training of special tactical EMS personnel.

Body Armor

✱ body armor vest made of tightly woven, strong fibers that offer protection against handgun bullets, most knives, and blunt trauma; also known as "bullet-proof vests."

Several years ago few EMS providers would have considered wearing body armor, or bullet-proof vests, while on duty. However, today more and more providers are taking "tactical patient care" seriously. To protect EMS personnel against danger, an increasing number of EMS agencies have chosen to supply body armor or to provide a sum of cash toward its purchase. Body armor manufacturers have responded by designing and marketing vests specifically for the EMS community.

Unlike conventional armor, body armor is soft. A series of fibers such as Kevlar™ are woven tightly together to form the vest. The tight weave and strength of the material offer protection from many handgun bullets, most knives, and blunt trauma. The number of layers of fiber determine the rating or "stopping power" of a vest. Most body armor is rated from level 1 (least protective) to level 3 (most protective). Specialty vests with steel inserts and other materials are available for use by the military or by SWAT teams.

Some critics of body armor claim that wearers may feel a false sense of security. They point out that body armor offers reduced protection when wet. They also note that it provides little or no protection against high-velocity bullets, such as those fired by a rifle, or from thin or dual-edged weapons. An ice pick, for example, can penetrate between the fibers of most vests.

Supporters of body armor feel that it should be viewed just like any other PPE offered to rescuers. They point to the new threats faced by emergency re-

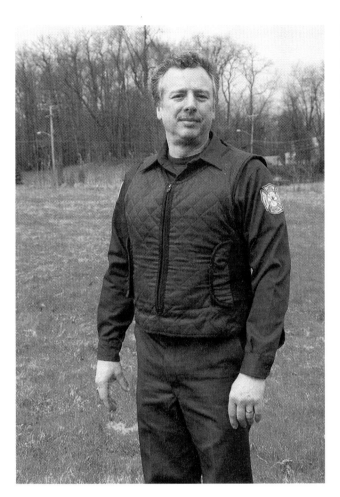

FIGURE 12-8 Over the past few years, an increasing number of EMS providers have started wearing body armor (bullet-proof vests) while on duty.

sponders, such as paramilitary groups, international terrorists, drug-related violence, and the widespread possession of handguns.

Whether you purchase or wear body armor is a personal decision (Figure 12-8). However, for it to be effective, you must follow several guidelines. They include:

- Keep in mind the limitations of body armor. Never do anything you wouldn't do without it.
- Remember that body armor doesn't cover the whole body. You can still get seriously injured or killed.
- Even though body armor can prevent many types of penetration, you can still experience severe cavitation.
- For body armor to work, it must be worn. The temptation not to wear it—especially in hot temperatures—can render even the best body armor useless.

Tactical EMS

As already mentioned, the provision of care in violent or tactically "hot" zones such as sniper situations often necessitates risks far beyond those found on most EMS calls. Medical personnel assigned to such incidents require special training and authorization. Like hazmat teams, they must don special equipment, function with compact gear, and, in most cases, work as medical adjuncts to the police or military.

The patient care offered by a Tactical Emergency Medical Service (**TEMS**) differs from routine EMS care in several ways. Differences include:

- A major priority is extraction of the patient from the hot zone.
- Care may be modified to meet tactical considerations.
- Trauma patients are more frequently encountered than medical patients.
- Treatment and transport interventions must almost always be coordinated with an incident commander.
- Patients must be moved to tactically cold zones for complete assessment, care, and transport.
- Metal clipboards, chemical agents, and other tools may be used as defensive weapons.

Local protocols, standing orders, and issues of medical direction must be re-solved before the employment of a TEMS unit. The units may be composed of EMTs, paramedics, and/or physicians who operate as part of a tactical law en-forcement team. Certification of SWAT-Medics and **EMT-Tacticals (EMT-Ts)** is offered by several organizations including the **CONTOMS**—Counter-Narcotics Tactical Operations—program and the National Tactical Officers Association (NTOA).

The training required of EMT-Ts or SWAT-Medics involves strenuous phys-ical activity, under a variety of conditions. In a CONTOMS program, medics may be exposed to scenarios or skills such as the following:

- Raids on clandestine drug laboratories
- Emergency medical care in barricade situations
- Wounding effects of weapons and booby traps
- Special medical gear for tactical operations
- Use of CS, OC or other riot-control agents
- Blank-firing weapons
- Helicopter operations
- Pyrotechnics (smoke and distraction devices)
- Operation under extreme conditions, darkness, and psychological stress
- Fire fighting and hazmat operations

In summoning or working with a TEMS unit, follow the same general ap-proaches and procedures recommended in Chapters 9, 10, and 11. If you have not had exposure to such a unit, find out more about EMT-Ts or SWAT-Medics from local law enforcement officials or from sites sponsored by CONTOMS on NTOA on the Internet.

EMS AT CRIME SCENES

A crime scene can be defined as a location where any part of a criminal act has occurred and where evidence relating to a crime may be found. The goal of per-forming EMS at a crime scene is to provide high-quality patient care while pre-serving evidence. NEVER jeopardize patient care for the sake of evidence. However, do not perform patient care with disregard of the criminal investiga-tion that will follow.

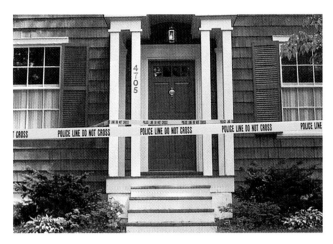

FIGURE 12-9 Police can remain on the scene of a crime for days, methodically searching for evidence. An EMS crew has a "platinum ten minutes" at the scene. During that time, they must protect themselves, treat the patient, AND preserve potential evidence, if at all possible.

EMS AND POLICE OPERATIONS

Often emergencies arise where police and EMS personnel respond to the same crisis. Both are there for specific purposes. The EMS crew has arrived on scene to treat patients and save lives. Law enforcement officers have come to protect the public and to solve a crime. These two primary goals sometimes create tensions between the two teams. For example, police and paramedics often work under different time constraints. As a paramedic, you have a limited time at the scene. The police, on the other hand, spend much more time at the location of a crime. In some major cases, police can remain on the scene for days or weeks as they methodically look for evidence (Figure 12-9).

The key to cooperation between EMS and law enforcement personnel is communication. You should become aware of the nature and significance of physical evidence at a crime scene and, if possible, keep that evidence intact. Police, on the other hand, should be aware that the first and foremost responsibility of a paramedic is to save the life of the victim. However, police and paramedics can usually reach a common ground. By preserving evidence, you can help the police to lock up a criminal before the person hurts, injures, or kills someone else. Remember: EMS personnel and law enforcement are really on the same side. Talk to each other.

Remember: EMS personnel and law enforcement are really on the same side. Talk to each other.

PRESERVING EVIDENCE

To prevent future violent injuries, be aware that anything on and around the patient may be evidence. You never know when a seemingly unimportant item may in fact be crucial evidence that could help solve a crime. Whenever in doubt, save or treat an object as evidence.

Whenever in doubt, save or treat an object as evidence.

If you are the first person on the scene of a crime, be aware that anything you touch, walk on, pick up, cut, wipe off, or move could be evidence. Developing an awareness of evidence will even affect the way you treat patients. You will need to observe the patient carefully and to disturb as little direct evidence as possible. For example, if clothing must be removed, never cut through a gunshot or knife wound. Instead, try to cut as far away from the wound as possible. Instead of placing the cut cloth or garment in a plastic bag, put it in a brown paper bag so condensation does not build up and destroy body fluid evidence.

Also, when examining a patient, remember that you may be at risk. The victim may have a concealed weapon, such as a knife or gun. Or the person who committed the crime may be intent on finishing it and reappear to attack the patient. As a result, your first responsibility is to protect yourself. If you have any

Brown paper bags allow evaporation and prevent mold from forming. This makes them ideal for crime scene evidence collection.

suspicions at all about the patient or the safety of the scene, wait for the police to frisk the patient and/or secure the scene.

Types of Evidence

Gathering evidence is a specialized and time-consuming job. While it is unrealistic to train EMS personnel in the details of police work, it is not unrealistic to ask them to develop an awareness of the general types of evidence that they may expect to encounter at a crime scene. Some of the main categories of evidence include: prints, blood and body fluids, particulate evidence, and your own observations at the scene.

Prints Prints include fingerprints, footprints, and tire prints. Of the three, fingerprints can be the most valuable source of evidence. No two people have identical fingerprints—the distinctive patterns left on a surface by the natural oils and moisture that form on a person's finger tips. The patterns can be compared to the millions of fingerprints already on file or compared to the fingerprints of a suspect charged with the crime.

As a paramedic, you have two concerns when it comes to fingerprints. First, try not to disturb any fingerprint evidence that may be present. Second, do not leave behind your own fingerprints at a crime scene.

The only way to preserve fingerprints is simply not to touch anything. Of course, this is impossible when treating a patient. However, you can and should minimize what you touch. If you must touch or move an item, remember to tell the police.

Because of BSI precautions, you will be wearing disposable gloves as a part of infection control. These gloves prevent you from leaving your own fingerprints. But they will not prevent you from smudging existing prints. Again, touch as little as possible. Also, bring in only the necessary equipment. The more equipment you have, the more evidence you have to disturb, including fingerprints.

Also, scan the approach to the scene and the scene itself for footprints or tire prints. These prints have value since they give the police an idea of what a perpetrator was wearing—e.g., sneakers vs. work boots—or the type of tread on a vehicle's tires. These patterns may be later matched to the footwear or vehicle used by an alleged perpetrator.

Blood and Body Fluids Blood and body fluids also give police a lot of information about a crime. For example, if the victim scratched or injured the perpetrator, blood samples might be found under the fingernails, on clothing, on hands, or elsewhere. By ABO blood typing these samples, the field of suspects can be narrowed down.

Identification of DNA (deoxyribonucleic acid) has been called "genetic fingerprinting." Matching the DNA found in blood samples or other body fluids to the DNA of a suspect is nearly 100% accurate. There is only one chance in several million that the DNA could be from someone else. The high cost of DNA testing prevents its widespread use. However, when performed, medical technologists need only a small sample to ascertain the genetic code of the person from which it came.

The way in which blood is splattered or dropped at the scene provides yet other clues for police. This so-called **blood spatter evidence** can indicate the type of weapon used, the position of the attacker in relation to the victim, and the direction or force used in the attack.

Preserving blood evidence can be performed in the following ways:

- Avoid mixing samples of blood whenever possible. Cross-contamination of blood will render blood evidence useless.

Content Review

TYPES OF EVIDENCE

- Prints—fingerprints, footprints, tire prints
- Blood and blood splatter
- Body fluids
- Particulate evidence
- On-scene EMS observations

If you must touch or move an item, remember to tell the police.

✱ **blood spatter evidence** the pattern that blood forms when it is splattered or dropped at the scene of a crime.

- Avoid tracking blood on your shoes. You will leave your own footprints, plus risk contaminating other blood evidence.

- If you must cut bloody clothing from a victim, place each piece in a separate brown paper bag. If the garment is wet, gently roll it in the paper bag to layer it. Place the entire contents in a second paper bag and then in a plastic bag for body fluid protection.

- Do not throw clothes stained with blood or other body fluids in a single pile or in a puddle of blood.

- Do not clean up or smudge blood spatter left at a scene.

- If you leave behind blood from a venipuncture, notify police.

- Because blood can be a biohazard, ask police whether the scene should be secured for evidence collection.

Particulate Evidence Particulate evidence, also known as microscopic or trace evidence, refers to evidence that cannot be readily seen by the human eye such as hairs or carpet and clothing fibers. Particulate evidence can help identify the actual crime scene, such as in cases where a body has been moved, or the DNA of the perpetrator. Minimal handling of a victim's clothes by EMS personnel may help to preserve this evidence.

 particulate evidence evidence such as hairs or fibers that cannot be readily seen with the human eye; also known as microscopic or trace evidence.

On-Scene Observations Everything that you and other members of the EMS crew see and hear can serve as evidence. Your observations of the scene will become part of the police record—and ultimately part of the court record. Be sure to look for and record the following information:

Everything that you and other members of the EMS crew see and hear can serve as evidence.

- Conditions at the scene—absence or presence of lights, locked or unlocked doors, open or closed curtains, and so on
- Position of the patient/victim
- Injuries suffered by the patient/victim
- Statements of persons at the scene
- Statements by the patient/victim
- Dying declarations
- Suspicious persons at, or fleeing from, the scene
- Presence and/or location of any weapons

If the victim is deceased by the time you arrive, any staff not immediately needed on the scene should leave to minimize the risk of disturbing evidence. If a gun is seen or found on the deceased victim, do not touch or move it unless it must be secured for the safety of others. Pick it up only as a last resort, and only touch it by the side grips or handles. The grips are coarse and will not generally leave good fingerprints. NEVER put anything into the barrel of the gun to lift or move it. The barrel of a gun can house the majority of the evidence used by the police—traces of gun powder, rifling patterns, and even flesh or blood from the victim.

NEVER put anything into the barrel of a gun to lift or move it.

Documenting Evidence

Record only the facts at the scene of a crime, and record them accurately. Otherwise, they might be thrown out of court as evidence. Use quotation marks to indicate the words of bystanders and any remarks made by the patient. Avoid opinions not relevant to patient care. If the patient has died, do not offer any judgments that might contradict later findings by the medical examiner. For example, a knife wound is not a knife wound until it is proven that a knife caused the laceration. Instead, describe the shape and anatomical location of the puncture or cut.

Record only the facts at the scene of a crime, and record them accurately.

Also keep in mind the protocols, local laws, and ethical considerations in reporting certain crimes such as child abuse, rape, geriatric abuse, domestic violence, and so on. (For more on reporting abuse and assault, see Chapter 4.) Finally, follow local policies and regulations regarding confidentiality surrounding any criminal case. Any offhand remarks that you make might later become testimony in a courtroom along with other documents that you prepare at the scene.

SUMMARY

Your first priority at any crime scene is your own safety. To protect your life and the lives of others, you need to develop a "crime scene awareness." Whenever you survey the scene of any call, keep in mind some of the telltale signs of potential violence such as a suspiciously darkened house, lack of activity, and so on. Do not needlessly expose yourself to dangers better left to professional emergency medical personnel such as SWAT-Medics or EMT-Ts. When you do treat the victim(s) at a crime scene, keep in mind that police and EMS personnel must work together to preserve the evidence that may lead to conviction of the perpetrator. Touch only those items or objects that pertain directly to patient care.

YOU MAKE THE CALL

Your ambulance receives a call for a 65-year-old male with chest pain. You arrive at the scene and scan for dangers. Detecting no visible hazards, you enter the patient's home and begin assessment. The patient describes the pain as crushing and points to the center of his chest. You observe labored breathing and begin care. You direct your partner to administer oxygen, while you look for a peripheral IV site.

While treatment progresses, the patient's son bursts through the door. He appears intoxicated and is obviously agitated at the presence of an ambulance. The patient whispers, "My son isn't quite right when he's drinking. You better be careful."

While you introduce yourself to the son, your partner slips away to radio the police. The dispatcher advises her that it could be a few minutes before the police can arrive on scene. Meanwhile, you tell the son why it is important that you start an IV. The son yells, "You're no doctor. Get away from my father. He needs to get to a hospital, not stay here in the living room. Get out of here before I throw you out."

1. What is your evaluation of this situation from a safety perspective?
2. What are your options?

See Suggested Responses at the back of this book.

FURTHER READING

Cohn, B.M., A.J. Azzara, R. Petrie: "EMS and Law Enforcement," in *Legal Aspects of Emergency Medical Services*. Philadelphia, PA: W.B. Saunders, Co., 1998.

DeLorenzo, R.A., R.S. Porter: *Weapons of Mass Destruction: Emergency Care*. Upper Saddle River, NJ: Prentice-Hall, 2000.

Dernocoeur, K.B.: *Streetsense: Communication, Safety, and Control*. Upper Saddle River: NJ: Brady Co., 1996, Third Edition.

Eliopilos, L.N.: *Death Investigator's Handbook: A Field Guide to Crime Scene Processing Forensic Evaluation, and Investigation Techniques*. Boulder, CO: Paladin Press, 1993.

Heiskell, L.E., P. Carlo: "Scoop and Run Versus Stay and Treat: Some Tactical Considerations," in *The Tactical Edge*, 1996, 14(3): 61–63.

Katz, S.M.: *Anytime Anywhere!: On Patrol with Nypd's Emergency Services Unit*. NY, NY: Pocket Books, 1997.

Reese, K., J. Jones, G. Kenepp, J. Krohmer: "Into the Frey: Integration of Emergency Medical Services and Special Weapons and Tactics (SWAT) Terms," in *Prehospital Disaster Med*, 1996, 11(3): 202–206.

ON THE WEB

Visit Brady's Paramedic Website at www.bradybooks.com/paramedic.

CHAPTER 13

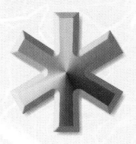

Rural EMS

Objectives

After reading this chapter, you should be able to:

*1. Identify situations and conditions unique to rural EMS. (pp. 467–469, 472–473)

*2. Discuss various challenges facing rural EMS providers. (pp. 467–469, 472–473)

*3. Describe some of the possible solutions to problems commonly faced by rural EMS units. (pp. 462–472)

*4. Differentiate between rural and urban EMS when considering treatment and response time. (pp. 467, 472–473)

*5. Identify important issues when faced with agricultural emergencies. (pp. 475, 477–479, 480)

*6. Review typical rural EMS scenarios, and identify what decisions a rural EMS provider needs to consider. (pp. 473–475, 482–483, 484–485)

*Note: The objectives for this chapter are not included in the DOT Paramedic curriculum.

CASE STUDY

It's a warm sunny afternoon in July when a call comes into your paramedic unit for "a man down in a farmyard." Dispatch has toned out the local volunteer BLS squad. However, because the call involves an unresponsive patient, the dispatcher has also requested backup from the nearest paramedic unit. Your unit, which lies over 29 miles away, receives the call.

It takes the local volunteer squad 5 minutes to assemble and get an ambulance en route to the farm, which lies at the edge of the squad's district. Your unit—a full time paid agency—is off the floor in less than 1 minute. Because both units must travel quite a distance, they race against the clock to reach the scene safely.

The BLS squad arrives at the farm just a few minutes ahead of your unit. Crew members meet the patient's wife at the door of the house. She says, "Please hurry. Follow me. I will show you where my husband is." The squad leader informs the wife that crew members will proceed as soon as they ensure that the scene is safe. By this time, the man's wife is frantic. She yells, "You must help my husband right now!"

At this point, your unit arrives on the scene and you assist the squad leader in calmly obtaining information. As the woman gestures toward a silo, you

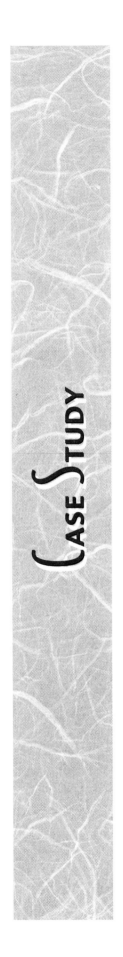

notice a man lying at its base. About a foot away from the patient, you see a ladder propped up against the silo. A rope runs up the ladder to the top of the silo.

When the squad leader asks the woman what may have happened, she replies: "My husband was going to clean the silo today. Everything seemed ok, until I heard someone yelling. When I looked out the window, my husband was having trouble climbing down the ladder. As he got near the ground, he seemed to keel over and fall."

The squad leader then finds out whether the woman's husband was using any hazardous materials and whether she has had any ill effects from being near the silo. She responds "no" to both questions. You and the squad leader agree that the scene is probably safe and relay this information to the dispatch center.

As you move toward the base of the silo, you note no apparent trauma to the victim. You ask the woman, "How far do you think your husband fell?" The patient's wife now says that he did not actually fall to the ground, but slumped forward to his current face-down position. Her comment corroborates your initial observation.

Because the patient is unresponsive, you assume control of the situation. You and your partner carefully log roll the patient to assess the airway. You note that the man is breathing, but his respirations are less than 8 per minute. He is diaphoretic, ashen, and unconscious. His pulse is slow and weak.

The down time is now 40 minutes. Because the patient must be ventilated, your partner assists breathing with a BVM. Meanwhile, you place a monitor on the patient and note a bradycardia. You establish an IV using aseptic techniques, while your partner obtains vitals. She reports blood pressure 60/p, pulse 40 BPM.

The patient is now receiving ventilations at 16–20 BPM. You order the airway secured with a number 8.0 mm ET tube. Using a landline, you report the situation to medical direction. The medical director orders 0.5 mg of atropine IV push (IVP). Because this is a rural setting, you realize the ambulance may experience communication black-outs. As a result, you must anticipate any problems that may arise en route to the hospital. In case the atropine does not help, you request orders for transcutaneous pacing (TCP) and/or additional doses of atropine according to advanced cardiac life support (ACLS) protocols.

After receiving approval from medical direction, you administer the prescribed atropine and load the patient into the ambulance. The total time of treatment prior to transport is 11 minutes. En route, you apply the TCP and achieve mechanical capture at 60 milliamperes (ma) on the rate of 70 BPM. The patient responds well to the treatment and is taken to a local hospital 33 miles away. At the hospital, he receives a temporary pacemaker. The patient is then transferred to the regional cardiac center for an internal pacemaker. The actions of the BLS and paramedic crews in this rural emergency have made the difference between life and death.

INTRODUCTION

Recent census data indicates that more than 53 million people in the United States live in rural areas. In fact, some states have rural populations of nearly 50 percent or more. In the West, states with large rural populations include Alaska, Montana, North Dakota, and South Dakota. In the South, they include Arkansas, Kentucky, Mississippi, North Carolina, South Carolina, and West Virginia. In the Northeast, they include Maine, New Hampshire, and Vermont.

People choose to live in rural areas for a variety of reasons. Their families have always lived there. They work at occupations such as farming, ranching, or mining. They like the solitude, open space, or recreational activities found in rural areas. Regardless of the reason, most rural dwellers face a similar problem—lack of easy access to the health care facilities found in most urban and suburban areas.

In the rural setting, resources such as full-service hospitals, fire departments, and EMS units are often as thinly distributed as the population. Specialty teams may be non-existent. One of the challenges for rural EMS providers is to ensure that their patients receive the same high-quality care as people living elsewhere in the nation. The following sections outline some of the obstacles and decisions typically faced by rural EMS providers.

One of the challenges for rural EMS providers is to ensure that their patients receive the same high-quality care as people living elsewhere in the nation.

PRACTICING RURAL EMS

In general, the United States government defines rural areas in terms of their sparse populations and distances from cities, towns, or villages. In relation to health care, rural areas can also be characterized by their higher percentage of people over age 65 and their lower physician-to-patient ratios. While one in five people in the United States live in rural settings, only about one in ten doctors choose to practice in these locations.

It has been found that rural residents experience a disproportionate number of serious injuries and chronic health conditions. Because of the greater distances to health care facilities, rural residents suffer a higher level of mortality associated with trauma and medical emergencies. In many cases, an EMS unit may provide the definitive care. In meeting the challenge of practicing rural EMS, paramedics and other health care personnel need to be aware of the special problems facing them.

Because of the greater distances to health care facilities, rural residents suffer a higher level of mortality associated with trauma and medical emergencies.

SPECIAL PROBLEMS

As already indicated in this book, the cost of medical care and the rise of HMOs have expanded the roles and responsibilities of EMS personnel in the 21st century (see Chapter 6). The need for non-emergent transports, especially in rural areas, has increased. The shortage of specialized doctors and well-equipped hospitals in rural areas has become an even more critical problem. In the years ahead, a growing number of patients may have to be transported to urban areas to receive the care unavailable to them in rural facilities.

In the case of natural disasters, such as tornadoes, floods, or hurricanes, the situation is equally serious. In such instances, EMS personnel may be the *only* available medical support until state or federal agencies can be transported into the area.

Regardless of the circumstances surrounding a call, rural EMS crews face a number of obstacles and challenges not found in most urban areas. If you currently work for a rural EMS unit, you may already be aware of some of these situations from first-hand experience. As a paramedic, you will assume an expanded leadership role in directing other EMS personnel on how best to handle or overcome the following special problems.

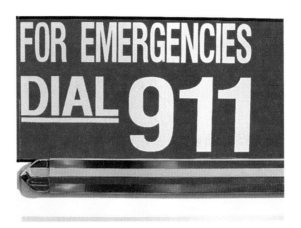

FIGURE 13-1 A universal access number, such as 911, is essential for rapid public access to the EMS system. However, many rural areas lack such a number, hampering communications and increasing response times.

Distance and Time

Rural EMS often relies on volunteer services. In responding to calls, volunteers must first travel varying distances to a squad building. Once aboard the ambulance, they then travel the distance to the patient and later the distance to the hospital. As a result, every decision that a paramedic makes in a rural setting needs to be made with the thought of distance in mind. (The "distance factor," one of the most critical aspects of rural EMS, will be discussed in more detail later in this chapter.)

Every decision that a paramedic makes in a rural setting needs to be made with the thought of distance in mind.

Communication Difficulties

In rural areas, poor or old communication equipment often hampers public access to EMS. A rural area, for example, may not have universal access to 911 (Figure 13-1). Lack of 911 service will delay response time or, in many cases, lead people to turn telephone operators into dispatchers.

Rural EMS crews can also be hampered by inadequate communications. Antiquated "fire phones" or "crash bars" might notify them of an emergency call, but crew members may have no way of communicating with each other en route to the service vehicle. Crews may also lack information from dispatch until they arrive at the squad building or are onboard the ambulance.

While traveling on the ambulance, rural EMS providers may experience dead spots where they cannot transmit (Figure 13-2). Frequencies can also be overloaded with static from highway departments and school buses. This impairs a medic's ability to communicate with other ambulance crews or with medical direction. As a result, rural paramedics must often think ahead, asking for orders in anticipation of medical conditions that might develop during a dead spot.

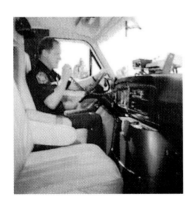

FIGURE 13-2 A rural paramedic must anticipate radio dead spots and request orders to treat any possible medical conditions that may arise during transport.

Rural paramedics must often think ahead, asking orders in anticipation of medical conditions that might develop during a radio dead spot.

Enrollment Shortages

Because many rural EMS providers work on a volunteer basis, units or squads can experience enrollment shortages. Volunteers must respond to calls from their jobs or homes. The greater distances and time involved in many rural EMS calls can take volunteers from their work or families for lengthy periods. This situation can impact upon their ability to earn a living or to raise their children. As a result, they often serve for only short stretches or resign entirely.

Training and Practice

Access to training and continuing education is not readily available in many rural areas. In addition, the cost and amount of time required for certification as a paramedic has increased. For the volunteer, this means increased personal expense and time away from home. The net effect can be EMS providers with a less advanced level of training than their paid urban counterparts.

This situation can be further complicated by the low volume of EMS calls in some rural areas. EMS providers simply do not have the opportunity to practice their skills on a consistent basis. Members of rescue squads may experience what has become known as **rust out,** or an inability to keep abreast of new technologies and standards. The networking opportunities or volume of calls simply do not exist.

✱ **rust out** an inability to keep abreast of new technologies and standards.

Inadequate Medical Support

As might be expected, rural areas sometimes have inadequate medical direction. Local physicians may lack the training in EMS operations or feel EMS operations should not be part of their job.

Rural areas also may not have the budgets to buy new equipment and ambulances. In addition, air medical transport may not always be readily available due to many factors such as distance, lack of landing areas, cost, or too few helicopters for a large area.

Finally, hospitals and rural EMS agencies may not always implement protocols or standards for prehospital providers. Roles may not be clearly defined, or hospitals may have varying protocols. A rural paramedic faced with the decision to transport a patient to two different hospitals may have to deal with two different sets of protocols for prehospital care. That means that volunteers must seek out and familiarize themselves with these protocols often on their own.

CREATIVE PROBLEM-SOLVING

To overcome the obstacles involved in the practice of rural EMS, agencies have turned to creative problem-solving. The following sections outline some of the possible solutions available to rural EMS providers.

Improved Communications

In recent years, some rural counties have been fortunate enough to receive grants to modernize or supplement their communications equipment. In other areas, rural counties have joined together to share in the cost of implementing 911 systems. As 911 systems enter rural areas, dispatchers gain valuable education in Medical Priority Dispatch and Medical-Assist Dispatch. Dispatchers with specialized training can provide life-saving instructions while rural crews are en route to emergencies.

Radio dead spots and crowded frequencies can be handled by requesting additional frequencies and/or by upgrading radio equipment. One possible solution is more powerful base station radios and towers. A group effort in the form of a 911 user advisory board or consortium of agencies can help reduce or eliminate the problem of radio traffic overcrowding. Such advisory boards or consortiums can also provide a forum for discussion of common communication concerns and other issues.

A technological innovation that promises to improve communications in rural areas is the cell phone. Through use of cell phones, rural paramedics can

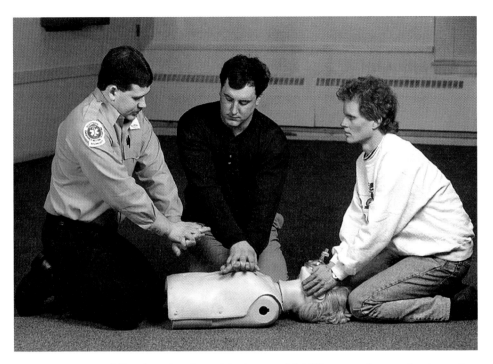

Figure 13-3 Public education is a critical part of fulfilling enrollment shortages in rural areas. As a paramedic, you should involve yourself in the training of techniques used by first responders such as CPR.

communicate with emergency room physicians or their medical directors. Another innovation currently under consideration is the designation of cells for EMS use only.

Recruitment and Certification

One of the most important ways to improve rural EMS centers is the effort to increase the number of trained paramedics in rural areas. Recognizing the problem of distance, units with paramedics onboard can intercept BLS crews that require advanced life support measures for their patients. Paramedic units can thus help ensure the highest level of service in rural counties.

The issues of recruitment and certification of paramedics in rural areas can be addressed through flexible training sessions and ongoing education. Agencies can pool their resources with neighboring squads to offer education to all their members.

To increase interest in volunteer EMS service, rural agencies can utilize "explorer" and "ride along" programs, when appropriate. Paramedics can serve as "recruiters" by taking the lead in training rural residents as CPR drivers or first responders (Figure 13-3). The goal is to involve them in ambulance service or quick response units as soon as possible. Once part of the EMS system, these volunteers can be encouraged to advance to the EMT and paramedic levels of training.

Some of the most important training advancements for rural areas have come through the use of computers and the Internet. Using the Internet, of course, means accessing valid sources of information. However, once these sources are identified, EMS personnel can use "distance learning" to develop an awareness of new standards and procedures. The Internet also provides rural

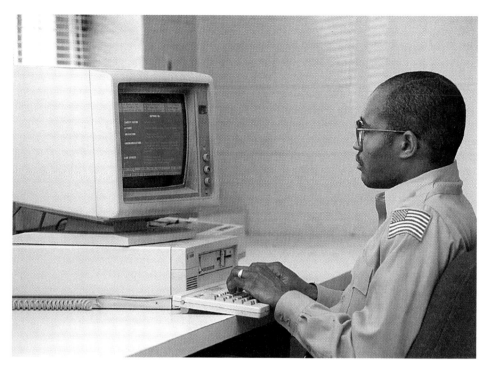

FIGURE 13-4   As a rural paramedic, your education should never end. You can overcome lack of access to classroom instruction through use of the Internet or computerized programs and simulations. You have a responsibility to provide patients with the same high-level care as your urban counterparts.

squads with a cost-effective way to interface with other agencies. Networking over the Internet can be an excellent way to promote creative problem-solving or to share new ideas.

Even without benefit of the Internet, agencies or units can purchase interactive CD-ROMS and EMS computer simulation programs. These programs allow crew members to maintain a high level of knowledge and skills. They also help EMTs or EMT-Intermediates to train as paramedics (Figure 13-4).

Improved Medical Support

The National Association of EMS Physicians provides numerous educational opportunities for physicians interested in learning more about the supervision and oversight of EMS operations. Conferences held by this organization offer courses in EMS medical direction. Although many doctors choose to practice in urban areas, some highly trained physicians live in rural areas. If you live in a rural area, you or an officer in your agency might approach such physicians and determine their willingness to serve as an Emergency Medical Director. If it is impossible to find a medical director among local physicians, you may need to search at the nearest urban hospital.

Regardless of where a paramedic lives, positive relationships with a hospital depend upon good communications. A medic should spend time at the hospitals that serve their districts and, when possible, request to sit in on relevant in-service training sessions provided for the hospital staff.

Rural paramedics should spend time at the hospitals that serve their districts and, when possible, request to sit in on relevant in-service training sessions provided for the hospital staff.

Ingenuity and Increased Responsibilities

Rural EMS requires ingenuity. For most rural agencies, it is a constant struggle to retain members, supplement budgets, update equipment, provide quality education programs, and network with other health care facilities. As a rural paramedic, you will be involved in most, if not all, of these aspects of rural EMS.

As a rural paramedic, you can expect your role to grow as counties attempt to fill the "health-care gap" between rural and urban areas. You may find yourself involved in hospital outreach programs such as **prompt care facilities,** or agencies that provide limited care and non-emergent medical treatment. In such cases, you may work under the direction of a physician or a physician's assistant (PA) and administer immunizations, wound care, and provide emergent transport as necessary.

Governments in some rural areas are also considering the involvement of paramedics in the public health system when not responding to emergency calls. Whatever the future may hold, you will be challenged as a rural paramedic to raise the standard of prehospital care offered to the rural residents who make up nearly one-quarter of the nation's population.

✳ **prompt care facilities** hospital agencies that provide limited care and non-emergent medical treatment.

TYPICAL RURAL EMS SITUATIONS AND DECISIONS

Rural paramedics must be highly skilled and highly practiced to compensate for the extended run times and more complicated logistics found in many rural settings.

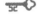

Rural paramedics must be highly skilled and highly practiced to compensate for the extended run times and more complicated logistics found in many rural settings. The following pages are designed to familiarize you with some of the unique factors a rural paramedic must consider. The scenarios that appear at the end of each section challenge you to consider some of the complex decisions faced by paramedics working in rural areas. In reviewing this material keep in mind one key point: Increased time and distance mean an increased chance of shock.

THE DISTANCE FACTOR

Every paramedic knows the axiom about the Golden Hour: Deliver the patient to a definitive health care center within an hour. In rural areas, however, you may find it impossible to meet this guideline. Consider this example. A patient lives 18 miles away from the squad building and 30 miles from the nearest hospital. If you travel at a rate of 60 miles an hour, you need 48 minutes just to get to the patient and to the hospital. That leaves you with 12 minutes to respond to the station and to manage and package the patient.

In rural settings, it is easy to travel even greater distances. As a result, you may spend far more time with the patient onboard the ambulance than at the scene itself. With this in mind, actions taken by a rural paramedic during transport can have a definitive impact upon the patient's outcome. During transport, for example, you could treat a CHF patient with nitrates, furosemide (Lasix), and morphine while providing assisted ventilations with a BVM. By the time you reach the hospital, the patient may be completely out of crisis. For this reason, you must keep accurate and complete documentation during any lengthy transport.

Another factor to consider during transport is the availability of emergency staff at the local hospital. In most urban areas, hospitals stay active all night. They have full-time emergency departments with around-the-clock staffing able to handle complicated procedures 24 hours a day seven days a week. Some rural hospitals, however, may only have a part-time emergency department with only one or two doctors on staff. In such cases, you may have to call the hospital from the patient's home to arrange for the necessary personnel to be in the building when you arrive. You many also have to make a judgment call on whether or not to transport a critically injured patient to a more distant full-time trauma center. In the case of cardiac problems, the availability of thrombolytic therapy might be the deciding factor.

In rural EMS, every decision depends upon the situation. Since paramedics live in a world of ACLS and PHTLS, you may have access to advanced equipment that is unavailable at your local hospital. A rural hospital under budget constraints, for example, may be unable to purchase equipment such as the Life Pack 12™. In such instances, you might decide with approval of medical direction to use your equipment at the local hospital or to transport the patient to a definitive treatment center at a more distant location.

In treating seriously ill or injured patients, keep in mind that you may see all phases of a patient's death before reaching a distant medical facility. Consider a motor vehicle patient with a serious head trauma. At first, your patient may be alert, conscious, and oriented. The patient then becomes agitated and aggressive. He or she may begin to have memory lapses and become more confused. You notice dilated pupils. If the transport is long enough, the patient will go into a decorticate posture, then a decerebrate posture. You face this situation knowing that there is little or nothing you can do to change patient outcome due to transport time.

Given scenarios such as the one just described, rural paramedics must know when and how to use air transport. The information in Table 13-1 provides general guidelines for when it is appropriate to consider using a helicopter to transport a patient to a medical facility. (For more on air transport, see Chapter 8.)

To assess that the effect of distance on the decisions made in many rural emergencies, consider the following scenario. (Questions appear at the end.)

> *In local hospitals with a part-time emergency department, you may have to call the hospital from the patient's home to arrange for the necessary personnel to be in the building when you arrive.*
>

Rural Scenario 1

You are a rural volunteer paramedic. It's a foggy night, and you're en route to conduct training at an outlying quick response unit (QRU). On your radio, you hear dispatch sending this same QRU to a car versus train collision 10 miles ahead of you.

In approximately 10 minutes, you arrive at a very foggy scene with many flashing lights. You determine that the QRU and its fire department have already arrived. You also see a vehicle in the ditch near a railroad crossing. The first responder unit recognizes you as a paramedic, and asks for your assistance. Crew members direct you to a 35-year-old male trapped behind the wheel of his vehicle.

Upon assessment, you find the patient alert and oriented, but very anxious. Your physical exam shows blunt chest trauma, decreased breath sounds on the left, a rigid painful abdomen, and several lacerations and abrasions on the head and arms. You record the following vital signs: HR 160; RR 32 and shallow; BP 90/60.

Fire department personnel inform you that it will take approximately 20 minutes to extricate the patient. A volunteer BLS ambulance will be on scene in 15 minutes. The closest hospital is a 20-bed, Level IV trauma facility located 30 miles east. The nearest Level II trauma center, with an ALS ambulance service, is 75 miles east and south of the scene.

1. Upon arrival on scene, you notice that the first responders with the QRU were not attempting to stabilize the cervical spine. They

Table 13-1	Use of Helicopters in Rural Emergencies

Consider putting a helicopter on standby if:

- The victim is in an unrestrained MVC.
- There is significant compartment intrusion (over 15 inches).
- You know that lengthy extrication is required.
- There is a fatality involved in the accident.
- The patient has been ejected from a vehicle.
- The victim has fallen over 20 feet.
- There is a pedestrian vs. a car collision or a motorcycle accident.

Consider requesting a helicopter to respond to the scene if:

- The medications and/or treatment required by the patient is at a higher level than the ground crew can provide.
- The ground transport to a trauma center is greater than 30 minutes.
- The terrain requires air rescue.
- The patient has any of the following conditions:
  - Multi-system trauma
  - Amputated limb
  - Second- and third-degree burns greater than or equal to 15% of the body surface area (10% for pediatric patients)
  - Signs of smoke or CO_2 inhalation with an altered LOC
  - Penetrating trauma to the head, neck, chest, and/or abdomen
  - Chest trauma with difficulty breathing
  - Head injury with an altered level of consciousness
  - Need for a hyperbaric chamber
  - HAPE or HACE (high-altitude pulmonary edema or high-altitude cerebral edema

Do NOT consider helicopter transport if:

- There is no appropriate landing zone available.
- The patient has a post-trauma cardiac arrest.
- Local policies do not allow prisoners to be transported due to the inability to provide adequate safety measures.

also were not using recommended BSI procedures. How and when would you correct this situation?

(After taking control of the scene, you correct any deficiencies that you might note right away. You would tell the first responders to stabilize the head and neck using manual stabilization and don the necessary gear.)

2. To which of the two trauma facilities would you transport this patient? Why?

(Because the patient is in decompensated shock with a possible pneumothorax and abdominal bleeding, the need for surgery is imminent. As a result, you should transport the patient to the Level II trauma center.)

3. What resources would you call upon to help ensure that this patient receives the highest level of care?

(Due to the mechanism of injury and distance to the appropriate hospital, you would request air transport as well as dispatch of the closest advanced life support unit. This will ensure that you receive the correct equipment on scene. Keep in mind that the foggy weather may make it impossible for the helicopter to land or necessitate intercept at a safer landing zone.)

4. Having no ALS equipment with you, are there any liability issues that might dictate your actions at the scene and during transport? Explain.

(You have a duty to act in this situation. As a result, there will be no liability solely for the fact that you do not have gear. Remember you are always a paramedic and, in this case, your knowledge is as important as your equipment. This does not cover, however, any harm that you may cause to the patient in your treatment. Because you provided treatment on this patient, you must fully document all your actions.)

AGRICULTURAL EMERGENCIES

Agriculture provides one of the major sources of income in the rural setting. Emergencies related to farming or ranching can range from equipment-related injuries to pesticide poisoning to any number of medical problems exacerbated by agricultural labor. When faced with an agricultural emergency, keep in mind the following considerations.

Safety

As in any emergency situation, you must place crew safety first. Interpret the situation described by the dispatcher, and think of all the scenarios that could be connected with this situation. In agricultural emergencies, many possibilities for injury exist. Potential dangers include livestock, chemicals, fuel tanks, fumes in storage bins and silos, and heavy or outdated farm equipment.

Farm Machinery If you live in an agricultural area, you must familiarize yourself with the range of equipment used on farms or ranches (Figures 13-5a to 13-5d). Farm equipment can be very different from a car, where a simple turn of the key shuts off the vehicle.

To prevent on-scene injuries, you need to make sure that farm equipment is both stable and locked down. Keep in mind that many types of farm equipment have fuel line shut-offs or power kill-switches. For this reason, it is important that you place personnel familiar with the equipment in charge of shutting off and locking down all machinery. Keep in mind this safety principle: **lock-out/tag-out.** After you shut off the equipment, you lock off the switch and place a tag on the switch stating why it is shut off. This prevents accidental retripping of switches.

Remember, too, that the possibility for injury exists even after the equipment has been turned off. Engines fueled by gasoline, diesel, or propane hold the potential for explosion. Equipment that is not properly stabilized or chained can still roll or turn over. When lifting equipment, the center of gravity can shift, increasing the pressure on either the patient or causing injury to crew members.

If you live in an agricultural area, you must familiarize yourself with the range of equipment used on farms or ranches.

* **lock-out/tag-out** locking off of a machinery switch, then placing a tag on the switch stating why it is shut off; method of preventing equipment from being accidentally restarted.

When dealing with equipment-related injuries, keep in mind this principle: lock-out/tag-out all switches or levers.

FIGURE 13-5a   Hay bale
stacker. (Mark Foster)

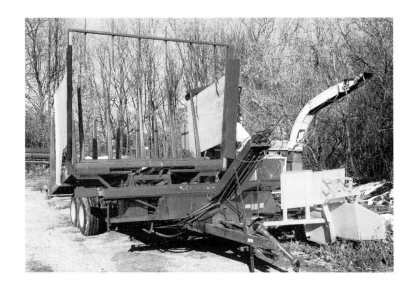

FIGURE 13-5b   Round hay
baler. (Mark Foster)

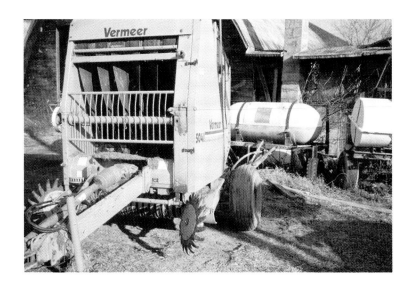

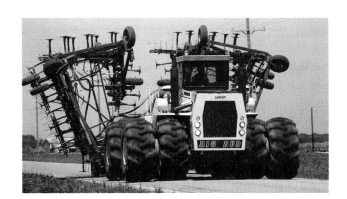

FIGURE 13-5c   Tractor with 72-inch planter, typical of
large commercial farms. (Grant Heilman, Grant Heilman
Photography, Inc.)

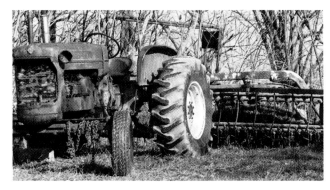

FIGURE 13-5d   Tractor and hay rake, typical of the old
equipment found on many rural farms. (Mark Foster)

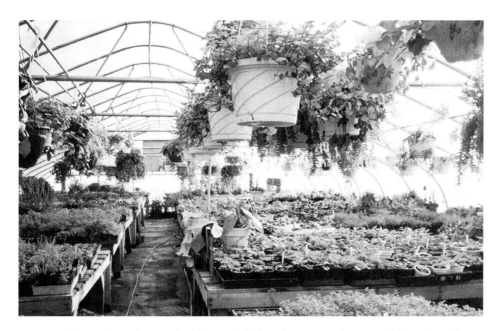

FIGURE 13-6   Greenhouses hold many hidden dangers such as pesticides, insecticides, and fertilizers. Remember that fertilizers possess nitrites. When mixed with diesel fuel, as in the Oklahoma bombing, they can form powerful explosives. (Mark Foster)

Hazardous Materials Hazardous materials can be found in many places on a farm or ranch (Figures 13-6 and 13-7). They exist in greenhouses, bins used to store pesticides, the equipment used to spray or dust crops, and the manure storage pits on large livestock facilities. For this reason, a self-contained breathing apparatus (SCBA) should be standard equipment on every rural EMS unit.

Be especially wary of rescues involving grain tanks and silos. Over time, grain and silage will ferment if stored long enough. During fermentation, crops release high levels of CO_2, **silo gas** (oxides of nitrogen), and methane. In rescues involving silos, you face the added risk of high angles, confined spaces, and the possibility of entombment under grain or silage. In such cases, determine whether any other agencies might be needed at the scene. Keeping in mind the distance factor, don't arrive at the scene to find out you lack the correct apparatus or support for the call. (For more on management of hazardous materials, see Chapter 11.)

✳ **silo gas** toxic fumes (oxides of nitrogen) produced by the fermentation of grains in a silo.

Potential for Trauma

Many farmers or ranchers work seven days a week, from sunrise to sunset. They endure extremes of heat, cold, and all kinds of weather conditions. They may spend a large part of the day in remote areas, far from telephones and help if injured.

The risk of serious agricultural accidents and injuries is increased by the equipment and machines routinely used by farmers. In some cases, farmers rely on old or outdated equipment because they cannot afford to replace it. They often wear little or no protective gear and may attempt to repair dangerous equipment themselves. All of these situations expose farm workers to equipment-related trauma. Depending on the type of machinery, the mechanism of injury could be crushing, twisting, tearing, penetrating, or a combination of mechanisms.

Equipment-related trauma is complicated by a number of factors related to agriculture. First, a wound may become contaminated by pesticides or manure.

In treating agricultural injuries, remember that a wound can become contaminated by pesticides or manure.

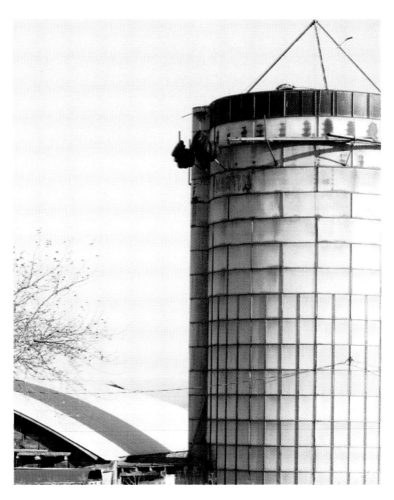

FIGURE 13-7   This old silo looks calm, but it possesses the potential for entombment in a confined space and exposure to toxic silo gas. (Mark Foster)

* **airbags** inflatable high-pressure pillows that when inflated can lift up to 20 tons, depending upon the make.

* **cribbing** wooden slates used to shore up heavy equipment.

* **compartment syndrome** condition that occurs when circulation to a portion of the body is cut off; after a period of time toxins can develop in the blood, leading to shock when circulation is restored.

Second, a patient may become easily trapped or entangled under heavy equipment, making extrication both difficult and time-consuming. Standard extrication devices used efficiently for automobiles may be unable to handle the weight of heavy farm equipment. In some cases, extrication equipment may be unavailable and crews will need to improvise using other farm equipment.

Lengthy extrications can worsen the patient's condition. You might use **airbags** (inflatable high-pressure pillows that when inflated can lift up to 20 tons) or **cribbing** (wooden slates used to shore up equipment) to relieve some of the equipment's weight. However, if extrication goes on too long, a patient may suffer from **compartment syndrome.** This occurs when circulation to a portion of the body is cut off. Over a period of time (usually hours), toxins develop in the blood, and when circulation is restored the patient goes into shock. This is a serious complication that can be fatal unless proper treatment is given in a timely manner. (For more on the treatment of shock, see Volume 4, Chapters 4 and 12 *Paramedic Care: Principles and Practices*.)

Mechanisms of Injury

Suspect many different mechanisms of injury in accidents involving agricultural equipment. For example, most farm machinery has spinning parts, such

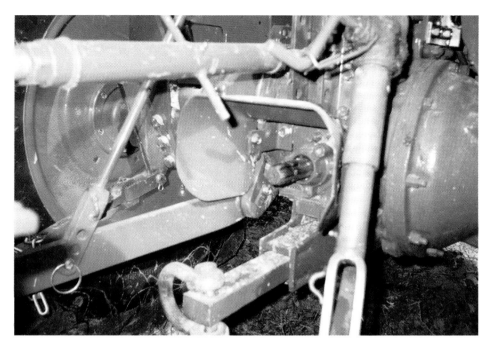

FIGURE 13-8   Tractor's PTO is a prime example of a possible mechanism for a wrap point injury. (Mark Foster)

as fans, power takeoff (PTO) shafts, augers, pulleys, and wheels. All of these have multiple **wrap points** in which an appendage can get caught and significantly twisted (Figure 13-8). The resulting injuries include sprains, strains, avulsions, fractures, and possible amputations. Other common mechanisms of injury include:

* **Pinch Points:** Pinch points occur when two objects come together and catch a portion of the patient's body in between them. This could be anything from a plow blade falling on somebody's foot to catching a hand in a log splitter (Procedure 13-1).
* **Shear Points:** Like pinch points, sheer points result when two objects come together. However, in this instance, the pinch points either meet or pass, causing amputation of a body part. An example of farm equipment able to cause a shear point is a sickle bar mower.
* **Crush Points:** Crush points develop when two or more objects come together with enough weight or force to crush the affected appendage. A common crush point mechanism of injury is a tractor rollover.

Emergency Medical Care

In general, provide the same emergency medical care to patients involved in agricultural emergencies as you would to any other patient with similar injuries. However, at all times, keep in mind the effect of time and distance on the potential for shock. A farmer involved in a minor accident, for example, may lie injured for hours in harsh weather conditions before someone suspects any trouble. In cases involving long response and/or transport times, any serious bleeding

✱ **wrap points** mechanisms of injury in which an appendage gets caught and significantly twisted.

In general, provide the same emergency medical care to patients involved in agricultural emergencies as you would to any other patient with similar injuries.

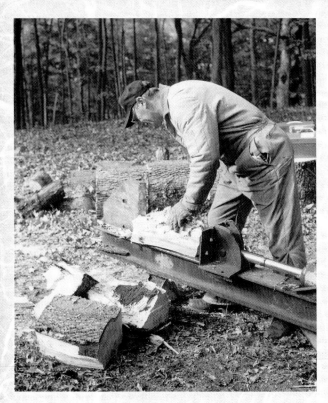

13-1a   Log splitter—a typical mechanism for a pinch-point injury in a rural setting. Note the absence of protective gear on the farmer, except for lightweight work gloves. (Mark Foster)

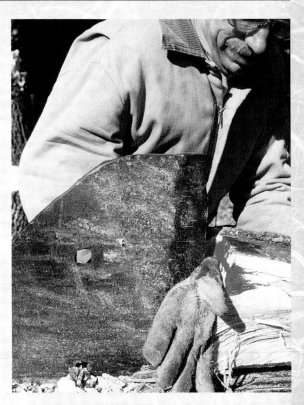

13-1b   Hand caught in pinch-point mechanism for injury, with the possibility of compartment syndrome. (Mark Foster)

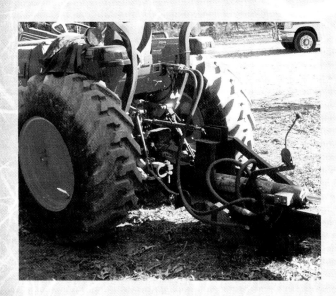

13-1c   Determine if machinery is operated by other equipment, in this case a tractor. If so, use the machinery to extricate the patient. Then lock-out/tag-out the appropriate levers or switches. (Mark Foster)

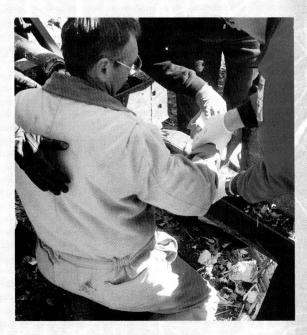

13-1d   Stabilize both fractures and circulatory injuries during extrication. (Mark Foster)

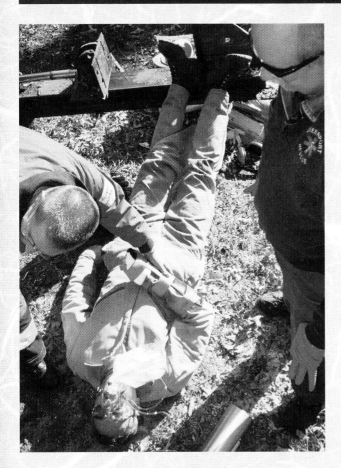

13-1e   Provide rapid treatment for shock, especially if the call for help was delayed for a lengthy period. (Mark Foster)

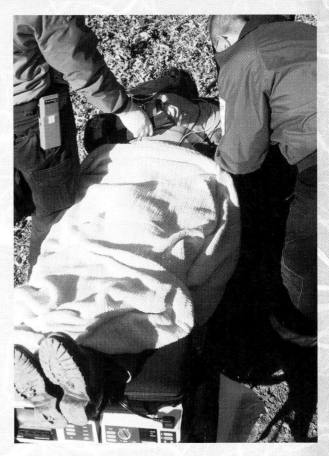

13-1f   Package and transport to the nearest appropriate medical facility, using the most effective means of transport. (Mark Foster)

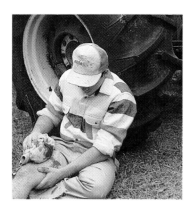

FIGURE 13-9 In rural settings, any serious bleeding injury can result in shock if distance delays treatment or transport.

injury can result in inadequate tissue perfusion if not treated promptly and effectively (Figure 13-9). In addition, because of unsanitary work conditions, sepsis or poisoning are very real possibilities.

To assess the decisions in an agricultural emergency, consider the following scenario.

Rural Scenario 2

It's a late afternoon on a warm day in May. You are the on-duty paramedic at a rural rescue squad. The squad's staff consists of a 24-hour paid paramedic and a supplemental BLS ambulance crew. Having just completed a call, you're in the bay of the squad building restocking your ALS bag and checking your gear. Suddenly a car enters the squad's parking lot, and a very anxious man jumps out. The man rushes up to you. He declares, "My father is trapped under a tractor. He's hurt real bad, and I don't know what to do."

You load the four-wheel drive quick response vehicle, and tell the man that you will follow him to the scene of the accident. However, he speeds off before you can get precise directions to the farm.

En route to the emergency, you contact the county dispatcher and request that she tone out the BLS crew and the local fire rescue squad. Although you still cannot report an address, the dispatcher begins to assemble emergency personnel.

You follow the man into a field, using the four-wheel drive vehicle to travel over the rough terrain. When you arrive at the site of the overturned tractor, you call county dispatch and provide your exact location before exiting the quick response vehicle. You also request that a helicopter be dispatched.

As you approach the scene, you see an elderly man trapped underneath a tractor from the waist down. Before beginning assessment, you ask the patient's son to make sure the tractor is shut down and the fuel shut-off switch is in place. You also look for fuel leaks, but find none.

Upon initial assessment, you observe that the patient has multiple contusions to his head and chest and an open humerus fracture on his right arm. Because of the position of the tractor, you are unable to access his lower extremities. The patient is unconscious, unresponsive, ashen, and diaphoretic. Vitals include: pulse 132, respirations 32 and shallow, blood pressure 130 over 88.

Ten minutes later, the fire and BLS crews arrive on the scene. The helicopter is still 30 minutes out.

1. What would have made this call go smoother in the response phase?

   (The best scenario would be to have the son ride in your vehicle. A car chase is never a good idea, especially when you do not have a clue where you are going. You should also specify the need for extrication, giving the crew time to assemble the necessary equipment.)

2. During the ten minutes you are alone, what care would you provide to the patient?

   You would protect the airway and use all appropriate ALS procedures such as IV and monitor to treat for shock. Just because you are alone, does not mean you cannot provide treatment.)

3. As the on-scene paramedic, what directions would you provide to BLS and fire crews?

   (Directions would be: treat for shock and rapid extrication.)

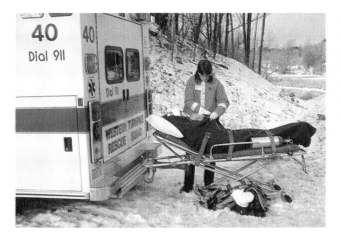

FIGURE 13-10 The recreational activities that draw people to rural settings for vacations, adventure, and sports activities also increase the chances for EMS involvement in environmental emergencies.

4. What steps might you take to reduce compartment syndrome?

   (The best treatment is rapid extrication. If you suspect compartment syndrome may have set in, be prepared to treat for septic shock.)

5. What details of this scenario are common to other calls you might make in a rural setting?

   (Details might include: use of volunteers, lengthy distances, patients located in isolated areas, the use of many organizations to facilitate the treatment of your patient, consideration of air transport, and so on.)

RECREATIONAL EMERGENCIES

Recreational activities have always drawn people to rural settings. Depending upon the season and the activity, the population in a rural community can swell dramatically as vacationers, sports enthusiasts, or "adventurer-seekers" arrive in an area. Small hill towns, for example, can grow to two or three times their size when a ski slope opens. Such a situation presents unique challenges to EMS units in the area (Figure 13-10). A ski slope, for instance, may have its own first aid station and ski patrol, but cannot usually provide advanced care or transport to a patient involved in a skiing accident.

As a rural paramedic, you need to be familiar with the recreational or wilderness pursuits in your area. If you live near a lake, local lifeguards can perform basic first aid and CPR, but they cannot abandon their beach patrol. Further treatment and transport falls to local EMS units. In such cases, a paramedic would need to be well-versed in the procedures and skills related to water emergencies.

If you live in a wilderness or mountainous area, you might need to be aware of the accidents commonly encountered by hunters, backpackers, mountaineers, rock climbers, or mountain bikers. You might decide to take courses to receive certification in wilderness rescue. You might also practice rescues in extreme weather conditions such as those found on New Hampshire's Mt. Washington, where harsh and unpredictable weather patterns can trap or injure even the most experienced climber. (For more information on treating environmental emergencies, see Volume 3, Chapter 10 of *Paramedic Care: Principles and Practice*.)

In wilderness rescues, distance and extrication time play an important part in your decisions. For example, if a rock climber is injured in the Shawangunks in New Paltz, New York, several hospitals lie within a 30-minute range. However, if the patient is injured on the second pitch of a three-pitch climb, evacuation will delay transport—especially if the injury occurs on a class 5.10 or 5.11 route.

A helicopter might seem the obvious choice of transport in wilderness rescues. However, you must take into account weather conditions, availability of suitable landing zones, and the time it will take a helicopter to arrive. In some instances, ground transport may be more efficient, even it means carrying a patient out in a basket stretcher. In other instances, a helicopter might be able to provide a higher level of care, depending upon regional and state protocols. For example, if a rock climber has sustained a severe head injury and if ground transport lacks protocols for rapid sequence intubation, the patient's needs might be better served with helicopter transport.

Keep in mind that the helicopter is not a panacea. It has specific uses, tied to distance and level of care. Indiscriminate use of air transport can sometimes add dangerous minutes to patient treatment or even carry the risk of further patient injury. For example, high-altitude sickness can be worsened by an increase in altitude due to unpressurized flight. Decompression syndrome patients are definitely candidates for low-altitude transport. (For more on diving-related injuries, see Volume 3, Chapter 10, of *Paramedic Care: Principles and Practice*.)

To assess the decisions in a recreational emergency, consider the following scenario.

Rural Scenario 3

Shifting his weight from side to side, Jim compensates for the boat's wake as he glides across New York's Hudson River. His girlfriend Renee is piloting Jim's new boat, while two of Jim's friends enjoy the ride. As Jim shifts to tack in the opposite direction, he catches a wave and drops into the water. Renee sees Jim fall and turns the boat around to pick up the skier. She does her best to bring the boat gently to him, but piloting is new to her. She realizes too late that the boat is going hit Jim and puts the motor in reverse.

When the boat strikes Jim, the motor sucks his legs into the propeller. Both of his legs become twisted in and around the shaft. Fearing the worst, Jim's friends jump into the water to hold up his head so that he does not drown. They then yell to the nearest boat for help. The owner of that boat uses his cell phone to call 911.

The 911 dispatcher receives the call. Using pre-arrival dispatch instructions, the dispatcher initiates bystander treatment and gathers the necessary information. Meanwhile, the dispatcher's partner tones out the local rescue squad and the fire department extrication team. Because of the seriousness of the situation, the dispatcher also tones out the nearest ALS unit where you serve as a paid 24-hour paramedic. Listening to other dispatches on the scanner, you had already begun to move closer to the scene. You now respond rapidly.

Upon arrival, you find that members of the rescue squad and fire department have entered the water to relieve the patient's exhausted friends. By this time, the patient is unconscious and unresponsive. He has a patent airway and does not have any trauma to his upper body. Post-extrication assessment reveals the following vitals: a weak, rapid pulse of 130; respirations 24 and shallow; blood pressure 90/PALP. Upon physical examination, you note that both legs have multiple fractures. Deep lacerations run from the patient's groin to his ankles. Included in the lacerations are two arterial bleeders.

1. What would be the appropriate BLS and ALS treatment for this patient?

    (BLS treatment includes high-flow O_2, removal of wet clothing, passive warming for hypothermia, and direct pressure on the lesser bleeders. ALS treatment includes airway management, manual tamponading of arterial bleeders, IV therapy with moderate fluid challenges, monitor, and rapid transport to a trauma center. Desired blood pressure should remain approximately 90/PALP.)

2. Would MAST pants be appropriate in this situation? Explain.

    (MAST pants would not be advised due to the fact that application will not tamponade arterial bleeding and will hide large blood loss inside the pants.)

3. What could be done to ensure better long-term management of this patient in the rural emergency setting?

    (Because saline does not carry oxygen, better long-term management would include moderate fluid challenges instead of large fluid challenges. Also, tamponading of specific arterial bleeding, rather than tamponading a large area, increases blood flow to the extremities. This makes the extremities more salvageable.)

4. Suppose air transport was unavailable. How would this change treatment provided by the paramedic?

    (The paramedic could transport the patient to the nearest local hospital for stabilization and possible blood transfusions. This action, of course, would depend on equipment and services rendered by the local hospital.)

5. How did the availability of universal access to a 911 number affect the outcome of this patient?

    (The 911 number provided rapid dispatch of all necessary equipment and personnel. It also allowed bystanders to be prompted by a highly trained dispatcher.)

SUMMARY

Rural EMS presents the paramedic and other health care personnel with special challenges such as lengthy distances, radio dead spots, shortages of EMS providers and medical directors, lack of around-the-clock emergency departments, less opportunity for skills practice, and more. To meet these challenges, many rural EMS units have turned to creative problem-solving. Counties have joined together to share in the cost of universal access to the 911 system. Squads have adopted flexible training sessions, making use of computerized instruction and networking through the Internet.

Paramedics play an important part in filling the "health-care gap" between rural and urban areas. They take a leading role in training rural residents as CPR drivers and first responders. They intercept volunteer BLS units traveling over long distances and provide definitive care. They develop the specialized skills and training to handle the agricultural and/or recreational emergencies unique to their county or district. Because distance often increases the contact time between paramedics and their rural patients, decisions about treatment and use of air transport literally make the difference between life and death.

You MAKE THE CALL

The stone quarry in your district was abandoned after it flooded several years ago. Since then, the county has used it as a water source and placed it off limits to recreational users. However, the quarry's clear water and high cliffs serve as a magnet to teenagers who want to go swimming. To you, the quarry holds nothing but trouble for the teens. It's isolated and filled with old rusted equipment. Nothing, not even a well-traveled road, lies near the quarry.

One hot sunny afternoon in August, three teenagers—John, Todd, and Stacey—decide to hike into a remote part of the quarry for a swim. Once at the quarry, Todd rushes to top of one of the 50-foot cliffs and jumps into the water. Misjudging the water's depth, he hits bottom. When Todd doesn't come up for air, Stacey realizes something is wrong. She and John dive into the water and pull Todd to shore.

The two teens now panic. Todd is breathing, but unconscious. Blood is pouring from a wound in his leg. Stacey tries to stop the bleeding by applying direct pressure. Meanwhile John races to get help. It takes him nearly 30 minutes to reach a telephone. Lacking a universal access number, he calls the local fire department, which in turn places a call to your volunteer ALS unit. By the time you get into your ambulance, 45 minutes have passed since the accident took place. Although it will only take you about 10 minutes to reach the quarry, you will still need to gain access to the patient at the distant location where the teens chose to swim.

1. What apparatus or support are you going to need to perform this rescue?
2. Based on the mechanisms of injury, what injuries should you suspect?
3. What will you do to stabilize this patient?
4. What factors made it impossible for you to adhere to the axiom of the Golden Hour?

See Suggested Responses at the back of this book.

FURTHER READING

Farabee, Charles R. ("Butch"), Jr.: *Death, Daring, and Disaster: Search and Rescue in the National Parks*. Boulder, CO: Roberts, Rinehart Publishers, 1998.

Tilton, Buck, M.S., and Frank Hubbel, D.O.: *Medicine for the Backcountry, Third Edition*. Merrillville, Indiana: ICS Books, Inc., 1999.

Wilkerson, James A., M.D.: *Medicine for Mountaineering & Other Wilderness Activities*, Fourth Edition. Seattle, Washington: The Mountaineers, 1992.

ON THE WEB

Visit Brady's Paramedic Website at www.bradybooks.com/paramedic.

Suggested Responses to "You Make the Call"

The following are suggested responses to the "You Make the Call" scenarios presented in each chapter of Paramedic Care, Volume 5, Special Considerations/Operations. Each represents an acceptable response to the scenario but should not be interpreted as the only correct response.

Chapter 1—Neonatology

1. *Should you stimulate this baby to breathe as soon as it is delivered? Why or why not?*

    You should not stimulate this baby to breathe, either while on the perineum, or immediately following delivery due to the presence of thick meconium. Quickly prepare equipment and visualize the airway with a laryngoscope. Suction the airway with a catheter or, preferably, insert an appropriately sized uncuffed ET tube. Apply suction to the ET tube with a suction adaptor. After a few seconds, the majority of the meconium should be removed from the airway. Discard the soiled tube and place a new one. This whole procedure should take no longer than 30–45 seconds. After securing the airway, stimulate the infant. The infant may require a brief trial of mechanical ventilation. Always administer 100% supplemental oxygen. Be sure to report the presence of thick meconium to the receiving staff.

2. *What is the major danger associated with this type of problem?*

    Meconium aspiration syndrome is a very serious problem in which the infant aspirates meconium. This often results in pulmonary infections and extended mechanical ventilation and NICU time. Taking time to aspirate the airway results in much better outcomes in neonates exposed to meconium *in utero*.

3. *Once you have stabilized this infant, where should it be transported?*

    This infant should be transported to a hospital with a neonatal intensive care unit with an available bed and mechanical ventilator.

Chapter 2—Pediatrics

1. *What are your assessment priorities for this patient?*

    You should immediately pick up on the fact that family dynamics in this case are stressed and that this is a potentially dangerous situation. The story is a little odd in that the neighbors called 911 because they heard "loud cries" coming from the house. Your assessment priorities are to assure your own safety and that of your partner. Identify an exit and be ready to leave if violence erupts. Leave your equipment until law enforcement personnel arrive. Your assessment should follow the standard approach taught in this book. Assess the airway, breathing, and circulation as well as other components of the initial assessment. Regardless of your suspicions, your primary responsibility is to care for the child. However, carefully monitor the environment and note any clues that might point to child abuse. The rule "eyes open, mouth shut" really applies here. Document your findings and prepare for transport.

2. *What interventions would you perform on scene and en route to the hospital?*

    This child should be transported if at all possible. Provide any indicated care including airway management, spinal immobilization, bandaging and splinting,

IV therapy, emotional support, and any other steps. Report your suspicions to hospital and law enforcement personnel. Do not spend a great deal of time quizzing the parents about the event as it may make them suspicious. The parents may refuse transport arguing that they will take the child to their doctor later. If this occurs, you should gently remind them that emergency care can't wait. The child may need tests that are only available at the ED. Try to gain the trust of the parents. If the family steadfastly refuses, inform the parents of the risks of refusing transport and have a refusal document signed by both parents and witnessed by a police officer. Remind the parents that they can call you back any time and you will immediately respond. If the child is "at risk" in your mind, and the parent(s) refuse transport, notify the appropriate agencies. Withdraw from the scene and arrange to meet the supportive personnel at a location a safe distance from the house. Remember, a good law enforcement officer can be very effective in convincing the parents to take the child to the ED. Employ this strategy early.

3. *Describe possible transport considerations, including a potential refusal of transport by the angry parents.*

As discussed in question 2, the ideal situation is for the child to be transported to an appropriate ED accompanied by the parents. If the situation turns ugly, the police may arrest one of the parents if the person becomes problematic. Following this, the mother can grant consent to treat and transport. If both refuse, document all actions. Have the informed refusal witnessed by a law enforcement officer. Again, as noted in question 2, assure the family that they can call EMS at anytime if they change their minds.

4. *What are the important factors in reporting this incident and documenting the call?*

You are so busy that many important details may escape your memory. It is best to immediately document the call in detail before taking the next assignment. Be sure to identify all personnel at the scene and the reason they were there. Remember, this information will be your primary reminder of what happened if and when you are called to court.

Chapter 3—Geriatric Emergencies

1. *What general impression do you have of this patient?*

The patient has fallen, leaving him at risk for head injury or fracture of the hip or pelvis. He may also have sustained blunt trauma to the chest or abdomen. A question exists as to how this patient fell. Alcohol use is prevalent among the elderly population, but the man could have experienced a syncopal episode or stroke.

2. *Do you suspect that this is an acute or chronic problem? Explain.*

Probably acute. The house is clean and well cared for, and the wife implied that he does the cleaning.

3. *Aside from the patient's presentation and response to your interventions, what other information must be included in your hospital report?*

The hospital staff needs to know that Mr. Jones is the primary caregiver for his disabled wife. Arrangement for her care must be made.

4. *What support do you provide for Mrs. Jones?*

Keep in mind the devastating effect of an ill spouse on an elderly patient. You could soon have two patients, instead of one. Provide Mrs. Jones with psychological support, and tell her that everything possible will be done for her husband. Ask if she can call anybody to help her. Assure her that you will make the hospital aware of her need for home care.

Chapter 4—Abuse and Assault

1. What do you suspect is taking place?

You suspect that the patient is a victim of child abuse.

2. What physical evidence do you have to support this suspicion?

The boy has bruises to both his upper arms and his back, all at different stages of healing.

3. What emotional evidence do you have to support this suspicion?

The boy is unusually quiet for his age and does not make any effort to contact his parents.

4. What other clues lead you to believe that abuse might be taking place?

The boy is in the care of parents involved in a domestic dispute and is dressed inappropriately for the circumstances.

5. What are your priorities in this case?

Your priorities are to assess the patient for physical injuries requiring immediate treatment, to alert the police officers to the possible abuse situation, to remove the patient to a medical facility appropriate for abused children, and to document your findings.

Chapter 5—The Challenged Patient

1. Why did the patient's doctor tell her that she is an increased risk of infection?

Cancer patients are at a high risk for infection if they have recently undergone chemotherapy. Chemotherapy can lead to neutropenia, which is a decrease in the white blood cells that help fight infection. For this reason, patients on chemotherapy do not have the ability to fight infection as well as a person with a normal neutrophil count.

2. What signs indicate that this patient has cancer?

The patient usually wears a wig to cover her head due to alopecia, she has lost her appetite, and she is vomiting. All of these conditions are side effects of chemotherapy. The patient has also recently had mastectomy, which is a treatment for breast cancer.

3. Is it necessary for all three of you to wear a mask? Explain.

It is important for your partner to wear a mask because he has an illness that is spread through the respiratory tract. It is important for your patient to wear a mask so she is not exposed to your germs or to any droplets that may have been left in the ambulance from the previous patient. Since you are healthy and you are not at risk for contracting a communicable disease from your patient, it is not necessary for you to wear a mask, but you may do so in order to reassure your patient.

4. Will you start a peripheral IV on this patient? Explain.

You will probably not start a peripheral IV on this patient. She most likely has a subcutaneous port since she is currently undergoing chemotherapy treatment. It will be accessed when she gets to the emergency department, based on the lack of a life-threatening emergency when presenting to you.

5. What information will you include in your patient report so the emergency department is prepared for this patient?

It is important to relay the neutropenic status of your patient to the emergency department so they can have a private room ready to decrease her exposure to other illnesses.

Chapter 6—Acute Interventions for the Chronic-Care Patient

1. What does the condition of the apartment tell you?

A messy, dirty apartment may indicate that the patient is on her own and has little support from family or friends. It may also show that she is receiving inadequate home care. These social factors may help you understand the patient's state of mind and interact with greater compassion.

2. *Why is it important to immediately interview the home care worker?*

The home care worker usually knows the patient well and can tell you exactly what is different, if anything, about the patient. If you don't fully understand the patient's baseline mental status and disability, you cannot adequately assess and compare your own findings.

3. *What are some of the causes of urinary incontinence?*

Causes include: seizures, spinal injury, abdominal trauma, and overdoses among others.

4. *How can you rule out spinal injury to this patient?*

You can't. The possibility of spinal injury in a patient with a pre-existing neurological deficit cannot be ruled out without knowing the exact nature of his or her baseline deficit. That decision is best left to the patient's own physician or the ED staff.

5. *Why do you think the patient denies a history of diabetes and seizures if she takes Tegretol and glucophage?*

Imagine how you would feel if confined to a wheelchair at age 18 for the rest of your life. Such patients can become unhappy, lonely, resentful, and bitter. They may also deny certain aspects of their disability in an attempt to feel better or to gain acceptance. In this case, since the patient exhibited no complicating factors related to diabetes or seizures, the crew decided not to argue with her. However, they had a responsibility to report all medications—and suspicions—as a part of their transfer of care.

6. *Why is it acceptable to defer the glucose test when patient medications indicate a possible blood sugar problem?*

The patient seems to be sensitive to her condition. Since she shows no signs of hypoglycemia, it is probably better to keep the patient calm than to argue with her about the test. If the crew had any doubts about their actions, they should, of course, consult with medical direction.

7. *Was there any need for an IV?*

No. The patient was showing no signs of shock, nor did she need to have any medications given.

8. *Should the patient have been placed on oxygen?*

Oxygen would not have hurt the patient in any way, but there was no indications for its use. The patient exhibited no shortness of breath, was in no distress, and had good skin color. (She was getting enough oxygen from room air.)

Chapter 7—Assessment-Based Management

No questions or answers for this chapter.

Chapter 8—Ambulance Operations

1. *Should you drive down the open eastbound right lane with your lights and siren on? Explain.*

No. It is strongly suggested that you do not pass other vehicles on the right with lights and siren because a motorist might hear the siren at the last minute and pull to the right directly into your vehicle.

2. *Should you enter the oncoming traffic by going around the left side of the vehicle that is currently stopped in the left hand, eastbound lane? Explain.*

Yes. But be very careful. Slow down to a crawl, and use lights and siren to alert all traffic as you approach.

3. *How can you best deal with this very dangerous intersection?*

Avoid the intersection, if possible. If it is not possible, enter each lane slowly, making eye contact with all drivers. Use your lights and siren as suggested in this chapter. Remember—most ambulance collisions take place in intersections. So be very careful in all such situations.

Chapter 9—Medical Incident Command

1. *What two roles in the Incident Management System will you and your partner fill?*

Local protocols will determine the roles of the two first responders. The most common IMS positions are Incident Commander and Triage Officer.

2. *How would you size-up the incident?*

Sample size-up: Fire in a nursing home, health-care facility. At least 30 major injuries and/or fatalities are anticipated, with another 38 patients in need of evacuation, evaluation, shelter, treatment, and transport.

3. *What additional resources would you anticipate, and what instructions would you provide for them?*

In addition to the resources supplied by the fire department, you would estimate 30 ambulances, plus wheelchair vans or convalescent units. You would instruct the units to stage in an area with good access routes to the main entrance and away from crews fighting the fire. You would also request off-duty EMS personnel for staffing assistance.

4. *How would you use the Incident Management System to organize this incident?*

Using IMS procedures, you decide to divide the incident into two divisions, North and South. Each division will have a manager and separate triage, treatment, and transport units. A Staging Officer will control the flow of ambulances and incoming personnel. A Safety Officer will monitor operations for potential dangers. The three divisions—Staging, North, and South—will report to an EMS Operations Section Chief, who reports to the unified incident command.

5. *What problems would you anticipate, and how would you protect against them?*

The South division will have many more critical patients than the North division. As a result, it will require greater medical resources. The North division will be primarily a relocation operation, but patients must still be evacuated for medical conditions that may have worsened during this event. Any fatalities will need to be collected in a Morgue set up at a separate location. Two ambulances should be dedicated to the Fire Operations section—one for rehabilitation of firefighters and one as a rapid intervention team in case fire or EMS personnel are injured.

Chapter 10—Rescue Awareness and Operations

1. *What are your immediate considerations as you size-up the scene?*

Immediate considerations include safety, hazards, number of patients, control of traffic and bystanders, and need for additional resources (implementation of the IMS).

2. *Why would you consider this a rescue operation?*

Because the patient is unconscious and entrapped in a potentially unstable vehicle/environment.

3. *What additional resources would you request?*

Additional resources might include police, fire department, another EMS unit, and possibly a low-angle rescue team to help move the patient up the embankment.

Chapter 11—Hazardous Materials Incidents

1. *What do you suspect has happened based on your quick scene size-up?*

You suspect hazardous materials are involved in the incident. The tractor-trailer is carrying a placard, it is leaking some kind of liquid, and occupants are drooling, tearing, sweating, and experiencing respiratory distress.

2. *What are your initial priorities?*

Your incident priorities include life safety, incident stabilization, and property conservation.

3. *How will you identify the substance involved in the accident?*

Identification of the substance can be performed through use of the placard, which indicates some kind of poison. An NAERG will identify the specific chemical. Based on the poison placard and the SLUDGE symptoms exhibited by the occupants of the truck, you suspect an organophosphate insecticide. Positive identification can be made using the shipping papers found with the driver of the truck or in the cab. You might also consult one or more of the computerized data banks or telephone hotlines mentioned in this chapter.

4. *What additional resources would you request?*

You will ask for a hazmat team and special fire apparatus. These units will be needed for entry, removal of the patient from the car, hazard control, and decontamination. You will also request three additional ambulances. Counting your unit, there will be one ambulance for each patient and one for the hazardous materials team.

5. *Is this a fast-break or a long-term incident? Explain.*

This is a fast-break incident. Two patients exhibiting critical symptoms have self-rescued and brought themselves to your ambulance.

6. *What are your first actions?*

Your first actions are to secure the scene, set up a perimeter to prevent further decontamination, and request assistance. Upon arrival of fire apparatus, available PPE can be donned, and two-step decontamination performed on the two occupants of the truck who are near your ambulance.

Chapter 12—Crime Scene Awareness

1. *What is your evaluation of this situation from a safety perspective?*

There is a significant potential for danger. The son's apparent intoxication combined with the patient's warning that he "isn't quite right when he's drinking" clearly indicate the need for immediate action.

2. *What are your options?*

The two immediate options both involve retreat. You either retreat with the patient or without the patient. In this case, both you and the son want the same thing—you to leave. However, unless you can calm down the son, you may have to leave the patient behind, at least temporarily. Even though this action may be tactically and legally correct, thoughts of abandonment charges can be haunting. You may try to buy some time until the police arrive, but your main priority is personal safety. You also know that further agitation may only worsen the patient's condition. No matter how unsatisfactory, you may have to leave the scene until the police arrive to take charge of the situation.

Chapter 13—Rural EMS

1. What apparatus or support are you going to need to perform this rescue?

As soon as the mechanism of injury and scene environment are known, additional personnel should be summoned. Because the water is surrounded by high cliffs and is remote, you should request a water rescue team. Following the request for adequate support and specialized rescue teams, you determine whether the patient should be transported by helicopter or ground unit. The transport time to the trauma center, the weather, the difficulty accessing the patient, and the overall time from the onset of the injury should be considered. It is best to ask for help that you may not need than to need help and realize it has not been requested.

2. Based on the mechanism of injury, what injuries should you suspect?

The victim jumped into the water from a 50-foot cliff and landed in water of unknown depth, but apparently shallow. The history that he "jumped" in the water instead of "dove" into the water indicates that the patient may have lower extremity injuries in addition to head and chest injuries. As the patient is unresponsive, it is likely that he has sustained a head injury. A chest injury is possible, as is the possibility of barotrauma if Todd held his breath when he jumped. If the patient landed on his feet, you should expect lower extremity injuries, including possible calcaneal fractures, lumbar spine fractures, and a cervical spinal injury. Always assume the worse and hope for the best.

3. What will you do to stabilize this patient?

Stabilization of this patient is primarily surgical. However, you can attempt "field stabilization" while rescue resources prepare for egress from the quarry. The airway should be controlled if the GCS is less than or equal to 8. Full spinal immobilization should occur. Special attention should be paid to the chest as the patient is at risk for direct trauma and barotrauma. The on-scene time could be prolonged. Therefore, initiate fluid therapy per protocols and splint any fractures. If the patient has a neuro deficit consistent with a spinal cord injury, consider beginning high-dose methylprednisolone therapy. Be sure to protect body temperature.

4. What factors made it impossible for you to adhere to the axiom of the Golden Hour?

The location, mechanism of injury, required rescue resources, distance to the trauma center, and many other factors indicate that this patient will not be in a trauma center within an hour, much less an operating room. You may have to provide extended care while extrication is carried out. You have to do the best you can with what you have available. This victim undertook a high-risk exposure with some knowledge that transport to a hospital might be quite prolonged. He has to accept those risks.

Glossary

acetylcholinesterase (AChE) enzyme that stops the action of acetylocholine, a neurotransmitter.

acrocyanosis cyanosis of the extremities.

active rescue zone area where special rescue teams operate; also known as the "hot zone" or "inner circle."

acute effects signs and/or symptoms rapidly displayed upon exposure to a toxic substance.

acute respiratory distress syndrome (ARDS) respiratory insufficiency marked by progressive hypoxemia, due to severe inflammatory damage.

advance directive legal document prepared when a person is alive, competent, and able to make informed decisions about health care. The document provides guidelines on treatment if the person is no longer capable of making decisions.

aeromedical evacuations transport by helicopter.

ageism discrimination against aged or elderly people.

airbags inflatable high-pressure pillows that when inflated can lift up to 20 tons, depending upon the make.

air-purifying respirator (APR) system of filtering a normal environment for a specific chemical substance using filter cartridges.

Alzheimer's disease a progressive, degenerative disease that attacks the brain and results in impaired memory, thinking, and behavior. It affects an estimated 4 million American adults.

aneurysm abnormal dilation of a blood vessel, usually an artery, due to a congenital defect or a weakness in the wall of the vessel.

anorexia nervosa eating disorder marked by excessive fasting.

anoxic hypoxemia an oxygen deficiency due to disordered pulmonary mechanisms of oxygenation.

antepartum before the onset of labor.

aortic dissection a degeneration of the wall of the aorta.

APGAR scoring a numerical system of rating the condition of a newborn. It evaluates the newborn's heart rate, respiratory rate, muscle tone, reflex irritability, and color.

aphasia absence or impairment of the ability to communicate through speaking, writing, or signing as a result of brain dysfunction; occurs when the individual suffers brain damage due to stroke or head injury.

asthma a condition marked by recurrent attacks of dyspnea with wheezing due to spasmodic constriction of the bronchi, often as a response to allergens, or by mucous plugs in the arterial walls.

autonomic dysfunction an abnormality of the involuntary aspect of the nervous system.

bacterial tracheitis bacterial infection of the airway, subglottic region; in children, most likely to appear after episodes of croup.

bend fractures fractures characterized by angulation and deformity in the bone without an obvious break.

biotransformation changing a substance in the body from chemical to another; in the case of hazardous materials, the body tries to create less toxic materials.

BIPAP bilevel positive airway pressure.

birth injury avoidable and unavoidable mechanical and anoxic trauma incurred by the newborn during labor and delivery.

blood splatter evidence the pattern that blood forms when it is splattered or dropped at the scene of a crime.

body armor vest made of tightly woven, strong fibers that offer protection against handgun bullets, most knives, and blunt trauma; also known as "bullet-proof vest."

brain ischemia injury to brain tissues caused by an inadequate supply of oxygen and nutrients.

branches functional levels within the IMS based upon primary roles and geographic locations.

bronchiectasis chronic dilation of a bronchus or bronchi, with a secondary infection typically involving the lower portion of the lung.

bronchiolitis viral infection of the medium-sized airways, occurring most frequently during the first year of life.

buckle fractures fractures characterized by a raised or bulging projection at the fracture site.

CAMEO® Computer-Aided Management of Emergency Operations; website developed by the EPA and NOAA as a source of information, skills, and links related to hazardous substances.

cardiogenic shock the inability of the heart to meet the metabolic needs of the body, resulting in inadequate tissue perfusion.

cataracts medical condition in which the lens of the eye loses its clearness.

cellulitis inflammation of cellular or connective tissue.

central IV line intravenous line placed into the superior vena cava for the administration of long-term fluid therapy.

cerumen ear wax.

C-FLOP mnemonic for the main functional areas within the IMS—command, finance/administration, logistics, operations, and planning.

chain of evidence legally retaining items of evidence and accounting for their whereabouts at all times to prevent loss or tampering.

CHEMTEL, Inc. Chemical Telephone, Incorporated; maintains a 24-hour, toll-free hotline at 800-255-3024; for collect calls and calls from other points of origin, dial 813-979-0626.

CHEMTREC Chemical Transportation Emergency Center; maintains a 24-hour, toll-free hotline at 800-424-9300; for collect calls and calls from other points of origin, dial 703-527-3887.

child abuse physical or emotional violence or neglect towards a person from infancy to eighteen years of age.

choanal atresia congenital closure of the passage between the nose and pharynx by a bony or membranous structure.

cleft lip congenital vertical fissure in the upper lip.

cleft palate congenital fissure in the roof of the mouth, forming a passageway between oral and nasal cavities.

closed incident an incident that is not likely to generate any further patients; also known as a contained incident or a stable incident.

cold zone location at a hazmat incident outside the warm zone; area where incident operations take place; also called the green zone or the safe zone.

colostomy a surgical diversion of the large intestine through an opening in the skin where the fecal matter is collected in a pouch; may be temporary or permanent.

command the individual or group responsible for coordinating all activities and who makes final decisions on the emergency scene; often referred to as the Incident Commander (IC) or Officer in Charge (OIC).

command post (CP) place where command officers from various agencies can meet with each other and select a management staff.

comorbidity having more than one disease at a time.

compartment syndrome condition that occurs when circulation to a portion of the body is cut off; after a period of time toxins can develop in the blood, leading to shock when circulation is restored.

concealment hiding the body behind objects that shield a person from view but that offer little or no protection against bullets or other ballistics.

conductive deafness deafness caused when there is a blocking of the transmission of the sound waves through the external ear canal to the middle or inner ear.

congenital present at birth.

congregate care living arrangement in which the elderly live in, but do not own, individual apartments or rooms and receive select services.

CONTOMS Counter-Narcotics Tactical Operations; program that manages the training and certification of EMT-Ts and SWAT-Medics.

cor pulmonale congestive heart failure secondary to pulmonary hypertension.

cover hiding the body behind solid and impenetrable objects that protect a person from bullets.

CPAP continuous positive airway pressure.

cribbing wooden slates used to shore up heavy equipment.

Critical Incident Stress Management (CISM) Team monitors the emotional status of all on-scene personnel and provides the necessary support.

croup laryngotracheobronchitis; a common viral infection of young children, resulting in edema of the sub-glottic tissues. Characterized by barking cough and inspiratory stridor.

cytochrome oxidase enzyme complex, found in cellular mitochondria, that enables oxygen to create the adenosine triphosphate (ATP) required for all muscle energy.

deafness the inability to hear.

delayed effects signs, symptoms, and/or conditions developed hours, days, weeks, months, or even years after the exposure.

DeLee suction trap a suction device that contains a suction trap connected to a suction catheter. The negative pressure that powers it can come either from the mouth of the operator or, preferably, from an external vacuum source.

delirium an acute alteration in mental functioning that is often reversible.

dementia a deterioration of mental status that is usually associated with structural neurological disease. It is often progressive and irreversible.

demobilized release of resources—personnel, vehicles, and equipment—for use outside the incident when they are no longer needed at the scene.

demographic pertaining to population makeup or changes.

demylenation destruction or removal of the myelin sheath of nerve tissue; found in Guillain–Barré syndrome.

deployment strategy used by an EMS agency to maneuver its ambulances and crews in an effort to reduce response times.

diabetic ketoacidosis complication of diabetes due to decreased insulin secretion or intake. It is characterized by high levels of blood glucose, metabolic acidosis, and, in advanced stages, coma. Often referred to as diabetic coma.

diabetic retinopathy slow loss of vision as a result of damage done by diabetes.

diaphragmatic hernia protrusion of abdominal contents into the thoracic cavity through an opening in the diaphragm.

disaster management management of incidents that generate large numbers of patients, often overwhelming resources and damaging parts of the infrastructure.

disentanglement process of freeing a patient from wreckage, to allow for proper care, removal, and transfer.

distributive shock marked decrease in peripheral vascular resistance with resultant hypotension. Examples include septic shock, neurogenic shock, and anaphylactic shock.

domestic elder abuse physical or emotional violence or neglect when an elder is being cared for in a home-based setting.

DOT KKK 1822D specs the manufacturing and design specifications produced by the Federal General Services Administrative Automotive Commodity Center.

ductus arteriosus channel between the main pulmonary artery and the aorta of the fetus.

due regard legal terminology found in the motor vehicle laws of most states that sets up a higher standard for the operators of emergency vehicles.

dysphagia inability to swallow or difficulty swallowing.

dysphoria an exaggerate feeling of depression or unrest, characterized by a mood of general dissatisfaction, restlessness, discomfort, and unhappiness.

eddies water that flows around especially large objects and, for a time, flows upstream around the downside of an obstruction; provides an opportunity to escape dangerous currents.

elderly a person age 65 or older.

Emergency Medical Services for Children (EMSC) federally funded program aimed at improving the health of pediatric patients who suffer from life-threatening illnesses and injuries.

emesis vomitus.

EMS Communications Officer notifies hospitals of incoming patients from an MCI; reports to the Transportation Officer and may also be called the EMS COM or MED COM.

EMT-Tacticals (EMT-Ts) EMS personnel trained to serve with a tactical Emergency Medical Services or a law enforcement agency.

enucleation removal of the eyeball after trauma or illness.

epiglottitis bacterial infection of the epiglottis, usually occurring in children older than age four. A serious medical emergency.

epistaxis nosebleed.

essential equipment equipment/supplies required on every ambulance.

exocrine disorder involving external secretions.

extrauterine outside the uterus.

Extrication group or branch responsible for removing patients from entanglements and transferring them to the treatment area; also known as Rescue.

extrication use of force to free a patient from entrapment.

Facilities Unit selects and maintains areas used for rehabilitation and command.

febrile seizures seizures that occur as a result of a sudden increase in temperature; occur most commonly between ages 6 months and 6 years.

fibrosis the formation of fiber-like connective tissue, also called scar tissue in an organ.

Finance/Administration responsible for maintaining records for personnel, time, and costs of resources/procurement; reports directly to the IC.

foreign body airway obstruction (FBAO) blockage or obstruction of the airway by an object that impairs respiration; in the case of pediatric patients, tongues, abundant secretions, and deciduous (baby) teeth are more likely to block airways.

functional impairment decreased ability to meet daily needs on an independent basis.

gangrene death of tissue or bone, usually from an insufficient blood supply.

geriatric abuse a syndrome in which an elderly person is physically or psychologically injured by another person.

geriatrics the study and treatment of diseases of the aged.

gerontology scientific study of the effects of aging and of age-related diseases on humans.

glaucoma group of eye diseases that results in increased intraocular pressure on the optic nerve; if left untreated, can lead to blindness.

global aphasia a combination of motor and sensory aphasia.

glomerulonephritis a form of nephritis, or inflammation of the kidneys; primarily involves the glomeruli, one of the capillary networks that are part of the renal corpuscles in the nephrons.

glottic function opening and closing of the glottic space.

gold standard ultimate standard of excellence

greenstick fractures fractures characterized by an incomplete break in the bone.

growth plate the area just below the head of a long bone in which growth in bone length occurs in the epiphyseal plate.

Guillain–Barré syndrome acute viral infection that triggers the production of autoantibodies, which damage the myelin sheath covering the peripheral nerves; causes rapid, progressive loss of motor function, ranging from muscle weakness to full-body paralysis.

hate crimes crimes committed against a person solely on the basis of the individual's actual or perceived race, color, national origin, ethnicity, gender, disability, or sexual orientation.

hazardous material (hazmat) any substance that causes adverse health effects upon human exposure.

Heat Escape Lessening Position (HELP) developed by Dr. John Hayward. It is an in-water, head-up tuck or fetal position designed to reduce heat loss by as much as 60%.

heatstroke life-threatening condition caused by a disturbance in temperature regulation; in the elderly, characterized by extreme fever and, in extreme cases, delirium or coma.

hemoptysis expectoration of blood arising from the oral cavity, larynx, trachea, bronchi, or lungs; characterized by sudden coughing with production of salty sputum with frothy bright red blood.

hepatomegaly enlarged liver.

herniation protrusion or projection of an organ or part of an organ through the wall of the cavity that normally contains it.

herpes zoster an acute eruption caused by a reactivation of latent varicella virus (chicken pox) in the dorsal root ganglia; also known as shingles.

hiatal hernia protrusion of the stomach upward into the mediastinal cavity through the esophageal hiatus of the diaphragm.

hospice program of palliative care and support services that addresses the physical, social, economic, and spiritual needs of terminally ill patients and their families.

hot zone location at a hazmat incident where the actual hazardous material and highest levels of contamination exist; also called the red zone or the exclusionary zone.

hyperbilirubinemia an excessive amount of bilirubin—the orange-colored pigment associated with bile—in the blood. In newborns, the condition appears as jaundice. Precipitating factors include maternal Rh or ABO incompatibility, neonatal septis, anoxia, hypoglycemia, and congenital liver or gastrointestinal defects.

hyperglycemia abnormally high concentration of glucose in the blood.

hypertrophy an increase in the size or bulk of an organ or structure; caused by growth rather than by a tumor.

hypochondriasis an abnormal concern with one's health, with the false belief of suffering from some disease, despite medical assurances to the contrary; commonly known as hypochondria.

hypoglycemia abnormally low concentration of glucose in the blood.

hypovolemic shock decreased amount of intravascular fluid in the body; often due to trauma that causes blood loss into a body cavity or frank external hemorrhage; in children, can be the result of vomiting and diarrhea.

immune senescence diminished vigor of the immune response to the challenge and rechallenge by pathogens.

Incident Management System (IMS) national system used for the management of multiple-casualty incidents, involving assumption of responsibility for command and designation and coordination of such elements as triage, treatment, transport, and staging; sometimes called the Incident Command System.

incontinence inability to retain urine or feces because of loss of sphincter control or cerebral or spinal lesions.

institutional elder abuse physical or emotional violence or neglect when an elder is being cared for by a person paid to provide care.

Intermittent Mandatory Ventilation (IMV) respirator setting where a patient-triggered breath does not result in assistance by the machine.

intracerebral hemorrhage bleeding directly into the brain.

intractable resistant to cure, relief, or control.

intrapartum occurring during childbirth.

isolette also known as an *incubator;* a clear plastic enclosed bassinet used to keep prematurely born infants warm. The temperature of an isolette can be adjusted regardless of the room temperature. Some isolettes also provide humidity control.

kyphosis exaggeration of the normal posterior curvature of the spine.

labrynthitis inner ear infection that causes vertigo, nausea, and an unsteady gait.

Liaison Officer coordinates all incident operations that involve outside agencies.

life-care community communities that provide apartments/homes for independent living and a range of services, including nursing care. Usually the elderly own their own homes.

local effects effects involving areas around the immediate site; should be evaluated based upon the burn model.

lock-out/tag-out locking off of a machinery switch, then placing a tag on the switch stating why it is shut off; method of preventing equipment from being accidentally restarted.

Logistics supports incident operations, coordinating procurement and distribution of all medical resources.

maceration process of softening a solid by soaking in a liquid.

Management Staff officers that handle public information, safety, outside liaisons, and critical stress debriefing; also known as the Command Staff.

Marfan's Syndrome hereditary condition of connective tissue, bones, muscles, ligaments, and skeletal structures characterized by irregular and unsteady gait, tall lean body type with long extremities, flat feet, stooped shoulders. The aorta is usually dilated and may become weakened enough to allow an aneurysm to develop.

material safety data sheets (MSDS) easily accessible sheets of detailed information about chemicals found at fixed facilities.

meconium dark green material found in the intestine of the full-term newborn. It can be expelled from the intestine into the amniotic fluid during periods of fetal distress.

Medical Supply Unit coordinates procurement and distribution of equipment and supplies at an MCI.

melena a dark, tarry stool caused by the presence of "digested" free blood.

Meniere's disease a disease of the inner ear characterized by vertigo, nerve deafness, and a roar or buzzing in the ear.

meningomyelocele hernia of the spinal cord and membranes through a defect in the spinal column.

mesenteric infarct death of tissue in the peritoneal fold (mesentery) that encircles the small intestine; a life-threatening condition.

minimum standards lowest or least allowable standards.

morgue area where deceased victims of an incident are collected.

Morgue Officer person who supervises the morgue; may report to the Triage Officer or the Treatment Officer.

motor aphasia occurs when the patient cannot speak but can understand what is said.

multiple casualty incident (MCI) incident that generates large numbers of patients and that often make traditional EMS response ineffective because of special circumstances surrounding the event; also known as a mass casualty incident.

muscoviscidosis cystyic fibrosis of the pancreas resulting in abnormally viscous mucoid secretion from the pancreas.

mutual aid agreements or plans for sharing departmental resources.

Myesthania gravis disease characterized by episodic muscle weakness triggered by an autoimmune attack of the acetylcholine receptors.

nasogastric tube/orogastric tube a tube that runs through the nose or mouth and esophagus into the stomach; used for administering liquid nutrients or medications or for removing air or liquids from the stomach.

neonatal abstinence syndrome (NAS) a generalized disorder presenting a clinical picture of CNS hyperirritability, gastrointestinal dysfunction, respiratory distress, and vague autonomic symptoms. It may be due to intrauterine exposure to heroin, methadone, or other less potent opiates. Non-opiate central nervous system depressants may also cause NAS.

neonate an infant from the time of birth to one month of age.

nephrons the functional units of the kidneys.

neutropenic a condition that results from an abnormally low neutrophil count in the blood (less than 2000/mm^3).

newborn a baby in the first few hours of its life, also called a *newly born infant.*

nocturia excessive urination during the night.

noncardiogenic shock types of shock that result from causes other than inadequate cardiac output.

old-old an elderly person age 80 or older.

omphalocele congenital hernia of the umbilicus.

open incident an incident that has the potential to generate additional patients; also known as an uncontained incident or an unstable incident.

Operations fulfills directions from command and does the actual work at an incident.

osteoarthritis a degenerative joint disease, characterized by a loss of articular cartilage and hypertrophy of bone.

osteoporosis softening of bone tissue due to the loss of essential minerals, principally calcium.

otitis media middle ear infection.

Parkinson's disease chronic, degenerative nervous disease characterized by tremors, muscular weakness and rigidity, and a loss of postural reflexes.

particulate evidence evidence such as hairs or fibers that cannot be readily seen with the human eye; also known as microscopic or trace evidence.

partner abuse physical or emotional violence from a man or woman towards a domestic partner.

peak load the highest volume of calls at a given time

PEEP positive end-expiratory pressure.

persistent fetal circulation condition in which blood continues to bypass the fetal respiratory system, resulting in ongoing hypoxia.

personal-care home living arrangement that includes room, board, and some supervision.

phototherapy exposure to sunlight or artificial light for therapeutic purposes. In newborns, light is used to treat hyperbilirubinemia or jaundice.

Pierre Robin syndrome unusually small jaw, combined with a cleft palate, downward displacement of the tongue, and an absent gag reflex.

pill-rolling motion an involuntary tremor, usually in one hand or sometimes in both, in which fingers move as if they were rolling a pin back and forth.

placard diamond-shaped graphic placed on vehicles to indicated hazard classification.

Planning provides past, present, and future information about an incident.

polycythemia an excess of red blood cells. In a newborn, the condition may reflect hypovolemia or prolonged intrauterine hypoxia.

polypharmacy multiple drug therapy in which there is a concurrent use of a number of drugs.

post partum depression the "let down" feeling experienced during the period following birth occurring in 70–80% of mothers.

presbycusis progressive hearing loss that occurs with aging.

pressure ulcer ischemic damage and subsequent necrosis affecting the skin, subcutaneous tissue, and often the muscle; result of intense pressure over a short time or low pressure over a long time; also known as pressure sore or bedsore.

primary area of responsibility (PAR) stationing of ambulances at specific high-volume locations.

primary contamination direct exposure of a person or item to a hazardous substance.

primary triage triage that takes place early in the incident, usually upon first arrival.

prompt care facilities hospital agencies that provide limited care and non-emergent medical treatment.

pruritus itching; often occurs as a symptom of some systemic change or illness.

Public Information Officer (PIO) collects data about the incident and releases it to the press or media.

rape Penile penetration of the genitalia or rectum without the consent of the victim.

Rapid Intervention Team ambulance and crew dedicated to stand by in case a rescuer becomes ill or injured.

recirculating currents movement of currents over a uniform obstruction; also known as a "drowning machine."

reportable collisions collisions that involve over $1,000 in damage or a personal injury.

reserve capacity the ability of an EMS agency to respond to calls beyond those handled by the on-duty crews.

retinopathy any disorder of the retina.

rust out an inability to keep abreast of new technologies and standards.

Safety Officer monitors all on-scene actions and ensures that they do not create any potentially harmful conditions.

scene-authority law legal state or local statue specifying who has ultimate authority at an MCI.

scrambling climbing over rocks and/or downed trees on a steep trail without the aid of ropes. This can be especially dangerous when the surface is wet or icy.

scree loose pebbles or rock debris that can form on the slopes or bases of mountains; sometimes used to describe debris in sloping dry stream beds.

secondary contamination transfer of a hazardous substance to a non-contaminated person or item via contact with someone or something already contaminated by the substance.

secondary triage triage that takes place after patients are moved to a treatment area to determine any change in status.

Section Chief officer who supervises major functional areas or sections; reports to the Incident Commander.

Sector interchangeable name for a branch, group, or division; does not, however, designate a functional or geographic area.

semi-decontaminated patient another name for field-decontaminated patient.

senile dementia general term used to describe an abnormal decline in mental functioning seen in the elderly; also called "organic brain syndrome" or "multi-infarct dementia."

sensorineural deafness   deafness caused by the inability of nerve impulses to reach the auditory center of the brain because of nerve damage either to the inner ear or to the brain.

sensorium   sensory apparatus of the body as a whole; also that portion of the brain that functions as a center of sensations.

sensory aphasia   occurs when the patient cannot understand the spoken word.

sexual assault   Unwanted oral, genital, rectal, or manual sexual contact.

shipping papers   documents routinely carried aboard vehicles transporting hazardous materials; ideally should identify specific substances and quantities carried; also known as bills of lading.

short haul   a helicopter extrication technique where a person is attached to a rope that is, in turn, attached to a helicopter. The aircraft lifts off with the person attached to it. Obviously this means the evacuation requires highly specialized skills.

shunt   surgical connection that runs from the brain to the abdomen for the purpose of draining excess CNS fluid and preventing increased intracranial pressure.

Shy-Drager syndrome   chronic orthostatic hypotension caused by a primary autonomic nervous system deficiency.

sick sinus syndrome   a group of disorders characterized by dysfunction of the sinoatrial node in the heart.

silent myocardial infarction   a myocardial infarction that occurs without exhibiting obvious signs and symptoms.

silo gas   toxic fumes (oxides of nitrogen) produced by the fermentation of grains in a silo.

singular command   process where a single individual is responsible for coordinating an incident; most useful in single-jurisdictional incidents.

span of control   number of people or tasks that a single individual can monitor.

Special Weapons and Tactics (SWAT) Team   a trained police unit equipped to handle hostage holders and other difficult law enforcement situations.

spondylosis   a degeneration of the vertebral body.

spotter   the person behind the left rear side of the ambulance who assists the operator in backing up the vehicle.

Staff Functions   officers who perform supervisory roles in the IMS rather than those who actually perform a task.

staging   location where ambulances, personnel, and equipment are kept in reserve for use at an incident.

Staging Officer   supervises the staging area and guards against premature commitment of resources and freelancing by personnel; reports to the branch director.

START   acronym for the most widely used disaster triage system; stands for **S**imple **T**riage **a**nd **R**apid **T**ransport.

status epilepticus   prolonged seizure or multiple seizures with no regaining of consciousness between them.

Stokes-Adams syndrome   a series of symptoms resulting from heart block, most commonly syncope. The symptoms result from decreased blood flow to the brain caused by the sudden decrease in cardiac output.

stoma   a permanent surgical opening in the neck through which the patient breathes.

strainers   a partial obstruction that filters, or strains, the water such as downed trees or wire mesh; causes an unequal force on the two sides.

stroke   injury or death of brain tissue resulting from interruption of cerebral blood flow and oxygenation; also known as brain attack.

subarachnoid hemorrhage   bleeding that occurs between the arachoid and dura mater of the brain.

substance abuse   misuse of chemically active agents such as alcohol, psychoactive chemicals, and therapeutic agents; typically results in clinically significant impairment or distress.

Sudden infant death syndrome (SIDS)   illness of unknown etiology that occurs during the first year of life, with the peak at ages 2–4 months.

synergism   a standard pharmacological principle in which two substances or drugs work together to produce an effect that neither of them can produce on its own.

system status management (SSM)   a computerized personnel and ambulance deployment system

systemic effects   effects that occur throughout the body after exposure to a toxic substance.

Tactical Emergency Medical Service (TEMS)   specially trained unit that extracts patients from tactically hot zones; provides on-site medical support to law enforcement personnel.

thyrotoxicosis   toxic condition characterized by tachycardia, nervous symptoms, and rapid metabolism due to hyperactivity of the thyroid gland.

tiered response system   system that allows multiple vehicles to arrive at an EMS call at different times, often providing different levels of care or transport

tinnitus   subjective ringing or tingling sound in the ear.

tracheostomy   a surgical incision that a surgeon makes from the anterior neck into the trachea; held open by a metal or plastic tube.

transient ischemic attacks (TIA)   reversible interruptions of blood flow to the brain; often seen as a precursor to a stroke.

Transportation Supervisor   coordinates operations with Staging Officer and the Transportation Supervisor; gets patients into the ambulance and routed to hospitals.

Trauma Intervention Programs (TIP)   a national non-profit organization that establishes and operates local chapters of citizen volunteers specially trained to provide assistance to anyone emotionally traumatized by a crisis event.

Treatment Group Supervisor   controls all actions in the Treatment Group/Sector.

Treatment Unit Leaders   EMS personnel who manage the various treatment units and who report to the Treatment Group Supervisor.

triage   act of sorting patients based upon the severity of their injuries.

turgor   ability of the skin to return to normal appearance after being subjected to pressure.

two-pillow orthopnea   the number of pillows—in this case, two—needed to ease the difficulty of breathing while lying down; a significant factor in assessing the level of respiratory distress.

UN number   a four-digit identification number specific to a given chemical; some UN numbers are assigned to a group of related chemicals, but with different characteristics, such the UN 1203 designation for diesel fuel, gasohol, gasoline, motor fuels, motor spirits, and petrol. (The letters *UN* stand for "United Nations." Sometimes the letters *NA* for "North America" appear with or instead of the UN designation.)

unified command   process in which managers from different jurisdictions—law enforcement, fire, EMS—coordinate their activities and share responsibility for command.

urosepsis   septicemia originating from the urinary tract.

urostomy   surgical diversion of the urinary tract to a stoma, or hole, in the abdominal wall.

vagal response   stimulation of the vagus nerve causing a parasympathetic response.

valsalva maneuver   forced exhalation against a closed glottis, such as with coughing. This maneuver stimulates the parasympathetic nervous system via the vagus nerve, which in turn slows the heart rate.

varicosities   an abnormal dilation of a vein or group of veins.

vertigo   the sensation of faintness or dizziness; may cause a loss of balance.

warm zone   location at a hazmat incident adjacent to the hot zone; area where a decontamination corridor is established; also called the yellow zone or contamination reduction zone.

weapons of mass destruction (WMD)   variety of chemical, biological, or nuclear devices used by terrorists to strike at government or high-profile targets; designed to create a maximum number of casualties.

wrap points   mechanisms of injury in which an appendage gets caught and significantly twisted.

Index

BLS (basic life support), 68, 96, 294
Body armor, 456–57
Body fluids, at crime scene, 460–61
Body surface area (BSA), 53–54, 125
Body temperature, 66
    effects of aging on, 165
    newborns, 10, 12, 19
        fevers, 31–32
    water rescues and, 384–85, 389, 390
Boiling point, 427
Bowel infarct, 182
Bowel obstruction, 182
BPD (bronchopulmonary dysplasia), 265–66
Bradycardia, 13, 17, 29
Bradydysrhythmias, 106
Brain attack, 175–76
Brain injuries. *See* Head injuries
Brain ischemia, 175
Branch Directors, 352–53
Branches, IMS and, 351, 352–53
Breathing. *See also* Respiratory system
    assessment, 59–61
Brochiolitis, 98–99
Bronchiectasis, 267
Bronchitis, 264
Bronchopulmonary dysplasia (BPD), 265–66
Broviac catheters, 274
BSA (body surface area), 53–54, 125
Buckle fractures, 124
Bullet-proof vests, 456–57
Burns
    chemical, 227
    on children, 119–20, 125–26
        child abuse and, 214–15
    on the elderly, 201–2
Bystanders, dangerous, 450

CAAMS (Commission on Accreditation of Air Medical Services), 334–35
CAAS (Commission on Accreditation of Ambulance Services), 320
Calcium chloride, 85
California Firescope, 343
CAMEO (Computer-Aided Management of Emergency Operations), 424
Cancer, 235–36, 284
    lung, 170
Capillary refill, 61, 62, 64
Caput succedaneum, 35
Carbamates, 432
Carbon monoxide, 432–33
Car collisions. *See* Motor vehicle collisions
Cardiac arrest. *See* Cardiopulmonary arrest
Cardiac conditions, in home health care setting, 276
Cardiac decompensation, 251
Cardiac dysrhythmias, 105–6, 172–73, 188
Cardiac syncope, 174
Cardiogenic shock, 101, 102, 104

Cardiomyopathy, 104–5
Cardiopulmonary (cardiac) arrest, 54, 81
    anticipating, 62–63
    hypoxia and, 21–22
    medications, 84–85
    in newborns, 35–36
Cardiovascular system, 54, 162–63
    assessment, 81–85
    disorders, of the elderly, 170–75
    elderly trauma management and, 198
Cars. *See* Motor vehicles
Cataracts, 155, 156
Catheters, 276–78. *See also specific catheters*
    complications involving, 277–78
Cave-ins, 395–96
Cell phones, in rural settings, 469–70
Cellulitis, 252
Center for Pediatric Medicine (CPEM), 42
Central IV (intravenous) lines, 133
Cerebral palsy, 228, 236–37
Cerebrovascular disease, 175–76
Certification, in rural settings, 470–71
Cerumen, 225
Cervical collar application, 392
Cervical spine (C-spine) immobilization, 86–89
Cervical spine injuries, 124, 202
C-FLOP (command, finance/administration, logistics, operations, and planning), 343
    command, 343–49
    finance/administration, 343, 351
    logistics, 343, 351
    operations, 343, 351
    planning, 343, 351
Chain of evidence, 220
Challenged patients, 222–43
    case study, 223–24
    with communicable diseases, 241–42
    culturally diverse, 240–41
    developmental disabilities, 232–34
    with financial challenges, 242
    mental and emotional impairments, 232
    pathological. *See* Chronic conditions
    physical impairments, 224–32
    terminally ill, 241
Chemical asphyxiants, 432–33
Chemical burns, 227
Chemicals, 394
Chemotherapy treatments, 236
CHEMTEL, Inc., 426
CHEMTREC (Chemical Transportation Emergency Center), 426
Chest, 53
Chest compressions, 95, 106
    newborn resuscitation and, 21–22
Chest injuries, 124
Chest pain, 149, 155, 171, 241
CHF (congestive heart failure), 173, 265
Chicken pox, 90

Dopamine, 24, 83, 86, 103
Dopamine hydrochloride, 85
DOT (Department of Transportation), 415, 420, 421
    KKK 1822D specs, 318, 319
Down syndrome, 233–34
Drain cleaners, 431
Drains, 280–81
Drownings, 119. *See also* Surface water rescues
Drug abuse, 193. *See also* Substance abuse
    by mothers, 23, 25
Drug-related crimes, 451–52
Drugs. *See* Medications
Drying, newborn resuscitation and, 15, 17
Ductus arteriosus, 6, 28
Due regard standard, 326–27
Dust masks, 373
Dysarthria, 230
Dysphagia, 149
Dysphoria, 195
Dysrhythmias, 105–6, 162, 172–73, 188

Earthquakes, 395
Eddies, 388
Education, continuing, 41–42
Eight-step decontamination process, 436
Elavil, 191
Elder abuse. *See* Geriatric abuse
Elderly, the, 140. *See also* Geriatrics
    assessment of, 154–59
    common complaints of, 149
    management of, 159
    pathophysiology of, 149–53
    population characteristics of, 140–41
    prevention strategies for, 146, 147
    resources for, 145–48
    societal issues of, 141–45
Electrical hazards, 398
Electrical therapy, 85–86
Electricity, 394
Elimination problems, of the elderly, 152–53
Embolus, 281
Emergencies. *See also specific emergencies*
    agricultural, 475–83
    environmental, 186–87
        for rescue operations, 407–9
    geriatric, 136–204
        trauma, 196–202
    neonatal, 26–36
    pediatric, 89–117
        general approach to, 43–55
        trauma, 117–26
    recreational, 483–85
    respiratory. *See* Respiratory emergencies
    trauma. *See* Trauma
Emergency lighting, 397
Emergency Medical Services for Children (EMSC), 42
Emesis, 259

Emotional abuse, of children, 216–17. *See also* Child abuse
Emotional impairments, 232
Emphysema, 264
EMSC (Emergency Medical Services for Children), 42
EMS Communications Officer, 361
EMT-Tacticals (EMT-Ts), 458
Endocrine system
    disorders, 179–80
    effects of aging on, 164, 179
End-organ perfusion, 62
Endotracheal intubation, 76–80
    anatomical and physiological concerns, 76–77
    indications for, 77
    of newborns, 17–18, 20–21
    techniques for, 78–80
Engine compartment, of vehicles, 400
Engulfment, 394
Entrapment, 401
Enucleation, 227
Environmental distractions, as factor in assessment, 296
Environmental emergencies, 186–87
    for rescue operations, 407–9
Environmental Protection Agency (EPA), 343, 416, 424
Epidemiology
    of the elderly, 140–45, 247–57
    of newborns, 5–6
Epiglottitis, 93, 94–95
Epinephrine, 14, 24, 29, 85, 86, 106
    subcutaneous, 103
Epistaxis, 174
Equipment, 297–98. *See also* Protective equipment; *and specific equipment*
    essential, for ambulances, 318, 320
    guidelines according to age and weight, 72, 73
    malfunction, in home health care setting, 248, 253–54
    for monitoring vital signs, 65–68
    standards, 320
Equipment-related trauma, 477–78
Escorts, 328
Esophageal obturator airways (EOA), 76
Esophageal-tracheal combitubes (ETC), 76
Esophageal varices, 181
Ethics, of caring for elderly patients, 143–45
Evacuations. *See also* Transport
    aeromedical, 331, 332. *See also* Air medical transport
    in hazardous terrain, 407
        high-angle, 403–4, 405–6
        low-angle, 404, 405–6
    immediate, 300
Evasion, at crime scene, 455
Evidence, 459–62
    documenting, 461–62
    types of, 460–61
Examinations. *See* Physical exam
Exocrine, 265

Medical hazmat operations, 427–28. *See also* Hazardous
    materials
Medical history, 293, 301
    of children, 63–64
    of elderly patients, 150, 155–58
        communication challenges, 155–57
        mental status, 157–58
    in home health care setting, 260–62
Medical incident command, 338–67
    case study, 340–41
    division of functions, 352–53
    functional groups within, 353–62
    regulations and standards, 343
    support, 349–51
Medical Supply Unit, 351
Medical therapy, in home health care setting, 267–74
Medicare, 145, 247, 283
    funding of home care, 1967-1997, 247
Medications. *See also specific medications*
    cardiopulmonary arrest, 84–85
    in the elderly, 149–50
    newborn resuscitation and, 21–23, 24
    for pain management, 255
    toxicological emergencies, 188–92
Melena, 181
Meniere's disease, 155
Meningitis, 102, 110
Meningomyelocele, 8
Mental illnesses, 232
Mental status, 56. *See also* Consciousness
    altered, 157–58, 251–52
    of elderly patients, 157–58
        in home health care setting, 260–61
Mesenteric infarct, 181, 182
Metabolic differences, 55
Metabolic disorders, in the elderly, 179–80
Metabolic emergencies, in children, 111–14
Methane, 477
Methylene chloride, 433
METTAG, 356
Minimum standards, 318
Mitigation, disasters and, 362
Mobility problems, of the elderly, 151–52
MOI. *See* Mechanisms of injury
Molestation, 218
Monitoring, at hazmat incidents, 424, 439
Morbidity, 41–43
Morgue, 357
Morgue Officer, 357
Mortality, 41–43
Motor aphasia, 230
Motor development, of infants and children, 45–49
Motor vehicle collisions (MVC), 117, 118–19, 341,
    399–402. *See also* Ambulance collisions
    hazards in highway operations, 396–99
    parking and loading ambulance, 328–30
    placards, 418, 420–22

    rescue strategies, 401–2
    risk of violence at, 448–49
Motor vehicles, 399–400
    basic constructions, 399–400
    bumpers, 398–99
    doors, 400–401
    firewall and engine compartment, 400
    glass, 400
    rolling, 399
    stabilization equipment, 402
    unstable, 399
Moving water surface rescues, 386–88
MSDS (material safety data sheets), 424, 425
Multi focal seizures, 31
Multiple casualty incidents (MCI), 341, 363–64. *See also*
    Incident Management System
    command at, 343–49
    common problems, 363
    preplanning, drills, and critiques, 363–64
Multiple sclerosis (MS), 238
Multiple-system failure, 149
Multi-vehicle responses, 328
Murder, 449–50
Muscoviscidosis, 237–38, 265
Muscular dystrophy (MD), 238, 266
Musculoskeletal disorders, in the elderly, 183–85
Musculoskeletal system, effects of aging on, 165
Mutual aid, 351
MVCs. *See* Motor vehicle collisions
Myasthenia gravis, 240, 251, 267
Myocardial infarctions (MI), 171–72, 198
Myoclonic seizures, 31

NAERG (North American Emergency Response Guide),
    423–24
Naloxone, 23, 24, 25, 27
Narcan (Naloxone), 23, 24, 25, 27
Narcotic depression, 23, 25
NAS (neonatal abstinence syndrome), 34
Nasogastric (NG) intubation, 21, 28, 80–81, 82, 278
Nasopharyngeal airways, 74
National Association for Search and Rescue, 407
National Association of EMS Physicians, 471
National associations, for the elderly, 148
National Fire Academy (Emmitsburg, Maryland), 343
National Fire Protection Association (NFPA), 320, 343,
    416, 420
704 System, 422
National Flight Nurses Association (NFNA), 319
National Flight Paramedics Association (NFPA), 319
National Home and Hospice Care Survey (NHHCS), 248
National Institute for Occupational Safety and Health
    (NIOSH), 320, 392
National Oceanic and Atmospheric Administration
    (NOAA), 424
National Tactical Officers Association (NTOA), 458
Nature of the illness (NOI), 56

Status asthmaticus, 98
Status epilepticus, 109, 110
Stokes-Adams syndrome, 174
Stokes baskets, 404–5, 406
Stoma, 132
Strainers, 386, 387, 388
Street gangs, 450–51
Street incidents, violent, 449–51
Strokes, 175–76
Structural collapses, 394–96
Stuttering, 230
Subarachnoid hemorrhage, 175
Submerged victims, 390
Substance abuse, 193–94
    factors contributing to, 193
    by mothers, 23, 25
Subtle seizures, 31
Suction catheters, 10, 71
Suctioning, 71
    newborn resuscitation and, 15, 17, 18
Sudden infant death syndrome (SIDS), 126–27
Suicide, 195–96
Supplemental oxygen, newborn resuscitation and, 19–20
Supplemental restraint systems (SRS) air bags, 399
Support, for incident command, 349–51
Supraventricular tachycardia, 105
Surface water rescues, 383–92
    flat water, 388–92
    moving water, 386–88
    rescue techniques, 385–86
    water temperature, 384–85
Surgically implanted medication delivery systems, 275
Surgical masks, 373
SWAT Team, 456, 458
Sweating, 165
Swift-water rescues, 386–88
Syncope, 174–75
Synergism, 431
Systemic changes, age-related, 161
Systemic effects, 430–31
System pathophysiology, in the elderly, 159–66
System status management (SSM), 322

Tachydysrhythmias, 105
Tachypnea, 59, 60
Tactical Emergency Medical Service (TEMS), 445, 458
Tactile stimulation, newborn resuscitation and, 15, 17
Tagging, in triage, 356–57
Tattoos, 451
Teaching Resource for Instructors in Prehospital Pediatrics (TRIPP), 42
Team leader, 297
TEMS (Tactical Emergency Medical Service), 445, 458
Terminally ill patients, 241, 285. *See also* Hospice care
Terrain rescue. *See* Hazardous terrain
Terrorism, 419–20
Texas catheters, 276–77

Thermoregulatory system. *See also* Body temperature
    effects of aging on, 165
Thorazine, 191, 194
Threshold limit value/ceiling level (TLV-CL), 428
Threshold limit value/short-term exposure limit (TLV/STEL), 428
Threshold limit value/time weighted average (TLV/TWA), 428
Thyroid disorders, 164, 180
Thyrotoxicosis, 34
Tiered response system, 322, 323
Tinnitus, 155, 226
TIP (Trauma Intervention Programs), 364
Tire prints, 460
Toddlers, 46–47
Tofranil, 191
Tonic seizures, 31
Topical absorption, of hazardous materials, 430
Toxic chemicals, 394
Toxic exposure, 114–17. *See also* Poisoning
Toxicological emergencies, in the elderly, 188–92
Toxicological terms, 428–29
Toxicology review, 429–33
Trace evidence, 461
Trach-button, 270
Tracheal suctioning, 17, 18, 20–21
Tracheostomies, 131–32, 269–71
    common complications, 270
    management, 270–71
Tracheostomy tubes, 131–32
Tracking log, 360
Traffic congestion, 322–23, 330
Traffic hazards, 330–31, 378, 397
    reducing, 397
Traffic redirection, 397
Training, 469
    continuing, 41–42
    hazmat incidents, 416–17
Transient ischemic attacks (TIA), 153, 173, 175
Transport. *See also* Air medical transport;
    Ambulances
    elderly trauma management and, 199, 200
    eruption of danger during, 446, 448
    guidelines for, 89
    at hazmat incidents, 418–19, 437
    in home health care setting, 262
    IMS and, 359–60
    of infants, 25, 55
    initial assessment and priority of, 63
    of obese patients, 231
    at rescue operations, 383, 404–7
    in rural settings, 468, 472–75
Transportation Department, U. S. *See* Department of Transportation
Transportation Supervisor, 359–60
Trauma
    equipment-related, 477–78